Lifestyle in Oral Health and Disease

S. R. Prabhu
Saman Warnakulasuriya
Sanjana Bhardwaj
Editors

Lifestyle in Oral Health and Disease

A Comprehensive Guide for Oral Healthcare Providers

Springer

Editors
S. R. Prabhu
School of Dentistry
University of Queensland
Brisbane, QLD, Australia

Sanjana Bhardwaj
Gates Foundation
Seattle, WA, USA

Saman Warnakulasuriya
Oral Medicine, Faculty of Dentistry
and Craniofacial Sciences
King's College London
London, UK

ISBN 978-3-032-05887-4 ISBN 978-3-032-05888-1 (eBook)
https://doi.org/10.1007/978-3-032-05888-1

This Springer imprint is published by the registered company Springer Nature Switzerland AG
The registered company address is: Gewerbestrasse 11, 6330 Cham, Switzerland

Dedicated to our teachers, mentors, families, and friends whose guidance and support have shaped our lives.

Foreword

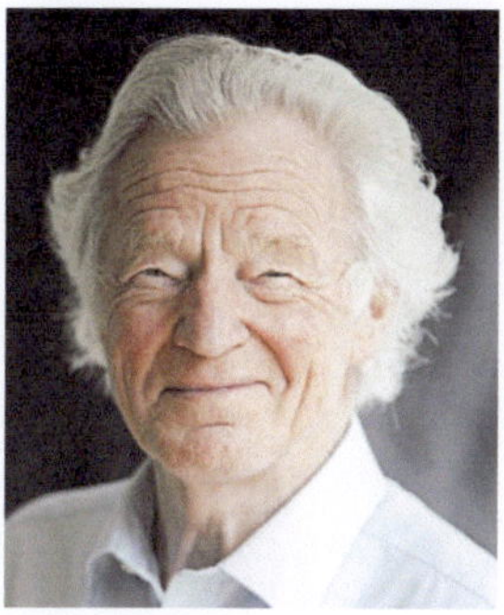

Lifestyle medicine is a transformative force in healthcare—one that champions the integration of non-drug therapies alongside, and at times in place of, conventional pharmaceutical treatments. Crucially, this approach extends beyond the individual. While the term *lifestyle* may imply a personal focus, it is now widely recognised that many health challenges are rooted in environmental factors. Physical and social environments, along with the exposome—the totality of environmental exposures—are increasingly acknowledged as having a greater impact than genetics in the development of common health conditions, particularly as populations age.

In *Lifestyle in Oral Health and Disease*, the editors draw from this evolving body of knowledge to explore the emerging discipline of lifestyle dentistry. This field emphasises the strong links between oral diseases and lifestyle behaviours. The chapters delve into the effects of smoking, alcohol misuse, recreational drug use, nutrition, stress, eating disorders, obesity, and other risk factors that significantly influence oral and dental health.

Authored by experts from diverse fields of dentistry and medicine, as well as from around the globe, this volume provides a comprehensive foundation for understanding and addressing oral diseases through evidence-based lifestyle interventions. The mission of lifestyle medicine, and by extension, lifestyle dentistry—represents a forward-thinking endeavour to benefit not only those seeking care but also the practitioners and systems that provide and support it.

This book serves as a valuable resource for anyone involved in the pursuit or delivery of oral healthcare.

Visiting Professor
Nuffield Department of Surgical Sciences
The University of Oxford
Oxford, UK

Sir Muir Gray

Preface

In an era where healthcare is increasingly characterised by the pursuit of integrated, preventative, and patient-centred approaches, *Lifestyle in Oral Health and Disease* emerges as both timely and essential. At the intersection of dentistry and lifestyle medicine, this volume illuminates a subject long overlooked: the profound influence of everyday behaviours on oral health and, in turn, on overall well-being.

Despite the well-documented health benefits of positive lifestyle choices, the crucial connection between oral health and behaviours such as nutrition, sleep, stress management, and substance use remains insufficiently understood in clinical practice. Oral healthcare professionals are often ill-equipped to comprehensively address these factors, leading to missed opportunities for prevention and holistic care.

This book presents an extraordinary collaboration of over 50 international experts, offering a rigorous, evidence-based examination of how habits, both beneficial and harmful, impact the mouth and body alike. Through 26 thoughtfully curated chapters, readers will discover not only the science behind lifestyle-related oral health concerns but also innovative perspectives on technology, behaviour change, and the evolving role of the clinician.

More than a reference, this work invites dental professionals to expand their roles—not just as healers of oral disease but as advocates for healthier lives. The insights presented here empower readers to integrate lifestyle-based strategies into their oral care, making dentistry a vital pillar in the pursuit of overall wellness.

We hope this book serves as a valuable resource and inspiration for clinicians, educators, and researchers alike. As the boundaries between disciplines continue to fade, *Lifestyle in Oral Health and Disease* reinforces the growing alliance between lifestyle medicine and lifestyle dentistry, two fields rooted in prevention, behavioural change, and whole-person care. This convergence reflects a broader shift towards integrated healthcare, where oral health is recognised not as separate from systemic health but as an essential component of it. This volume stands as a testament to the power of collaboration, curiosity, and the shared goal of improving lives through knowledge, compassion, and innovation.

Brisbane, QLD, Australia — S. R. Prabhu
London, UK — Saman Warnakulasuriya
Seattle, WA, USA — Sanjana Bhardwaj

Acknowledgements

We are deeply honoured by Sir Muir Gray CBE, FRCPS (Glas), FCLIP, Visiting Professor at Oxford University, for contributing the Foreword to this volume. His thoughtful reflections eloquently highlight the essential integration of lifestyle disease prevention within dental practice. We extend our profound thanks to the chapter contributors whose dedication, scholarship, and collaborative spirit have brought this book to life. Their efforts have added richness and depth to each chapter, and we are sincerely grateful for their expertise. We also express warm appreciation to our international colleagues for generously sharing their clinical photographs, which have significantly enhanced the scientific and visual merit of this work. We have endeavoured to acknowledge all copyrighted material used throughout the book.

We are especially grateful to the exceptional team at *Springer Nature* for their professional editorial support and stewardship throughout the publishing process. Their commitment to excellence is reflected in both the print and digital editions of this book.

S. R. Prabhu
Saman Warnakulasuriya
Sanjana Bhardwaj

Contents

Editors and Contributors

About the Editors

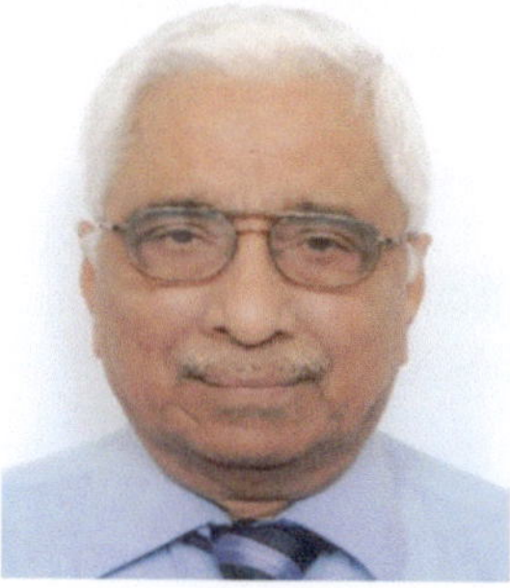

S. R. Prabhu BDS; MDS (Oral Path); FFDRCSI (Oral Med); FDSRCS(Edin); FDSRCPS(Glasgow); FDSRCS(Eng.); FFGDP RCS(UK); MOMed RCS(Edin); FICD is an Honorary Associate Professor at the School of Dentistry in Brisbane and a globally recognized expert in oral and maxillofacial pathology and oral medicine. With academic and leadership roles in India, Kenya, Sudan, Trinidad and Tobago, Malaysia, Saudi Arabia, the UAE, and Australia, he has helped shape dental education internationally. He is a Fellow of all four Royal Colleges of Surgeons in the UK and Ireland, a former international advisor for the Caribbean and UAE regions, and an examiner for the membership examinations of the Royal College of Surgeons of Edinburgh. In collaboration with the University of Alabama at Birmingham School of Dentistry, he has conducted HIV/AIDS education workshops for oral healthcare professionals across Asia and the Caribbean. He has published numerous articles in peer-reviewed journals and edited several books on various topics related to oral diseases, published by renowned international academic publishers. He currently serves on the editorial board of the *International Dental Journal* (IDJ), published by the FDI World Dental Federation, Geneva.

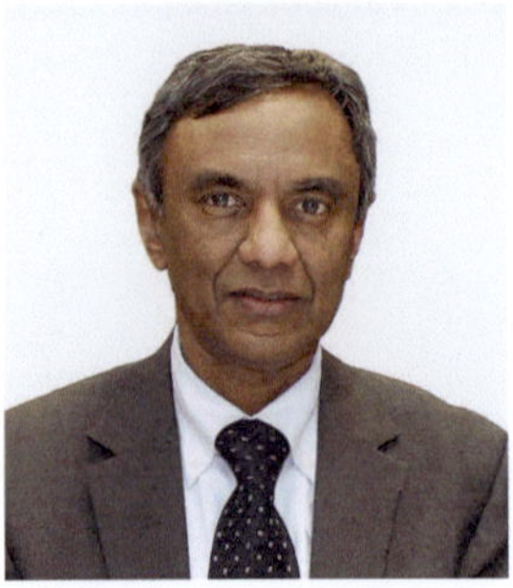

Saman Warnakulasuriya OBE, FDS RCS, PhD is an Emeritus Professor of Oral Medicine and Experimental Pathology at King's College London, UK. He served as the Chairman of the Oral Medicine Division at King's College Hospital and Guy's Hospital, London, from 2005 to 2015. He has significantly contributed to cancer epidemiology, oral medicine, and experimental pathology. He is also the Director of the WHO Collaborating Centre for Oral Cancer. He has participated in several expert panels for the International Agency for Research on Cancer (IARC), where he evaluated carcinogenic substances and lifestyle habits. He received the IADR Distinguished Scientist Award in Oral Medicine and Pathology in 2014 and the IADR Distinguished Scientist Award in Global Oral Health in 2022. He was honored with an OBE by Her Majesty the Queen for his services to Medicine. He was elected a Fellow of King's College London (FKC) for his sustained and significant contributions to the College.

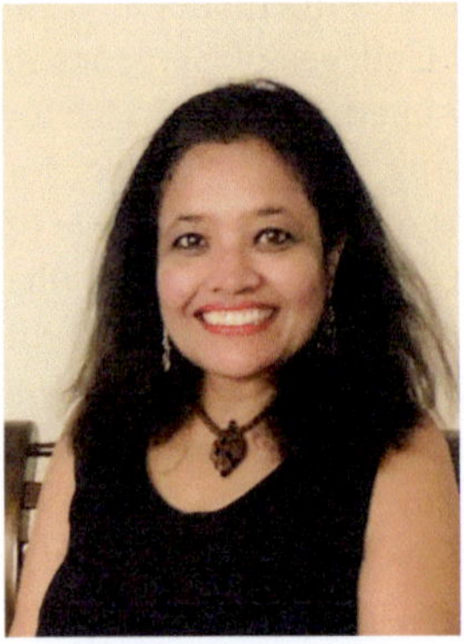

Sanjana Bhardwaj MBBS, MD, MPH, FFPH leads policy and advocacy work at the Gates Foundation in Duvall, USA, focusing on family planning, maternal and child health, nutrition, and primary healthcare systems. Before joining the foundation, she worked with the United Nations, leading child survival and development efforts across Bangladesh, India, Papua New Guinea, Nigeria, and South Africa. She also worked in academia, teaching and overseeing the development of a Master of Public Health degree course in health behavior at the University of the West Indies. Her areas of interest encompass reproductive, maternal, newborn, and child health and well-being, adolescent health, HIV, emergency healthcare, digital health, public health education, evidence-based policy advocacy, and program design. Her work has been published in peer-reviewed journals and has received service awards and certificates for her contributions.

Contributors

Rahena Akhter BDS, PhD Sydney Dental School, Faculty of Medicine and Health, The University of Sydney, Camperdown, NSW, Australia

Sadeq Ali Al-Maweri Department of Preclinical Oral Health Sciences, College of Dental Medicine, QU Health, Qatar University, Doha, Qatar

Ramesh Balasubramaniam Discipline of Oral Medicine, UWA Dental School, The University of Western Australia, Nedlands, WA, Australia

Elis Ângela Batistella College of Dentistry, University of Saskatchewan Saskatoon, SK, Canada

Shilpa Bhandi College of Dental Medicine, Roseman University of Health Sciences, South Jordan, UT, USA

Sanjana Bhardwaj Gates Foundation, Washington, USA

João T. S. Botelho Egas Moniz Centre for Interdisciplinary Research, Egas Moniz School of Health and Science, Almada, Portugal

Vickie Cai Sydney Dental School, Faculty of Medicine and Health, The University of Sydney, Camperdown, NSW, Australia

Rebecca Chen Sydney Dental School, Faculty of Medicine and Health, The University of Sydney, Camperdown, NSW, Australia

Ananda P. Dasanayake Department of Epidemiology & Health Promotion, New York University, New York, NY, USA

Loc Giang Do School of Dentistry, Faculty of Health, Medicine, and Behavioural Sciences, The University of Queensland, Brisbane, QLD, Australia

Sangeeta Gajendra Department of Community Dentistry, Eastman Institute for Oral Health, Rochester, NY, USA

Gerado Marcelo Gilligan Department of Oral Medicine, Facultad de Odontología, Universidad Nacional de Córdoba, Córdoba, Argentina

Yet Ching Goh Department of Oral and Maxillofacial Clinical Sciences, Faculty of Dentistry, Universiti Malaya, Kuala Lumpur, Malaysia

Diep Hong Ha School of Dentistry, Faculty of Health, Medicine, and Behavioural Sciences, The University of Queensland, Brisbane, QLD, Australia

Esam Saleh Halboub Department of Maxillofacial Surgery and Diagnostic Sciences, College of Dentistry, Jazan University, Jazan, Saudi Arabia

Faiez Najeeb Hattab Oskar-Maria-Graf-Ring, Munich, Germany

Anupama Ivaturi Department of Human-Centred Computing, Faculty of IT, Monash University, Clayton, VIC, Australia

Sonali Kohli Sir H N Reliance Foundation Hospital, Mumbai, India

Sachin Kulkarni Dental School, Sydney University, Sydney, NSW, Australia

Jeronimo Pablo Lazos Department of Oral Medicine, Facultad de Odontología, Universidad Nacional de Córdoba, Córdoba, Argentina

Frank W. Licari College of Dental Medicine, Roseman University of Health Sciences, South Jordan, UT, USA

Patrícia Lyra Egas Moniz Center for Interdisciplinary Research, Egas Moniz School of Health and Science, Almada, Portugal

Vanessa Machado Egas Moniz Center for Interdisciplinary Research, Egas Moniz School of Health and Science, Almada, Portugal

Sam Manger College of Medicine and Dentistry, James Cook University, Douglas, QLD, Australia

Luc Martens Paediatric Dentistry, ELOHA (Equal Lifelong Oral Health for All) Research Group, Oral Health Sciences, Ghent, Belgium

Richard McGowan New York University Health Sciences Library, New York, NY, USA

Scott McIntosh Department of Public Health Sciences and Eastman Institute for Oral Health, University of Rochester Medical Center, Rochester, NY, USA

José João Mendes Egas Moniz Center for Interdisciplinary Research, Egas Moniz School of Health and Science, Almada, Portugal

Paula Moynihan Adelaide Dental School, The University of Adelaide, Adelaide, SA, Australia

Arvind Muthukrishnan Department of Oral Medicine and Radiology and Special Care Dentistry, Saveetha Dental College and Hospital, Saveetha Institute of Medical and Technical Sciences, Chennai, India

Rene Panico Department of Oral Medicine, Facultad de Odontología, Universidad Nacional de Córdoba, Córdoba, Argentina

Shankargouda Patil College of Dental Medicine, Roseman University of Health Sciences, South Jordan, UT, USA

Eduardo David Piemonte Department of Oral Medicine, Facultad de Odontología, Universidad Nacional de Córdoba, Córdoba, Argentina

S. R. Prabhu School of Dentistry, University of Queensland, Brisbane, QLD, Australia

Abhirami Premarajan Department of Oral and Maxillofacial Pathology and Oral Microbiology, Dr. D. Y. Patil Dental College and Hospital, Dr. D. Y. Patil Vidyapeeth, Pune, Maharashtra, India

Sivaprakash Rajsekaran Paediatric Dentistry, ELOHA (Equal Lifelong Oral Health for All) Research Group, Oral Health Sciences, Ghent, Belgium

Cameron L. Randall Department of Oral Health Sciences, University of Washington School of Dentistry, Seattle, WA, USA

Kannan Ranganathan Department of Oral and Maxillofacial Pathology, Ragas Dental College, Chennai, Tamil Nadu, India

Dulip Ratnasoma First Physicians Group, Sarasota, FL, USA

Rajkumar Sanahan National Drug Dependence Treatment Centre, All India Institute of Medical Sciences, New Delhi, India

Siddharth Sarkar National Drug Dependence Treatment Centre, All India Institute of Medical Sciences, New Delhi, India

Gargi Sarode Department of Oral and Maxillofacial Pathology and Oral Microbiology, Dr. D. Y. Patil Dental College and Hospital, Dr. D. Y. Patil Vidyapeeth, Pune, Maharashtra, India

Sachin Sarode Department of Oral and Maxillofacial Pathology and Oral Microbiology, Dr. D. Y. Patil Dental College and Hospital, Dr. D. Y. Patil Vidyapeeth, Pune, Maharashtra, India

Jaya Seneviratne Periodontology, School of Dentistry, The University of Queensland, Brisbane, QLD, Australia

Christopher Sexton The University of Queensland, Poche Centre for Indigenous Health and The University of Queensland, School of Dentistry, Brisbane, QLD, Australia

Nandita Shenoy Department of Oral Medicine and Radiology, Manipal College of Dental Sciences, Mangalore, Manipal Academy of Higher Education, Manipal, Karnataka, India

Meena Singh Department of Epidemiology & Health Promotion, New York University, New York, NY, USA

Pankaj Singh APP-NEA, New York, NY, USA

Advanced Dentistry of Long Island, Woodbury, NY, USA

Latasha Treger Slavin Global Health Visions, Gauteng, South Africa

Nicole Stormon The University of Queensland, School of Dentistry and Queensland Health, Metro North Health, Community and Oral Health, Brisbane, QLD, Australia

Supeetha Suntharamoorthy Discipline of Oral Medicine, UWA Dental School, University of Western Australia, Nedlands, WA, Australia

John Rong Hao Tay National Dental Centre Singapore, Singapore, Singapore

Aruni Tilakaratne Department of Restorative Dentistry, Faculty of Dentistry, Universiti Malaya, Kuala Lumpur, Malaysia

Wanninayake Mudiyanselage Tilakaratne Department of Oral and Maxillofacial Clinical Sciences, Faculty of Dentistry, Universiti Malaya, Kuala Lumpur, Malaysia

Tamanna Tiwari Department of Primary Dental Care, School of Dentistry, University of Minnesota, Minneapolis, MN, USA

Saman Warnakulasuriya Faculty of Dentistry, Oral and Craniofacial Sciences, King's College London, and WHO Collaborating Centre for Oral Cancer, London, UK

Lasanthini Weerakkody Discipline of Oral Medicine, UWA Dental School, The University of Western Australia, Nedlands, WA, Australia

Sue-Ching Yeoh Dental School, Sydney University, Sydney, NSW, Australia

1 Healthy Lifestyle Behaviours

Sam Manger

1.1 Health: A Biopsychosocial–Cultural Concept

At first reflection on what health means, this seemingly simple question and concept that underlies the field of lifestyle medicine (LM) is in reality a complex philosophical and practical question that has profound implications on the practice of contemporary health professionals.

The conceptualisation of health has evolved significantly over time and across cultures to encompass multiple dimensions of well-being. The well-known definition established by the World Health Organization (WHO) in 1948 described health as 'a state of complete physical, mental and social well-being and not merely the absence of disease or infirmity' [1]. Whilst this definition remains relevant, the phrase 'complete well-being' has been questioned over the decades as idealistic and therefore impractical [1].

Multiple alternative concepts of health have been explored since then to consider health on a more practical dynamic spectrum, as well as a growing recognition of the additional determinants of health and the relevance of how health impacts the ability to live one's life. The biopsychosocial–cultural model of health, first proposed by George Engel in 1977, recognises that health outcomes are determined by, and hence cannot be understood in isolation of, the complex interaction of biological, psychological, social and cultural factors [2]. In 1987, Aaron Antonovsky introduced the term 'salutogenesis' (the study of the origins [genesis] of health [saluto]) in his proposed Salutogenic Model of Health, which emphasised focusing attention on the origins of and assets for positive health, such as meaning and a sense of coherence, which in turn helps one mobilise resources to cope with stressors and helps determine one's movement on the health and disease continuum [3].

S. Manger (✉)
College of Medicine and Dentistry, James Cook University, Douglas, QLD, Australia
e-mail: sam.manger@jcu.edu.au

S. R. Prabhu et al. (eds.), *Lifestyle in Oral Health and Disease*,
https://doi.org/10.1007/978-3-032-05888-1_1

In the first International Conference on Health Promotion in Ottawa in 1986, the WHO provided further exploration of their original definition to include these more positive concepts: 'To reach a state of complete physical, mental and social well-being, an individual or group must be able to identify and to realize aspirations, to satisfy needs, and to change or cope with the environment. Health is, therefore, seen as a resource for everyday life, not the objective of living. Health is a positive concept emphasizing social and personal resources, as well as physical capacities' [4]. This additional focus on capability rather than incapability was neatly summarised by Sigmund Freud's response to defining health as 'the capacity to love and work' [5].

Importantly, this holistic understanding of health aligns more synchronously with concepts proposed by First Nation Australians. In 1989, the National Aboriginal Health Working Party proposed a definition on Aboriginal health as 'not just the physical well-being of an individual but refers to the social, emotional and cultural well-being of the whole Community in which each individual is able to achieve their full potential as a human being thereby bringing about the total well-being of their Community. It is a whole of life view' [6]. This understanding broadens our concept of health to acknowledge the intertwined relationship between the community, an individual and a culture.

Overall however, there does not seem to be one agreed definition of health [7]. What does this practically mean then for the 'health' professional? First, it means we must acknowledge that health is not a persistent absolute state, but rather a dynamic continuum or the 'progressive realisation of a worthy ideal', to paraphrase US author Earl Nightingale. Second, that it entails multiple interacting biopsycho-social–cultural and spiritual risks and protective factors that influence an individual and a community and hence each of these needs to be considered in diagnosis, assessment and management. Third, that health is seen as a biopsychosocial–cultural and spiritual resource that can be cultivated to enhance the positive capability for life. And finally, that involving the patient or community in identifying what health means to them may be necessary in achieving it.

This biopsychosocial–cultural–spiritual approach forms the philosophical and practical foundation of lifestyle medicine and lifestyle dentistry, which seeks to address the lifestyle, social and cultural roots of illness and health in the prevention, management and, when possible, reversal of chronic disease and optimisation of the human state.

1.2 Contemporary Trends in Chronic Disease and Lifestyle Behaviours

Recent and concerning trends in chronic disease burden and lifestyle behaviours highlight the need to assess and intervene in the lifestyle and social factors. The global burden of disease has shifted dramatically over the past century, with non-communicable chronic diseases (NCDs) now accounting for approximately 71% of all deaths worldwide and over 90% of deaths in Australia [8]. In Australia, type 2 diabetes mellitus (T2DM) and cardiovascular disease exemplify these concerning trends. Between the years 2000 and 2020, the prevalence of T2DM increased almost 2.8-fold [9]; now, approximately 5% of Australians are diagnosed with T2DM and 16% are in pre-diabetic states [9], though studies indicate the true disease burden of T2DM is likely an underrepresentation as 1 in 3 diabetic people may be underdiagnosed [10]. Furthermore, the American College of Cardiology released a statement in 2019 summarising a 16-year study from 2000 to 2016, that indicated that the proportion of young people (<40 years) having a heart attack has been increasing, rising by 2% each year for the last 10 years [11].

The WHO Global Burden of Disease (GBD) study identified that almost all major NCDs such as cardiovascular diseases, metabolic diseases such as T2DM, cancers, respiratory diseases and neurological and psychiatric diseases share many common lifestyle-related risk and protective factors, including nutrition, physical activity, tobacco use, alcohol consumption, stress, sleep and social connection [8]. The European Prospective Investigation into Cancer and Nutrition (EPIC) study found that improvements in four simple lifestyle behaviours could prevent 93% of type 2 diabetes cases, 81% of heart attacks, 50% of strokes and 36% of all cancers [12]. Similarly, a global analysis of type 2 diabetes risk and diet across 184 countries revealed that 11 dietary factors predicted over 70% of diabetes cases, with poor carbohydrate quality (e.g. excess refined grains, insufficient whole grains) emerging as the leading driver [13]. In a UK study of over 400,000 people, sleep duration of ≤5 h and ≥9 h are both associated with a 25% higher risk of all-cause mortality compared to 7 h of sleep [14]. In other nations, such as the USA [15], there has been a doubling in the number of adults sleeping ≤6 h in a 24-h period from 1985 to 2012 indicating a concerning trend of modern lifestyles. The health impacts of loneliness and social isolation are widely recognised. Large observational meta-analyses of over 300,000 people indicated a 50% increased likelihood of survival for participants with stronger social relationships, concluding that the influence of social relationships on risk for mortality is comparable with well-established risk factors for mortality [16].

An estimated 95% of Australian adults do not consume sufficient amounts of fruit or vegetables, 63% are overweight or have obesity, 56% are insufficiently physically active, 76% are doing insufficient strengthening activities, 17% consume harmful levels of alcohol, 60% report at least one chronic sleep symptom and 16% of Australians are experiencing social loneliness with particularly worsening trends in young people [17, 18]. The trends in lifestyle behaviours are not all negative; however, with age-standardised daily smoking rates falling from 25.6% in 1989–1990 to 14.7% in 2014–2015 [17].

Social determinants of health, including education, housing, employment and access to healthcare, significantly influence an individual's capacity to adopt and maintain health-promoting behaviours. For example, food insecurity may limit access to nutritious foods, whilst neighbourhood design can either facilitate or impede physical activity. Addressing these upstream determinants is essential for creating environments that support healthy lifestyle choices, hence the relatively recent growth of clinical approaches such as 'social prescribing'. Social prescribing is the practice where healthcare professionals connect patients to non-clinical community-based services and activities to improve their health and wellbeing, addressing social determinants of health and strengthening community connections [19].

Healthcare systems and leading clinical guidelines increasingly recognise the value of lifestyle interventions as foundational components of chronic disease management. This shift is reflected in updated clinical guidelines, such as the 2021 Royal Australian and New Zealand College of Psychiatrists' clinical practice guidelines for mood disorders that highlight lifestyle approaches as 'first-line, foundational and essentially non-negotiable for all patients' [20]. In addition, the recommendation for lifestyle approaches as first line in cardiovascular and metabolic diseases has been present for some time though it is becoming evident that lifestyle and social assessment and interventions are also not limited to chronic disease management. In 2022 a large systematic review analysed the impact of structured lifestyle programmes during the antenatal period on total adverse maternal and neonatal outcomes, reducing risk by 25% and 56%, respectively [21]. Furthermore, of relevance to the field of surgery and dentistry, perioperative lifestyle interventions significantly reduce the adverse risks of surgery including pain, disability and infection, and reduce total length of hospital stay [22].

Surveys indicate a strong desire and acceptability of lifestyle medicine and a preference for non-pharmacological treatment approaches in chronic physical and mental disease management [23, 24]. However, data reviewing how consistently and effectively lifestyle assessments and interventions are done in practice demonstrate room for improvement, with studies showing nutrition, weight, exercise, smoking, lifestyle, prevention and alcohol were together given at a rate of only 8 per 100 encounters and <4% of primary care consults including clinical treatment advice on diet and exercise [25, 26].

1.3 The Pillars of Lifestyle Medicine: *Nutrition, Physical Activity, Sleep, Social Connection, Social Prescribing, Substance Reduction, Mind–Body Approach and Nature Prescriptions*

Lifestyle Medicine (LM) is a rapidly growing field in clinical practice and research over the past 25 years that focuses on the role of modifiable lifestyle and social factors in preventing, managing and reversing chronic disease. It is the formal evidence-based application of nutrition, movement, sleep, mind–body practices, reduced substance use, social connectedness, connection with the natural world and social prescribing combined with behaviour change science, health coaching and new models of care and technology to lead to whole-of-person well-being [27]. An LM approach strongly aligns with the quintuple aim of healthcare: better health outcomes, lower cost, improved patient satisfaction, improved provider wellbeing and advancement of health equity [28]. Health equity is inherent in the provision of lifestyle medicine and social prescribing as the burden of chronic disease disproportionately affects populations of need.

Lifestyle assessment and interventions can be considered core and foundational components of care based on their evidence of effect on mental, physical and social well-being; the understanding of the physiological and psychological mechanisms of action; and their strong safety profile (however, more intensive lifestyle approaches should be monitored by appropriately trained professionals). LM strategies can be provided at relatively low cost across a range of settings and age groups with diverse clinical and demographic characteristics and can be delivered alone or in conjunction with established therapies. It is worth noting that the target of lifestyle approaches is not a 'one size fits all' and there are many healthy approaches available that can be adapted following common principles in diverse cultures and backgrounds.

The role of lifestyle factors in prevention is clear and in the past 25 years multiple randomised controlled trials have demonstrated the role of LM in contributing to the reversal of pathophysiological processes, potentially contributing to disease remission in conditions such as atherosclerotic heart disease, type 2 diabetes and major depression disorder, cognitive impairment and a range of other disorders [29–31]. Furthermore, these interventions have been shown to be particularly cost-effective in health economic evaluations [32].

Common principles of these lifestyle interventions include a reduction of ultra-processed foods and higher consumption of nutrient-rich whole foods; increasing physical activity and literacy in the areas of aerobic, strength and balance training; improving sleep quality, quantity and consistency; reduced substance and pathological social media use; improved social and natural world connections; tailored mind–body interventions; and social prescription. Lifestyle interventions such as nutrition are not limited to specific ratios of macronutrients, but rather include a wide number of biopsychosocial and cultural factors including quality and quantity of the produce, the order/timing/intervals of food intake, the unique biopsychosocial profile of the person consuming the food, the cognitive, emotional and behavioural concepts and practices around food, the social and cultural context and sharing of food, and the ecological impacts. This is also true for physical activity and mind–body interventions that do not have to only be the 'traditional' forms most common in some modern cultures such as running, weights and swimming but systematic reviews also demonstrate the physical, social and psychological benefits of diverse forms of movement such as physical games, dance, tai chi and yoga, relaxation therapies, mindfulness, breathwork and prayer [33, 34].

Lifestyle approaches impact mental and physical well-being through multiple pathways and with short- and long-term effects. There are several closely linked physiological pathways explaining why and how lifestyle approaches can affect physical, mental and cognitive health [35]. These include modulation of pathways involved in reduced inflammation, the gut microbiota, oxidative stress, mitochondrial function, vagal tone and blood pressure, insulin sensitivity, improved immune function, collagen and other soft tissue integrity, endorphin release, endocannabinoid system regulation, tryptophan–kynurenine metabolism, the hypothalamic–pituitary axis, autonomic nervous system function, neuronal health, epigenetic regulation and increased telomerase expression, *which extends chromosomal telomere length, a common indicator of biological age and disease risk* and a variety of systemic repair mechanisms [35–38]. As an example of the profound impact of lifestyle interventions, Neufer et al. in 2015 stated 'physical activity challenges homeostasis in virtually every organ system and activates acute and long-term compensatory mechanisms to preserve and/or re-establish homeostasis' [38]. Lifestyle interventions are also mutually supportive, for example physical activity also supports other lifestyle behaviours such as improved sleep and social connection and has other psychological benefits, such as increased self-esteem and a sense of accomplishment [39].

Lifestyle-based healthcare is not a single intervention but rather several interacting layers that involve lifestyle domains combined with implementation. The more each of these aspects are cultivated within an individual's life, environments and healthcare, the greater the opportunity for earlier intervention, potential to prevent disease progression and relapse, enhancing resilience against adverse internal or external events and improving mental, physical and social well-being. Hence, this field holds significant potential to improve the mental and physical well-being of individuals and communities but is yet to be fully realised in both clinical service implementation and research.

1.4 Behaviour Change and Health Coaching in Supporting Healthy Lifestyles

Behavioural science can be defined as 'an interdisciplinary approach to the study of human behaviour encompassing disciplines including psychology, sociology, anthropology and economics and the interaction between these' [40]. What influences human behaviour is a complex theme; however, several developed frameworks can be used to answer the fundamental question: 'What conditions internal to individuals and in their social and physical environment need to be in place for a specified behavioural goal to be achieved?'

The science of behaviour change relevant to human health is a large and expanding field but can be split into two broad categories. First relates to the clinical behaviour change skills a health professional may use in an individual or group-based clinical setting, often referred to as 'health coaching' [41]. A number of frameworks and skills can be integrated into clinical care to motivate and support people adopting and sustaining healthy lifestyle and social interventions. These include but are not limited to: motivational interviewing that aims to strengthen a therapeutic relationship and motivate change in patients that are ambivalent [42]; strengths-based coaching that focuses on the innate strengths of individuals, families and communities to enable self-empowerment and self-determination [43]; and established behaviour change frameworks such as the Transtheoretical Domains Framework (TDF) *and Capability–Opportunity–Motivation (COM-B) framework* [44]. The second category includes the use of behaviour change principles that inform the modification of built environments, ranging from the placement of food in a pantry to the architectural design of a clinical waiting area.

There are hundreds of behaviour change theories and models, though common and integral aspects to effective patient–clinician communication and behavioural activation include cultivating a therapeutic relationship, engaging patients in decision making, curiosity and empathy [45]. Evidence demonstrates the foundational importance of strong therapeutic relationships using these principles [45]. Strong therapeutic relationships make substantial and consistent contributions to patient success in treatment. Some authors report that the quality of the client–therapist alliance in mental health, which commonly requires behavioural activation, is a reliable predictor of positive clinical outcomes independent of the variety of psychotherapy approaches [46].

For the seemingly 'unmotivated' patient, it is worth considering whether they are unmotivated to address any or all aspects of their life, or just the ones the therapist has focussed on, for example, 'diet and exercise'. Is it possible to engage them in any aspect of what they do want from their own life, health and well-being, turning it from a disease-specific approach to a human-centric approach, and what does quality of life look like for them? This can be very wide ranging, like attending classes or catching up with an old mate, which acts as the initial keystone step to positive health experiences and an ongoing journey. Some people are obviously not immediately motivated and this must be accepted. In these settings it is important to perform our job well, develop a strong therapeutic relationship, advise of risks and benefits of behaviours, provide education, support, organise follow-up and, if needed, provide harm minimisation strategies. As therapists, focussing on those that do not change can lead to burnout and loss of hope, and hence having realistic expectations about the complexity of human behaviour and practicing self-compassion can help.

1.5 Models of Care and Implementation of Lifestyle Medicine

The assessment and prescription of lifestyle and social approaches is not merely limited to the practice of individual health professionals. In fact, how a health service or 'model of care' is delivered can either significantly hinder or enhance the provision of effective and efficient lifestyle-based healthcare. Since the early 2000s, the field of implementation science has emerged to provide structure and guidance via theories, models and frameworks for the systematic uptake of research findings and other evidence-based practices into routine practice to improve the quality and effectiveness of health services and care [47]. One of the foundational goals of implementation science is to identify the core components that help to understand and explain how and why implementation succeeds or fails. Theories, methods and frameworks can be used to guide programme implementation and are typically more like 'common-sense' checklists of factors relevant to various aspects of implementation, but generally no one method works for all settings.

Like clinical assessment and prescriptions, the 'service assessment and implementation' requires the combination of understanding principles in assessing the needs and assets of a setting, and then adapting these to create a unique yet structured programme plan. Common principles across multiple frameworks in implementation science include an initial observation/assessment phase where the population needs and service gaps are understood, and an analysis of enablers (strengths, assets), barriers, settings, stakeholders, creative co-design to identify potential solutions, implementation, evaluation (qualitative and quantitative), promotion/dissemination and, if desired, scaling [48].

There are a wide variety of unique and innovative programmes and models that are the fruit of these principles, each suited to their setting (primary, community, tertiary) and population needs. These include, but certainly are not limited to: developing interdisciplinary teamwork and a needs-based workforce, for example, health coaches and peer support workers, specialised lifestyle-disease/health clinics, and group consults; hosting health events; utilising digital technology, staff well-being programmes, community-based programmes, and cultural and rural health programmes; optimising the built environment; and more [47–49]. Digital technology has a wide range of potential uses in clinical practice (e.g. artificial intelligence, behaviour change tools, biometric devices 'wearables', telehealth, decision support software, online programmes), administration (scheduling, medical records, data analysis, automation) and research (data collection, remote monitoring, evaluation) [50].

The success and sustainability of any lifestyle medicine programme is dependent on initial implementation planning followed over the long term by automating processes and embedding programmes and funding into the culture and priorities of a service. Collaboration and coordination to encourage a team-based approach with early stakeholder engagement to improve the odds of success is a common requirement, including from the lived experience/patient and executive/leadership positions. Programmes or services that are implemented should be congruent with pre-existing priorities and strengths of that population, culture, or service [49].

1.6 The Beneficial Impact of Practising Lifestyle Medicine on the Health Professional

Unfortunately, the well-being of the health practitioners is often a distant third priority after the health of our patients and the operation of the service. Rates of burnout, psychological distress, chronic disease and substance use are concerningly high in the health profession indicating that the evolution of our services must also include the focus on the well-being of its providers [51]. In 2023, a survey of 482 LM health professionals found that 90% reported practising LM had positively impacted their professional satisfaction due to providing a sense of meaning, improved patient outcomes and satisfaction, pleasure in the job and improving their own personal quality of life, and it was overall associated with a 43% decrease in the odds of experiencing burnout [52].

Whilst less mentally and physically healthy providers can still and do deliver excellent care, evidence indicates that on average low levels of physicians' wellbeing can lead to suboptimal performing healthcare systems whereas physicians with higher levels of wellbeing tend to provide better patient care (e.g. satisfaction, adherence to treatment and interpersonal aspects of patient care) [53]. Moreover, health professionals who model healthy behaviour have greater confidence in their ability to provide diet and exercise counselling and are more likely to counsel their patients about exercise, diet and smoking [54]. Furthermore, patients become more receptive to health promotion counselling from physicians who demonstrate healthy behaviours themselves [55].

It is crucial for service managers, decision makers and all staff to consider how to create opportunity for well-being practices at work and create a culture whereby provider well-being is recognised and supported.

1.7 Future Opportunities in Lifestyle Medicine Clinical Practice and Research

In the past 10 years, a number of seminal studies have demonstrated the substantial role of LM in chronic disease management, specifically in mood disorders, metabolic disease, heart disease and opportunistic health optimisation in areas such as antenatal and presurgical care. However, in truth, the field of LM is still very much in its infancy. For the motivated health professional, the field of LM offers many career and 'change' opportunities. There is still a significant amount of high-quality clinical research to be done across a range of health or disease targets that remain understudied, such as autoimmune disease, oncology, neurological disease, men and women's health and severe mental illness. Research in the implementation and evaluation of LM models of care is also urgently needed to demonstrate and scale best practice care that more effectively addresses the biopsychosocial–cultural and spiritual determinants of health.

References

1. van Druten VP, Bartels EA, van de Mheen D, de Vries E, Kerckhoffs APM, Nahar-van Venrooij LMW. Concepts of health in different contexts: a scoping review. BMC Health Serv Res. 2022;22(1):389. https://doi.org/10.1186/s12913-022-07702-2.
2. Bolton D, Gillett G. The biopsychosocial model 40 years on. In: The biopsychosocial model of health and disease: new philosophical and scientific developments. Cham: Palgrave Pivot; 2019.
3. Mittelmark MB, Bauer GF. Salutogenesis as a theory, as an orientation and as the sense of coherence. In: Mittelmark MB, Bauer GF, Vaandrager L, et al., editors. The handbook of salutogenesis. 2nd ed. Cham: Springer; 2022.
4. Ottawa charter for health promotion. Health Promot Int. 1986;1(4):405. https://doi.org/10.1093/heapro/1.4.405.

5. Werbart A, Bergstedt A, Levander S. Love, work, and striving for the self in balance: anaclitic and introjective patients' experiences of change in psychoanalysis. Front Psychol. 2020;11:144. https://doi.org/10.3389/fpsyg.2020.00144.
6. Senior T. The aboriginal definition of health. Br J Gen Pract. 2023;73(733):369. https://doi.org/10.3399/bjgp23X734637.
7. Huber M, Knottnerus JA, Green L, van der Horst H, Jadad AR, Kromhout D, Leonard B, Lorig K, Loureiro MI, van der Meer JW, Schnabel P, Smith R, van Weel C, Smid H. How should we define health? BMJ. 2011;343:d4163. https://doi.org/10.1136/bmj.d4163.
8. GBD 2019 Australia Collaborators. The burden and trend of diseases and their risk factors in Australia, 1990–2019: a systematic analysis for the Global Burden of Disease Study 2019. Lancet Public Health. 2023;8(8):e585–99. https://doi.org/10.1016/S2468-2667(23)00123-8.
9. Australian Institute of Health and Welfare. Diabetes: Australian facts [Internet]. Canberra: Australian Institute of Health and Welfare; 2024. [cited 2025 Mar 19]. Available from: https://www.aihw.gov.au/reports/diabetes/diabetes.
10. Galicia-Garcia U, Benito-Vicente A, Jebari S, et al. Pathophysiology of type 2 diabetes mellitus. Int J Mol Sci. 2020;21(17):6275. https://doi.org/10.3390/ijms21176275.
11. Yang J, Biery DW, Singh A, Divakaran S, DeFilippis EM, Wu WY, et al. Risk factors and outcomes of very young adults who experience myocardial infarction: the partners YOUNG-MI registry. Am J Med. 2020;133(5):605–612.e1. https://doi.org/10.1016/j.amjmed.2019.10.020.
12. Ford ES, Bergmann MM, Kröger J, Schienkiewitz A, Weikert C, Boeing H. Healthy living is the best revenge: findings from the European Prospective Investigation Into Cancer and Nutrition-Potsdam study. Arch Intern Med. 2009;169(15):1355–62. https://doi.org/10.1001/archinternmed.2009.237.
13. O'Hearn M, Lara-Castor L, Cudhea F, et al. Incident type 2 diabetes attributable to suboptimal diet in 184 countries. Nat Med. 2023;29(4):982–95. https://doi.org/10.1038/s41591-023-02278-8.
14. Tao F, Cao Z, Jiang Y, Fan N, Xu F, Yang H, et al. Associations of sleep duration and quality with incident cardiovascular disease, cancer, and mortality: a prospective cohort study of 407,500 UK biobank participants. Sleep Med. 2021;81:401–9. https://doi.org/10.1016/j.sleep.2021.03.015.
15. Ford ES, Cunningham TJ, Croft JB. Trends in self-reported sleep duration among US adults from 1985 to 2012. Sleep. 2015;38(5):829–32. https://doi.org/10.5665/sleep.4684.
16. Holt-Lunstad J, Smith TB, Layton JB. Social relationships and mortality risk: a meta-analytic review. PLoS Med. 2010;7(7):e1000316. https://doi.org/10.1371/journal.pmed.1000316.
17. Australian Institute of Health and Welfare. Australia's health 2018. Canberra: AIHW, Australian Government; 2018. https://doi.org/10.25816/5ec1e56f25480.
18. Reynolds AC, Appleton SL, Gill TK, Adams RJ. Chronic insomnia disorder in Australia. A Report to the Sleep Health Foundation; 2019.
19. Calderón-Larrañaga S, Greenhalgh T, Finer S, Clinch M. What does social prescribing look like in practice? A qualitative case study informed by practice theory. Soc Sci Med. 2024;343:116601. https://doi.org/10.1016/j.socscimed.2024.116601.
20. Malhi GS, Bell E, Bassett D, Boyce P, Bryant R, Hazell P, et al. The 2020 Royal Australian and New Zealand College of Psychiatrists clinical practice guidelines for mood disorders. Aust N Z J Psychiatry. 2021;55(1):7–117. https://doi.org/10.1177/0004867420979353.
21. Teede HJ, Bailey C, Moran LJ, Bahri Khomami M, Enticott J, Ranasinha S, et al. Association of antenatal diet and physical activity-based interventions with gestational weight gain and pregnancy outcomes: a systematic review and meta-analysis. JAMA Intern Med. 2022;182(2):106–14. https://doi.org/10.1001/jamainternmed.2021.6373.
22. McIsaac DI, Gill M, Boland L, Hutton B, Branje K, Shaw J, et al. Prehabilitation in adult patients undergoing surgery: an umbrella review of systematic reviews. Br J Anaesth. 2022;128(2):244–57. https://doi.org/10.1016/j.bja.2021.11.014.
23. Richardson K, Petukhova R, Hughes S, et al. The acceptability of lifestyle medicine for the treatment of mental illness: perspectives of people with and without lived experience of mental illness. BMC Public Health. 2024;24:171. https://doi.org/10.1186/s12889-024-17683-y.

24. Litterbach E, Holmes-Truscott E, Pouwer F, Speight J, Hendrieckx C. 'I wish my health professionals understood that it's not just all about your HbA1c!'. Qualitative responses from the second Diabetes MILES–Australia (MILES-2) study. Diabet Med. 2020;37(6):971–81. https://doi.org/10.1111/dme.14199.
25. Britt H, Miller GC, Henderson J, Bayram C, Harrison C, Valenti L, et al. General practice activity in Australia 2015–16. In: Bettering the Evaluation and Care of Health (BEACH). Sydney: Sydney University Press; 2016.
26. Beattie J, Binder M, Harrison C, Miller GC, Pedler D. Lifestyle risk factors and corresponding levels of clinical advice and counselling in general practice. Aust Fam Physician. 2017;46(10):751–5.
27. Lippman D, Stump M, Veazey E, et al. Foundations of lifestyle medicine and its evolution. Mayo Clin Proc Innov Qual Outcomes. 2024;8(1):97–111. https://doi.org/10.1016/j.mayocpiqo.2023.11.004.
28. Nundy S, Cooper LA, Mate KS. The quintuple aim for health care improvement: a new imperative to advance health equity. JAMA. 2022;327(6):521–2. https://doi.org/10.1001/jama.2021.25181.
29. Lean ME, Leslie WS, Barnes AC, et al. Primary care-led weight management for remission of type 2 diabetes (DiRECT): an open label, cluster-randomised trial. Lancet. 2018;391(10120):541–51. https://doi.org/10.1016/S0140-6736(17)33102-1.
30. Ornish D, Scherwitz L, Billings JH, et al. Intensive lifestyle changes for reversal of coronary heart disease. JAMA. 1998;280(23):2001–7. https://doi.org/10.1001/jama.280.23.2001.
31. Jacka FN, O'Neil A, Opie R, et al. A randomised controlled trial of dietary improvement for adults with major depression (the 'SMILES' trial). BMC Med. 2017;15(1):23. https://doi.org/10.1186/s12916-017-0791-y.
32. Chatterton ML, Mihalopoulos C, O'Neil A, et al. Economic evaluation of a dietary intervention for adults with major depression (the "SMILES" trial). BMC Public Health. 2018;18:599. https://doi.org/10.1186/s12889-018-5504-8.
33. Brinsley J, Schuch F, Lederman O, Girard D, Smout M, Immink MA, et al. Effects of yoga on depressive symptoms in people with mental disorders: a systematic review and meta-analysis. Br J Sports Med. 2021;55(17):992–1000. https://doi.org/10.1136/bjsports-2019-101242.
34. Prieto LA, Haegele JA, Columna L. Dance programs for school-age individuals with disabilities: a systematic review. Adapt Phys Act Q. 2020;37(3):349–76. https://doi.org/10.1123/apaq.2019-0117.
35. Marx W, Lane M, Hockey M, Aslam H, Berk M, Walder K, et al. Diet and depression: exploring the biological mechanisms of action. Mol Psychiatry. 2021;26(1):134–50. https://doi.org/10.1038/s41380-020-00925-x.
36. Horn J, Mayer DE, Chen S, Mayer EA. Role of diet and its effects on the gut microbiome in the pathophysiology of mental disorders. Transl Psychiatry. 2022;12(1):164. https://doi.org/10.1038/s41398-022-01922-0.
37. Schutte NS, Malouff JM. A meta-analytic review of the effects of mindfulness meditation on telomerase activity. Psychoneuroendocrinology. 2014;42:45–8. https://doi.org/10.1016/j.psyneuen.2013.12.017.
38. Neufer PD, Bamman MM, Muoio DM, Bouchard C, Cooper DM, Goodpaster BH, et al. Understanding the cellular and molecular mechanisms of physical activity-induced health benefits. Cell Metab. 2015;22(1):4–11. https://doi.org/10.1016/j.cmet.2015.05.011.
39. Kandola A, Ashdown-Franks G, Hendrikse J, Sabiston CM, Stubbs B. Physical activity and depression: towards understanding the antidepressant mechanisms of physical activity. Neurosci Biobehav Rev. 2019;107:525–39. https://doi.org/10.1016/j.neubiorev.2019.09.040.
40. Curtis K, Fulton E, Brown K. Factors influencing application of behavioural science evidence by public health decision-makers and practitioners, and implications for practice. Prev Med Rep. 2018;12:106–15. https://doi.org/10.1016/j.pmedr.2018.08.012.
41. Conn S, Curtain S. Health coaching as a lifestyle medicine process in primary care. Aust J Gen Pract. 2019;48(10):677–80. https://doi.org/10.31128/AJGP-07-19-4984.

42. Bischof G, Bischof A, Rumpf HJ. Motivational interviewing: an evidence-based approach for use in medical practice. Dtsch Arztebl Int. 2021;118(7):109–15. https://doi.org/10.3238/arztebl.m2021.0014.
43. van Zyl LE, Roll LC, Stander MW, Richter S. Positive psychological coaching definitions and models: a systematic literature review. Front Psychol. 2020;11:793. https://doi.org/10.3389/fpsyg.2020.00793.
44. Atkins L, Francis J, Islam R, O'Connor D, Patey A, Ivers N, et al. A guide to using the theoretical domains framework of behaviour change to investigate implementation problems. Implement Sci. 2017;12(1):77. https://doi.org/10.1186/s13012-017-0605-9.
45. Norcross JC, Wampold BE. Evidence-based therapy relationships: research conclusions and clinical practices. Psychotherapy (Chic). 2011;48(1):98–102. https://doi.org/10.1037/a0022161.
46. Ardito RB, Rabellino D. Therapeutic alliance and outcome of psychotherapy: historical excursus, measurements, and prospects for research. Front Psychol. 2011;2:270. https://doi.org/10.3389/fpsyg.2011.00270.
47. Armstrong R, Sales A. Welcome to implementation science communications. Implement Sci Commun. 2020;1:1. https://doi.org/10.1186/s43058-020-00018-4.
48. Nilsen P. Making sense of implementation theories, models and frameworks. Implement Sci. 2015;10:53. https://doi.org/10.1186/s13012-015-0242-0.
49. Waltz TJ, Powell BJ, Matthieu MM, Damschroder LJ, Chinman MJ, Smith JL, et al. Use of concept mapping to characterize relationships among implementation strategies and assess their feasibility and importance: results from the Expert Recommendations for Implementing Change (ERIC) study. Implement Sci. 2015;10:109. https://doi.org/10.1186/s13012-015-0295-0.
50. Butcher CJ, Hussain W. Digital healthcare: the future. Future Healthc J. 2022;9(2):113–7. https://doi.org/10.7861/fhj.2022-0046.
51. O'Connor K, Muller Neff D, Pitman S. Burnout in mental health professionals: a systematic review and meta-analysis of prevalence and determinants. Eur Psychiatry. 2018;53:74–99. https://doi.org/10.1016/j.eurpsy.2018.06.003.
52. Pollard KJ, Gittelsohn J, Patel P, Lianov L, Freeman K, Staffier KL, et al. Lifestyle medicine practitioners implementing a greater proportion of lifestyle medicine experience less burnout. Am J Health Promot. 2023;37(8):1121–32. https://doi.org/10.1177/08901171231182875.
53. Scheepers RA, Boerebach BC, Arah OA, Heineman MJ, Lombarts KM. A systematic review of the impact of physicians' occupational well-being on the quality of patient care. Int J Behav Med. 2015;22(6):683–98. https://doi.org/10.1007/s12529-015-9473-3.
54. Wallace JE, Lemaire JB, Ghali WA. Physician wellness: a missing quality indicator. Lancet. 2009;374(9702):1714–21. https://doi.org/10.1016/S0140-6736(09)61424-0.
55. Oberg EB, Frank E. Physicians' health practices strongly influence patient health practices. J R Coll Physicians Edinb. 2009;39(4):290–1. https://doi.org/10.4997/JRCPE.2009.422.

Lifestyle Risk Factors for Oral Diseases: An Overview

2

Loc Giang Do and Diep Hong Ha

2.1 Introduction

Despite improvements in living conditions in most countries, oral diseases remain the most prevalent chronic conditions, affecting 3.5 billion people worldwide [1]. Oral diseases significantly impact the quality of life and society. There are gaps in oral health both between and within countries. Preventing oral diseases requires concerted efforts from all levels of government and organisations.

Most oral diseases are non-communicable and chronic. Lifestyle factors increase the risk of developing certain oral diseases and are important proximal determinants of oral health. Individual lifestyle factors can directly affect oral tissues, initiating or progressing oral diseases; modifying these can improve oral health. Higher-level determinants influence lifestyle risk factors, including socioeconomic and commercial elements that shape individual lifestyle choices. Understanding the contributing factors, oral health consequences and potential interventions related to lifestyle risk factors is crucial for preventing chronic oral diseases and enhancing population oral health. This chapter explores the conceptual pathways linking upstream factors to lifestyle risk factors and oral health. It also examines the contributing factors, affected oral conditions and potential interventions related to the primary lifestyle risk factors impacting oral health.

L. G. Do (✉) · D. H. Ha
School of Dentistry, Faculty of Health, Medicine, and Behavioural Sciences, The University of Queensland, Brisbane, QLD, Australia
e-mail: l.do@uq.edu.au; d.ha@uq.edu.au

S. R. Prabhu et al. (eds.), *Lifestyle in Oral Health and Disease*,
https://doi.org/10.1007/978-3-032-05888-1_2

2.2 Socioecological Determinants and the Pathways to Oral Health

Lifestyle factors are individual constructs that can directly influence health (see Chap. 1). A healthy lifestyle is described as: 'a way of living that lowers the risk of being seriously ill or dying early' and 'a way of living that helps you enjoy more aspects of your life' [2]. In contrast, risky lifestyles can increase the likelihood of diseases and injuries. Much scientific research has investigated approaches to improve individual lifestyle factors to prevent oral diseases.

Since lifestyle factors are primary causes of oral diseases, targeting these factors at the individual level seems intuitive. This approach has often been the primary focus in health prevention and management, including oral health. Individual-level lifestyle interventions have demonstrated some success and are generally accepted by healthcare professionals and organisations. However, there is significant variation in the characteristics of those who benefit most from these interventions, which drives inequalities in population health [3]. A deeper understanding of the upstream causes of these lifestyle risk factors is crucial.

A socioecological approach rather than an individual one to studying early childhood development may be superior [4]. An individual approach focuses on simple cause-and-effect relationships, while a socioecological approach emphasises feedback structures among multilevel systems that interact to influence individual behaviours. Do et al. conducted a scoping review to develop a socioecological framework for oral health [5]. This was based on Bronfenbrenner's socioecological model [4], which suggests that behaviours affect and are influenced by the interactions of factors at different levels, nested within higher levels of a complex dynamic system: the microsystem, mesosystem, exosystem and macrosystem.

Figure 2.1 demonstrates the pathways through which lifestyle factors are formed and affect oral diseases. The *microsystem* (the individual's immediate surroundings that directly interact with them) includes biological, psychosocial and socioeconomic factors. The *mesosystem* (formed by interactions of several microsystems) encompasses health support and cultural and socioeconomic factors in the environment surrounding individuals. The *exosystem* includes elements of the local social environment that shape and constrain behaviours. The *macrosystem* comprises the social, physical and cultural environments, national health policies and commercial determinants of health. Based on this model, oral lifestyle factors are individual actions influenced by the immediate environment, external health information, public policies, marketing and advertising, cultural values and general socioeconomic conditions [3, 6]. It should be noted that higher-level factors can define environments and even set the direction for lower-level factors.

A comprehensive understanding of the systems is necessary to inform actions that improve lifestyle alongside the implementation and sustainability of effective solutions at various levels within the system. It must move beyond merely persuading individuals to change their health habits [7]. These solutions must address the

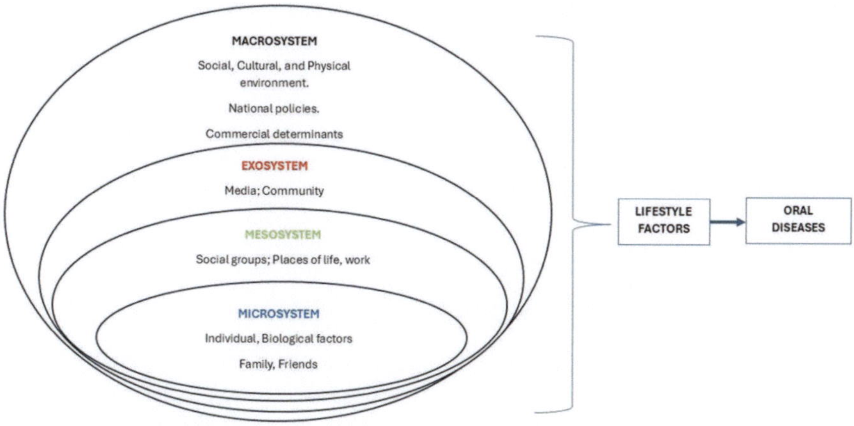

Fig. 2.1 Structural determinants of lifestyle risk factors and their pathways to oral conditions. (Adapted from Do et al. [5])

multifaceted determinants of oral health inequities to make healthy individual lifestyle choices readily accessible in the immediate environment. Such understanding is often lacking, making it challenging to develop effective, efficient and equitable policies and practices that enhance lifestyle factors and prevent oral diseases.

2.3 Overview of Key Lifestyle Factors Affecting Oral Health

Multiple lifestyle risk factors for oral diseases have been identified and researched. Several oral diseases are influenced by various lifestyle factors, which are impacted by numerous contributing elements at different levels (Table 2.1). Therefore, potential interventions must be comprehensive and broader than those that directly target lifestyle factors.

2.3.1 Dietary Patterns

The role of sugars and carbohydrates in tooth decay has been identified [16, 17] (see Chap. 13). Dietary patterns are established early in life, influenced by multiple factors [13, 18], and can have lifelong effects on oral health [19]. The intake of free sugars is recommended to remain below 10% of energy intake [8]. Behavioural interventions can significantly impact the reduction of sugar intake [20]. Commercial factors are crucial in the population's consumption of foods and drinks containing sugars [21]. National policies like sugar taxation can help reduce population-level sugar intake in both low- and high-income countries [22].

Table 2.1 Common lifestyle risk factors and their effect on oral conditions

Lifestyle factor	Contributing factors	Oral conditions	Potential interventions
Dietary patterns [8]	Health policy Regulations on food marketing Commercial determinants Socioeconomic status Cultural factors Media influences School environment Parental/family influence	Dental caries Oral mucosal conditions Oral cancer	Regulating food marketing National dietary policies Nutrition education and awareness programmes
Smoking [9, 10]; illicit recreational drugs [11]	Tobacco policy Illicit drug policy Commercial determinants Socioeconomic status Cultural factors Media influences Parental/family influence	Periodontal diseases Oral mucosal conditions Oral cancer	National tobacco policy Public place regulations on smoking Education and awareness programmes
Alcohol consumption [12]	Alcohol policy Commercial determinants Socioeconomic status Cultural factors Media influences Parental/family influence	Oral mucosal conditions Oral cancer Orofacial trauma	National alcohol policy Public place regulations on drinking Education and awareness programmes
Oral hygiene behaviours and practices [13]	Socioeconomic status Cultural factors Media influences Parental/family influence	Dental caries Periodontal diseases Oral mucosal conditions	Improving dental access Education and awareness programmes
Betel nut chewing [14]	Cultural factors Socioeconomic status Parental/family influence	Oral mucosal conditions Oral cancer	Education and awareness programmes
Access to fluoride [15]	Public health policy Availability of dental services Socioeconomic status Media influences	Dental caries	National policy on fluoride Improving dental access Education and awareness programmes

2.3.2 Tobacco Smoking and Illicit Recreational Drug Use

The evidence linking smoking to periodontal diseases, oral mucosal conditions and oral cancer has been well established [23, 24] (see Chap. 4). Multiple factors, including cultural, social, material and psychosocial influences, affect smoking rates in populations [25, 26]. Cannabis has also been associated with an elevated risk of periodontal disease [11] (see Chap. 11). The tobacco industry's motivations for sales are significant commercial determinants of smoking and, consequently, health [27]. The effectiveness of global tobacco control varies based on national policies regarding taxation and public place restrictions [28].

2.3.3 Alcohol Abuse

Alcohol abuse is a known risk factor for multiple oral conditions [24] (See Chap. 10). A strong commercial determinant drives alcohol consumption [27]. Social and cultural factors significantly influence alcohol use within a socioecological framework [29].

2.3.4 Poor Oral Hygiene Practices

Poor oral hygiene is a direct causal factor for multiple oral diseases [23, 30, 31] (See Chap. 22). This is one of the most significant lifestyle factors influencing oral health. Oral health education can help address this issue [32, 33]. However, the availability of oral hygiene products, such as toothbrushes and toothpaste, can be affected by factors beyond individual control. People with limited capacity need assistance to maintain their oral hygiene status [34].

2.3.5 Betel Nut Chewing

Betel nut chewing is a cultural lifestyle factor impacting oral health [35] (see Chap. 7). This factor has strong cultural causes, so it needs to be appropriately addressed [14]. There should be a combination of population approaches and individual health campaigns.

2.3.6 Access to Fluoride

Fluoride is the cornerstone of preventive programmes against dental caries [15, 36] (see Chap. 15). The WHO names fluoride as an essential medicine [1]. A national policy is needed to guide the profession, industry and public on the appropriate use of various forms of fluoride [37]. Water fluoridation is an effective and safe mode of fluoride delivery. Due to the passive delivery of fluoride through drinking water,

water fluoridation does not require individual lifestyle changes. Furthermore, water fluoridation can mitigate the adverse effects of other lifestyle factors, such as sugar consumption [38]. However, public policy and funding are necessary to establish and maintain a water fluoridation programme.

2.4 Conclusion

Lifestyle risk factors can influence oral health. However, reducing the impact of those risk factors requires addressing the upstream determinants. Most lifestyle risk factors cannot adequately be addressed by targeting individual behaviours alone. It is more effective to create an environment that enables health. Broader socioeconomic and commercial determinants must be addressed alongside behavioural change programmes.

References

1. WHO. The Bangkok Declaration–No health without oral health. Geneva: World Health Organization; 2025.
2. WHO. Healthy living: what is a healthy lifestyle? Copenhagen: WHO Regional Office for Europe; 1999.
3. Alvaro C, Jackson LA, Kirk S, McHugh TL, Hughes J, Chircop A, Lyons RF. Moving Canadian governmental policies beyond a focus on individual lifestyle: some insights from complexity and critical theories. Health Promot Int. 2011;26(1):91–9.
4. Bronfenbrenner U, Morris P. The ecology of developmental processes. In: Lerner R, editor. Theoretical models of human development. 5th ed. New York: Wiley; 1998.
5. Do LG, Song YH, Du M, Spencer AJ, Ha DH. Socioecological determinants of child oral health-a scoping review. Community Dent Oral Epidemiol. 2022;51:1024.
6. Braun W. The system archetypes. Harvard; 2002.
7. Baum F, Fisher M. Why behavioural health promotion endures despite its failure to reduce health inequities. Sociol Health Illn. 2014;36(2):213–25.
8. WHO. Guideline: sugars intake for adults and children. Geneva: World Health Organization; 2015.
9. Do LG, Slade GD, Roberts-Thomson KF, Sanders AE. Smoking-attributable periodontal disease in the Australian adult population. J Clin Periodontol. 2008;35(5):398–404.
10. Morphett K, Hyland A, Sellars D, Gartner C. The environmental impact of tobacco products: time to increase awareness and action. Addiction. 2023;118(3):396–8.
11. Thomson WM, Poulton R, Broadbent JM, Moffitt TE, Caspi A, Beck JD, et al. Cannabis smoking and periodontal disease among young adults. JAMA. 2008;299(5):525–31.
12. Iftikhar A, Islam M, Shepherd S, Jones S, Ellis I. What is behind the lifestyle risk factors for head and neck cancer? Front Psychol. 2022;13:960638.
13. Lioret S, Campbell KJ, McNaughton SA, Cameron AJ, Salmon J, Abbott G, Hesketh KD. Lifestyle patterns begin in early childhood, persist and are socioeconomically patterned, confirming the importance of early life interventions. Nutrients. 2020;12(3):724.
14. Das A, Orlan E, Duncan K, Thomas H, Ndumele A, Ilbawi A, Parascandola M. Areca nut and betel quid control interventions: halting the epidemic. Subst Use Misuse. 2020;55(9):1552–9.
15. NHMRC. Information paper—water fluoridation: dental and other human health outcomes. Canberra: National Health and Medical Research Council; 2017.

16. Moynihan PJ, Kelly SA. Effect on caries of restricting sugars intake: systematic review to inform WHO guidelines. J Dent Res. 2014;93(1):8–18.
17. Sheiham A, James WP. A new understanding of the relationship between sugars, dental caries and fluoride use: implications for limits on sugars consumption. Public Health Nutr. 2014;17(10):2176–84.
18. Ha DH, Do LG, Spencer AJ, Thomson WM, Golley RK, Rugg-Gunn AJ, et al. Factors influencing early feeding of foods and drinks containing free sugars-a birth cohort study. Int J Environ Res Public Health. 2017;14(10):1270.
19. Feldens CA, Dos Santos IF, Kramer PF, Vítolo MR, Braga VS, Chaffee BW. Early-life patterns of sugar consumption and dental caries in the permanent teeth: a birth cohort study. Caries Res. 2021;55(5):505–14.
20. Abdel Rahman A, Jomaa L, Kahale LA, Adair P, Pine C. Effectiveness of behavioral interventions to reduce the intake of sugar-sweetened beverages in children and adolescents: a systematic review and meta-analysis. Nutr Rev. 2018;76(2):88–107.
21. Schram A, Labonte R, Baker P, Friel S, Reeves A, Stuckler D. The role of trade and investment liberalization in the sugar-sweetened carbonated beverages market: a natural experiment contrasting Vietnam and The Philippines. Glob Health. 2015;11(1):41.
22. Hajishafiee M, Kapellas K, Listl S, Pattamatta M, Gkekas A, Moynihan P. Effect of sugar-sweetened beverage taxation on sugars intake and dental caries: an umbrella review of a global perspective. BMC Public Health. 2023;23(1):986.
23. Genco RJ, Borgnakke WS. Risk factors for periodontal disease. Periodontol 2000. 2013;62(1):59–94.
24. Morse DE, Psoter WJ, Cleveland D, Cohen D, Mohit-Tabatabai M, Kosis DL, Eisenberg E. Smoking and drinking in relation to oral cancer and oral epithelial dysplasia. Cancer Causes Control. 2007;18(9):919–29.
25. Jenkins CN, Dai PX, Ngoc DH, Kinh HV, Hoang TT, Bales S, et al. Tobacco use in Vietnam. Prevalence, predictors, and the role of the transnational tobacco corporations. JAMA. 1997;277(21):1726–31.
26. Stronks K, van de Mheen HD, Looman CW, Mackenbach JP. Cultural, material, and psychosocial correlates of the socioeconomic gradient in smoking behavior among adults. Prev Med. 1997;26(5 Pt 1):754–66.
27. McHardy J. The WHO FCTC's lessons for addressing the commercial determinants of health. Health Promot Int. 2021;36(Supplement_1):i39–52.
28. Gartner C, Hall WD. Mixed progress in global tobacco control. PLoS Med. 2024;21(4):e1004392.
29. Sudhinaraset M, Wigglesworth C, Takeuchi DT. Social and cultural contexts of alcohol use: influences in a social-ecological framework. Alcohol Res. 2016;38(1):35–45.
30. Mascarenhas AK. Oral hygiene as a risk indicator of enamel and dentin caries. Community Dent Oral Epidemiol. 1998;26(5):331–9.
31. Selwitz RH, Ismail AI, Pitts NB. Dental caries. Lancet. 2007;369(9555):51–9.
32. Mouatt B. Encouraging healthier lifestyles–1. Children and their teeth. J Fam Health Care. 2007;17(1):11–3.
33. Moynihan P, Tanner LM, Holmes RD, Hillier-Brown F, Mashayekhi A, Kelly SAM, Craig D. Systematic review of evidence pertaining to factors that modify risk of early childhood caries. JDR Clin Trans Res. 2019;4(3):202–16.
34. Vermaire JH, Kalf SM, Schuller AA. Oral health and oral health behaviour of adolescents with mild or borderline intellectual disabilities compared with a national representative sample of 17-year-olds in The Netherlands. J Appl Res Intellect Disabil. 2021;34(2):615–23.
35. Ko AM, Wu PW, Lin WT, Lee CH. Betel-quid addictive use disorders and Oral potentially malignant disorders and Oral cancer in south, southeast, and East Asia: a systematic review and meta-analysis. Oral Dis. 2025;31:1517–30.

36. Marinho VC. Cochrane reviews of randomized trials of fluoride therapies for preventing dental caries. Eur Arch Paediatr Dent. 2009;10(3):183–91.
37. Do LG. Guidelines for use of fluorides in Australia: update 2019. Aust Dent J. 2020;65(1):30–8.
38. Ha D, Spencer AJ, Moynihan P, Thomson WM, Do LG. Excess risk of dental caries from higher free sugars intake combined with low exposure to water fluoridation. J Dent Res. 2021;100(11):1243–50.

Non-Communicable Diseases and Oral Health: A Two-Way Relationship

3

José João Mendes, Patrícia Lyra, Vanessa Machado, and João T. S. Botelho

3.1 Introduction

According to the World Health Organization (WHO), non-communicable diseases (NCDs), commonly known as chronic diseases, result from a combination of genetic, physiological, environmental and behavioural factors [1]. In 2021, NCDs were responsible for the deaths of approximately 43 million people [1], 73% of whom were in low- and middle-income countries (LMICs). Between 2022 and 2025, NCDs are projected to account for most of the global burden [2]. NCDs include diseases that affect the mouth and disrupt oral health.

Oral health refers to the condition of the mouth, teeth and orofacial structures, enabling individuals to perform essential functions such as eating, breathing and speaking [3]. Its integral role in general health may vary across different stages of life and serves as a pillar for the social endeavours of individuals [4, 5]. The disruption of oral homeostasis leads to the development of oral diseases and chronic, progressive conditions of the oral cavity from childhood to adulthood, causing negative aesthetic, functional, emotional and social impacts, which significantly affect the quality of life [6]. These conditions are among the most prevalent NCDs worldwide, with caries and periodontal diseases ranking as the two most common, both having severe economic and social implications [7, 8]. Like other NCDs, oral diseases are driven by inadequate lifestyle behaviours, particularly those related to oral hygiene and preventive measures.

Behavioural lifestyle factors significantly influence health trajectories, affecting both the risk and progression of chronic diseases, including those related to the oral cavity. Key lifestyle components such as dietary habits, tobacco and alcohol consumption, physical activity (PA) levels and stress management contribute to

J. J. Mendes · P. Lyra · V. Machado · J. T. S. Botelho (✉)
Egas Moniz Centre for Interdisciplinary Research, Egas Moniz School of Health and Science, Almada, Portugal
e-mail: jmendes@egasmoniz.edu.pt; plyra@egasmoniz.edu.pt; vmachado@egasmoniz.edu.pt; jbotelho@egasmoniz.edu.pt

S. R. Prabhu et al. (eds.), *Lifestyle in Oral Health and Disease*,
https://doi.org/10.1007/978-3-032-05888-1_3

systemic inflammation, immune function and metabolic equilibrium—elements that directly impact oral health. Furthermore, oral hygiene practices and access to dental care are crucial determinants mediating the relationship between lifestyle and disease. The collective effect of these behaviours determines oral health outcomes and represents critical intervention points for mitigating the overall burden of non-communicable diseases (NCDs). Understanding these interconnections underscores the importance of adopting a preventive, health-promoting approach that transcends traditional medical and dental boundaries.

Recognising the complex relationship between lifestyle choices and oral health is crucial for addressing the impact of oral diseases within the broader context of non-communicable diseases (NCDs). The modifiable risk factors not only influence the development and progression of oral diseases but also reflect wider systemic health issues, underscoring the necessity for integrated preventive measures. This chapter explores the influence of lifestyle on oral health and disease, emphasising the importance of incorporating oral health into broader NCD prevention frameworks. It advocates for interdisciplinary strategies that address lifestyle factors at their roots and promote a unified vision of health.

3.2 Global Burden of Oral Health Conditions

According to the most recent Global Burden of Disease Study (GBD) 2021, oral diseases are estimated to affect around 3.69 billion people worldwide [9], which aligns with the WHO report of 2022 diseases [5]. The GBD report indicates that untreated dental caries of permanent teeth and severe periodontitis were the most common oral conditions. Additionally, edentulism, severe periodontitis and lip and oral cavity cancer contributed the highest burden, as demonstrated by their counts of Disability-Adjusted Life Years and associated age-standardised rates. Overall, this updated large-scale study shows that the slight variations in the prevalence of oral conditions over the last three decades suggest that both past and present strategies to manage these issues have not been effective, indicating the need for alternative methods [9].

The total cost of dental diseases in 2015 and 2019 was estimated at $544.41 billion, comprising $356.80 billion in direct costs and $187.61 billion in indirect costs [10]. Periodontitis alone was estimated to result in a loss of $154.06B in the USA and €158.64B in Europe in 2018 [11].

The persistent global burden and economic impact of oral diseases underscore the urgent need to address their underlying determinants, particularly lifestyle-related factors [12]. Oral health is influenced by clinical care, daily behaviours and broader social determinants [13]. Echoing the sentiment that 'oral health is indeed health', the Bangkok Declaration on Oral Health is a call for stakeholders to collectively work towards universal health coverage for oral health by 2030. Member States must develop tailored national roadmaps that integrate oral health into broader health strategies, where these socio-political factors stand out as key determinants of health in a wider socio-environmental milieu [14]. This is the main common ground that oral diseases and NCDs share; in other words, limited access to preventive care, disparities in health literacy and socioeconomic inequities further exacerbate the burden, particularly in low- and middle-income countries (LMICs) [6, 15].

3.3 Overview of NCDs and Oral Health

In an extensive umbrella review of systematic reviews, meta-analytic estimates of the association between oral diseases and NCDs were appraised [16]. Overall, 28 NCDs were strongly associated with oral diseases, despite unfavourable methodological inconsistencies, yet with reasonably robust consistency. Among those NCDs are five types of cancer, diabetes mellitus, cardiovascular diseases, depression, neurodegenerative conditions, rheumatic diseases, inflammatory bowel disease, gastric *Helicobacter pylori*, obesity and asthma. The explanation for this extensive range of orosystemic links is based on biological mechanisms that have been widely studied (see Sect. 3.2) and common lifestyle factors that hinder a healthy lifestyle, synonymous with a lifestyle that fosters NCDs.

There is robust evidence supporting associations between oral diseases and various NCDs. For instance, dental caries have been linked to iron deficiency, while tooth loss has shown significant associations with cognitive impairment, dementia and lung cancer. Additionally, edentulism has been associated with an increased risk of pancreatic cancer and endodontic infections with elevated levels of systemic inflammation, as indicated by serum C-reactive protein (CRP).

Periodontal disease, in particular, demonstrates strong associations with an increased risk of several systemic conditions, including cancer, cardiovascular disease, diabetes mellitus, adverse pregnancy outcomes, reduced longevity, neurodegenerative disorders (e.g. cognitive decline and dementia), polycystic ovary syndrome (PCOS), psoriasis, altered haematological parameters (e.g. mean corpuscular haemoglobin) and elevated systemic inflammatory markers (e.g. CRP).

When considering oral diseases as outcomes, individuals with mental health disorders exhibited a higher prevalence of dental caries and tooth loss. Other associations include dental trauma in individuals with special needs, denture stomatitis and periodontal disease in patients with diabetes, greater tooth loss and periodontitis in individuals with cardiovascular disease, mouth breathing and increased gingival bleeding in patients with asthma, and edentulism in individuals with obesity.

Furthermore, risk factors for periodontal disease include lower levels of physical activity, rheumatoid arthritis, PCOS, non-alcoholic fatty liver disease, medication-related osteonecrosis of the jaw, ankylosing spondylitis, inflammatory bowel disease, obstructive sleep apnoea and *Helicobacter pylori* infection. These findings underscore the bidirectional and multifactorial relationship between oral and systemic health.

Remarkably, two types of oral treatments showed strong scientific evidence for improving systemic health: one linking gum treatment to reduced body inflammation and another connecting root canal treatment to benefits for cardiovascular health [16]. Additionally, some studies suggested that gum treatments may help with heart conditions, diabetes, pregnancy complications, breathing problems and inflammation.

For instance, the effectiveness of periodontal therapy in reducing systemic inflammation and enhancing renal function markers in individuals with chronic kidney disease or diabetes has already been demonstrated [17, 18]. Indeed, treating chronic oral infections has been shown to alleviate the inflammatory burden on the kidneys, potentially slowing the progression of chronic kidney disease [19]. Furthermore, in the context of diabetes, addressing oral infections has been shown to improve glycaemic control in individuals with the condition [18]. Conversely, treating NCDs has positively impacted oral health, with tissue healing and infection resolution in diabetes patients contributing to the enhancement of oral health [20].

3.4 Biological Mechanisms Linking NCDs and Oral Health

Oral diseases and other systemic NCDs share molecular and immunological links. Commensal microorganisms are known to maintain oral microbial homeostasis by coexisting with potentially pathogenic species. However, the disruption of this equilibrium due to dysbiotic processes, such as in the case of caries and periodontitis (both biofilm-mediated diseases), can result in the overgrowth of potentially pathogenic microorganisms, leading to an increase in virulence. This can, in turn, heighten health risks and exacerbate disease development. Therefore, oral infections, particularly periodontitis, can influence the progression and pathogenesis of systemic diseases through various mechanisms [21].

Indeed, periodontitis represents a substantial source of inflammation [22]. In cases of untreated periodontal infection, there exists the possibility of the spread of periodontal bacteria and their by-products (e.g. gingipains from *Porphyromonas gingivalis*) locally via saliva or other fluids (such as crevicular fluid) or to extra-oral areas through various routes, including haematogenous [23], oropharyngeal [24] and orodigestive routes [25].

In healthy subjects, transient bacteraemia is generally resolved through the immune system's capacity to recognise these pathogens as foreign intruders via their antigens, thus instigating an immune response. On the one hand, the activation of monocytes and macrophages is initiated in response to the infection, with the concomitant release of cytokines, growth factors and acute-phase proteins by host cells to facilitate the repair of tissue and organ damage [21]. On the other hand, oral pathogens release endotoxins, including oxidative waste products [26], lipopolysaccharides [27], acute-phase proteins and cytokine signalling molecules, to coordinate their activities with other bacteria. These endotoxins have been shown to trigger inflammatory responses from antibodies [28], macrophages [29] and monocytes.

Similarly, inflammatory mediators recruited locally to the periodontal tissues can disseminate into the bloodstream, causing a low-grade systemic inflammatory burden [30–33]. Both scenarios may induce peripheral chronic inflammation and immune activation in distant organs, thereby triggering a sequence of inflammatory biomarkers, including interleukin (IL)-1, IL-6, IL-1β, C-reactive protein (CRP), tumour necrosis factor-alpha (TNF-α), fibrinogen and neutrophils [30, 34]. This underlying chronic inflammation often increases environmental stress on host cells, potentially causing dysfunction, inefficiency, or cell death [30]. Furthermore, oral pathogens may contribute to carcinogenesis by inducing genetic mutations in the host cells, transforming them into cancerous or aberrant forms [31, 32]. Therefore, oral pathogens can infect and damage multiple organs or selectively target specific ones, as organs provide a rich and ideal protective environment that shields them from immune detection and attack [21]. Ultimately, in cases of immune impairment or in the presence of underlying health conditions, bacteraemia and the disruption of normal cellular functions drive disease progression, including sepsis, endocarditis, or the colonisation of distant tissues [33]. This can, in turn, result in the onset or exacerbation of extra-oral inflammatory pathologies.

Additionally, as previously mentioned, several shared risk factors have been identified that link non-communicable diseases (NCDs) and oral health. These factors include smoking, alcohol use, unhealthy diets, sedentary behaviour and environmental pollution. As previously outlined by the World Health Organization [5], NCDs and oral health are closely linked, and, therefore, a common risk factor approach is more desirable and rational compared to disease-specific approaches. If a risk factor is common to several diseases, it can be addressed across disease boundaries [34].

Overall, periodontitis is a significant oral infection that can influence the host's susceptibility to systemic disease in three ways: through shared risk factors, subgingival biofilms functioning as reservoirs of Gram-negative bacteria, and the periodontium serving as a reservoir of inflammatory mediators.

Furthermore, the existing body of research on the relationship between dental caries and systemic diseases remains limited [35]. Current evidence primarily associates metabolic diseases, such as diabetes and obesity, with dental caries. These conditions share common environmental factors, including a hyperglycaemic state and a high-carbohydrate, sugar-rich diet [36].

In the context of dental caries, the root canal space and marginal periodontium have been identified as the primary pathways for the systemic spread of oral microbiota [37]. Host factors and microbial pathogenic traits contribute to caries progression, increasing the risk of oral-systemic dissemination. Key factors include systemic diseases and medications that reduce saliva production [38, 39], the expression of *Streptococcus mutans adhesin* for collagen binding [40], oral microbiota dysbiosis [41] and genetic predispositions that link dental caries with systemic diseases through shared mechanisms.

Further human and animal studies are needed to investigate the potential systemic effects of untreated dental caries and the mechanistic role of oral microbial inflammation in these associations through parallel mechanisms to the systemic spread of periodontitis [42].

3.5 Lifestyle Factors

Lifestyle behaviours are a fundamental and modifiable determinant of health, lying at the intersection of oral diseases and other NCDs. A broad spectrum of daily behaviours—such as dietary habits, physical exercise, smoking, stress management and oral care—not only influence the onset and progression of oral health issues but are also intricately linked to systemic diseases like cardiovascular disease, diabetes, respiratory conditions and certain cancers. Understanding these shared risk factors is crucial for developing integrated prevention and health promotion strategies. Taking periodontitis as an example, good oral hygiene remains a fundamental aspect that accounts for personal care and regular professional support demand; it is essential to acknowledge that dental plaque accounts for only 20% of its direct risk [43]. Other factors, including individual host characteristics, the environment, and chronic diseases, also play a significant role in disease development, emphasising the multifaceted nature of oral health within the broader context of lifestyle and systemic well-being.

3.5.1 Diet and Body Mass Index (BMI)

Diet is perhaps the most universally significant lifestyle factor, impacting nearly every facet of health [44–47]. Beyond its systemic functions, diet influences the onset, progression and treatment outcomes of oral diseases [47–49]. Nutrients influence immune function, tissue repair and inflammatory responses, which are key processes in the pathogenesis and healing of periodontal tissues.

Diet's pivotal role in health throughout one's life is primarily linked to two types of nutrients: micronutrients and macronutrients. Micronutrients, such as vitamins and trace elements, are crucial for tissue regeneration and immune defence. For example, vitamin A is known to maintain epithelial integrity, although its effects on periodontal health are still not well defined [47, 50]. Vitamin C is vital in collagen production and has been shown to help reduce gingival inflammation and promote wound healing [51, 52]. Vitamin E, found in nuts and seeds, stabilises cell membranes and reduces inflammation; however, its specific effects on the periodontium require further research [47, 53, 54]. Its antioxidant properties are significant for smokers, as their increased oxidative stress leads to more substantial tissue damage [55].

Carbohydrates, proteins and fats, which are macronutrients, also play several roles in maintaining oral health. Diets rich in refined carbohydrates and frequency, mainly sucrose, encourage plaque buildup and heighten the risk of developing caries and periodontitis [48, 49, 56, 57]. On the one hand, dental caries and periodontal disease are primarily linked to sugars because bacteria break them down, resulting in the production of acid that leads to the demineralisation of the tooth surface [49]. On the other hand, xylitol, a substitute sweetener, may help reduce the presence of periodontal pathogens, such as *P. gingivalis* [58, 59]. Maintaining good oral hygiene practices and undergoing regular non-surgical cleanings can improve periodontal health. However, in the absence of brushing, chewing xylitol or mannitol gum significantly reduces gingivitis scores compared to chewing a gum base [60].

Additionally, minerals and trace elements such as calcium, magnesium, iron, zinc and fluoride are essential for maintaining oral health. Calcium is a key component of teeth and bones. A deficiency in dietary calcium may also impact periodontal health. Co-supplementation with dietary calcium and vitamin D has been found to reduce the severity of periodontitis and enhance the results of periodontal therapy [61, 62]. Magnesium is essential for bone metabolism, and its deficiency has been linked to impaired healing; however, further evidence is needed [63]. Iron's antioxidant properties suggest it may help reduce periodontal inflammation, particularly in anaemic individuals with a reduced antioxidant capacity [64]. Zinc plays a role in tissue repair, keratinocyte migration, and the scavenging of reactive oxygen species [65, 66]. Notably, zinc deficiency may exacerbate diabetes-related periodontitis, and supplementation could enhance the effectiveness of periodontal therapy [67, 68]. Fluoride, well known for its role in preventing dental caries [69], also contributes to periodontal stability by strengthening enamel resistance and providing antibacterial effects [70]. Additionally, fluoride supplementation may reduce root resorption during orthodontic treatment [71].

Beyond the importance of maintaining a balanced macro- and micronutrient intake, keeping an adequate and healthy weight is crucial for overall health. In recent decades, the global prevalence of overweight and obesity has increased substantially, reaching 41.5% [72]. This trend is concerning, as individuals with a normal body mass index (BMI) typically exhibit higher metabolic rates compared to those with obesity, who often present a reduced resting metabolic rate [73]. The link between body mass index (BMI) and oral health, particularly dental caries and periodontitis, remains a topic of controversy. While some studies report no clear relationship [74–77], others indicate a higher incidence of caries among overweight and obese individuals [78], especially children [74, 79] and adolescents [75, 80], possibly due to dietary and lifestyle factors. A meta-analysis by Chen et al. [81] reinforced this association in primary dentition, whereas other research suggests that BMI is a contributing, but not exclusive, risk factor for caries. Furthermore, advanced caries has also been shown to negatively impact nutrition and reduce BMI [82].

To effectively integrate nutrition into oral health strategies, a concerted effort is required involving healthcare professionals, public health systems, educational institutions and community organisations. Initiatives that educate individuals about the importance of a balanced diet for oral and overall health from an early age can promote lifelong healthy habits. Policy measures such as sugar taxes, enhanced food labelling, and restricting the marketing of unhealthy foods to children can facilitate changes at the population level. The effect of an unbalanced diet on oral health is discussed in Chap. 12.

3.5.2 Physical Activity and Exercise

Physical activity (PA), a term encompassing a wide range of activities including daily living, leisure, occupation, sports and active transportation [83, 84], is widely recognised as a key factor in preventing various non-communicable diseases (NCDs). Additionally, engaging in regular exercise enhances multiple physical abilities and contributes positively to overall human health, which is not limited to cognitive improvement [85], maintenance of cardiovascular physiology [86], or fat reduction [86].

Evidence from meta-analytical studies indicates that physically active individuals have significantly lower odds ratios for periodontitis compared to their sedentary counterparts, suggesting a potential protective role for exercise in maintaining periodontal health [87]. Similarly, Chan et al. reported that regular physical activity is associated with lower levels of clinical attachment loss and gingival inflammation, particularly when combined with a healthy diet [88].

Physical activity may influence other aspects of oral health through its effects on salivary composition. Saliva plays a crucial role in maintaining oral homeostasis, and exercise-induced changes in salivary biomarkers, such as increases in immunoglobulin A, α-amylase, and cortisol, reflect physiological stress responses and immune modulation. Moderate-to-intense physical activity alters salivary protein profiles, which may affect mucosal immunity and susceptibility to oral diseases [89].

The biological mechanisms underpinning this relationship are multifactorial; however, altering immune markers is considered the primary mechanism involved [90]. Physical activity reduces systemic inflammation, as evidenced by lower levels of circulating inflammatory biomarkers such as C-reactive protein [91]. Since periodontitis is driven by an exaggerated host inflammatory response to oral biofilms, the systemic anti-inflammatory effects of exercise may mitigate periodontal tissue destruction. Moreover, exercise improves insulin sensitivity [92], modulates immune function and reduces stress—factors known to influence the progression of periodontal disease [93].

3.5.3 Smoking Habits

Smoking remains one of the most detrimental lifestyle choices, significantly affecting both oral and overall health [94]. It is a well-established risk factor for periodontal disease, oral cancer, tooth loss and delayed recovery after dental treatments. Additionally, smoking plays a significant role in the development of cardiovascular disease, chronic obstructive pulmonary disease and various types of cancer [95, 96]. The inflammatory and immunosuppressive properties of tobacco smoke worsen both systemic and localised disease processes, creating a compounded burden [97, 98]. Initiatives aimed at reducing tobacco use through public policy, cessation support and education can significantly lessen the risks to both oral and general health [99].

In terms of oral health, smoking is closely linked to a higher risk and increased severity of gum disease, tooth loss, slower healing of wounds and oral cancer. Nicotine's vasoconstrictive and immunosuppressive properties hinder blood flow to the gums and weaken the body's defence mechanisms, enabling harmful bacteria to thrive and accelerate tissue damage [97, 98]. Additionally, smokers tend to have a diminished response to periodontal treatments and surgical procedures 1 year after [100].

Smoking is often associated with other risky lifestyle choices, such as inadequate nutrition, lack of physical activity and poor oral care. This combination of unhealthy habits increases the likelihood of developing multiple chronic conditions. Additionally, smoking rates tend to be higher among socioeconomically disadvantaged groups, highlighting it as both a public health concern and an issue of social equity. From a policy standpoint, controlling tobacco use remains one of the most cost-efficient measures in global health. Interventions such as imposing taxes, regulating packaging, banning advertisements, and offering support for quitting have effectively decreased tobacco consumption in numerous nations [101, 102]. Dental practitioners can significantly contribute to cessation counselling by using regular appointments as opportunities to educate and intervene with patients [103]. A detailed discussion on the effects of smoking on oral health is presented in Chap. 4.

3.5.4 Stress

Chronic psychological stress is increasingly recognised as a significant factor in the development of NCDs, including oral health issues [104]. Hormonal changes triggered by stress, particularly the rise in cortisol levels, can lead to immune system imbalances, increased systemic inflammation, behavioural shifts such as teeth grinding, tobacco or alcohol consumption and poor oral hygiene practices [105–108]. In terms of oral health, stress is strongly associated with conditions like periodontitis, canker sores and temporomandibular joint disorders [104]. Additionally, stress contributes to cardiovascular diseases, digestive issues and mental health problems like anxiety and depression [109, 110].

Chronic stress is a critical yet often overlooked factor affecting oral and systemic health. The body's stress response, controlled by the hypothalamic–pituitary–adrenal (HPA) axis, increases cortisol production, which has both immunosuppressive and pro-inflammatory effects. This hormonal imbalance can trigger or worsen NCDs, such as high blood pressure, heart disease and mental health disorders like depression and anxiety. In oral health, stress is associated with a higher risk of periodontal disease, teeth grinding, temporomandibular disorders and recurring canker sores [104]. Stress-related behaviours further increase the risk, such as neglecting oral hygiene, making poor dietary choices, smoking and drinking alcohol [111]. In periodontal disease, elevated stress markers have been linked to poorer clinical outcomes and a diminished response to treatment. The interaction between stress, mental health and oral health creates a complex, two-way feedback loop. For example, individuals with noticeable oral disease or tooth loss may feel socially embarrassed, experience lower self-esteem and withdraw socially, which can increase psychological distress. This cyclical relationship highlights the need to include mental health support in comprehensive healthcare strategies.

Efforts to reduce stress should be multifaceted, involving psychological counselling, mindfulness practices, stress management education and community support networks. Healthcare providers, including dental professionals, should be trained to identify signs of psychosocial stress and refer patients as needed. Incorporating mental health literacy into oral health promotion can lead to more comprehensive and compassionate care models. Chapter 20 presents more information on the impact of stress on oral health.

3.6 Integrated Healthcare Approaches

To effectively address the challenge of oral diseases within the broader context of NCDs, it is necessary to transition from a fragmented approach to healthcare to a cohesive model that integrates oral health with overall systemic health. The established connections between oral diseases and various NCDs highlight the importance of interdisciplinary cooperation, the integration of primary care and community-driven initiatives to achieve comprehensive and lasting health improvements. Moreover, addressing oral health inequalities is crucial, as they are deeply intertwined with broader social determinants and extend beyond common behavioural risks [112].

The link between oral health and overall health necessitates a collaborative approach involving professionals from various healthcare sectors, including doctors, dentists, nurses, nutritionists and public health specialists [34]. Effective teamwork necessitates pre-professional and professional preparation, equipping oral health professionals with skills beyond clinical expertise [113]. Interprofessional collaboration, including patient family members and caregivers, is crucial for optimal oral health outcomes, particularly in geriatric care [114]. The connection between oral and systemic health underscores the importance of healthcare providers collaborating with oral health professionals to ensure quality care [115]. Despite longstanding recommendations for interdisciplinary training and collaboration, progress has been slow. There is a critical need for new initiatives to redesign health professionals' curricula, addressing the growing population of medically complex older adults and the limited oral health information in medical education.

Additionally, research that connects medical and dental fields can strengthen evidence-based guidelines, promoting a more cohesive healthcare system. Integrating oral health into primary care is essential for a more patient-focused healthcare model. Since oral diseases share risk factors with major systemic conditions, primary care providers should routinely evaluate oral health as part of overall patient assessments. Similarly, dentists should be trained to recognise signs of systemic diseases and refer patients for necessary medical care. Initiatives such as shared electronic health records, interdisciplinary training and the co-location of dental and medical services can enhance communication among professionals, streamline patient care and reduce the fragmented nature of healthcare delivery.

Community-based strategies are essential for promoting oral health and preventing non-communicable diseases at a population level. Public health approaches should address the social determinants of oral health through a common risk factor approach rather than focusing solely on changing individual behaviours [116]. Effective oral health promotion requires multifaceted strategies: education, behaviour change, service access and policy integration [117]. Recognising the link between oral and general health, a paradigm shift towards a public health approach is needed, integrating various health professionals to address non-communicable diseases [118]. Comprehensive, multilevel interventions that combine behavioural practices, educational interventions and dietary modifications are crucial for improving oral health outcomes across diverse populations [119]. These strategies should extend beyond traditional dental settings and emphasise the importance of preventive care in achieving oral health equity.

3.7 Future Directions and Recommendations

The increasing acknowledgement of the complex link between oral health and NCDs demands a progressive approach to research, public health strategies and policy advocacy [5, 120]. Although significant advancements have been made in understanding the shared risk factors and this bidirectional relationship, critical gaps persist [5]. Addressing these challenges requires a concerted effort to advance research, implement comprehensive public health initiatives and advocate for policy reforms that integrate oral health into broader healthcare frameworks.

Further research is needed to elucidate causal mechanisms, refine risk assessment models and develop targeted interventions. Longitudinal studies examining the temporal relationships between oral inflammation and systemic diseases, as well as the effects of lifestyle modifications on disease progression, are crucial [16]. Additionally, emerging areas such as the role of the oral microbiome in systemic health, personalised medicine approaches in dentistry and the development of non-invasive biomarkers for early disease detection hold significant promise [121, 122].

Leveraging artificial intelligence and big data analytics with caution and in an ethical way can further enhance predictive modelling and precision healthcare strategies in oral disease prevention and management [123, 124]. Public health strategies must adopt a more integrated and preventive approach to reduce the burden of oral diseases and their systemic implications. Programmes promoting early childhood oral health, community-based fluoride interventions and initiatives targeting sugar consumption and tobacco use are critical. Furthermore, enhancing public awareness through educational campaigns that emphasise the interconnection between oral and overall health can drive behavioural changes at the individual and community levels [125]. Strengthening healthcare workforce training to include interdisciplinary competencies in dental and medical education is also crucial to fostering a more holistic approach to patient care [5].

A shift in healthcare policy is also needed to align oral health with broader health agendas. Policymakers must prioritise oral health within universal health coverage frameworks, ensuring equitable access to preventive and therapeutic dental care [126, 127]. Strategies such as integrating oral health screenings into routine medical visits, expanding insurance coverage for dental services and incentivising interdisciplinary collaboration can bridge existing gaps in care [128]. Additionally, regulatory efforts to address social determinants of health—such as improving access to nutritious food, clean water and comprehensive health education—can have far-reaching effects on both oral and systemic disease prevention [112, 129]. Global health organisations, professional societies and advocacy groups are pivotal in driving these policy changes and ensuring oral health is recognised as a fundamental component of overall well-being.

References

1. Non communicable diseases. https://www.who.int/news-room/fact-sheets/detail/noncommunicable-diseases. Accessed 17 Mar 2025.
2. Vollset SE, Ababneh HS, Abate YH, Abbafati C, et al. Burden of disease scenarios for 204 countries and territories, 2022–2050: a forecasting analysis for the Global Burden of Disease Study 2021. Lancet. 2024;403:2204–56. https://doi.org/10.1016/S0140-6736(24)00685-8.
3. WHO. Pudlowski oral health WHO. In: Oral health. https://www.who.int/health-topics/oral-health/#tab=tab_1.
4. Sischo L, Broder HL. Oral health-related quality of life: what, why, how, and future implications. J Dent Res. 2011;90:1264–70. https://doi.org/10.1177/0022034511399918.
5. World Health Organization. Global oral health status report: towards universal health coverage for oral health by 2030. World Health Organization; 2022.
6. Peres MA, Macpherson LMD, Weyant RJ, Daly B, Venturelli R, Mathur MR, Listl S, Celeste RK, Guarnizo-Herreño CC, Kearns C, Benzian H, Allison P, Watt RG. Oral diseases: a global public health challenge. Lancet. 2019;394:249–60. https://doi.org/10.1016/S0140-6736(19)31146-8.
7. Listl S, Galloway J, Mossey PA, Marcenes W. Global economic impact of dental diseases. J Dent Res. 2015;94:1355–61. https://doi.org/10.1177/0022034515602879.
8. Watt RG, Daly B, Allison P, Macpherson LMD, Venturelli R, Listl S, Weyant RJ, Mathur MR, Guarnizo-Herreño CC, Celeste RK, Peres MA, Kearns C, Benzian H. Ending the neglect of global oral health: time for radical action. Lancet. 2019;394:261–72. https://doi.org/10.1016/S0140-6736(19)31133-X.
9. Bernabe E, Marcenes W, Abdulkader RS, Abreu LG, Afzal S, Alhalaiqa FN, Al-Maweri S, Alsharif U, Anyasodor AE, Arora A, Asgary S, Ashraf T, Balasubramanian M, Banakar M, Barrow A, Bashiri A, Belay SA, Belgaumi UI, Berhie AY, Bhardwaj P, Bhaskar S, Bijani A, Bouaoud S, Cao Y, Chaurasia A, Chen MX, Chu D-T, Cruz-Martins N, Dadras O, Dai X, Diaz D, Du M, Ekholuenetale M, Ekundayo TC, El Tantawi M, Elhadi M, Fagbamigbe AF, Farshidfar N, Fatehizadeh A, Fischer F, Folayan MO, Gaewkhiew P, Gajdács M, Golechha M, Gupta B, Gupta S, Hagins H, Halboub ES, Hamidi S, Hariyani N, Hay SI, Heidari M, Herrera-Serna BY, Heyi DZ, Hostiuc S, Humphrey KM, Ibitoye SE, Ilic MD, Isola G, Kandaswamy E, Kantar RS, Kaur N, Kemmer L, Khader YS, Khateri S, Kisa A, Krishan K, Kruger E, Lalloo R, Li A, Lim SS, Mestrovic T, Mokdad AH, Moreira RS, Morrison SD, Murray CJL, Natto ZS, Nayak BP, Nguyen T, Nguyen VT, Omotayo AO, Padron-Monedero A, Patel J, Patil S, Pawar S, Petcu I-R, Qattea I, Rahman M, Ratan ZA, Riad A, SM, SNC, Sabour S, Saheb Sharif-Askari F, Sahebkar A, Sakshaug JW, Samy AM, Sarode

SC, Sawhney M, Schwendicke F, Shaikh MA, Tadakamadla SK, Tesler R, Thiyagarajan A, Tovani-Palone MR, Umair M, Unnikrishnan B, Valadan Tahbaz S, Varma SA, Vukovic AP, Wang C, Wickramasinghe ND, Yadav L, Yiğit A, Zare I, Zhang Z-J, Kassebaum NJ. Trends in the global, regional, and national burden of oral conditions from 1990 to 2021: a systematic analysis for the Global Burden of Disease Study 2021. Lancet. 2025;405:897–910. https://doi.org/10.1016/S0140-6736(24)02811-3.

10. Righolt AJ, Jevdjevic M, Marcenes W, Listl S. Global-, regional-, and country-level economic impacts of dental diseases in 2015. J Dent Res. 2018;97:501–7. https://doi.org/10.1177/0022034517750572.
11. Botelho J, Machado V, Leira Y, Proença L, Chambrone L, Mendes JJ. Economic burden of periodontitis in the United States and Europe – an updated estimation. J Periodontol. 2021. https://doi.org/10.1002/JPER.21-0111.
12. Jin LJ, Lamster IB, Greenspan JS, Pitts NB, Scully C, Warnakulasuriya S. Global burden of oral diseases: emerging concepts, management and interplay with systemic health. Oral Dis. 2016;22:609–19. https://doi.org/10.1111/odi.12428.
13. Tellez M, Zini A, Estupiñan-Day S. Social determinants and oral health: an update. Curr Oral Health Rep. 2014;1:148–52. https://doi.org/10.1007/s40496-014-0019-6.
14. Samaranayake L, Phantumvanit P, Varenne B. Bangkok declaration on oral health: a clarion call for action by all stakeholders. Int Dent J. 2025;75:381–2. https://doi.org/10.1016/j.identj.2025.03.003.
15. Chidzonga MM, Carneiro LC, Kalyanyama BM, Kwamin F, Oginni FO. Determinants of oral diseases in the African and Middle East region. Adv Dent Res. 2015;27:26–31. https://doi.org/10.1177/0022034515581645.
16. Botelho J, Mascarenhas P, Viana J, Proença L, Orlandi M, Leira Y, Chambrone L, Mendes JJ, Machado V. An umbrella review of the evidence linking oral health and systemic noncommunicable diseases. Nat Commun. 2022;13:7614. https://doi.org/10.1038/s41467-022-35337-8.
17. Delbove T, Gueyffier F, Juillard L, Kalbacher E, Maucort-Boulch D, Nony P, Grosgogeat B, Gritsch K. Effect of periodontal treatment on the glomerular filtration rate, reduction of inflammatory markers and mortality in patients with chronic kidney disease: a systematic review. PLoS One. 2021;16:e0245619. https://doi.org/10.1371/journal.pone.0245619.
18. Simpson TC, Clarkson JE, Worthington HV, MacDonald L, Weldon JC, Needleman I, Iheozor-Ejiofor Z, Wild SH, Qureshi A, Walker A, Patel VA, Boyers D, Twigg J. Treatment of periodontitis for glycaemic control in people with diabetes mellitus. Cochrane Database Syst Rev. 2022;2022:CD004714. https://doi.org/10.1002/14651858.CD004714.pub4.
19. Maringhini S, Zoccali C. Chronic kidney disease progression—a challenge. Biomedicines. 2024;12:2203. https://doi.org/10.3390/biomedicines12102203.
20. Spampinato SF, Caruso GI, De Pasquale R, Sortino MA, Merlo S. The treatment of impaired wound healing in diabetes: looking among old drugs. Pharmaceuticals. 2020;13:60. https://doi.org/10.3390/ph13040060.
21. Murray PE, Coffman JA, Garcia-Godoy F. Oral pathogens' substantial burden on cancer, cardiovascular diseases, Alzheimer's, diabetes, and other systemic diseases: a public health crisis—a comprehensive review. Pathogens. 2024;13:1084. https://doi.org/10.3390/pathogens13121084.
22. Li X, Kolltveit KM, Tronstad L, Olsen I. Systemic diseases caused by oral infection. Clin Microbiol Rev. 2000;13:547–58. https://doi.org/10.1128/CMR.13.4.547.
23. Loos BG. Systemic markers of inflammation in periodontitis. J Periodontol. 2005;76:2106–15. https://doi.org/10.1902/jop.2005.76.11-S.2106.
24. Mammen MJ, Scannapieco FA, Sethi S. Oral-lung microbiome interactions in lung diseases. Periodontology. 2000;83:234–41. https://doi.org/10.1111/prd.12301.
25. Arimatsu K, Yamada H, Miyazawa H, Minagawa T, Nakajima M, Ryder MI, Gotoh K, Motooka D, Nakamura S, Iida T, Yamazaki K. Oral pathobiont induces systemic inflammation and metabolic changes associated with alteration of gut microbiota. Sci Rep. 2014;4:4828. https://doi.org/10.1038/srep04828.

26. Irfan M, Delgado RZR, Frias-Lopez J. The oral microbiome and cancer. Front Immunol. 2020;11:591088. https://doi.org/10.3389/fimmu.2020.591088.
27. De Jongh CA, De Vries TJ, Bikker FJ, Gibbs S, Krom BP. Mechanisms of Porphyromonas gingivalis to translocate over the oral mucosa and other tissue barriers. J Oral Microbiol. 2023;15:2205291. https://doi.org/10.1080/20002297.2023.2205291.
28. Franciotti R, Pignatelli P, Carrarini C, Romei FM, Mastrippolito M, Gentile A, Mancinelli R, Fulle S, Piattelli A, Onofrj M, Curia MC. Exploring the connection between Porphyromonas gingivalis and neurodegenerative diseases: a pilot quantitative study on the bacterium abundance in oral cavity and the amount of antibodies in serum. Biomolecules. 2021;11:845. https://doi.org/10.3390/biom11060845.
29. Fan X, Zheng S, Chen C, Lin L, Wang H, Shen Y, Pan Y, Li C. Sialidase facilitates Porphyromonas gingivalis immune evasion by reducing M1 polarization, antigen presentation, and phagocytosis of infected macrophages. Front Cell Infect Microbiol. 2023;13:1173899. https://doi.org/10.3389/fcimb.2023.1173899.
30. Thoden Van Velzen SK, Abraham-Inpijn L, Moorer WR. Plaque and systemic disease: a reappraisal of the focal infection concept. J Clin Periodontol. 1984;11:209–20. https://doi.org/10.1111/j.1600-051X.1984.tb02211.x.
31. Issrani R, Reddy J, Dabah THE-M, Prabhu N. Role of oral microbiota in carcinogenesis: a short review. J Cancer Prev. 2022;27:16–21. https://doi.org/10.15430/JCP.2022.27.1.16.
32. Sun J, Tang Q, Yu S, Xie M, Xie Y, Chen G, Chen L. Role of the oral microbiota in cancer evolution and progression. Cancer Med. 2020;9:6306–21. https://doi.org/10.1002/cam4.3206.
33. Del Giudice C, Vaia E, Liccardo D, Marzano F, Valletta A, Spagnuolo G, Ferrara N, Rengo C, Cannavo A, Rengo G. Infective endocarditis: a focus on oral microbiota. Microorganisms. 2021;9:1218. https://doi.org/10.3390/microorganisms9061218.
34. Sheiham A, Watt RG. The common risk factor approach: a rational basis for promoting oral health. Community Dent Oral Epidemiol. 2000;28:399–406. https://doi.org/10.1034/j.1600-0528.2000.028006399.x.
35. Cepeda MS, Weinstein R, Blacketer C, Lynch MC. Association of flossing/inter-dental cleaning and periodontitis in adults. J Clin Periodontol. 2017;44:866–71. https://doi.org/10.1111/jcpe.12765.
36. Chi DL, Luu M, Chu F. A scoping review of epidemiologic risk factors for pediatric obesity: implications for future childhood obesity and dental caries prevention research. J Public Health Dent. 2017;77:S8–31. https://doi.org/10.1111/jphd.12221.
37. Scannapieco FA. The oral microbiome: its role in health and in oral and systemic infections. Clin Microbiol Newsl. 2013;35:163–9. https://doi.org/10.1016/j.clinmicnews.2013.09.003.
38. Pedersen AML, Bardow A, Nauntofte B. Salivary changes and dental caries as potential oral markers of autoimmune salivary gland dysfunction in primary Sjögren's syndrome. BMC Clin Pathol. 2005;5:4. https://doi.org/10.1186/1472-6890-5-4.
39. Hu K-F, Chou Y-H, Wen Y-H, Hsieh K-P, Tsai J-H, Yang P, Yang Y-H, Lin C-HR. Antipsychotic medications and dental caries in newly diagnosed schizophrenia: a nationwide cohort study. Psychiatry Res. 2016;245:45–50. https://doi.org/10.1016/j.psychres.2016.07.047.
40. Lemos JA, Palmer SR, Zeng L, Wen ZT, Kajfasz JK, Freires IA, Abranches J, Brady LJ. The biology of Streptococcus mutans. Microbiol Spectr. 2019;7:7.1.03. https://doi.org/10.1128/microbiolspec.GPP3-0051-2018.
41. Tanner ACR, Kressirer CA, Rothmiller S, Johansson I, Chalmers NI. The caries microbiome: implications for reversing dysbiosis. Adv Dent Res. 2018;29:78–85. https://doi.org/10.1177/0022034517736496.
42. Sabharwal A, Stellrecht E, Scannapieco FA. Associations between dental caries and systemic diseases: a scoping review. BMC Oral Health. 2021;21:472. https://doi.org/10.1186/s12903-021-01803-w.
43. Lang NP, Bartold PM. Periodontal health. J Clin Periodontol. 2018;45:S9–S16. https://doi.org/10.1111/jcpe.12936.

44. Palmer CA, Burnett DJ, Dean B. It's more than just candy: important relationships between nutrition and oral health. Nutr Today. 2010;45:154–64. https://doi.org/10.1097/NT.0b013e3181e98969.
45. Palmer CA, Boyd L. Diet and nutrition in oral health. 3rd ed. Pearson; 2016.
46. Ritchie CS, Kinane DF. Nutrition, inflammation, and periodontal disease. Nutrition. 2003;19:475–6. https://doi.org/10.1016/S0899-9007(02)01043-2.
47. Dodington DW, Fritz PC, Sullivan PJ, Ward WE. Higher intakes of fruits and vegetables, β-carotene, vitamin C, α-tocopherol, EPA, and DHA are positively associated with periodontal healing after nonsurgical periodontal therapy in nonsmokers but not in smokers. J Nutr. 2015;145:2512–9. https://doi.org/10.3945/jn.115.211524.
48. Hujoel P. Dietary carbohydrates and dental-systemic diseases. J Dent Res. 2009;88:490–502. https://doi.org/10.1177/0022034509337700.
49. Edgar WM. Extrinsic and intrinsic sugars: a review of recent UK recommendations on diet and caries. Caries Res. 1993;27:64–7. https://doi.org/10.1159/000261605.
50. Gunther S. Vitamin A acid: clinical investigations with 405 patients. Cutis. 1976;17:287–90.
51. Crescini A, Nieri M, Buti J, Baccetti T, Mauro S, Pini Prato GP. Short- and long-term periodontal evaluation of impacted canines treated with a closed surgical–orthodontic approach. J Clin Periodontol. 2007;34:232–42. https://doi.org/10.1111/j.1600-051X.2006.01042.x.
52. Padayatty SJ, Katz A, Wang Y, Eck P, Kwon O, Lee J-H, Chen S, Corpe C, Dutta A, Dutta SK, Levine M. Vitamin C as an antioxidant: evaluation of its role in disease prevention. J Am Coll Nutr. 2003;22:18–35. https://doi.org/10.1080/07315724.2003.10719272.
53. Culmsee K, Gruber AD, Von Samson-Himmelstjerna G, Nolte I. Quantification of MDR-1 gene expression in canine tissues by real-time reverse transcription quantitative polymerase chain reaction. Res Vet Sci. 2004;77:223–9. https://doi.org/10.1016/j.rvsc.2004.03.001.
54. Kim JE, Shklar G. The effect of vitamin E on the healing of gingival wounds in rats. J Periodontol. 1983;54:305–8. https://doi.org/10.1902/jop.1983.54.5.305.
55. Pacht ER, Kaseki H, Mohammed JR, Cornwell DG, Davis WB. Deficiency of vitamin E in the alveolar fluid of cigarette smokers. Influence on alveolar macrophage cytotoxicity. J Clin Invest. 1986;77:789–96. https://doi.org/10.1172/JCI112376.
56. Saido M, Asakura K, Masayasu S, Sasaki S. Relationship between dietary sugar intake and dental caries among Japanese preschool children with relatively low sugar intake (Japan Nursery School SHOKUIKU Study): a nationwide cross-sectional study. Matern Child Health J. 2016;20:556–66. https://doi.org/10.1007/s10995-015-1854-3.
57. Frostell G, Birkhed D, Edwardsson S, Goldberg P, Petersson L-G, Priwe C, Winholt A-S. Effect of partial substitution of invert sugar for sucrose in combination with Duraphat® treatment on caries development in preschool children: the Malmö study. Caries Res. 1991;25:304–10. https://doi.org/10.1159/000261381.
58. Park E, Na HS, Kim SM, Wallet S, Cha S, Chung J. Xylitol, an anticaries agent, exhibits potent inhibition of inflammatory responses in human THP-1-derived macrophages infected with Porphyromonas gingivalis. J Periodontol. 2014;85:e212–23. https://doi.org/10.1902/jop.2014.130455.
59. Kim S, Park MH, Song YR, Na HS, Chung J. Aggregatibacter actinomycetemcomitans-induced AIM2 inflammasome activation is suppressed by xylitol in differentiated THP-1 macrophages. J Periodontol. 2016;87:e116–26. https://doi.org/10.1902/jop.2016.150477.
60. Keukenmeester R, Slot D, Rosema N, Van Loveren C, Van Der Weijden G. Effects of sugar-free chewing gum sweetened with xylitol or maltitol on the development of gingivitis and plaque: a randomized clinical trial. Int J Dental Hyg. 2014;12:238–44. https://doi.org/10.1111/idh.12071.
61. Garcia MN, Hildebolt CF, Miley DD, Dixon DA, Couture RA, Anderson Spearie CL, Langenwalter EM, Shannon WD, Deych E, Mueller C, Civitelli R. One-year effects of vitamin D and calcium supplementation on chronic periodontitis. J Periodontol. 2011;82:25–32. https://doi.org/10.1902/jop.2010.100207.

62. Adegboye ARA, Christensen LB, Holm-Pedersen P, Avlund K, Boucher BJ, Heitmann BL. Intake of dairy products in relation to periodontitis in older Danish adults. Nutrients. 2012;4:1219–29. https://doi.org/10.3390/nu4091219.
63. Staudte H, Kranz S, Völpel A, Schütze J, Sigusch BW. Comparison of nutrient intake between patients with periodontitis and healthy subjects. Quintessence Int. 2012;43:907–16.
64. Chakraborty S, Tewari S, Sharma RK, Narula SC, Ghalaut PS, Ghalaut V. Impact of iron deficiency anemia on chronic periodontitis and superoxide dismutase activity: a cross-sectional study. J Periodontal Implant Sci. 2014;44:57. https://doi.org/10.5051/jpis.2014.44.2.57.
65. Rostan EF, DeBuys HV, Madey DL, Pinnell SR. Evidence supporting zinc as an important antioxidant for skin. Int J Dermatol. 2002;41:606–11. https://doi.org/10.1046/j.1365-4362.2002.01567.x.
66. Mirastschijski U, Haaksma CJ, Tomasek JJ, Ågren MS. Matrix metalloproteinase inhibitor GM 6001 attenuates keratinocyte migration, contraction and myofibroblast formation in skin wounds. Exp Cell Res. 2004;299:465–75. https://doi.org/10.1016/j.yexcr.2004.06.007.
67. Pushparani DS. Zinc and type 2 diabetes mellitus with periodontitis- a systematic review. Curr Diabetes Rev. 2015;10:397–401. https://doi.org/10.2174/1573399810666141121161514.
68. Pushparani DS. Serum zinc and β D glucuronidase enzyme level in type 2 diabetes mellitus with periodontitis. Curr Diabetes Rev. 2016;12:449–53. https://doi.org/10.2174/1573399811666150724094525.
69. Maguire A. ADA clinical recommendations on topical fluoride for caries prevention. Evid Based Dent. 2014;15:38–9. https://doi.org/10.1038/sj.ebd.6401019.
70. Seppa L, Forss H, Øgaard B. The effect of fluoride application on fluoride release and the antibacterial action of glass lonomers. J Dent Res. 1993;72:1310–4. https://doi.org/10.1177/00220345930720090901.
71. Karadeniz EI, Gonzales C, Nebioglu-Dalci O, Dwarte D, Turk T, Isci D, Sahin-Saglam AM, Alkis H, Elekdag-Turk S, Darendeliler MA. Physical properties of root cementum: part 20. Effect of fluoride on orthodontically induced root resorption with light and heavy orthodontic forces for 4 weeks: a microcomputed tomography study. Am J Orthod Dentofacial Orthop. 2011;140:e199–210. https://doi.org/10.1016/j.ajodo.2011.05.017.
72. Wong MCS, Huang J, Wang J, Chan PSF, Lok V, Chen X, Leung C, Wang HHX, Lao XQ, Zheng Z-J. Global, regional and time-trend prevalence of central obesity: a systematic review and meta-analysis of 13.2 million subjects. Eur J Epidemiol. 2020;35:673–83. https://doi.org/10.1007/s10654-020-00650-3.
73. Mcmurray RG, Soares J, Caspersen CJ, Mccurdy T. Examining variations of resting metabolic rate of adults: a public health perspective. Med Sci Sports Exerc. 2014;46:1352–8. https://doi.org/10.1249/MSS.0000000000000232.
74. Willershausen B, Moschos D, Azrak B, Blettner M. Correlation between oral health and body mass index (BMI) in 2071 primary school pupils. Eur J Med Res. 2007;12:295–9.
75. Thippeswamy HM, Kumar N, Acharya S, Pentapati KC. Relationship between body mass index and dental caries among adolescent children in South India. West Indian Med J. 2011;60:581–6.
76. Kim Y, Kim J. Body mass index and oral health status in Korean adults: the Fifth Korea National Health and Nutrition Examination Survey. Int J Dent Hyg. 2017;15:172–8. https://doi.org/10.1111/idh.12207.
77. Idrees M, Hammad M, Faden A, Kujan O. Influence of body mass index on severity of dental caries: cross-sectional study in healthy adults. Ann Saudi Med. 2017;37:444–8. https://doi.org/10.5144/0256-4947.2017.444.
78. Kantovitz KR, Pascon FM, Rontani RMP, Gavião MBD. Obesity and dental caries–a systematic review. Oral Health Prev Dent. 2006;4:137–44.
79. Khattak O, Iqbal A, Chaudhary FA, Syed J, Alsharari T, Vundavalli S, Aljahdali BAS, AlZahrani AEA, Issrani R, Sultan SE. Evaluating a linkage between obesity and the occurrence of dental caries among school going children in Sakaka, Al Jouf, Kingdom of Saudi Arabia. PeerJ. 2022;10:e13582. https://doi.org/10.7717/peerj.13582.

80. Modéer T, Blomberg CC, Wondimu B, Julihn A, Marcus C. Association between obesity, flow rate of whole saliva, and dental caries in adolescents. Obesity. 2010;18:2367–73. https://doi.org/10.1038/oby.2010.63.
81. Chen D, Zhi Q, Zhou Y, Tao Y, Wu L, Lin H. Association between dental caries and BMI in children: a systematic review and meta-analysis. Caries Res. 2018;52:230–45. https://doi.org/10.1159/000484988.
82. Silva MJ, Kilpatrick NM, Craig JM, Manton DJ, Leong P, Ho H, Saffery R, Burgner DP, Scurrah KJ. A twin study of body mass index and dental caries in childhood. Sci Rep. 2020;10:568. https://doi.org/10.1038/s41598-020-57435-7.
83. Chodzko-Zajko WJ, Proctor DN, Fiatarone Singh MA, Minson CT, Nigg CR, Salem GJ, Skinner JS. Exercise and physical activity for older adults. Med Sci Sports Exerc. 2009;41:1510–30. https://doi.org/10.1249/MSS.0b013e3181a0c95c.
84. Garber CE, Blissmer B, Deschenes MR, Franklin BA, Lamonte MJ, Lee I-M, Nieman DC, Swain DP. Quantity and quality of exercise for developing and maintaining cardiorespiratory, musculoskeletal, and neuromotor fitness in apparently healthy adults: guidance for prescribing exercise. Med Sci Sports Exerc. 2011;43:1334–59. https://doi.org/10.1249/MSS.0b013e318213fefb.
85. Fernandes RM, Correa MG, Dos Santos MAR, Almeida APCPSC, Fagundes NCF, Maia LC, Lima RR. The effects of moderate physical exercise on adult cognition: a systematic review. Front Physiol. 2018;9:667. https://doi.org/10.3389/fphys.2018.00667.
86. De Souza DC, Matos VAF, Dos Santos VOA, Medeiros IF, Marinho CSR, Nascimento PRP, Dorneles GP, Peres A, Müller CH, Krause M, Costa EC, Fayh APT. Effects of high-intensity interval and moderate-intensity continuous exercise on inflammatory, leptin, IgA, and lipid peroxidation responses in obese males. Front Physiol. 2018;9:567. https://doi.org/10.3389/fphys.2018.00567.
87. Ferreira RDO, Corrêa MG, Magno MB, Almeida APCPSC, Fagundes NCF, Rosing CK, Maia LC, Lima RR. Physical activity reduces the prevalence of periodontal disease: systematic review and meta-analysis. Front Physiol. 2019;10:234. https://doi.org/10.3389/fphys.2019.00234.
88. Chan CCK, Chan AKY, Chu CH, Tsang YC. Physical activity as a modifiable risk factor for periodontal disease. Front Oral Health. 2023;4:1266462. https://doi.org/10.3389/froh.2023.1266462.
89. Ntovas P, Loumprinis N, Maniatakos P, Margaritidi L, Rahiotis C. The effects of physical exercise on saliva composition: a comprehensive review. Dent J (Basel). 2022;10:7. https://doi.org/10.3390/dj10010007.
90. Gleeson M, Bishop NC, Stensel DJ, Lindley MR, Mastana SS, Nimmo MA. The anti-inflammatory effects of exercise: mechanisms and implications for the prevention and treatment of disease. Nat Rev Immunol. 2011;11:607–15. https://doi.org/10.1038/nri3041.
91. Ford ES. Does exercise reduce inflammation? Physical activity and C-reactive protein among U.S. adults. Epidemiology. 2002;13:561–8. https://doi.org/10.1097/00001648-200209000-00012.
92. Bird SR, Hawley JA. Update on the effects of physical activity on insulin sensitivity in humans. BMJ Open Sport Exerc Med. 2017;2:e000143. https://doi.org/10.1136/bmjsem-2016-000143.
93. D'Aiuto F, Gable D, Syed Z, Allen Y, Wanyonyi KL, White S, Gallagher JE. Evidence summary: the relationship between oral diseases and diabetes. Br Dent J. 2017;222:944–8. https://doi.org/10.1038/sj.bdj.2017.544.
94. Bergström J, Preber H. Tobacco use as a risk factor. J Periodontol. 1994;65:545–50. https://doi.org/10.1902/jop.1994.65.5s.545.
95. Fabbri LM. Smoking, not COPD, as the disease. N Engl J Med. 2016;374:1885–6. https://doi.org/10.1056/NEJMe1515508.
96. Sin DD, Man SP. Impact of cancers and cardiovascular diseases in chronic obstructive pulmonary disease. Curr Opin Pulm Med. 2008;14:115–21. https://doi.org/10.1097/MCP.0b013e3282f45ffb.

97. Lee J, Taneja V, Vassallo R. Cigarette smoking and inflammation: cellular and molecular mechanisms. J Dent Res. 2012;91:142–9. https://doi.org/10.1177/0022034511421200.
98. Arnson Y, Shoenfeld Y, Amital H. Effects of tobacco smoke on immunity, inflammation and autoimmunity. J Autoimmun. 2010;34:J258–65. https://doi.org/10.1016/j.jaut.2009.12.003.
99. Winn DM. Tobacco use and oral disease. J Dent Educ. 2001;65:306–12. https://doi.org/10.1002/j.0022-0337.2001.65.4.tb03400.x.
100. Leite FRM, López R, Pajaniaye JB, Nascimento GG. Effect of smoking exposure on non-surgical periodontal therapy: 1-year follow-up. J Dent Res. 2023;102:280–6. https://doi.org/10.1177/00220345221135100.
101. Jha P, Chaloupka FJ, Corrao M, Jacob B. Reducing the burden of smoking world-wide: effectiveness of interventions and their coverage. Drug Alcohol Rev. 2006;25:597–609. https://doi.org/10.1080/09595230600944511.
102. Hoffman SJ, Tan C. Overview of systematic reviews on the health-related effects of government tobacco control policies. BMC Public Health. 2015;15:744. https://doi.org/10.1186/s12889-015-2041-6.
103. Holliday R, Hong B, McColl E, Livingstone-Banks J, Preshaw PM. Interventions for tobacco cessation delivered by dental professionals. Cochrane Database Syst Rev. 2021;2021:CD005084. https://doi.org/10.1002/14651858.CD005084.pub4.
104. Vasiliou A, Shankardass K, Nisenbaum R, Quiñonez C. Current stress and poor oral health. BMC Oral Health. 2016;16:88. https://doi.org/10.1186/s12903-016-0284-y.
105. Duran-Pinedo AE, Solbiati J, Frias-Lopez J. The effect of the stress hormone cortisol on the metatranscriptome of the oral microbiome. NPJ Biofilms Microbiomes. 2018;4:25. https://doi.org/10.1038/s41522-018-0068-z.
106. Spector AM, Postolache TT, Akram F, Scott AJ, Wadhawan A, Reynolds MA. Psychological stress: a predisposing and exacerbating factor in periodontitis. Curr Oral Health Rep. 2020;7:208–15. https://doi.org/10.1007/s40496-020-00282-2.
107. Acharya S, Pentapati KC. Work stress and oral health-related quality of life among Indian information technology workers: an exploratory study. Int Dent J. 2012;62:132–6. https://doi.org/10.1111/j.1875-595X.2011.00104.x.
108. Sekiguchi A, Kawashiri S, Hayashida H, Nagaura Y, Nobusue K, Nonaka F, Yamanashi H, Kitamura M, Kawasaki K, Fukuda H, Iwasaki T, Saito T, Maeda T. Association between high psychological distress and poor oral health-related quality of life (OHQoL) in Japanese community-dwelling people: the Nagasaki Islands Study. Environ Health Prev Med. 2020;25:82. https://doi.org/10.1186/s12199-020-00919-9.
109. Madison A, Kiecolt-Glaser JK. Stress, depression, diet, and the gut microbiota: human–bacteria interactions at the core of psychoneuroimmunology and nutrition. Curr Opin Behav Sci. 2019;28:105–10. https://doi.org/10.1016/j.cobeha.2019.01.011.
110. Cohen BE, Edmondson D, Kronish IM. State of the art review: depression, stress, anxiety, and cardiovascular disease. Am J Hypertens. 2015;28:1295–302. https://doi.org/10.1093/ajh/hpv047.
111. Deinzer R, Granrath N, Spahl M, Linz S, Waschul B, Herforth A. Stress, oral health behaviour and clinical outcome. Br J Health Psychol. 2005;10:269–83. https://doi.org/10.1348/135910705X26858.
112. Watt RG, Sheiham A. Integrating the common risk factor approach into a social determinants framework. Community Dent Oral Epidemiol. 2012;40:289–96. https://doi.org/10.1111/j.1600-0528.2012.00680.x.
113. Nowjack-Raymer RE. Teamwork in prevention: possibilities and barriers to integrating oral health into general health. Adv Dent Res. 1995;9:100–5. https://doi.org/10.1177/08959374950090020101.
114. Kaufman LB, Henshaw MM, Brown BP, Calabrese JM. Oral health and interprofessional collaborative practice. Dent Clin N Am. 2016;60:879–90. https://doi.org/10.1016/j.cden.2016.05.007.

115. Genco RJ, Genco FD. Common risk factors in the management of periodontal and associated systemic diseases: the dental setting and interprofessional collaboration. J Evid Based Dent Pract. 2014;14:4–16. https://doi.org/10.1016/j.jebdp.2014.03.003.
116. Watt RG. Strategies and approaches in oral disease prevention and health promotion. Bull World Health Organ. 2005. https://doi.org/10.1590/S0042-96862005000900018.
117. Cabrera M, Bedi R, Lomazzi M. The public health approach to oral health: a literature review. Oral. 2024;4:231–42. https://doi.org/10.3390/oral4020019.
118. Wolf TG, Cagetti MG, Fisher J-M, Seeberger GK, Campus G. Non-communicable diseases and oral health: an overview. Front Oral Health. 2021;2:725460. https://doi.org/10.3389/froh.2021.725460.
119. Chamut S, Alhassan M, Hameedaldeen A, Kaplish S, Yang AH, Wade CG, Alghamdi S, Chamut D, Novy BB, Chandel T. Every bite counts to achieve oral health: a scoping review on diet and oral health preventive practices. Int J Equity Health. 2024;23:261. https://doi.org/10.1186/s12939-024-02279-0.
120. WHO. Oral health resolution. Genéve, Switzerland; 2021. https://apps.who.int/gb/ebwha/pdf_files/WHA74/B148_REC1_EXT-en.pdf.
121. Belibasakis GN, Bostanci N, Marsh PD, Zaura E. Applications of the oral microbiome in personalized dentistry. Arch Oral Biol. 2019;104:7–12. https://doi.org/10.1016/j.archoralbio.2019.05.023.
122. Steigmann L, Kačarević ŽP, Khoury J, Nagy K, Feres M. Integration of precision medicine into the dental care setting. Front Dent Med. 2024;5:1398897. https://doi.org/10.3389/fdmed.2024.1398897.
123. Ducret M, Mörch C-M, Karteva T, Fisher J, Schwendicke F. Artificial intelligence for sustainable oral healthcare. J Dent. 2022;127:104344. https://doi.org/10.1016/j.jdent.2022.104344.
124. Khoury ZH, Ferguson A, Price JB, Sultan AS, Wang R. Responsible artificial intelligence for addressing equity in oral healthcare. Front Oral Health. 2024;5:1408867. https://doi.org/10.3389/froh.2024.1408867.
125. Benzian H, Greenspan JS, Barrow J, Hutter JW, Loomer PM, Stauf N, Perry DA. A competency matrix for global oral health. J Dent Educ. 2015;79:353–61. https://doi.org/10.1002/j.0022-0337.2015.79.4.tb05891.x.
126. Wang TT, Mathur MR, Schmidt H. Universal health coverage, oral health, equity and personal responsibility. Bull World Health Organ. 2020;98:719–21. https://doi.org/10.2471/BLT.19.247288.
127. Listl S, Quiñonez C, Vujicic M. Including oral diseases and conditions in universal health coverage. Bull World Health Organ. 2021;99:407. https://doi.org/10.2471/BLT.21.285530.
128. Harnagea H, Lamothe L, Couturier Y, Esfandiari S, Voyer R, Charbonneau A, Emami E. From theoretical concepts to policies and applied programmes: the landscape of integration of oral health in primary care. BMC Oral Health. 2018;18:23. https://doi.org/10.1186/s12903-018-0484-8.
129. Slavkin HC, Dubois PA, Kleinman DV, Fuccillo R. Science-informed health policies for oral and systemic health. J Healthc Leadersh. 2023;15:43–57. https://doi.org/10.2147/JHL.S363657.

4 Tobacco Smoking and Oral Health

Sangeeta Gajendra and Scott McIntosh

4.1 Introduction

According to the American Lung Association, a burning cigarette produces more than 7000 chemicals, of which 69 are carcinogens [1] that may affect public health in several ways [2]. In addition to general health, smoking tobacco has direct detrimental effects on oral health. Both smoking combustible products and emerging nicotine products continue to remain an ongoing major global public health problem. Tobacco smoking increases the risk of oral diseases and conditions, including but not limited to oral cancer, mucosal lesions, periodontal disease and dental caries. Dental office visits have long been recognised as providing an excellent opportunity for providing cessation intervention, a frequently visited 'point of care'. However, an overall lack of knowledge of and training in tobacco use prevention and cessation among oral health professionals remains an issue. Increased efforts are needed to increase tobacco use screening and cessation interventions in the dental office. Routine and brief tobacco cessation interventions that oral health care providers can provide can include educational, behavioural and pharmacological interventions and referral to adjunctive evidence-based tobacco cessation treatment. Gajendra et al. have presented a review of the effects of tobacco product use on oral health and the role of dentists in cessation [3].

This chapter provides an overview of the ill effects of tobacco smoking on oral health and the role of oral health care providers in the management and treatment of tobacco dependence. This can essentially be translated into clinical practice to

S. Gajendra (✉)
Department of Community Dentistry, Eastman Institute for Oral Health, Rochester, NY, USA
e-mail: Sangeeta_Gajendra@urmc.rochester.edu

S. McIntosh
Department of Public Health Sciences and Eastman Institute for Oral Health, University of Rochester Medical Center, Rochester, NY, USA
e-mail: scott_mcintosh@urmc.rochester.edu

S. R. Prabhu et al. (eds.), *Lifestyle in Oral Health and Disease*,
https://doi.org/10.1007/978-3-032-05888-1_4

deliver counselling successfully and implement tobacco use cessation strategies in the dental office. The scope of this chapter primarily includes combustible products, such as cigarettes, cigars, little cigars, bidis and waterpipes (also known as hookahs).

4.2 The Global Burden of Tobacco Smoking

According to the World Health Organization (WHO), 20.9% of all persons aged 15 years and over used some form of tobacco on a current basis in 2022, where 80% of these were current smokers with a prevalence of current tobacco smoking of 16.7% [4]. Globally, there are 1.1 billion smokers and over 8 million die each year due to smoking. The global target for the total population is predicted to fall short of meeting the overall global target of 18.4% by an absolute 1.3% by the current year (2025) [5]. While current cigarette smoking has decreased to the lowest level in over 60 years, current tobacco product use among adults has not changed much since 2017.

Tobacco smoking imposes a significant economic burden on a country, including the health care costs associated with treating smoking-related diseases and lost productivity. The total global economic cost of smoking is estimated at around $US 1.85 trillion [6]. Comprehensive strategies, such as price increases, smoke-free policies, high-impact media campaigns and cessation support, are critical to prevent and reduce tobacco product use, nicotine addiction and their associated adverse health outcomes.

4.3 Types of Smoked Tobacco Products

Cigarettes Cigarette smoking remains the most popular method of using tobacco for nicotine delivery. Other various smoked tobacco products include cigars, bidis, waterpipes and others. Tobacco has been used as far back as 12,300 years ago [7], with combustible cigarettes being the most popular method of use. Modern-day cigarettes typically contain 10–14 mg of nicotine, 1–1.5 mg of which is absorbed into the body [1]. Nicotine, which drives tobacco addiction, is the primary reinforcing component of tobacco. Nicotine is generally delivered through the lungs, as well as through the skin and mucous membranes. Cigarette smoking is a significant public health issue. According to the Centers for Disease Control and Prevention (CDC), in 2022, an estimated 11.6% of US adults currently smoked cigarettes, including 13% of men and 10% of women. Interestingly, nearly 9 out of 10 adults who smoke cigarettes daily first try smoking by age 18 [8].

Cigars and Little Cigars In a recent systematic review by Vargees et al. (2023), cigars have evolved from traditional cigars to now encompassing other products such as little cigars and cigarillos (LCCs), which are available in many flavours and prices [9]. Increases in product choices, accompanied by varying regulations and pricing, result in widespread use by diverse populations and age groups. LCCs are more prevalent among youth, young adults and persons who identify as Black/African American and are often used with other tobacco products, alcohol and cannabis. Cigars and LCCs generate smoke similar to that of cigarettes.

Bidis A bidi stick is a type of cigarette made from uncured tobacco, rolled into a leaf (flavoured and unflavoured) and tied with a string at one end. Although not legally sold in the United States, bidis dominate the smoking market in India. Indian medicinal systems, such as Ayurveda, prescribe inhalation of the fumes of medicinal herbs rolled in leaves, which facilitated the acceptance of the bidi in various sub-cultures [10]. Higher odds of bidi smoking have been observed among males, older age groups and among those with lower socioeconomic status (SES) [11].

Based on the nicotine content, it has been proposed that the equivalent for one pack-year of cigarettes (or 20 cigarettes per day per year) be taken as 43 bidis per day per year. However, each bidi stick has an average of 0.46 times the nicotine of commercial cigarettes; longer abstinence from bidis as compared to cigarettes is required to observe the return of nicotine levels to normal due to deeper puffing [12].

Waterpipes (Hookah) Waterpipe use, a traditional way of smoking that originated in India, is also known as hookah, shisha, narghile, argileh and hubble-bubble [13]. The device usually consists of a bowl, a pipe, a water jar and a saucer to hold the ashes. Tobacco, usually shisha tobacco, is heated via charcoal above the bowl. The smoke then descends from the bowl through a pipe, which is cooled and humidified by the water in the jar. The smoke is then inhaled through a hose.

The popularity of the waterpipe is increasing worldwide, particularly among young adults. In a recent systematic review [14], the prevalence ever of waterpipe smoking among 10–24-year-olds (mainly in the United States) was 18.16% (95% confidence interval [CI], 18.03–18.29), whereas the prevalence of current (30-day) use was 6.43% (95% CI, 6.34–6.50). The age of initiation of waterpipe smoking varied. Prevalence was highest among males, those in high- and middle-income groups and among university students. Common risk factors of waterpipe smoking include concomitant cigarette smoking, alcohol and substance use. Waterpipe smoking can result in increased susceptibility to smoking among those who were never smokers.

4.4 Health Hazards of Tobacco Smoking

More than16 million citizens in the United States fare living with a smoking-related disease. In addition to the costs in terms of human morbidity and mortality, smoking places a significant financial burden on Americans, as smoking-attributable health care spending exceeds $170 billion per year [15]. The evidence base supporting tobacco as a risk factor for non-communicable diseases such as cardiovascular diseases and cancer has been strong for decades. Smoking is linked with lung diseases, impacts the immune system and increases susceptibility to infections. Smoking increases the risk and severity of pulmonary infections because of structural damage to the upper airways and a decrease in pulmonary immune function [16].

The evidence base is also strong and growing regarding the association between smoking and infectious diseases, including HIV, tuberculosis and COVID-19 due to the alteration of the structural, functional and immunologic host defences [17, 18].

Evidence has shown that cigar use, particularly with more frequent and deeper inhalation, is associated with cardiovascular and pulmonary toxicity and higher all-cause and cancer-related mortalities [19]. The inhaled smoke from the waterpipe contains toxic and hazardous materials, including nicotine, tar, polyaromatic hydrocarbons and heavy metals, all of which are associated with lung diseases and cancer [20]. Regular use is associated with respiratory symptoms, a decrease in pulmonary function and an increased risk for lung diseases such as chronic obstructive pulmonary disease (COPD), increased risk for cardiovascular disease and cancer.

Second-Hand Smoke and Third-Hand Smoke Second-hand smoke (SHS; smoke exhaled from a user, coming off the tip of a cigarette and/or the undissipated airborne smoke near a smoker) is another measurable nicotine delivery vector. Relatedly, third-hand smoke (particulates from ambient smoke that have settled onto surfaces, such as clothing, furniture, drapes and carpets) also represents a vector of exposure. Exposure to second-hand smoke (SHS) or passive smoking is a risk factor for a variety of adverse health effects. SHS exposure in children due to parental smoking has been shown to have a detrimental impact on paediatric lung function, body mass index (BMI) and physical fitness [21]. A study reviewed the effects of SHS on various diseases among both adults and children. The diseases mainly studied for adults were lung cancer, ischaemic heart disease, stroke, asthma, chronic obstructive pulmonary disease, diabetes and breast cancer. In children, the burden from lower respiratory tract infection, otitis media, asthma, sudden infant death syndrome and low birth weight were investigated. The authors concluded that many hazards due to SHS exposure are well known, and morbidity and mortality attributable to SHS have been studied widely. Yet, there are gaps, as many diseases and geographic regions are understudied [22].

4.5 Impact of Tobacco Smoking on Oral Health

Smoked tobacco products, including cigarettes, cigars, little cigars, bidis and hookah, are significant risk factors for oral cancer, oral mucosal lesions, periodontal disease, implant failure, salivary gland hypofunction and dental caries, among other oral diseases and conditions.

Oral Cancer Globally, oral cancer (including the lips, oral cavity, salivary glands and oropharynx) ranks eleventh among all newly diagnosed cancers, accounting for 550,804 new cases with an estimated 264,392 deaths reported in 2022 [23]. In the United States, an estimated 58,450 new cases were reported in 2024, with a 5-year relative survival rate of 69% from 2014 to 2020 [22]. Oral squamous cell carcinoma (OSCC), caused by smoked or smokeless tobacco, accounts for more than 90% of all oral cancers [24].

Cigarettes, cigars, little cigars, bidis, waterpipes and other combusted tobacco products contain a complex mixture of tumour promoters, co-carcinogens and various toxicants that exacerbate the effects of the carcinogens [25]. Jiang et al. proposed a plausible carcinogenic pathway attributing smoked tobacco as the major risk factor for OSCC [26]. Tobacco and its toxic metabolites cause epigenetic alterations in oral epithelial cells, inhibit multiple systemic immune functions of the host, and induce oxidative stress, releasing reactive oxygen species that lead to OSCC. Sadri et al. found that smokers were 4.65 (95% CI = 3.19–6.77) times more likely to have oral cancer [27].

Smoking and alcohol have a synergistic effect on oral cancer development. Mello et al. conducted a systematic review of 33 studies and found that alcohol and tobacco smoking synergistically increased the risk for oral cancer (odds ratio [OR] = 4.74; 95% CI = 3.51–6.40) [28]. Other smoked tobacco forms have also been implicated in causing premalignant lesions and oral cancer, such as waterpipe smoking [29, 30] and bidis [31]. The risk for oral cancer increases with the number of smoked tobacco products per day, duration of smoking and age of onset of smoking. Thus, smokers who are at high risk for oral cancer need to be identified early to prevent the onset of this disease. It is imperative to understand the relationship between smoking and oral cancer so that targeted public health initiatives can be used to reduce the risk of oral cancer.

Mariano et al. found that people exposed to second-hand smoke (SHS) were 1.51 (95% CI = 1.20–1.91) times more likely to have oral cancer. When the duration of exposure exceeded 10–15 years, the risk increased, with an odds ratio (OR) of 2.07 (95% CI = 1.54–2.79). This study supports a causal relationship between SHS and oral cancer, providing guidance for the development of policies and interventions [32].

Oral Mucosal Lesions Tobacco use has been strongly associated with mucosal lesions such as leucoplakia, smokeless tobacco keratosis at the site of tobacco placement, nicotinic stomatitis, smoker's melanosis [33], and erythroplakia [34]. Leucoplakia, particularly associated with tobacco, should be further investigated with a biopsy for the presence of epithelial dysplasia or carcinoma. Malignant transformation occurs in about 3–6% of leucoplakias, increasing in prevalence with more prolonged exposure to smoking [35]. Among smokers, epithelial dysplasia may appear clinically as either white or red, depending on whether it is associated with hyperkeratosis or epithelial atrophy, respectively. It is termed carcinoma *in situ* when it does not invade the connective tissue and is only restricted to the entire thickness of epithelium [33]. Black hairy tongue is a condition predominantly seen among heavy smokers, when the dorsal surface of the tongue has a hair-like appearance as a result of filiform papillae undergoing hypertrophy and retardation of the normal rate of desquamation [33]. Management of oral mucosal lesions requires a thorough examination of the lesions and an assessment of all relevant risk factors.

Periodontal Disease and Dental Implants Periodontal disease is a chronic, inflammatory, destructive but preventable disease in which smoking is considered the strongest modifiable risk factor. As early as the 1940s, studies have found a relationship between tobacco use and periodontal disease. Pipe and cigar smokers have higher gingival recession, tooth loss and pocket depths compared to non-smokers (NS) [36]. Leite et al. conducted a systematic review and concluded that tobacco smoking increases the risk for periodontitis by 85% (risk ratio [RR] = 1.85; 95% CI = 1.5–2.2). Only original prospective longitudinal studies were included in this review. Thus, they could positively conclude that smoking has a major impact on the incidence and progression of periodontitis and should be assessed along with other risk factors of periodontitis [37].

Increased gingival microvascular density with considerable gingival inflammation, suppressed angiogenesis due to local immune suppression and oxidative stress leading to periodontal disease and complications are seen in tobacco smokers [38]. A cross-sectional pilot study [39] involving cigarette smokers (CS), e-cigarette smokers (EC), dual smokers (DS) and non-smokers (NS) found that the levels of inflammatory mediators and oxidative stress were statistically significantly higher in EC compared to NS, as well as in DS compared to EC. Systematic reviews have determined that smokers have an 80% and 85% higher risk of periodontitis than quitters and never-smokers [37, 40]. A meta-analysis of longitudinal studies also found smokers have 2.6 (95% CI = 2.29–2.96) times higher risk of tooth loss [41].

Several studies, including systematic reviews, have proven that tobacco smoking has an adverse effect on dental implants. Smoking has been attributed as the primary risk factor for implant failure, with the risk being more than 100% higher than in non-smokers in both the maxillary and mandibular teeth [42, 43]. Waterpipe smoking had similar outcomes [44].

The pattern of tobacco smoking and dose–response data (including smoking intensity, duration, pack years and time since quitting) are crucial to estimating the burden of oral diseases due to tobacco smoking. Clearly, more exposure (time, quantity, intensity of use) to the carcinogens and toxicants of smoking leads to more morbidity and mortality. The dose–response effect between cigarette smoking and implant failure was investigated. Patients who smoked more than 20 cigarettes per day had a significantly higher risk of implant failure than non-smokers (implant-based: RR = 2.45, CI = 1.42–4.22; and patient-based: RR = 4.0, CI = 2.72–5.89) [45]. Smoking can impair health through both systemic and local routes. The heat from smoking tobacco and its toxic by-products, such as nicotine, carbon monoxide and hydrogen cyanide, may impair healing after oral surgery. This is also observed after surgical procedures involving implants due to arteriolar vasoconstriction and decreased blood flow [46]. Patients need to be advised to stop smoking to improve the success rate of implants.

Effects on Salivary Glands There is a paucity of studies on tobacco smoking and its impact on salivary glands. Tobacco smoking has been associated with increased sialolithiasis (stones within salivary ducts) formation and decreased salivary flow rate. In a cross-sectional study of 947 cases and 3788 controls, a statistically significant association was observed between smoking and sialolithiasis with an odds ratio of 1.31 (95% CI = 1.08–1.59). Patients who smoked had thicker saliva with reduced salivary flow [47], decreased salivary pH [48], and altered secretory immunoglobulin A (sIgA) levels [49] as compared to non-smokers. All these factors could lead to an increase in periodontal disease and dental caries.

Dental Caries Dental caries is a multifactorial, chronic, microbial disease. Factors such as poor eating habits, oral hygiene and compliance with treatment have been implicated in its aetiology. Studies have demonstrated a relationship between smoking and caries-causing bacteria. *Streptococcus mutans*, a bacteria present in the mouth, is a major agent that promotes dental caries. Nicotine in cigarettes may be the leading cause of an ecological imbalance by increasing colonisation and metabolism of *Streptococcus mutans*. Smoking influences saliva by lowering its neutralising capacity, altering its chemical composition and bacterial components, and thus promoting the formation of a caries-susceptible environment [50].

Several epidemiological studies have linked tobacco use and increased dental caries prevalence [50–53]. In the United States, national estimates found that 40–50% of adults aged 20–64 years had untreated dental decay, specifically among non-Hispanic Black, Mexican American, or poor, those with high school education or lower and current smokers. Smokers aged 65 years or more were twice as likely to have untreated caries than never smokers [52]. Smokers had higher decayed, missing, filled teeth (DMFT) scores than non-smokers in studies conducted in Italy and Finland [54, 55]. In a prospective open cohort 3-year study of 22,009 patients in Portugal, 36.6% had dental caries with smoking as a risk (odds ratio = 1.84; 95% CI = 1.64–2.07). The study also found that smoking prevention could lead to a 7% potential reduction in dental caries [53]. Undoubtedly, smoking increases the risk of dental caries and needs to be addressed among dental patients.

The introduction of new combustible tobacco products in the United States and around the world has made it crucial to determine the impact of socioeconomic factors on tobacco product use and oral health. This will help in designing targeted interventions in concert with the regulation of tobacco products to reduce tobacco-related diseases. Profound oral health disparities are seen in specific subpopulations. Among smokers, untreated decay, tooth loss and periodontal disease are disproportionately higher among racial and ethnic minorities, low-income individuals, those with limited education, those with public dental insurance, or those without any dental insurance [56]. Thus, oral diseases and other oral health-related issues should be part of the discussion when considering quitting.

4.6 The Role of Oral Health Providers in Tobacco Smoking Cessation

Quitting tobacco use greatly reduces the risk of developing many diseases. Nicotine dependence is a chronic condition that warrants interventions by all health care providers, including oral health care providers. A systematic review found that those who quit after a smoking cessation programme have a similar risk of periodontal disease as those who never smoked (RR = 0.97; 95% CI = 0.87–1.08) [57]. Multiple attempts are often necessary to achieve abstinence. A national survey conducted in 2015 in the United States found that 68% of adult smokers wanted to stop smoking, 55% made a past-year quit attempt, and about 7% quit. The study also found that a health professional had advised 57.2% to quit, and 31.2% used cessation counselling and/or medication when trying to quit [58].

The dental office is an excellent venue for providing cessation intervention as 46.6% of patients who smoke make an annual visit to the dentist [52]. The entire dental team needs to be involved, as dental hygienists and assistants are front-line professionals in educating patients about their oral health. Patients tend to pay more attention to educational messages about their oral health. Unfortunately, smokers have lower rates of dental care utilisation compared to non-smokers [59]. A common risk factor management approach that incorporates interprofessional collaboration should be employed in dental settings. Smoking cessation intervention (screening, education, referral) and interventions for diet, sugar consumption and weight control will help in reducing not only oral diseases but also systemic conditions such as diabetes, heart disease and cancer. Understanding how social determinants of health and oral health disparities intersect with smoking can inform more targeted interventions and public health strategies.

A statewide survey of dental professionals reported that although they asked and documented tobacco use (hygienists: 80%; dentists: 73%), they did not as frequently assist with cessation (hygienists: 27–49%; dentists: 10–31%) [60]. Findings suggest that more efforts are needed to engage dental professionals in tobacco cessation with a focus on increasing dental providers' relevant knowledge, skills and sense of professional responsibility. Brief counselling using the 5As model and nicotine replacement therapy (NRT) was used by dental hygienists in a randomised controlled trial. The study found that a statistically higher percentage of intervention participants had made a quit attempt of at least 1 week at 3 months (15% in the intervention group vs. 9% in the controls) and at 6 months (10% in the intervention group vs. 5% in the controls). This feasibility study has demonstrated the potential of dental hygienists in providing smoking cessation advice [61].

The most recent Surgeon General's Report of 2020 on smoking cessation [15] concluded that proven smoking cessation treatments are widely available. However, gaps exist in the utilisation of programmes, policies and resources that can improve cessation rates and help smokers quit. The Report also stated that there exists conclusive evidence that can serve as the foundation for the development and dissemination of evidence-based clinical practice guidelines. This will help in increasing the delivery of clinical interventions for smoking cessation.

Tobacco cessation in dental settings is both feasible and effective. The evidence is compelling for the effectiveness of tobacco cessation involving brief behavioural interventions complemented by pharmacological treatment and referral to state Quitlines and Quitsites. The electronic health record system integrated with tobacco cessation education and referrals, along with automated clinical reminders, can be a powerful tool. Behavioural interventions for tobacco cessation can be easily incorporated within routine oral examinations. Tobacco cessation interventions provided by oral health care providers can be classified into three categories, which can be used alone or in combination: (1) brief educational, (2) behavioural and (3) pharmacological.

Brief Educational Interventions Brief clinical (often office-based) interventions involve raising awareness about the harmful effects of tobacco products on general health. The 5As model is the most recognised and widely accepted framework for brief smoking cessation interventions and is based on the 'Stages of Change' model. It proposes that smokers should be given a brief intervention to address smoking at every visit. This model consists of Asking (about use), Advising (to quit), Assessing (willingness to quit), Assisting (with quit attempts) and Arranging (follow-up plans). For patients who are not ready to make a quit attempt in the next 30 days, oral health providers may use the 5Rs strategy [62]: Relevance (of quitting to person's goals), Risks (of continued use), Rewards (of quitting), Roadblocks (to success) and Repetition (of this advice).

Although the 5As model is a widely accepted framework for brief interventions, it has limitations, including time and expertise. A systematic review [63] conducted to determine if dental professionals could help people quit with advice and support revealed that all studies used behavioural programmes aimed at boosting motivation and offered advice to help people quit. Behavioural programmes involving dental professionals help people quit smoking, especially when combined with medication. A shortened three-step model can include Ask, Advise and Refer (to evidence-based treatment, such as a tobacco cessation Quitline) [62].

Behavioural Interventions Behavioural interventions aim to motivate, guide and assist smokers to quit. A meta-analysis by Hartmann-Boyce et al. found that behavioural interventions such as any form of counselling along with guaranteed financial incentives provided the most motivation to quit for 6 months or longer [65]. Behavioural support provided by dental professionals is beneficial for smoking cessation at 6 months compared to brief or no intervention. Multiple-session programmes have a higher quit rate than single-session programmes [64].

Telephone Quitlines are a cost-effective, evidence-based approach for providing behavioural counselling across large geographical areas and populations [66, 67]. Quitlines available throughout the United States (1-800-QUIT-NOW: www.smoke-free.gov) offer counselling and often free nicotine replacement therapy. Quitlines increase overall quit rates by approximately 60% compared to minimal counselling, no counselling, or self-help [62]. Health care providers are more likely to provide smoking cessation interventions if state Quitlines are available as a referral source.

Pharmacotherapy Smoking cessation advice for even a few minutes increases long-term smoking abstinence rates by 5%, which can be increased by 50–70% by combining with pharmacotherapy (e.g. nicotine replacement therapy) for cravings and withdrawal symptoms [68, 69]. Medications include nicotine replacement therapies (NRTs), varenicline, cytisine and bupropion SR.

Nicotine Replacement Therapy (NRT) NRTs are the most used cessation aids. NRT aims to reduce the desire for smoking by increasing nicotine levels in the bloodstream [70]. Several types of NRTs are available: over-the-counter (Gum, Lozenge and Patch) and prescription (Nasal Spray). The Nicotine Inhaler has been discontinued at the time of this writing. The Nicotine Patch delivers a steady dose of nicotine, maintaining a consistent blood nicotine level. To achieve this with other forms of NRT, the products must be taken regularly throughout the day rather than just for symptom relief. However, when using a combination medication approach, the nicotine patch can be combined with one of the others, which, in those cases, can be used for additional symptom relief.

Bupropion SR Bupropion is widely used as an antidepressant and separately as a smoking cessation aid. The mechanism of action is not fully understood, but it weakly inhibits the release of norepinephrine and dopamine. Additionally, it has some action on nicotinic and serotonin receptors [71]. It can be combined with NRTs.

Varenicline (CHANTIX/CHAMPIX) Varenicline is a prescription smoking cessation medication used in combination with education and counselling. Studies have shown varenicline to have more efficacy than bupropion SR and nicotine patches in the short term (e.g. 8 weeks). It acts as a partial agonist of the alpha-4-beta-2 nicotinic acetylcholine receptors and inhibits the activation of the dopaminergic pathway, which is associated with withdrawal symptoms during cessation attempts [72].

Cytisine Cytisine is a plant-based alkaloid and has been used in Eastern Europe for smoking cessation since 1964. It acts as a partial agonist of alpha-4-beta-2 nicotinic acetylcholine receptors and inspired the development of varenicline [73]. Oral cytisine has a shorter half-life (4.8 hours vs. 17 hours) and treatment course (3.5 weeks vs. 12 weeks) than varenicline [74].

Combination Therapy Combination therapy of drugs with distinct mechanisms of action or therapeutic properties helps achieve therapeutic synergism [75]. For tobacco cessation, this typically means combining nicotine replacement therapies (NRTs) with each other or with other evidence-based front-line medications approved by the FDA for cessation. A systematic review involving 3200 participants found that combination nicotine replacement therapy (NRT) had a statistically significantly higher quit rate at 6 months or longer compared to single or no NRT [76]. The only FDA-approved combination therapy for smoking cessation is bupropion SR and nicotine patches [77], although the CDC recommends combinations among the NRTs.

4.7 Barriers to Smoking Cessation Interventions

Oral health care providers need to address barriers to successful quitting. In a study of the self-reported obstacles to quitting among young adult smokers [78], researchers found low SES smokers reported several barriers such as the cost of classes or programmes, craving or withdrawal from nicotine, loss of a way to handle stress, and friends' smoking status. The risk of gaining weight was statistically significant between individuals with low socioeconomic status (SES) and those with high SES [78].

Barriers can also exist from the perspective of oral health providers. Carr and Ebbert [79] cited several barriers; while 61.5% of dentists believed that their patients do not expect tobacco cessation services and resources, 58.5% of patients felt these services/resources should be provided. Barriers included concerns about patient resistance, lack of knowledge, time constraints, inadequate financial reimbursement and poor coordination between dentistry and tobacco cessation services. Another systematic review [80] found that dental practitioners lacked satisfactory knowledge, confidence and training and were unaware of existing referral pathways. Dental hygienists have reported greater levels of activity and confidence, fewer barriers and longer consultation times compared to dentists. However, rates of assisting and referring patients were significantly lower compared to advising [81].

Effective public health policies and laws are needed to reduce the impact of tobacco use. The World Health Organization Framework Convention on Tobacco Control (WHO-FCTC; ratified by 180 countries to date) provides a global response to the tobacco epidemic [82]. To guide the implementation of effective interventions at the country level, the WHO introduced the MPOWER measures in 2007, which include *m*onitoring tobacco use and prevention policies, *p*rotecting people from tobacco smoke, *o*ffering help to quit tobacco, *w*arning about the dangers of tobacco, *e*nforcing bans on tobacco advertising, promotion and sponsorship and *r*aising taxes on tobacco [83]. Since its implementation, 107 countries have adopted at least one

MPOWER policy at the best-practice level and 74 countries have introduced laws enforcing smoke-free indoor public buildings and workplaces. However, additional efforts are needed as the morbidity and mortality rates of tobacco use continue to remain high.

Adequate reimbursement for tobacco cessation services is essential to incentivise health professionals, including dental professionals, to promote tobacco cessation. Considering the prohibitive costs associated with tobacco-related illnesses, both publicly financed insurance (such as Medicaid and Medicare in the United States) and private insurance (individual-purchased and employer-sponsored) should cover tobacco cessation programmes.

Coverage for tobacco cessation in the dental office would be beneficial because adults are more likely to visit a dentist annually for routine preventive care. Dental providers should be aware of reimbursement rates for tobacco cessation by both publicly and privately funded insurance. There is strong evidence that comprehensive, barrier-free insurance coverage would reduce smoking and smoking-related morbidity, mortality and cost.

4.8 Clinical Implications

Smoking tobacco has detrimental effects on overall health, including oral health. Smokers exhibit significantly higher rates of oral cancer, oral mucosal lesions, periodontal disease, dental caries and implant failure. Several systematic reviews and longitudinal studies provide strong evidence showing that smoking cigarettes and other tobacco products causes oral cancer, periodontal disease and implant failure [24, 37, 42]. Additionally, smoking tobacco has been linked to an increased prevalence of salivary gland hypofunction [47] and dental caries [51].

Dental practice settings provide a unique opportunity to provide tobacco cessation assistance. Free evidence-based treatment options for oral health care providers include telephone Quitlines, Quitsites, telehealth, brief educational interventions, behaviour counselling and pharmacotherapy. Research has shown that some common barriers faced by dentists include a lack of time and training. Considering the myriads of roles oral health care providers can play in tobacco cessation, more education (conferences, workshops) and research is needed to facilitate smoking cessation in dental practices.

Dental treatment involves several visits to the dental office, providing multiple 'teachable moments' for the dental team to address patient smoking. Every patient should be screened for smoking at every dental visit. Electronic health record systems should be integrated with evidence-based tobacco cessation resources, automated clinical reminders and easy referrals. The entire dental team needs to promote smoking cessation to ensure successful quit attempts.

4.9 Conclusion

Smoking tobacco products has a deleterious effect on oral health. Efforts need to be focused on reducing the prevalence of smoking. This can be accomplished in the dental office. Establishing accessible and comprehensive training, including continuing education programmes, is crucial to integrating dental health professionals into a multidisciplinary cessation approach.

References

1. American Lung Association. What's in a cigarette? 2020 [updated July 13, 2020]. Available from: https://www.lung.org/quit-smoking/smoking-facts/whats-in-a-cigarette.
2. World Health Organization. Fact sheet on ingredients in tobacco products. Geneva: WHO Press; 2015. Available from: https://www.who.int/publications/i/item/fact-sheet-on-ingredients-in-tobacco-products.
3. Gajendra S, McIntosh S, Ghosh S. Effects of tobacco product use on oral health and the role of oral healthcare providers in cessation: A narrative review. Tob Induc Dis [Internet]. 2023;21:12.
4. World Health Organization. The World Health Organization global report on trends in prevalence of tobacco use 2000–2030. Geneva: WHO Press; 2024. Available from: https://www.who.int/publications/i/item/9789240039322.
5. Arrazola RA, Husten CG, Cornelius ME, Armour BS. Notes from the field: tobacco product use among adults — United States, 2017–2023. MMWR Morb Mortal Wkly Rep. 2025;74:118–21.
6. Vulovic V. Economic costs of tobacco use. Chicago: Tobacconomics, Health Policy Center, Institute for Health Research and Policy, University of Illinois at Chicago; 2019.
7. Tobacco Free Life. History of tobacco. 2021. Available from: https://tobaccofreelife.org/tobacco/tobacco-history/.
8. Centers for Disease Control and Prevention. Burden of cigarette use in the U.S. Online: Centers for Disease Control and Prevention; 2022. Available from: https://www.cdc.gov/tobacco/campaign/tips/resources/data/cigarette-smoking-in-united-states.html#:~:text=In%202022%2C%20an%20estimated%2011.6,every%20day%20or%20some%20days.
9. Vargees C, Stroup AM, Niznik T, Dunn D, Wyatt R, Hoetger C, et al. Patterns of use, perceptions, and cardiopulmonary health risks of cigar products: a systematic review. BMC Public Health. 2023;23(1):2357.
10. Lal P. Bidi – a short history. Curr Sci. 2009;96(10):1335–7.
11. Mbulo L, Palipudi KM, Smith T, Yin S, Munish VG, Sinha DN, Gupta PC, Swasticharan L. Patterns and related factors of bidi smoking in India. Tob Prev Cessat. 2020;6:28.
12. Datta R, Singh S, Joshi A, Marwah V. Concept of BIDI years: relevance to the perioperative period. Lung India. 2022;39(4):337–42.
13. Zheng Z, Xie Z, Li D. Discussion of waterpipe tobacco smoking on reddit. Heliyon. 2022;8(9):e10635.
14. Bhargava S, Das S, Priya H, Mishra D, Shivabasappa S, Sood A, et al. The burden and correlates of waterpipe (hookah) smoking among adolescents and youth: A systematic review. Subst Use Misuse. 2024;59(1):29–40.
15. The United States Department of Health and Human Services. Smoking cessation. A report of the surgeon general. In: Department of Health and Human Services, Centers for Disease Control and Prevention, National Center for Chronic Disease Prevention and Health Promotion, editor. Atlanta: Office on Smoking and Health; 2020.
16. Huttunen R, Heikkinen T, Syrjänen J. Smoking and the outcome of infection. J Intern Med. 2011;269(3):258–69.

17. Jiang C, Chen Q, Xie M. Smoking increases the risk of infectious diseases: A narrative review. Tob Induc Dis. 2020;18:60.
18. Umnuaypornlert A, Kanchanasurakit S, Lucero-Prisno DEI, Saokaew S. Smoking and risk of negative outcomes among COVID-19 patients: a systematic review and meta-analysis. Tob Induc Dis. 2021;19(09):1.
19. Vargees C, Stroup AM, Niznik T, Dunn D, Wyatt R, Hoetger C, et al. Patterns of use, perceptions, and cardiopulmonary health risks of cigar products: a systematic review. BMC Public Health [Internet]. 2023;23(1):2357.
20. Darawshy F, Rmeileh AA, Kuint R, Berkman N. Waterpipe smoking: a review of pulmonary and health effects. Eur Respir Rev. 2020;30(160):200374.
21. Pavić I, Topalušić I, Poljičanin T, Hofmann Jaeger O, Žaja S, Stipić Marković A. Secondhand smoke exposure and its impact on pediatric lung function, aerobic fitness, and body mass: evidence from a cross-sectional study. Children (Basel). 2024;11(10):1250.
22. Carreras G, Lugo A, Gallus S, Cortini B, Fernández E, López MJ, Soriano JB, López-Nicolás A, Semple S, Gorini G, TackSHS Project Investigators. Burden of disease attributable to second-hand smoke exposure: A systematic review. Prev Med. 2019;129:105833.
23. Bray F, Laversanne M, Sung H, Ferlay J, Siegel RL, Soerjomataram I, Jemal A. Global cancer statistics 2022: GLOBOCAN estimates of incidence and mortality worldwide for 36 cancers in 185 countries. CA Cancer J Clin. 2024;74(3):229–63.
24. Chamoli A, Gosavi AS, Shirwadkar UP, Wangdale KV, Behera SK, Kurrey NK, Kalia K, Mandoli A. Overview of oral cavity squamous cell carcinoma: risk factors, mechanisms, and diagnostics. Oral Oncol. 2021;121:105451.
25. Hecht SS. Biochemistry, biology, and carcinogenicity of tobacco-specific N-nitrosamines. Chem Res Toxicol. 1998;11(6):559–603.
26. Jiang X, Wu J, Wang J, Huang R. Tobacco and oral squamous cell carcinoma: a review of carcinogenic pathways. Tob Induc Dis. 2019;17:29.
27. Sadri G, Mahjub H. Tobacco smoking and oral cancer: a meta-analysis. J Res Health Sci. 2007;7(1):18–23.
28. Mello FW, Melo G, Pasetto JJ, Silva CAB, Warnakulasuriya S, Rivero ERC. The synergistic effect of tobacco and alcohol consumption on oral squamous cell carcinoma: a systematic review and meta-analysis. Clin Oral Investig. 2019;23(7):2849–59.
29. Munshi T, Heckman CJ, Darlow S. Association between tobacco waterpipe smoking and head and neck conditions: a systematic review. J Am Dent Assoc. 2015;146(10):760–6.
30. Patil S, Awan KH, Arakeri G, Aljabab A, Ferrari M, Gomes CC, Gomez RS, Brennan PA. The relationship of "shisha" (water pipe) smoking to the risk of head and neck cancer. J Oral Pathol Med. 2019;48(4):278–83.
31. Rahman M, Sakamoto J, Fukui T. Bidi smoking and oral cancer: a meta-analysis. Int J Cancer. 2003;106(4):600–4.
32. Mariano LC, Warnakulasuriya S, Straif K, Monteiro L. Secondhand smoke exposure and oral cancer risk: a systematic review and meta-analysis. Tob Control. 2021;31:tobaccocontrol-2020-056393.
33. Mirbod SM, Ahing SI. Tobacco-associated lesions of the oral cavity: part I. Nonmalignant lesions. J Can Dent Assoc. 2000;66(5):252–6.
34. Villa A, Villa C, Abati S. Oral cancer and oral erythroplakia: an update and implication for clinicians. Aust Dent J. 2011;56(3):253–6.
35. Silverman S Jr. Oral cancer. 4th ed. Hamilton: B.C. Decker; 1998.
36. Krall EA, Garvey AJ, Garcia RI. Alveolar bone loss and tooth loss in male cigar and pipe smokers. J Am Dent Assoc (1939). 1999;130(1):57–64.
37. Leite FRM, Nascimento GG, Scheutz F, López R. Effect of smoking on periodontitis: a systematic review and meta-regression. Am J Prev Med. 2018;54(6):831–41.
38. Silva H. Tobacco use and periodontal disease—the role of microvascular dysfunction. Creative Commons Attribution (CC BY) license (https://creativecommons.org/licenses/by/40/). 2021;10:441.

39. Ye D, Gajendra S, Lawyer G, Jadeja N, Pishey D, Pathagunti S, Lyons J, Veazie P, Watson G, McIntosh S, Rahman I. Inflammatory biomarkers and growth factors in saliva and gingival crevicular fluid of e-cigarette users, cigarette smokers, and dual smokers: A pilot study. J Periodontol. 2020;91(10):1274–83.
40. Alwithanani N. Periodontal disease and smoking: systematic review. J Pharm Bioallied Sci. 2023;(Suppl 1):S64–71.
41. Souto MLS, Rovai ES, Villar CC, Braga MM, Pannuti CM. Effect of smoking cessation on tooth loss: a systematic review with meta-analysis. BMC Oral Health. 2019;19(1):245.
42. Fan YY, Li S, Cai YJ, Wei T, Ye P. Smoking in relation to early dental implant failure: a systematic review and meta-analysis. J Dent. 2024;151:105396.
43. Mustapha AD, Salame Z, Chrcanovic BR. Smoking and dental implants: a systematic review and meta-analysis. Medicina (Kaunas). 2021;58(1):39.
44. Akram Z, Javed F, Vohra F. Effect of waterpipe smoking on peri-implant health: a systematic review and meta-analysis. J Investig Clin Dent. 2019;10(3):e12403.
45. Naseri R, Yaghini J, Feizi A. Levels of smoking and dental implants failure: a systematic review and meta-analysis. J Clin Periodontol. 2020;47(4):518–28.
46. Levin L, Schwartz-Arad D. The effect of cigarette smoking on dental implants and related surgery. Implant Dent. 2005;14(4):357–61.
47. Petrušić N, Posavac M, Sabol I, Mravak-Stipetić M. The effect of tobacco smoking on salivation. Acta Stomatol Croat. 2015;49(4):309–15.
48. Grover N, Sharma J, Sengupta S, Singh S, Singh N, Kaur H. Long-term effect of tobacco on unstimulated salivary pH. J Oral Maxillofac Pathol: JOMFP. 2016;20(1):16–9.
49. Arbabi-Kalati F, Salimi S, Nabavi S, Rigi S, Miri-Moghaddam M. Effects of tobacco on salivary antioxidative and immunologic systems. Asian Pac J Cancer Prev. 2017;18(5):1215–8.
50. Wu J, Li M, Huang R. The effect of smoking on caries-related microorganisms. Tob Induc Dis. 2019;17:32.
51. Jiang X, Jiang X, Wang Y, Huang R. Correlation between tobacco smoking and dental caries: A systematic review and meta-analysis. Tob Induc Dis. 2019;17:34.
52. Centers for Disease Control and Prevention (CDC). Behavioral risk factor surveillance system survey data. Atlanta: U.S. Department of Health and Human Services, Centers for Disease Control and Prevention; 2020.
53. de Araújo Nobre M, Maló P. Prevalence of periodontitis, dental caries, and peri-implant pathology and their relation with systemic status and smoking habits: results of an open-cohort study with 22009 patients in a private rehabilitation center. J Dent. 2017;67:36–42.
54. Campus G, Cagetti MG, Senna A, Blasi G, Mascolo A, Demarchi P, et al. Does smoking increase risk for caries? A cross-sectional study in an Italian military academy. Caries Res. 2011;45(1):40–6.
55. Bernabé E, Delgado-Angulo EK, Vehkalahti MM, Aromaa A, Suominen AL. Daily smoking and 4-year caries increment in Finnish adults. Community Dent Oral Epidemiol. 2014;42(5):428–34.
56. Centers for Disease Control and Prevention. Oral health surveillance report: trends in dental caries and sealants, tooth retention, and edentulism, United States, 1999–2004 to 2011–2016. Atlanta: Centers for Disease Control and Prevention, US Department of Health and Human Services; 2019.
57. Leite FRM, Nascimento GG, Baake S, Pedersen LD, Scheutz F, López R. Impact of smoking cessation on periodontitis: a systematic review and meta-analysis of prospective longitudinal observational and interventional studies. Nicotine Tob Res. 2019;21(12):1600–8.
58. Babb S, Malarcher A, Schauer G, Asman K, Jamal A. Quitting smoking among adults — United States, 2000–2015. MMWR Morb Mortal Wkly Rep. 2019;2017(65):1457–64.
59. Bloom B, Adams PF, Cohen RA, Simile C. Smoking and oral health in dentate adults aged 18–64. NCHS Data Brief. 2012;85:1–8.
60. Chaffee BW, Urata J, Couch ET, Silverstein S. Dental professionals' engagement in tobacco, electronic cigarette, and cannabis patient counseling. JDR Clin Trans Res. 2020;5(2):133–45.

61. Binnie VI, McHugh S, Jenkins W, Borland W, Macpherson LM. A randomised controlled trial of a smoking cessation intervention delivered by dental hygienists: a feasibility study. BMC Oral Health. 2007;7:5.
62. U.S. Public Health Service (USPHS). A clinical practice guideline for treating tobacco use and dependence: 2008 update. A U.S. Public Health Service report. Am J Prev Med. 2008;35(2):158–76.
63. Dawson GM, Noller JM, Skinner JC. Models of smoking cessation brief interventions in oral health. N S W Public Health Bull. 2013;24(3):131–4.
64. Holliday R, Hong B, McColl E, Livingstone-Banks J, Preshaw PM. Interventions for tobacco cessation delivered by dental professionals. Cochrane Database Syst Rev. 2021;2(2):CD005084.
65. Hartmann-Boyce J, Livingstone-Banks J, Ordóñez-Mena JM, Fanshawe TR, Lindson N, Freeman SC, et al. Behavioural interventions for smoking cessation: an overview and network meta-analysis. Cochrane Database Syst Rev. 2021;1:CD013229.
66. Fellows JL, Bush T, McAfee T, Dickerson J. Cost effectiveness of the Oregon quitline "free patch initiative". Tob Control. 2007;16 Suppl 1(Suppl 1):i47–52.
67. Ossip-Klein DJ, McIntosh S. Quitlines in North America: evidence base and applications. Am J Med Sci. 2003;326(4):201–5.
68. Stassen LF, Hammarfjord O. Smoking cessation and the role of the dental practitioner. J Ir Dent Assoc. 2015;61(2):90–2.
69. Krist AH, Davidson KW, Mangione CM, Barry MJ, Cabana M, Caughey AB, et al. Interventions for tobacco smoking cessation in adults, including pregnant persons: US Preventive Services Task Force recommendation statement. JAMA. 2021;325(3):265–79.
70. Aubin HJ, Luquiens A, Berlin I. Pharmacotherapy for smoking cessation: pharmacological principles and clinical practice. Br J Clin Pharmacol. 2014;77(2):324–36.
71. Huecker MR, Saadabadi A. Bupropion. In: StatPearls [Internet]. Treasure Island: StatPearls Publishing; 2021. Available from: https://www.ncbi.nlm.nih.gov/books/NBK470212/.
72. Kalkhoran S, Benowitz NL, Rigotti NA. Prevention and treatment of tobacco use: JACC health promotion series. J Am Coll Cardiol. 2018;72(9):1030–45.
73. Karnieg T, Wang X. Cytisine for smoking cessation. CMAJ: Can Med Assoc J = journal de l'Association medicale canadienne. 2018;190(19):E596.
74. Jeong SH, Newcombe D, Sheridan J, Tingle M. Pharmacokinetics of cytisine, an α4 β2 nicotinic receptor partial agonist, in healthy smokers following a single dose. Drug Test Anal. 2015;7(6):475–82.
75. Lehár J, Krueger AS, Avery W, Heilbut AM, Johansen LM, Price ER, et al. Synergistic drug combinations tend to improve therapeutically relevant selectivity. Nat Biotechnol. 2009;27(7):659–66.
76. Stead LF, Perera R, Bullen C, Mant D, Lancaster T. Nicotine replacement therapy for smoking cessation. Cochrane Database Syst Rev. 2008;(1):CD000146.
77. Ebbert JO, Hays JT, Hurt RD. Combination pharmacotherapy for stopping smoking: what advantages does it offer? Drugs. 2010;70(6):643–50.
78. Carlson S, Widome R, Fabian L, Luo X, Forster J. Barriers to quitting smoking among young adults: the role of socioeconomic status. Am J Health Promot. 2018;32(2):294–300.
79. Carr AB, Ebbert JO. Interventions for tobacco cessation in the dental setting. Cochrane Database Syst Rev. 2006;(1):CD005084.
80. Goel D, Chaudhary PK, Khan A, Patthi B, Singla A, Malhi R, et al. Acquaintance and approach in the direction of tobacco cessation among dental practitioners-a systematic review. Int J Prev Med. 2020;11:167.
81. Edwards D, Freeman T, Roche AM. Dentists' and dental hygienists' role in smoking cessation: an examination and comparison of current practice and barriers to service provision. Health Promot J Austr. 2006;17(2):145–51.

82. World Health Organization. WHO framework convention on tobacco control (WHO FCTC). Online; 2003.
83. World Health Organization. WHO report on the global tobacco epidemic. Protect people from tobacco epidemic. Geneva: WHO Press; 2023. Available from: https://iris.who.int/bitstream/handle/10665/372043/9789240077164-eng.pdf?sequence=1.

Electronic Cigarette Use (Vaping) and Oral Health

5

Elis Ângela Batistella and Saman Warnakulasuriya

5.1 Introduction

Electronic nicotine delivery systems, commonly known as e-cigarettes or vaping devices, have rapidly gained popularity as they are marketed as safer alternatives to tobacco smoking and aids for smoking cessation [1]. Despite claims of reduced harm compared to combustible cigarettes, the long-term adverse health effects of e-cigarette use remain largely unknown. While research on the cardiovascular and respiratory impacts of vaping has garnered attention, one area that is often overlooked is its effect on oral health.

Oral health is an integral component of overall well-being, with conditions such as periodontal disease, dental caries and oral cancer affecting the quality of life and serving as indicators of systemic health problems. The use of tobacco, in all its forms, has been widely documented as a significant risk factor for various oral diseases, with traditional smoking being a major contributor to periodontal disease, tooth loss and oral cancer [2]. e-Cigarettes, which deliver nicotine and other chemicals via an aerosolised vapour, have been assumed to pose a lesser threat to oral health compared to traditional cigarettes. However, growing evidence suggests that vaping may also have adverse effects on the oral cavity, though the exact nature and extent of these effects remain unclear [3].

This chapter examines the impact of e-cigarette use on oral health, focusing on its effects on oral tissues, including the periodontium, dentition and oral mucosa. It explores the composition and delivery mechanisms of e-cigarettes, analysing how substances such as nicotine, propylene glycol (PG) and flavouring agents may

E. Â. Batistella (✉)
College of Dentistry, University of Saskatchewan, Saskatoon, SK, Canada

S. Warnakulasuriya
Faculty of Dentistry, Oral and Craniofacial Sciences, King's College London, and WHO Collaborating Centre for Oral Cancer, London, UK
e-mail: s.warne@kcl.ac.uk

S. R. Prabhu et al. (eds.), *Lifestyle in Oral Health and Disease*,
https://doi.org/10.1007/978-3-032-05888-1_5

contribute to oral health issues. Additionally, we summarise the evidence from clinical and laboratory studies investigating the oral health consequences of vaping. Yet, there remains a gap in formal guidelines and education surrounding the oral health implications of vaping. We conclude with recommendations for dental practitioners and public health policymakers, emphasising the need for increased awareness and research in this emerging field.

5.2 The Rise of e-Cigarettes: An Overview

e-Cigarettes first entered the market in their modern form in China in 2003 and were later introduced to Europe and the United States of America (USA) as a safer alternative to traditional tobacco smoking. By vaporising a nicotine solution, they mimicked the sensation of smoking without combustion's harmful byproducts. Initially marketed as smoking cessation tools, e-cigarettes gained global popularity, especially with the introduction of customisable nicotine levels and a variety of appealing flavours.

In the USA, over 3 million high school students used e-cigarettes in 2020 [4], a sharp increase from previous years. This trend extended globally, with significant uptake among young people drawn to discreet, flavourful devices. High nicotine concentrations, combined with enticing flavours, raised concerns about addiction, with many young users viewing e-cigarettes as a safer alternative to smoking, potentially leading to long-term nicotine dependence.

5.3 The Public Health Debate

e-Cigarettes have sparked an ongoing public health debate. As e-cigarette use grew, regulatory bodies worldwide began addressing public health concerns. In the USA, the Food and Drug Administration (FDA) started regulating e-cigarettes as tobacco products in 2009, finalising rules for premarket review and advertising restrictions in 2016. However, multiple e-cigarette brands with smart vape features are currently illegally marketed in the USA without U.S. FDA authorisation [5].

Countries have adopted varied approaches—India, Australia and Brazil have banned e-cigarettes due to their addictive potential and concerns about lung health, while the United Kingdom (UK) and New Zealand see them as tools for harm reduction in smoking cessation. In the USA, since the introduction of e-cigarettes, both nicotine-containing electronic cigarettes and cannabis-containing electronic cigarettes have seen a rapid rise in popularity [6].

Despite the ban in some countries, authorities struggle to regulate the use of e-cigarettes, in particular, due to the black market. Consequently, e-cigarettes have gradually entered the market through various forms of marketing strategies to consumers, and can be easily accessible to younger populations, such as children and adolescents.

5.4 Youth as a Target

The appeal to young users poses significant health challenges due to e-cigarettes' composition, which often includes flavouring agents and nicotine, sold in devices with sophisticated, modern designs. New 'smart' vapes present additional challenges, as they have digital displays and can include animations that display when puffing, built-in games, reward systems for vaping such as points and rankings, touchscreens, photo wallpapers and Bluetooth connectivity and are sold at a price similar to e-cigarettes [5].

Adolescents consider e-cigarettes as high-tech, accessible and convenient, especially in places where smoking cigarettes is not allowed. A recent study with young vapers revealed that the most commonly reported reason for vaping was a perception that vaping is safer than traditional smoking. In contrast, the participants' perceptions of vaping-related oral health risks were relatively low [7].

Increasingly, robust marketing and advertising to the public utilise celebrities and appealing flavours (e.g. chocolate, strawberry, cotton candy, and bubble gum) to make e-cigarettes especially attractive and appealing to children and adolescents. Much of the marketing for vaping has been promoted through the Internet and social media outlets such as YouTube [8]. A study analysed the extent to which synthetic nicotine e-cigarette brands have implemented FDA health warning requirements and evaluated the association between health warnings and user engagement on Instagram. Overall, 87% of sampled posts did not adhere to FDA health warning requirements in tobacco promotions [9]. The authors also observed that posts with health warnings and a larger warning size received less user engagement. Health warnings may lessen user engagement, which could deter youth uptake and use of synthetic nicotine products.

Concern is raised when national surveys conducted in Canada [2] and the USA [4] reveal that young non-smokers are becoming dependent on vaping. The Canadian Student Tobacco, Alcohol, and Drugs Survey conducted between 2020 and 2022 revealed that 17% of students in grades 7–12 reported using a vaping product (referred to as an e-cigarette in the survey) within the last 30 days. Over half of students in grades 7 to 12 (59%) thought it would be "fairly easy" or "very easy" to get a cigarette if they wanted one. Among students who used cannabis, 54% reported vaping liquid cannabis and 34% reported vaping dried cannabis in the past 12 months [2].

5.5 The 'Smoking-Cessation Tool' Marketing

The manufacturers and supporters argue that e-cigarettes are a less harmful alternative to smoking and may aid in quitting smoking traditional cigarettes. Public Health England has noted their potential for harm reduction but cautions against the unknown long-term effects of vaping. Critics, however, focus on the risks of nicotine addiction in adolescents and the potential health impacts on oral health, lung function and cardiovascular health.

Studies suggest e-cigarettes can help smokers reduce the habit of smoking [10]. However, among smokers who have attempted to stop without professional support, those who use e-cigarettes are more likely to report continued abstinence than those who used a licensed nicotine replacement therapy product bought over the counter or no aid to cessation. This difference persists after adjusting for a range of smoker characteristics, such as nicotine dependence [10].

Among smokers in the USA who used e-cigarettes to help quit, 12.9% successfully attained long-term abstinence. However, there was no difference compared with matched non-e-cigarette users. Furthermore, fewer e-cigarette users were abstinent from nicotine products in the long term, and approximately two-thirds of e-cigarette users who successfully quit smoking continued to use e-cigarettes. These results suggest e-cigarettes may not be an effective cessation aid for adult smokers and, instead, may contribute to continuing nicotine dependence [11, 12].

It remains uncertain whether the rise of e-cigarette technology will lead individuals to switch entirely from combustible products to exclusive e-cigarette use, or if dual usage of both will continue [13].

5.6 Composition and Mechanism of e-Cigarettes

Understanding the composition of e-cigarettes and the mechanism of use is essential for evaluating their health impacts, including oral health. Key components of e-cigarettes (Fig. 5.1) include the following:

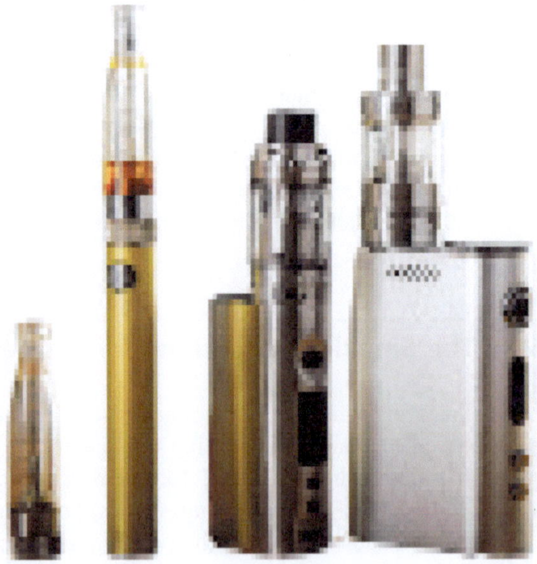

Fig. 5.1 Examples of e-cigarette systems

Mouthpiece and Tank/Cartridge: The mouthpiece allows the user to inhale the vapour, while the tank or cartridge holds the e-liquid, which may be transparent for easy monitoring.

Atomiser (Heating Element): The atomiser contains a coil, typically made from stainless steel or nickel, and a wick that vaporises the e-liquid. The operating temperature of the coil is essential, as high temperatures can create harmful chemicals, while low temperatures may lead to poor vapour quality.

e-Liquid (Vape Juice): e-Liquids may contain:

- *Nicotine*: The addictive component, available in varying concentrations. Nicotine salts allow for smoother, higher doses. Vapes can contain higher levels of nicotine than cigarettes. A disposable vape with 20 mg/mL of nicotine and 2 mL of e-liquid contains 40 mg of nicotine, which is equivalent to about 20–40 cigarettes, hence its highly addictive potential.
- *Propylene Glycol (PG)*: A colourless, odourless liquid that provides the throat akin to smoking. PG may irritate the oral and respiratory systems.
- *Vegetable Glycerin (VG)*: A thicker, sweeter liquid that produces larger vapour clouds but may contribute to residue build-up in the mouth.
- *Flavourings*: Flavours enhance the vaping experience, but certain chemicals like diacetyl have been linked to lung damage. Like menthol and other additives incorporated to smoked tobacco products by the tobacco industry to make it especially attractive to youth [14], flavourings are used to make e-cigarettes more appealing. Flavourings can be used to create a product identity and increase social acceptance when aromatic vapours are released, reducing the impact of the vapour to non-smokers. Some flavours (e.g. mint) may produce the sensation of freshness and cleanliness. In contrast, aromatic flavours (e.g. vanilla, almond, green apple) can give a pseudo sense that the product is healthy since it lacks the traditional tobacco smoke. The flavouring's sweetening effect encourages more frequent vaping, increasing exposure to potentially harmful substances.
- *Battery*: A rechargeable lithium-ion battery powers the device, providing energy to heat the liquid and produce vapour.

  e-Cigarettes are activated by inhalation or pressing a button, which triggers the device, sending power from the battery to the atomiser. Then, the atomiser heats the coil, vaporising the e-liquid into an aerosol. The vapour is inhaled through the mouthpiece, mimicking smoking. Formaldehyde and acrolein are toxic compounds that can be formed when e-liquids are overheated, which can irritate the respiratory and the lining mucosa of the oral cavity and pharynx. Aldehydes and volatile organic compounds can irritate and pose long-term oral and respiratory health risks. Trace metals such as nickel, chromium, and lead can leach from the heating elements, posing significant toxicity risks. Other products, such as tetrahydrocannabinol, dry herbs, and oily compounds, can also be vaporised by vapers, which may cause lung problems.

5.7 The Impact of Vaping on Oral Health

The rising popularity of e-cigarettes has raised significant concerns regarding their potential impact on oral health. Evidence suggests that vaping can negatively affect oral health.

Direct Effects of e-Cigarette Vapours on Oral Tissues: While e-cigarettes lack harmful combustion byproducts like tar and carbon monoxide, the vaporised chemicals can still interact with oral tissues, damaging dental and gingival tissues. Nicotine constricts blood vessels, which reduces blood flow to the gingiva. This impaired circulation can hinder tissue healing, making the gingiva more susceptible to infections and inflammation. The lowered bleeding on probing index found on some vapers as compared to non-vapers highlights the potential of e-cigarette use to alter oral tissue biology [15, 16]. Nicotine reduces saliva production, which is crucial for neutralising acids and maintaining oral health. This decrease can disrupt the oral microbiome, increasing the risk of periodontal disease and dental caries. Nicotine also affects blood vessels, impairing tissue repair. A study found that e-cigarettes may significantly hinder oral wound healing by affecting epithelial keratinisation and altering the oral microbiome. As a result, vaping is not safe for patients undergoing oral surgery [17].

Some flavouring chemicals, such as diacetyl (used for buttery flavours), have been associated with respiratory damage when inhaled in large quantities [18]. Although diacetyl is banned in many e-liquids, other flavouring agents may irritate oral tissues, leading to mouth sores, inflammation and an environment conducive to bacterial growth and plaque accumulation. While studying the effect of flavouring agents on dental surfaces, researchers observed a fourfold increase in microbial adhesion to enamel, a twofold increase in biofilm formation and a 27% reduction in enamel hardness. Flavouring agents can also pose risks to oral health as toxic substances can be released from flavour compounds when heating e-liquids [14, 19].

5.8 Oral Diseases/Disorders Related to the Use of e-Cigarettes: Evidence from Clinical Studies

This section summarises key clinical studies on the direct impact of vaping on oral health, with a focus on xerostomia, dental caries, periodontal disease, oral ulcers and oral cancer.

Xerostomia (Dry Mouth): Xerostomia is a common complaint among e-cigarette users. The use of e-cigarettes might lead to xerostomia by the action of PG and VG (which are hygroscopic), together with an increase in biofilm volume and a reduced salivary flow [10, 20]. Nicotine suppresses saliva production, while PG's moisture-absorbing properties exacerbate this condition. Saliva is essential in maintaining oral health by neutralising acids, washing away food particles and providing antimicrobial benefits. Reduced saliva flow increases the risk of harmful bacterial growth, dental caries, halitosis and oral infections, such as oral candidiasis (thrush). In severe cases, chronic dry mouth can cause difficulty in speaking, swallowing, and eating.

A study conducted in 2021 comparing the effects of e-cigarettes, cannabis and combustible tobacco found that e-cigarette users experienced a higher incidence of dry mouth than non-smokers, though less than traditional smokers [21]. PG was linked to increased dryness. Another study conducted in 2023 found that the prevalence of xerostomia among e-cigarette users was higher than in combustible tobacco users [22]. Chronic dry mouth can lead to various oral issue and contribute to overall oral discomfort.

Dental Caries: Dental caries is caused by the demineralisation of dental enamel and dentin due to acids produced by bacteria. Factors such as the composition of e-liquids and aerosols play a significant role in the development of dental caries. The high sugar content in many flavoured e-liquids can provide a food source for cariogenic bacteria. Specifically, cariogenic sugars such as sucrose, fructose and glucose, as well as aldehydes and sugary flavours like menthol, cinnamon and strawberry in e-liquids, may contribute to tooth decay. These substances are harmful to commensal (beneficial) oral bacteria, such as *Streptococcus gordonii*, *Streptococcus mitis*, *Streptococcus intermedius* and *Streptococcus oralis*, while encouraging the growth of cariogenic pathogens like *Streptococcus mutans*, which is responsible for dental caries [23].

The thicker consistency of vegetable glycerin can also contribute to plaque buildup, which increases the risk of dental caries and periodontal disease when combined with the sugar-like residue left in the mouth. Chemicals in e-liquids, including nicotine and flavouring agents, may negatively affect dentition, increasing the risk of developing dental caries [24]. e-Cigarettes can also alter saliva factors that are responsible for maintaining oral health and caries control [25]. The maintenance of oral environment pH is related to both the buffering activity of saliva and the constant salivary flow, which enables buffering of acids produced by oral bacteria that cause dental caries, or acids present in food and beverages [26].

e-Liquids often contain flavourings and sweeteners, which may increase the risk of dental caries and dysbiosis. Research on the mechanistic effects of e-liquids on biofilm formation and the growth of oral commensal streptococcal communities found that flavouring agents inhibit the growth of oral streptococci in a bactericidal mode [27]. Thus, flavoured, rather than unflavoured, e-liquids may be more contributory to biofilm formation and the growth of oral commensal bacteria, creating a favourable environment for cariogenic bacteria.

In 2024, Khattak et al. [7] conducted a study involving 142 young users of e-cigarettes. The researchers conducted intraoral examinations to assess the Decayed, Missing and Filled Teeth (DMFT) index and other relevant indices. Around 66% reported daily Electronic Cigarette (ECs) use, with 80.3% initiating vaping before the age of 18 years. The mean DMFT was 5.66 (standard deviation [SD] = 2.20). DMFT scores were notably lower among non-daily vapers (mean = 4.2; SD = 1.76) than those vaping over 19 times daily (mean = 8.2; SD = 0.95). Participants who started vaping ≤12 months ago had a lower DMFT (mean = 3.2; SD = 0.94) compared to those vaping for over 2 years (mean = 8.2; SD = 1.08). Although most participants (76.1%) reported brushing daily, poor oral hygiene (29.6%) and severe dental staining were prevalent.

Periodontal Disease: Periodontal disease, which includes gingivitis and periodontitis, is a well-known consequence of smoking [28]. Recent studies have begun to investigate whether e-cigarette use poses similar risks to periodontal health. While some studies have reported no significant association between e-cigarette smoking and periodontal disease [16, 29], others have found that the clinical attachment loss of recruited vaping participants after six months was significantly worse in the e-cigarette smokers' group [30]. Additionally, oral microbiome dysbiosis has been observed among cigarette smokers and smokeless tobacco users compared to non-users. Dysbiosis refers to an imbalance in bacterial composition, changes in bacterial metabolic activities, or a shift in bacterial distribution [31].

In a study involving young vapers, gingival bleeding and plaque accumulation were observed in 47.2% and 35.3%, respectively [7]. Significant changes have been identified in the oral microbiome of e-cigarette smokers that are in line with those seen in cigarette smokers and patients with periodontal disease [32, 33]. Another study suggested that e-cigarette use may promote an inflammatory environment that supports the development and progression of periodontal disease, similar to the effects of traditional smoking [15].

Oral Ulcers: The occurrence of oral ulcers in e-cigarette users has also been reported in the literature [34, 35]. Kotha et al. described a case series of young adults with the chief complaint of ulcers on the oral mucosa. All patients were regular or social vapers. This observation prompts further exploration into vaping as a potential aetiological factor for recurrent aphthous stomatitis, a common form of oral ulcers [34]. Another report described a case of a patient with a severe, necrotic-looking oral ulcer on the hard palate attributed to the use of e-cigarettes [35]. The aetiological mechanism behind these findings is the aim of further investigation.

Oral Cancer: Even though e-cigarettes do not produce tar or carbon monoxide like traditional cigarettes, they contain chemicals such as formaldehyde, acetaldehyde and acrolein, all classified as carcinogens by the International Agency for Research on Cancer [36]. While the concentration of these chemicals is lower than in traditional cigarette smoke, chronic exposure may still pose a risk for oral cancers.

Oral cancer has already been diagnosed in e-cigarette users [37], but an association between both remains to be established. Several toxic substances are found in e-cigarettes [38]. Nicotine, for instance, has been shown to mediate cell proliferation and tumour progression in smoking-related cancers [39], and certain flavouring chemicals (e.g. diacetyl) have been linked to respiratory diseases [18].

Studies comparing e-cigarette aerosol to tobacco smoke have reported that e-cigarettes emit toxic carbonyl compounds generated from thermal decomposition. These substances can have adverse health effects despite their levels being lower than those in tobacco cigarette smoke [40]. However, considerable levels of potential carcinogens, including toxic metals (cadmium, chromium, copper, lead, manganese and nickel), several organic compounds including carbonyls (e.g. acrolein from glycerol/glycerin) and potentially harmful compounds such as silicate beads, tin and flavourings as well as propylene oxide (from propylene glycol) and lipid-like compounds that are not present in traditional tobacco cigarettes can be found in these vaping aerosols [41–45]. Despite the theoretical risk, there is currently limited direct evidence linking e-cigarette use to oral cancer. Still, e-cigarette use is far from harmless [46] and presents several oral health risks, primarily due to the chemicals in e-liquids and their long-term exposure [46]. Thus, e-cigarette vaping carries significant risks and should not be encouraged.

A recent study [47] reported the effects of vaping versus smoking on the oral cell methylome of healthy young vapers and smokers relative to non-users. The Keck School of Medicine research at the University of Southern California focused on DNA methylation. This biochemical modification regulates gene expression and can contribute to disease when disrupted [47]. The authors examined the DNA methylation patterns in young adults who vape and found chemical alterations in their DNA similar to those observed in smokers. These changes, which are associated with cancer development, raise significant concerns regarding the health risks of e-cigarette use [47].

Notably, changes in the hypermethylated in cancer 1 (HIC1) gene, a well-known tumour suppressor gene, indicate a potential cancer risk from vaping. Unique methylation patterns in vapers suggest distinct chemical exposures from e-cigarettes [47]. The findings emphasise the need for further research, public health interventions and stricter vaping regulations to protect vulnerable populations, especially young people.

Braillon and Lang have suggested that the International Agency for Research on Cancer should evaluate the carcinogenic risk of e-cigarettes based on the currently available evidence from animal, in vitro and human studies [48]. Further research is needed to determine the potential cancer risks of vaping. Long-term studies on the oral cancer risk among vapers would help evaluate the potential harm to humans.

5.9 The Lung Effects of e-Cigarette Use

Our current knowledge of the harmful effects of vaping on humans is primarily based on its toxic effects on pulmonary tissues. e-Cigarette-induced lung adenocarcinoma and bladder urethral hyperplasia have been reported in a study conducted by Tang et al. involving mice [49]. Cancer risk and main oncogenic molecular mechanisms triggered by e-cigarettes have been evaluated by Vivarelli et al. These included epithelial–mesenchymal transition (EMT), redox stress/mitochondrial toxicity and DNA breaks/fragmentation potentially involved in cancer risk associated with e-cigarette use [50].

Vape pens, like e-cigarettes, aerosolise substances but typically contain tetrahydrocannabinol (THC) oil or concentrates instead of nicotine. Unlike nicotine-based products, THC extracts are mixed with oils, terpenes and tocopheryl acetate rather than propylene glycol or glycerol due to its hydrophobicity. While FDA-approved for oral use, these substances may pose risks when inhaled. Lipids in aerosols have been linked to severe respiratory effects. Potentially hazardous additives and contaminants, including the industrial chemical tributyl phosphine oxide and caffeine, have been detected in vaping products [38].

In 2021, an American Thoracic Society (ATS) workshop [51] was convened to identify and prioritise research and regulatory needs in response to the e-cigarette or vaping product use associated with lung injury outbreaks and to prevent similar instances of disease related to e-cigarette or vaping product use. e-Cigarette and vaping product use-associated lung injury (EVALI) has affected over 2700 individuals in the USA, causing 27 deaths [51]. Inhaling aerosolised compounds has been linked to respiratory conditions such as bronchitis, lipoid pneumonia and pneumonitis [39]. Cases of hypersensitivity pneumonitis and acute respiratory distress syndrome have also been reported [52]. A review of 38 studies found that cinnamon, strawberry and menthol flavours caused significant inflammatory and cytotoxic effects. While diacetyl and cinnamaldehyde are known to be harmful, the safety of other flavouring agents remains uncertain, emphasising the need for further research [18].

5.10 Oral Health Management and Recommendations

As vaping rises, it is increasingly important to address its potential risks to oral health. Despite being marketed as a safer alternative to smoking, e-cigarettes can negatively impact the periodontium, dentition and oral tissues. Regular dental check-ups are essential for detecting early signs of issues such as periodontal disease, dry mouth and dental caries. Dental professionals should inquire about vaping habits, including the frequency, type of e-liquids and duration of use, as this information helps assess individual risks and provide tailored advice for oral health maintenance.

Dry mouth is a common concern that increases the risk of dental caries and periodontal disease. Thus, oral health professionals can recommend frequent hydration and the use of saliva substitutes. Furthermore, users should be cautious when choosing e-liquids, as some flavourings and sweeteners can promote bacterial growth, leading to plaque accumulation, cavities, and periodontal issues. Thus, to reduce these risks, vapers should refrain from using sweetened flavours and oily e-liquids that contain harmful chemicals.

Those using e-cigarettes for smoking cessation should be encouraged to quit both habits. A step-down approach to nicotine use can be recommended to gradually reduce dependence, in addition to other measures, such as behavioural counselling and nicotine replacement therapy. There is a current need for developing interactive web-based educational programmes for oral health professionals on the health risks of vaping, similar to programmes available on smoking cessation [53].

On a broader scale, public health campaigns should continue to educate the public about the risks associated with e-cigarette use. Health professionals, particularly dentists and oral hygienists, must be equipped with the knowledge to counsel patients on the oral health implications of vaping. Collaboration among public health authorities, dental professionals and policymakers is crucial for providing users with the necessary information and support to make informed decisions about their oral and overall health. Public health efforts should focus on smoking cessation, raising awareness of vaping's possible oral health risks and preventing tobacco and e-cigarette use altogether. Further research is needed to understand vaping's long-term oral health effects and develop prevention strategies.

5.11 Conclusion

This chapter explores the rise in e-cigarette use and its effects on oral health. While some consider e-cigarettes as less harmful than traditional smoking, they still pose several risks. Key oral health concerns include periodontal disease, xerostomia and dental caries, with the potential for oral carcinogenesis still being investigated. These issues arise from nicotine's impact on blood flow, the dehydrating effects of propylene glycol, and the bacterial growth fostered by certain e-liquid flavourings and the potentially harmful chemicals that contact the oral mucosa. Some other harmful components are yet to be identified. We also encourage dental professionals not to advocate e-cigarette use as a means of smoking cessation.

The lack of long-term data limits the available evidence on the oral health effects of e-cigarettes. Future research should aim to understand the prolonged impact of vaping, focusing on e-liquid ingredients like flavouring sweeteners and cannabis oil and examining the impact on vulnerable groups such as adolescents and pregnant and lactating women. Public health strategies should focus on educating e-cigarette users about the oral health risks associated with vaping and encourage preventive care, such as regular dental visits, staying hydrated, maintaining proper oral hygiene and supporting alternative safe smoking cessation efforts.

Conflict of Interest Statement The authors have no conflict of interest to declare.

Declarations. Competing Interests The authors declare no competing interests.

Sources of Funding None.

References

1. Isik Andrikopoulos G, Farsalinos K, Poulas K. Electronic Nicotine Delivery Systems (ENDS) and their relevance in oral health. Toxics. 2019;7(4):61. https://doi.org/10.3390/toxics7040061.
2. Health Canada. Summary of results for the Canadian Student Tobacco, Alcohol and Drugs Survey 2021–22. 2025. https://www.canada.ca/en/health-canada/services/canadian-student-tobacco-alcohol-drugs-survey/2021-2022-summary.html. Accessed 16 Jan 2025.
3. Glantz SA, Nguyen N, Oliveira da Silva AL. Population-based disease odds for e-cigarettes and dual use versus cigarettes. NEJM Evidence. 2024;3(3) https://doi.org/10.1056/EVIDoa2300229.
4. Wang TW, Neff LJ, Park-Lee E, Ren C, Cullen KA, King BA. E-cigarette use among middle and high school students – United States, 2020. MMWR Morb Mortal Wkly Rep. 2020;69(37):1310–2. https://doi.org/10.15585/mmwr.mm6937e1.
5. Marynak K, Crane E, VanFrank B. Vaping. JAMA. 2025;333(6):536. https://doi.org/10.1001/jama.2024.25255.
6. Frohe T, Leeman RF, Patock-Peckham J, Ecker A, Kraus S, Foster DW. Correlates of cannabis vape-pen use and knowledge among U.S. college students. Addictive Behaviors Reports. 2018;7:32–9. https://doi.org/10.1016/j.abrep.2017.11.004.
7. Khattak O, Chaudhary FA, Sakoor A, et al. Oral health status, self-perceptions, and risk awareness among young adult users of electronic cigarettes in Pakistan. Tob Induc Dis. 2024;22(November):1–12. https://doi.org/10.18332/tid/194963.
8. Paek HJ, Kim S, Hove T, Huh JY. Reduced harm or another gateway to smoking? Source, message, and information characteristics of e-cigarette videos on YouTube. J Health Commun. 2014;19(5):545–60. https://doi.org/10.1080/10810730.2013.821560.
9. Wu J, Trifiro BM, Ranker LR, et al. Health warnings on Instagram advertisements for synthetic nicotine e-cigarettes and engagement. JAMA Netw Open. 2024;7(9):e2434434. https://doi.org/10.1001/jamanetworkopen.2024.34434.
10. Holliday R, Chaffee BW, Jakubovics NS, Kist R, Preshaw PM. Electronic cigarettes and oral health. J Dent Res. 2021;100(9):906–13. https://doi.org/10.1177/00220345211002116.
11. Friesen R, McGaw T, Peters E, Lai H. A retrospective analysis of referral patterns to a university oral medicine clinic. Oral Surg Oral Med Oral Pathol Oral Radiol. 2019;128(4):381–5. https://doi.org/10.1016/j.oooo.2019.04.007.
12. Chen R, Pierce JP, Leas EC, et al. Use of electronic cigarettes to aid long-term smoking cessation in the united states: prospective evidence from the PATH Cohort Study. Am J Epidemiol. 2020;189(12):1529–37. https://doi.org/10.1093/aje/kwaa161.
13. Brown J, Beard E, Kotz D, Michie S, West R. Real-world effectiveness of e-cigarettes when used to aid smoking cessation: a cross-sectional population study. Addiction. 2014;109(9):1531–40. https://doi.org/10.1111/add.12623.
14. Ebersole J, Samburova V, Son Y, et al. Harmful chemicals emitted from electronic cigarettes and potential deleterious effects in the oral cavity. Tob Induc Dis. 2020:18(May). https://doi.org/10.18332/tid/116988.
15. Fathi A, Salehi S, Sadeghi S, Atash R, Monirifard R, Farahmand S. Electronic cigarettes and peri-implantitis: an umbrella review. J Oral Implantol. 2024;50(6):653–8. https://doi.org/10.1563/aaid-joi-D-24-00157.
16. Shabil M, Khatib MN, Ballal S, et al. The impact of electronic cigarette use on periodontitis and periodontal outcomes: a systematic review and meta-analysis. BMC Oral Health. 2024;24(1):1197. https://doi.org/10.1186/s12903-024-05018-7.
17. Majid OW. Preliminary evidence of impaired oral wound healing in e-cigarette users: a call for perioperative vaping cessation. Evid Based Dent. 2024;25(2):63–4. https://doi.org/10.1038/s41432-024-00982-z.
18. Effah F, Taiwo B, Baines D, Bailey A, Marczylo T. Pulmonary effects of e-liquid flavors: a systematic review. J Toxicol Environ Health Part B. 2022;25(7):343–71. https://doi.org/10.1080/10937404.2022.2124563.

19. Irusa KF, Vence B, Donovan T. Potential oral health effects of e-cigarettes and vaping: a review and case reports. J Esthetic Restor Dent. 2020;32(3):260–4. https://doi.org/10.1111/jerd.12583.
20. Ferrazzo KL, Ortigara GB, Bonzanini LIL. Harmful effects of electronic cigarette on oral soft tissues mediated by dysbiosis: State of the art. Oral Dis. 2024;30(4):2719–21. https://doi.org/10.1111/odi.14735.
21. Chaffee BW, Halpern-Felsher B, Cheng J. E-cigarette, cannabis and combustible tobacco use: associations with xerostomia among California adolescents. Community Dent Oral Epidemiol. 2023;51(2):180–6. https://doi.org/10.1111/cdoe.12721.
22. Guo X, Hou L, Peng X, Tang F. The prevalence of xerostomia among e-cigarette or combustible tobacco users: a systematic review and meta-analysis. Tob Induc Dis. 2023;21(February):1–11. https://doi.org/10.18332/tid/156676.
23. Gaur S, Agnihotri R. The role of electronic cigarettes in dental caries: a scoping review. Scientifica (Cairo). 2023;2023:1–9. https://doi.org/10.1155/2023/9980011.
24. Irusa KF, Finkelman M, Magnuson B, Donovan T, Eisen SE. A comparison of the caries risk between patients who use vapes or electronic cigarettes and those who do not. J Am Dent Assoc. 2022;153(12):1179–83. https://doi.org/10.1016/j.adaj.2022.09.013.
25. Hasan NWM, Baharin B, Mohd N, Rahman MA, Hassan N. Comparative effects of e-cigarette smoking on periodontal status, salivary pH, and cotinine levels. BMC Oral Health. 2024;24(1):861. https://doi.org/10.1186/s12903-024-04650-7.
26. Baliga S, Muglikar S, Kale R. Salivary pH: a diagnostic biomarker. J Indian Soc Periodontol. 2013;17(4):461. https://doi.org/10.4103/0972-124X.118317.
27. Xu CP, Palazzolo DL, Cuadra GA. Mechanistic effects of e-liquids on biofilm formation and growth of oral commensal streptococcal communities: effect of flavoring agents. Dent J (Basel). 2022;10(5):85. https://doi.org/10.3390/dj10050085.
28. Warnakulasuriya S, Dietrich T, Bornstein M. Oral health risks of tobacco use and effects of cessation. Int Dent J. 2010;60(1):7–30.
29. Thiem DGE, Donkiewicz P, Rejaey R, et al. The impact of electronic and conventional cigarettes on periodontal health – a systematic review and meta-analysis. Clin Oral Investig. 2023;27(9):4911–28. https://doi.org/10.1007/s00784-023-05162-4.
30. Xu F, Aboseria E, Janal MN, et al. Comparative effects of e-cigarette aerosol on periodontium of periodontitis patient. Front Oral Health. 2021:2. https://doi.org/10.3389/froh.2021.729144.
31. Chattopadhyay S, Malayil L, Chopyk J, et al. Oral microbiome dysbiosis among cigarette smokers and smokeless tobacco users compared to non-users. Sci Rep. 2024;14(1):10394. https://doi.org/10.1038/s41598-024-60730-2.
32. Xu F, Pushalkar S, Lin Z, et al. Electronic cigarette use enriches periodontal pathogens. Mol Oral Microbiol. 2022;37(2):63–76. https://doi.org/10.1111/omi.12361.
33. Chopyk J, Bojanowski CM, Shin J, et al. Compositional differences in the oral microbiome of e-cigarette users. Front Microbiol. 2021:12. https://doi.org/10.3389/fmicb.2021.599664.
34. Kotha A, Mandapati SR, Rudraraju H. Potential association between vaping and recurrent Aphthous stomatitis: a case series. Cureus. 2024;26 https://doi.org/10.7759/cureus.70238.
35. Cant A, Collard B, Cunliffe D. Electronic cigarettes: necrotic ulcer. Br Dent J. 2017;222(4):226. https://doi.org/10.1038/sj.bdj.2017.150.
36. IARC Working Group. IARC Working Group on the Evaluation of carcinogenic risks to humans. personal habits and indoor combustions, vol. 100. IARC Monogr Eval Carcinog Risks Hum; 2012.
37. Klawinski D, Hanna I, Breslin NK, Katzenstein HM, Indelicato DJ. Vaping the venom: oral cavity cancer in a young adult with extensive electronic cigarette use. Pediatrics. 2021;147(5) https://doi.org/10.1542/peds.2020-022301.
38. Tehrani MW, Newmeyer MN, Rule AM, Prasse C. Characterizing the chemical landscape in commercial e-cigarette liquids and aerosols by liquid chromatography–high-resolution mass spectrometry. Chem Res Toxicol. 2021;34(10):2216–26. https://doi.org/10.1021/acs.chemrestox.1c00253.

39. Schaal C, Chellappan SP. Nicotine-mediated cell proliferation and tumor progression in smoking-related cancers. Mol Cancer Res. 2014;12(1):14–23. https://doi.org/10.1158/1541-7786.MCR-13-0541.
40. Bekki K, Uchiyama S, Ohta K, Inaba Y, Nakagome H, Kunugita N. Carbonyl compounds generated from electronic cigarettes. Int J Environ Res Public Health. 2014;11(11):11192–200. https://doi.org/10.3390/ijerph111111192.
41. Williams M, Villarreal A, Bozhilov K, Lin S, Talbot P. Metal and silicate particles including nanoparticles are present in electronic cigarette cartomizer fluid and aerosol. PLoS One. 2013;8(3):e57987. https://doi.org/10.1371/journal.pone.0057987.
42. Kamilari E, Farsalinos K, Poulas K, Kontoyannis CG, Orkoula MG. Detection and quantitative determination of heavy metals in electronic cigarette refill liquids using Total Reflection X-ray Fluorescence Spectrometry. Food Chem Toxicol. 2018;116:233–7. https://doi.org/10.1016/j.fct.2018.04.035.
43. Hess CA, Olmedo P, Navas-Acien A, Goessler W, Cohen JE, Rule AM. E-cigarettes as a source of toxic and potentially carcinogenic metals. Environ Res. 2017;152:221–5. https://doi.org/10.1016/j.envres.2016.09.026.
44. Lisko JG, Tran H, Stanfill SB, Blount BC, Watson CH. Chemical composition and evaluation of nicotine, tobacco alkaloids, pH, and selected flavors in E-cigarette cartridges and refill solutions. Nicotine Tob Res. 2015;17(10):1270–8. https://doi.org/10.1093/ntr/ntu279.
45. Varlet V, Farsalinos K, Augsburger M, Thomas A, Etter JF. Toxicity assessment of refill liquids for electronic cigarettes. Int J Environ Res Public Health. 2015;12(5):4796–815. https://doi.org/10.3390/ijerph120504796.
46. Chhina MS. Are e-cigarettes a safer alternative to reduce incidences of oral cancer? Evid Based Dent. 2024;25(1):13–4. https://doi.org/10.1038/s41432-023-00956-7.
47. Tommasi S, Brocchieri L, Tornaletti S, Besaratinia A. Epigenomic dysregulation in youth vapers: implications for disease risk assessment. Am J Respir Cell Mol Biol. 2025;72(2):206–18. https://doi.org/10.1165/rcmb.2024-0207OC.
48. Braillon A, Lang AE. The International Agency for Research on Cancer and e-cigarette carcinogenicity: time for an evaluation. Eur J Epidemiol. 2023;38(4):391. https://doi.org/10.1007/s10654-023-00993-7.
49. Shong TM, Wu XR, Lee HW, et al. Electronic-cigarette smoke induces lung adenocarcinoma and bladder urothelial hyperplasia in mice. Proc Natl Acad Sci. 2019;116(43):21727–31. https://doi.org/10.1073/pnas.1911321116.
50. Vivarelli F, Granata S, Rullo L, et al. On the toxicity of e-cigarettes consumption: focus on pathological cellular mechanisms. Pharmacol Res. 2022;182:106315. https://doi.org/10.1016/j.phrs.2022.106315.
51. Rebuli ME, Rose JJ, Noël A, et al. The e-cigarette or vaping product use–associated lung injury epidemic: pathogenesis, management, and future directions: an official American Thoracic Society workshop report. Ann Am Thorac Soc. 2023;20(1):1–17. https://doi.org/10.1513/AnnalsATS.202209-796ST.
52. Sommerfeld CG, Weiner DJ, Nowalk A, Larkin A. Hypersensitivity pneumonitis and acute respiratory distress syndrome from e-cigarette use. Pediatrics. 2018;141(6):e20163927. https://doi.org/10.1542/peds.2016-3927.
53. Keat RM, Fricain JC, Catros S, et al. The dentist's role in smoking cessation management – a literature review and recommendations: Part 1. Dent Update. 2018;45(3):197–206. https://doi.org/10.12968/denu.2018.45.3.197.

Smokeless Tobacco and Oral Health

6

Arvind Muthukrishnan and Nandita Shenoy

6.1 Introduction

Tobacco, *Nicotiana tabacum* and *Nicotiana rustica*, is consumed in two forms: smoking tobacco (ST) and smokeless tobacco (SLT). The carcinogenic properties of SLT are due to tobacco-specific nitrosamines (TSNAs) and nicotine in its unionised form. There is considerable geographic variation in nitrosamine content among various SLT preparations. Commercial SLT forms in the Indian subcontinent, such as gutka, Zarda and khaini, have higher TSNA concentrations. In addition to tobacco, SLT also contains metals like arsenic, which is toxic. SLT use causes changes in oral soft tissues and dental structures, including teeth and periodontium. Healthcare professionals and policymakers should formulate and implement an SLT cessation programme to prevent potentially malignant disorders and oral cancer. Early intervention and prevention of SLT-induced oral health changes would significantly reduce morbidity, mortality and economic burdens on the healthcare sector.

6.2 Smokeless Tobacco (SLT)

SMT (Smokeless Tobacco) refers to a category of non-combusted tobacco products that can be used orally or nasally, encompassing a variety of products. It is defined as any finely cut, ground, powdered or leaf tobacco intended for placement in the

A. Muthukrishnan (✉)
Department of Oral Medicine and Radiology and Special Care Dentistry, Saveetha Dental College and Hospital, Saveetha Institute of Medical and Technical Sciences, Chennai, India
e-mail: arvindm@saveetha.com

N. Shenoy
Department of Oral Medicine and Radiology, Manipal College of Dental Sciences, Mangalore, Manipal Academy of Higher Education, Manipal, Karnataka, India
e-mail: Nandita.shenoy@manipal.edu

S. R. Prabhu et al. (eds.), *Lifestyle in Oral Health and Disease*,
https://doi.org/10.1007/978-3-032-05888-1_6

oral cavity. The Comprehensive Smokeless Tobacco Health Education Act (CSTHEA), established by the Centres for Disease Control and Prevention (CDC), defines smokeless tobacco as any finely cut, ground, powdered or leaf tobacco designed for oral use [1]. SLT is a broad category of uncombusted tobacco products characterised by the absorption of nicotine and other chemicals across mucous membranes [2].

The key feature of smokeless tobacco is that it is not burned or heated and then inhaled like cigarettes, cigars or hookahs [3]. Instead, nicotine and other chemicals are absorbed through the lining of the mouth [4, 5]. Consumers chew tobacco in their mouths and spit out the juice that builds up, while the nicotine and other constituents are absorbed through the lining of the oral cavity [6].

6.2.1 Types of SLT Products

SLT products encompass a range of items, including chewing tobacco, snuff, gutka, betel quid with tobacco, khaini, mishri, Zarda and others [7]. These products differ in ingredients and methods of use across various regions in the world (Table 6.1).

Table 6.1 Global landscape of smokeless tobacco products

SLT type	Ingredients	Primary regions
Betel quid	Paan + areca nut + tobacco	South Asia, South Asian diaspora (UK, etc.)
Khaini	Tobacco + lime	North India
Mishri	Burnt tobacco	Maharashtra, India
Zarda	Boiled tobacco	Bangladesh, Arab countries
Gudakhu	Tobacco + molasses	Central India
Mava	Tobacco + lime + areca nut	Bhavnagar, India
Naswar	Tobacco + lime	Pakistan, Afghanistan, Eastern Europe
Nass	Tobacco + ash + cottonseed oil	Former USSR countries
Shammah	Tobacco + ash + lime	Saudi Arabia, Yemen
Toombak	Tobacco + sodium bicarbonate	Sudan
Gutka	Tobacco + areca nut + lime + flavouring agents	India, Southeast Asia, South Asian diaspora
Snuff (Dry/Moist)	Finely cut or powdered tobacco	USA, Canada
Snus	Pouched moist tobacco	Sweden, Norway, USA
Chewing tobacco	Loose leaf, plug, twist tobacco	USA, parts of Europe
Dissolvable tobacco	Tobacco-based strips, lozenges	USA
Nicotine pouches	Tobacco-free synthetic nicotine	USA, Sweden, Norway, Eastern Europe

6.2.2 Packaging and Branding of SLT

The packaging and branding of smokeless tobacco (SLT) products can make them appealing to young people, contributing to the initiation of use. Packaging influences the perception of harm associated with these products as part of marketing and promotion strategies. Packaging and storage conditions play critical roles in influencing chemical absorption rates, retaining harmful constituents and enhancing the attractiveness and addictiveness of SLT products [8]. Furthermore, packaging and storage conditions affect moisture content, pH levels, product freshness and the stability of additives, all of which directly impact the absorption of chemicals such as nicotine and tobacco-specific nitrosamines (TSNAs). Even slight variations in pH can lead to significant differences in the unprotonated nicotine content, thereby influencing the harmful potential of SLT products [9].

Moist snuffs are often sold in cans or tins designed to maintain moisture and optimal pH levels, increasing nicotine absorption. Loose-leaf chewing tobacco is typically sold in pouches or bags, which may not preserve specific moisture or pH levels as effectively [10]. Snus is generally sold in small pouches, focusing on maintaining moisture, pH and product freshness, which can impact nicotine delivery and chemical stability. Gutka is often packaged in small sachets that may or may not be airtight, impacting the degradation rate and chemical absorption [11, 12].

6.3 Geographic Variations in the Availability of Smokeless Tobacco Products

Smokeless tobacco (SLT) poses a significant global health burden, with diverse and culturally ingrained products affecting millions across South Asia, Africa, Europe and the Americas. The ingredients of smokeless tobacco (SLT) products vary significantly across different geographical regions, reflecting diverse cultural practices and preferences [13]. SLT use is prevalent worldwide, with a more significant burden in South and Southeast Asia. In some regions, SLT use is more common than smoking, particularly among women [14]. SLT products vary widely across different regions. In South Asia and Southeast Asia, everyday products include betel quid (paan), gutka, khaini, mava, mishri, Zarda and Gudakhu, each containing a mixture of tobacco, areca nut, lime and other additives. In the Middle East, Shammahs and Naswar are popular, with ingredients such as tobacco, slaked lime and ash. Africa has products like Tombac and various forms of snuff, while the former USSR region uses Nass made of tobacco, ash, cotton and sesame/cotton seed oil [15]. In North America, common forms of tobacco include moist snuff, loose-leaf chewing tobacco, plug/twist chewing tobacco, dry snuff and snus. Europe primarily uses snus, especially in Sweden, where it is manufactured through a pasteurisation process to reduce harmful nitrosamines. Other regions have unique products, such as Iq'mik in Alaska, maras in Turkey, Tuibur in northeastern India, Khiwam in Iran and Afghanistan and red tooth powder in parts of Africa. The composition and preparation methods of each product contribute to its distinct characteristics and associated health risks [16]. The global burden of SLT use is given in Table 6.1.

6.3.1 Key Differences in Ingredients and Processing

Indian smokeless tobacco (SLT) products often undergo fermentation, which can affect the production of tobacco-specific nitrosamines (TSNAs). These products are frequently combined with additives such as areca nuts and powdered lime, increasing their toxicity. In contrast, Swedish snus is pasteurised, minimising TSNA formation. Many SLT products, especially in South Asia, include various additives like lime, spices, molasses and flavourings, which can influence the pH of the product and the absorption of nicotine and other chemicals [17].

The type of tobacco used in SLT products varies across regions, with air-cured, fire-cured and boiled tobacco being common. The moisture content and pH significantly affect the absorption of nicotine and other chemicals, with even slight variations in pH leading to substantial differences in the unprotonated nicotine content. The geographical variation in SLT products reflects different cultural practices and varying levels of risk due to differences in chemical content, manufacturing processes and additives [18].

6.3.2 Chemical Composition of Smokeless Tobacco

Smokeless tobacco (SLT) products contain nicotine, a volatile alkaloid that serves as the main addictive component, influencing the central nervous system and elevating dopamine levels in the brain. Nicotine is absorbed through the oral mucosa. Additionally, SLT products contain carcinogenic tobacco-specific nitrosamines (TSNAs), such as N-nitrosonornicotine (NNN) and 4-(methylnitrosamino)-1-(3-pyridyl)-1-butanone (NNK), with levels varying widely among different brands. These products may also include harmful chemicals, such as heavy metals like arsenic, flavourings, sugars and other additives [19]. The contents of nicotine, TSNAs and other chemicals can differ significantly based on the specific product, packaging, moisture content and pH [20].

6.4 Harmful Effects of SLT

In Scandinavian countries, a smokeless tobacco product is linked to an increased risk of type 2 diabetes. These products highlight the significant health risks associated with smokeless tobacco use across different regions [21].

Carcinogenesis: SLT contains multiple carcinogens, including TSNAs, that damage DNA and lead to the development of oral cancer. These compounds can cause genotoxicity and cytotoxicity [22].

Reactive oxygen species (ROS): SLT generates reactive oxygen species (ROS), which cause damage to DNA, RNA and fibroblasts [23]. Inflammation and immune response: Chronic irritation from SLT induces inflammation in the oral mucosa, activating T cells and macrophages while releasing prostaglandins [24]. Cytokines such as interleukin-6, interferon-alpha, tumour necrosis factor-α (TNF-α) and transforming growth factor-beta are produced at the sites of irritation and contribute to oral submucous fibrosis (OSF) and malignancy [25].

Direct contact with the oral tissues of smokeless tobacco (SLT) products can cause irritation and inflammation. SLT contains numerous carcinogenic compounds, including tobacco-specific nitrosamines (TSNAs), which contribute to the development of oral cancer. Additionally, SLT can induce the production of reactive oxygen species (ROS) in the oral cavity, causing DNA damage and contributing to cancer and oral submucous fibrosis. While nicotine, the primary addictive substance in tobacco, is not directly carcinogenic, it encourages continuous use and exposure to other harmful chemicals [26].

6.5 The Impact of Nicotine on *Streptococcus mutans* Virulence

Nicotine significantly enhances the virulence of *Streptococcus mutans*, a key bacterium in the development of dental caries, by increasing its biofilm formation and metabolic activity, particularly under anaerobic conditions. It upregulates virulence-related proteins and extracellular polysaccharides, facilitating both sucrose-independent and sucrose-dependent attachment to tooth enamel. This results in a more cariogenic strain of S. mutans, with elevated lactic acid production and other glycolytic intermediates. Studies have shown that *S. mutans* isolates from smokers produce significantly more biofilms than nonsmokers, indicating increased bacterial tolerance [27].

6.6 SLT Use: Vulnerable Populations

Age, Gender and Socioeconomic Status: SLT use varies by age, gender and socioeconomic class. There is a higher prevalence among men, those in marginalised areas and specific communities. Young people and teenagers often use SLT due to peer pressure and easy availability [28].

Cultural and Regional Variations: The types of SLT products and their usage patterns vary across regions. The use of SLT is a deep-rooted issue in some developing nations and is observed among immigrants in the USA and Europe [29].

6.7 Oral Health Consequences of Smokeless Tobacco Use

Oral potentially malignant disorder (OPMD): In India and some other regions of Southeast Asia, betel quid, which often contains tobacco, is associated with oral cancer and genotoxic effects. Shammah, a smokeless tobacco product used in the Middle East, is also strongly linked to oral cancer. The use of chewing tobacco is strongly associated with the development of oral potentially malignant disorders (OPMDs). OPMDs are tissue 'fields' with distinct clinical appearances, some of which may progress to cancer over time. The term OPMD marks a shift from previous terminology, such as 'precancer' or 'premalignant', recognising that these are disorders associated with field changes due to environmental carcinogens. Their malignant potential varies, as not all cases progress to oral malignancy; non-homogeneous leukoplakia carries a higher risk than homogeneous forms. Clinically, OPMDs present diverse features, including colour variations (white, red, or mixed), topographic changes (smooth, verrucous, granular, etc.) and varying sizes. They are predominantly diagnosed in middle-aged or elderly male patients. These are a group of lesions and conditions that have a variably increased risk of developing cancers of the lip and oral cavity. An expert Working Group at the WHO Collaborating Centre on Cancer has endorsed this terminology [30].

Tobacco Pouch Keratosis: Tobacco pouch keratosis is a lesion at the site where smokeless tobacco (SLT) is placed in the mouth, presenting as a greyish-white, wrinkled area. It is most commonly found in the buccal mucosa and gingival sulcus but can also occur on the inner aspect of the lower lip (Fig. 6.1a) and the floor of the mouth. This condition develops due to the direct and prolonged contact of SLT with oral tissues, which can be irritating. Initially, the keratotic changes may be localised, but with prolonged use, the lesion may progress to more defined conditions, such as leukoplakia or erythroplakia [31].

While tobacco pouch keratosis is not cancerous, it is regarded as a precursor to more serious conditions, such as oral cancer. Variations in its appearance may occur, including pigmented lesions (Fig. 6.1b) and discrete elevated keratinised striae, which are sometimes described as a 'pumice pattern.' If the person quits the habit or changes the position where the quid is held, the condition may reverse without progressing to malignancy. It is also referred to as a 'tobacco and lime user's lesion' due to the lime content in some products. The risk of developing tobacco pouch keratosis and its potential to progress to malignancy depends on the type of SLT product used, the frequency and duration of use and other factors [31].

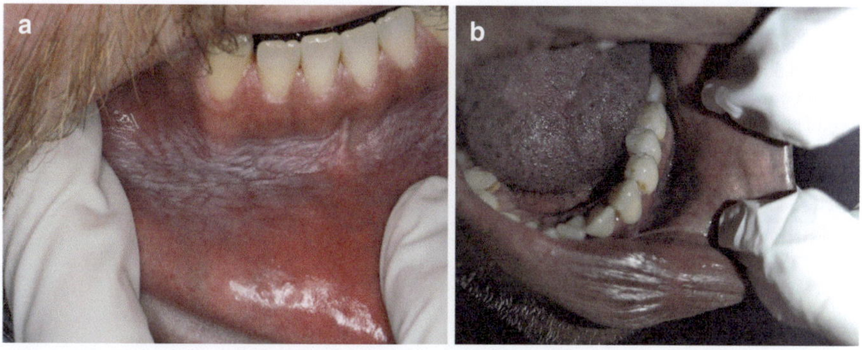

Fig. 6.1 (**a** and **b**). Tobacco pouch keratosis shows a white, wrinkled and thickened mucosal patch in the labial vestibule due to the prolonged contact of SLT with the mucosa (**a**). The left buccal vestibule shows a pigmented patch associated with the placement of SLT (**b**). (**a** is courtesy of Professor Nagamani Narayana, UNMC, Nebraska, USA)

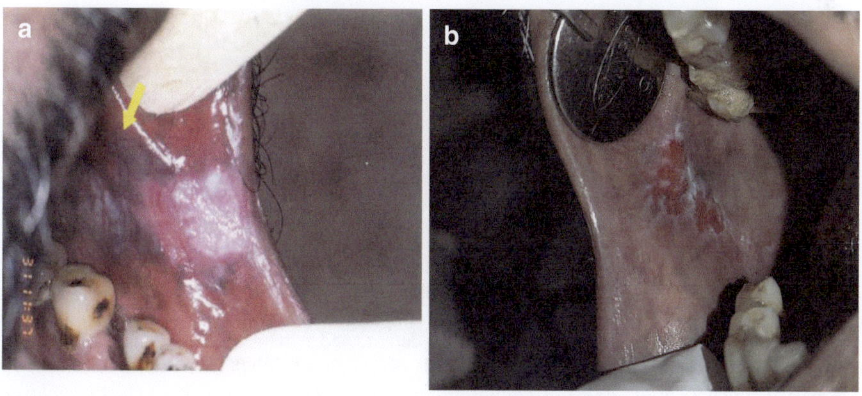

Fig. 6.2 (**a** and **b**) A well-defined white patch of homogeneous leukoplakia on the left commissure in an Indian beedi smoker. Note the pigmented areas (arrow) commonly observed in habitual smokers posterior to the leukoplakia (**a**). A mixed white and erythematous lesion with irregular surfaces of erythroleukoplakia is seen on the right buccal mucosa (**b**). (**a** is reproduced with permission from Ramdas K, Lucas E, Thomas G et al. 2008). *A Digital Manual for the Early Diagnosis of Oral Neoplasia*. Lyon: IARC. Available from http://screening.iarc.fr/atlasoral.pho?lang=1)

Leukoplakia: Leukoplakia is a predominantly white plaque of questionable risk, having excluded other known diseases or disorders that do not carry an increased risk for cancer [30]. Smokeless tobacco (SLT) use is strongly associated with the development of leukoplakia, an oral potentially malignant disorder (OPMD) [31]. Clinically, leukoplakia presents as a non-scrapable, asymptomatic homogeneous white plaque (Fig. 6.2a) or a mixed white and red non-scrapable lesion called erythroleukoplakia (Fig. 6.2b). Non-homogeneous leukoplakia appears as speckled, nodular or verrucous forms (Fig. 6.3). Non-homogeneous leukoplakia carries a

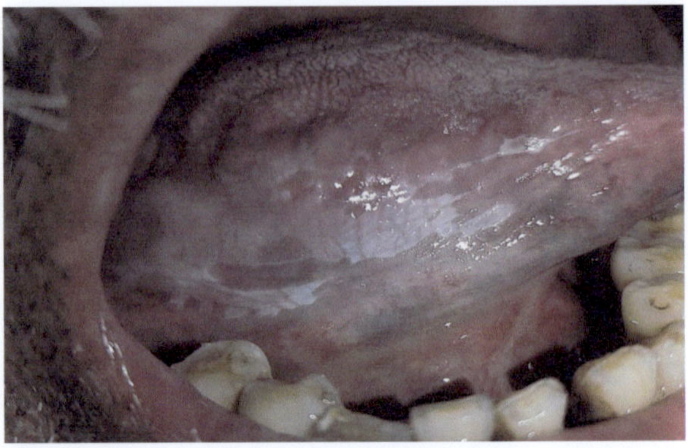

Fig. 6.3 Nonhomogeneous Leukoplakia on the right lateral border of the tongue, presenting as a well-defined, white, fissured, non-scrapable patch. The lesion is irregular, with no signs of ulceration or induration

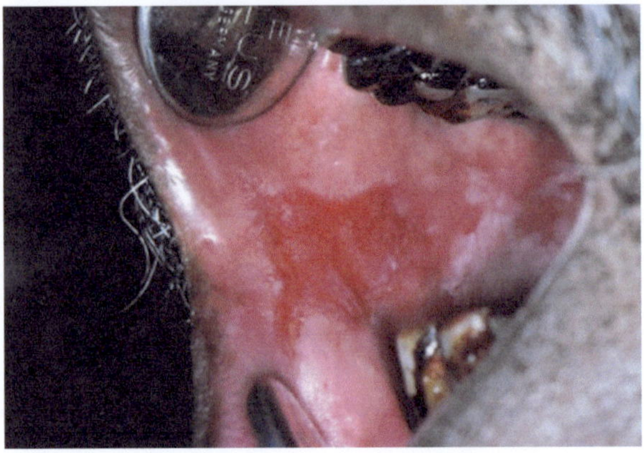

Fig. 6.4 Erythroplakia shows a bright, sharply demarcated patch on the right buccal mucosa. Prolonged use of SLT has also caused stained teeth. (Reproduced with permission from Ramdas K, Lucas E, Thomas G et al. 2008). *A Digital Manual for the Early Diagnosis of Oral Neoplasia*. Lyon: IARC. Available from http://screening.iarc.fr/atlasoral.pho?lang=1)

higher risk of malignant transformation. A positive association exists between SLT use and the occurrence of oral leukoplakia. Leukoplakias are reported to be six times more common among SLT users compared to non-tobacco users. In the Pan-American Health Organisation (PAHO) region, oral leukoplakia was the only OPMD associated with SLT use in the studies reviewed. However, the quality of the evidence for this association was considered very low due to the heterogeneity of the results [32].

Erythroplakia Erythroplakia is a predominantly fiery red patch that cannot be clinically or pathologically attributed to any other disease. It appears as a sharply demarcated, flat or depressed erythematous area with a matte surface, often presenting as a solitary lesion (Fig. 6.4). Patients experience pain and a burning sensation. A systematic review focusing on South Asia assessed the risk of developing OPMDs among SLT users. The review highlighted that SLT use is a significant risk factor for

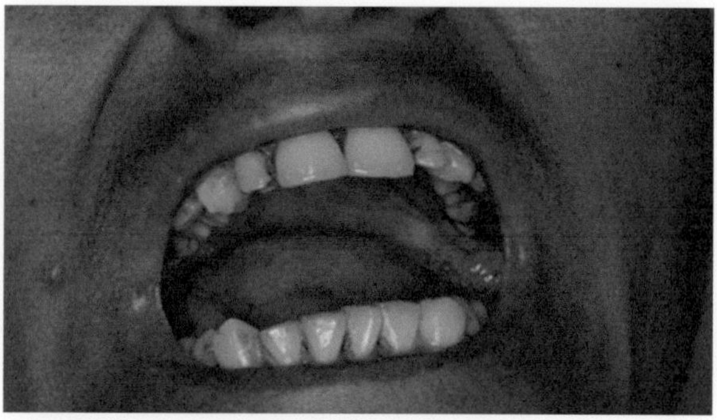

Fig. 6.5 Clinical presentation of oral submucous fibrosis (OSMF) showing restricted mouth opening. A vertical skin fold on the cheek is also seen

erythroplakia [33, 34]. Given its potential for malignant transformation, erythroplakia requires careful clinical evaluation and histopathological confirmation.

Oral Submucous Fibrosis (OSMF): OSMF is a chronic and insidious disease primarily associated with areca nut use, particularly in South and Southeast Asian countries. Chewing areca nut and its derivatives is a significant risk factor for this disorder. OSMF is characterised by a generalised fibrosis of the submucosal tissues of the oral mucosa, resulting in marked rigidity leading to progressive inability to open the mouth (Fig. 6.5) and difficulty in protruding the tongue. OSMF is highly prevalent in the Indian subcontinent. Commercially available products like gutka contain SLT and areca nut. However, SLT alone does not induce submucous fibrosis. Areca nut is the causative agent of OSMF. Other terms used to describe OSMF include idiopathic scleroderma of the mouth, juxtaepithelial fibrosis and sclerosing stomatitis [35, 36].

Oral Cancer: Oral cancer is significantly linked to smokeless tobacco (SLT) use. The International Agency on Research for Cancer (IARC) classifies SLT as a carcinogenic agent. Oral cancers associated with SLT include squamous cell carcinoma (SCC) and verrucous carcinoma (VC). SCC tumours appear as red granular or exophytic ulcerative-infiltrative areas with distinct rolled borders, with induration (Fig. 6.6). The buccal mucosa is commonly affected, with up to 80% involvement at the site of tobacco placement. The lateral margins of the tongue and the floor of the mouth are also high-risk sites. Late-stage symptoms encompass limited mouth opening, tongue rigidity and lymph node metastasis [37].

Verrucous Carcinoma (VC): VC is a variant of squamous cell carcinoma (SCC) linked to the use of smokeless tobacco (SLT), accounting for up to 16% of oral cancers in some populations [38]. VC commonly presents as an exophytic verrucous growth with finger-like projections (Fig. 6.7) overgrowth. The development of VC is associated with SLT use, particularly when combined with areca nuts in products such as gutka. Although VC has a high potential for local recurrence, it is less likely to metastasise to lymph nodes compared to squamous cell carcinoma (SCC). However, SLT can lead to multifocal tumours, necessitating careful monitoring of

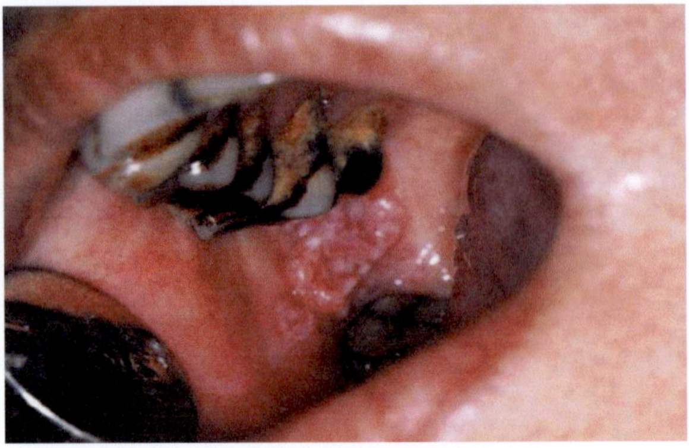

Fig. 6.6 Oral carcinoma presenting as an exophytic growth in the posterior right buccal mucosa in a 48-year-old woman who chewed betel quid for 30 years. Note the tobacco stains and the heavy calculus deposits in the right maxillary molars. (Reproduced with permission from Ramdas K, Lucas E, Thomas G et al. 2008). *A Digital Manual for the Early Diagnosis of Oral Neoplasia*. Lyon: IARC. Available from http://screening.iarc.fr/atlasoral.pho?lang=1)

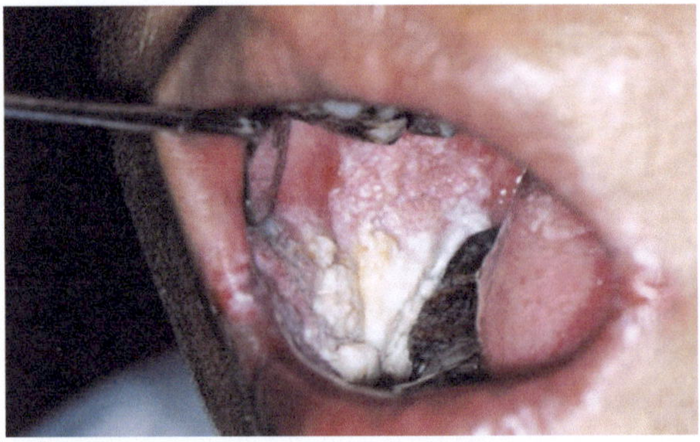

Fig. 6.7 Verrucous carcinoma of the right buccal mucosa. Note the extensive verrucous growth extending from the commissure to the posterior aspect of the right buccal mucosa. Note the heavy tobacco stains on the lower molars. (Reproduced with permission from Ramdas K, Lucas E, Thomas G et al. 2008). *A Digital Manual for the Early Diagnosis of Oral Neoplasia*. Lyon: IARC. Available from http://screening.iarc.fr/atlasoral.pho?lang=1)

individuals with a history of SLT use. Despite being more indolent than SCC, VC remains a serious condition that requires timely diagnosis and treatment.

Effects on Dental Hard Tissues: Smokeless tobacco can lead to brown-to-black tooth discolouration. Enamel, dentin and tooth roots can become stained. Patients with prostheses, whether removable or fixed, often report stains and discolouration. Chronic chewing over the long term can result in pathological tooth wear, including abrasion and attrition. The content of sweetening agents in commercially available SLT varies. The sugar content in SLT may have a cariogenic effect on teeth.

Effects on the Gingival and Periodontal Tissues: Smokeless tobacco (SLT) users often experience a gingival recession, exposing tooth-root surfaces. SLT use also raises the risk of periodontal pocket formation, plaque accumulation and calculus formation, which can lead to periodontitis. Moreover, there is a heightened risk of periodontal inflammation, including gingivitis, among SLT users [39]. SLT can cause damage to the periodontium, contributing to overall periodontal health issues. These effects highlight the significant oral health risks associated with SLT use.

Other Oral Health Consequences: Smokeless tobacco (SLT) use can lead to halitosis or bad breath. Additionally, SLT use can reduce salivation and mucus production, disrupting the normal oral microflora and increasing susceptibility to pathogens [40].

6.8 Prevention and Control

Healthcare providers should assess patients' tobacco use and actively implement prevention, cessation and treatment programmes. Public health interventions are necessary to control smokeless tobacco (SLT) use and promote oral health. Regulatory measures, including standards for ingredients and flavours, are essential to reducing the appeal and harm of SLT products. Educating the public, particularly children and teenagers, about the dangers of SLT is crucial [41].

6.9 Research and Future Directions

Future research on smokeless tobacco (SLT) and oral health should focus on several key areas to better understand and mitigate the harmful effects of SLT. Research is needed to understand the mechanisms by which SLT-induced harm occurs. This includes studying the specific chemicals and compounds in various SLT products and their impact on oral tissues and exploring the genetic and molecular pathways involved in the development of oral potentially malignant disorders (OPMDs) and oral cancer. More longitudinal studies are required to assess the progression of oral lesions and the effectiveness of interventions. Additionally, research should explore the association between smokeless tobacco and metabolic disorders. Investigations should be conducted into how SLT affects the oral microbiome and its role in disease development. Further research should be done to inform the development of evidence-based tobacco product standards and regulations.

Evaluating the effectiveness of current tobacco control measures and cessation programmes is crucial for enhancing prevention and treatment strategies and innovating new interventions. Studies should focus on populations with high rates of SLT use, particularly in South and Southeast Asia, as well as among immigrant groups in Europe, the USA and Australia [42, 43]. It is essential to identify effective ways to communicate the risks of SLT to various populations, especially youth, and to understand the reasons behind SLT use to inform targeted prevention efforts.

Regarding product standards and regulations, the research should aim to establish standards for carcinogens and toxicants in SLT products, develop regulations based on the effects of flavourings and create strategies to reduce the attractiveness of SLT products to youth. Monitoring and regulating nicotine and other harmful chemicals in SLT products are also crucial.

References

1. Arain SS, Kazi TG, Afridi HI, Talpur FN, Kazi AG, Brahman KD, et al. Correlation of arsenic levels in smokeless tobacco products and biological samples of oral cancer patients and control consumers. Biol Trace Elem Res. 2015;168:287–95.
2. Chaturvedi P. Resource Centre for Tobacco Free India. [Internet]. Available from: www.rctfi.org/. Accessed on Feb 2025.
3. International Agency for Research on Cancer. IARC monographs on the evaluation of carcinogenic risks to humans. Betel-quid and areca nut chewing and some areca-nut derived nitrosamines, vol. 85. Lyon: IARC; 2004.
4. Walsh PM, Epstein JB. The oral effects of smokeless tobacco. J Can Dent Assoc. 2000;66:22–5.
5. Guha N, Warnakulasuriya S, Vlaanderen J, Straif K. Betel quid chewing and the risk of oral and oropharyngeal cancers: a meta-analysis with implications for cancer control. Int J Cancer. 2014;135:1433–43.
6. Gupta PC, Ray CS. Smokeless tobacco and health in India and South Asia. Respirology. 2003;8:419–31.
7. Muthukrishnan A, Warnakulasuriya S. Oral health consequences of smokeless tobacco use. Indian J Med Res. 2018;148(1):35–40.
8. Gupta PC. Mouth cancer in India: a new epidemic? J Indian Med Assoc. 1999;97:370–3.
9. Birdsey J, Cornelius M, Jamal A, et al. Tobacco product use among U.S. middle and high school students – National Youth Tobacco Survey, 2023. MMWR Morb Mortal Wkly Rep. 2023;72(44):1173–82.
10. Saxena S, Sharma P, Khan S, Gupta N, Singh L. Smokeless tobacco use and public health nutrition. Public Health Nutr. 2022;26(1):46–55.
11. Javed F, Chotai M, Mehmood A, Almas K. Oral mucosal disorders associated with habitual gutka usage: a review. Oral Surg Oral Med Oral Pathol Oral Radiol Endod. 2010;109:857–64.
12. John RM, Sung HY, Max W. Economic cost of tobacco use in India, 2004. Tobacco Control. 2009;18:138–43.
13. Gupta PC, Mehta HC. Cohort study of all-cause mortality among tobacco users in Mumbai, India. Bull World Health Organ. 2000;78:877–83.
14. Gupta PC, Pednekar MS, Parkin DM, Sankaranarayanan R. Tobacco-associated mortality in Mumbai (Bombay) India. Results of the Bombay Cohort Study. Int J Epidemiol. 2005;34(6):1395–402.
15. Gupta C, Bhonsle RB, Mehta FS, Pindborg JJ. Mortality experience in relation to tobacco chewing and smoking habits from a 10-year follow-up study in Ernakulam District, Kerala. Int J Epidemiol. 1984a;13:184–7.
16. Gupta PC, Mehta FS, Pindborg JJ. Mortality among reverse chutta smokers in south India. BMJ. 1984b;289:865–6.
17. International Agency for Research on Cancer (IARC). Monographs on the evaluation of the carcinogenic risk of chemicals to humans, vol 37. Tobacco habits other than smoking; betel quid and areca nut chewing; and some related nitrosamines. Lyon: IARC; 1985.
18. Bhonsle RB, Murti PR, Gupta PC, Mehta FS. Reverse dhumti smoking in Goa. An epidemiologic study of 5449 villagers for oral precancerous lesions. Indian J Cancer. 1976;13:301–5.

19. Sankaranarayanan R, Mathew B, Jacob BJ, et al. Early findings from a community-based, cluster-randomised, controlled oral cancer screening trial in Kerala, India. The Trivandrum Oral Cancer Screening Study Group. Cancer. 2000;88:664–73.
20. Rao DN, Desai PB. Risk assessment of tobacco, alcohol and diet in cancers of base tongue and oral tongue – a case control study. Indian J Cancer. 1998;35:65–72.
21. Rao DN, Ganesh B, Rao RS, Desai PB. Risk assessment of tobacco, alcohol and diet in oral cancer – a case-control study. Int J Cancer. 1994;58:469–73.
22. Nandakumar A, Thimmasetty KT, Sreeramareddy NM, et al. A population-based case-control investigation on cancers of the oral cavity in Bangalore, India. Br J Cancer. 1990;62:847–51.
23. Balaram P, Sridhar H, Rajkumar T, et al. Oral cancer in southern India: the influence of smoking, drinking, paan-chewing and oral hygiene. Int J Cancer. 2002;98:440–5.
24. Znaor A, Brennan P, Gajalakshmi V, et al. Independent and combined effects of tobacco smoking, chewing and alcohol drinking on the risk of oral, pharyngeal and esophageal cancers in Indian men. Int J Cancer. 2003;105:681–6.
25. Nandakumar A, Anantha N, Pattabhiraman V, et al. Importance of anatomical subsite in correlating risk factors in cancer of the oesophagus – report of a case – control study. Br J Cancer. 1996;73:1306–11.
26. Nayar D, Kapil U, Joshi YK, et al. Nutritional risk factors in esophageal cancer. J Assoc Phys India. 2000;48:781–7.
27. Huang R, Li M, Gregory RL. Effect of nicotine on growth and metabolism of Streptococcus mutans. Eur J Oral Sci. 2012;120(4):319–25.
28. GATS. Global Adult Tobacco Survey-2 Factsheet India 2016–17. Available from: https://www.who.int/tobacco/surveillance/survey/gats/GATS_India_2016-_FactSheet.pdf
29. World Health Organization. Ministry of Health & Family Welfare Government of India. Global Adult Tobacco Survey: GATS-2 India 2016–17. 2018. Available from: https://mohfw.gov.in/sites/default/files/GlobaltobacoJune2018.pdf. Accessed on 20 Feb 2025.
30. Warnakulasuriya S, Kujan O, Aguirre-Urizar JM, Bagan JV, González-Moles MA, Kerr AR, et al. Oral potentially malignant disorders: a consensus report from an international seminar on nomenclature and classification, convened by the WHO Collaborating Centre for Oral Cancer. Oral Dis. 2021;27:1862–80.
31. Kerr AR. Diagnostic adjuncts for oral cavity squamous cell carcinoma and oral potentially malignant disorders. In: Warnakulasuriya S, Greenspan JS, editors. Textbook of oral cancer prevention, diagnosis and management. Cham: Springer; 2020. p. 99–117.
32. Pedroso CM. Pan-American prevalence of smokeless tobacco use and association with oral potentially malignant disorders and head and neck cancer: a systematic review and meta-analysis. Oral Surg Oral Med Oral Pathol Oral Radiol. 2023;136(3):322–32.
33. Khan Z, Khan S, Christianson L, et al. Smokeless tobacco and oral potentially malignant disorders in South Asia: a protocol for a systematic review. Syst Rev. 2016;5:142.
34. Warnakulasuriya S, Kerr AR. Oral submucous fibrosis: a review of the current management and possible directions for novel therapies. Oral Surg Oral Med Oral Pathol Oral Radiol. 2016;122:232–41.
35. Kerr AR, Warnakulasuriya S, Mighell AJ, Dietrich T, Nasser M, Rimal J, Jalil A, Bornstein MM, Nagao T, Fortune F, Hazarey VH, Reichart PA, Silverman S, Johnson NW. A systematic review of medical interventions for oral submucous fibrosis and future research opportunities. Oral Dis. 2011;17(Suppl 1):42–57.
36. Hazarey VK, Johnson NW. Oral submucous fibrosis: a historical perspective. In: Warnakulasuriya S, Ranganathan K, editors. Oral submucous fibrosis. Textbooks in contemporary dentistry. Cham: Springer; 2023. p. 3–16. https://doi.org/10.1007/978-3-031-12855-4_1.
37. Braakhuis BJ, Leemans CR, Brakenhoff RH. Expanding fields of genetically altered cells in head and neck squamous carcinogenesis. Semin Cancer Biol. 2005;15(2):113–20. https://doi.org/10.1016/j.semcancer.2004.08.004.

38. Rekha KP, Angadi PV. Verrucous carcinoma of the oral cavity: a clinico-pathologic appraisal of 133 cases in Indians. Oral Maxillofac Surg. 2010;14:211–8.
39. Warnakulasuriya S, Dietrich T, Bornstein MM, Casals Peidró E, Preshaw PM, Walter C, et al. Oral health risks of tobacco use and effects of cessation. Int Dent J. 2010;60:7–30.
40. Trivedy CR, Craig G, Warnakulasuriya S. The oral health consequences of chewing areca nut. Addict Biol. 2002;7:115–25.
41. Moller IJ, Pindborg JJ, Effendi I. The relation between betel chewing and dental caries. Scand J Dent Res. 1977;85:64–70.
42. Richter P, Hodge K, Stanfill S, Zhang L, Watson C. Surveillance of moist snuff: total nicotine, moisture, pH, unionized nicotine, and tobacco-specific nitrosamines. Nicotine Tob Res. 2008;10:1645–52.
43. Stepanov I, Hecht SS, Ramakrishnan S, Gupta PC. Tobacco-specific nitrosamines in smokeless tobacco products marketed in India. Int J Cancer. 2005;116:16–9.

Areca Nut (Betel Quid) Chewing and Oral Health

7

Kannan Ranganathan

7.1 Introduction

Areca nut (AN) consumption is linked to significant and profound health implications, including oral health problems, cancer, cardiovascular and metabolic issues and neurological and addiction concerns. It is the fourth most abused substance globally, the others being alcohol, tobacco and caffeine. Arecoline stimulates salivation and produces a mild euphoria, contributing to the habit's popularity. Areca nut contains psychoactive compounds that lead to dependency [1–3]. Dependency mechanisms involve neurochemical reinforcement, tolerance development, social and cultural conditioning and psychological reinforcement. The cumulative impact of these health risks renders the habit detrimental to health.

Areca nut is widely used in Asia, the Pacific Islands and in South Africa. With approximately 600 million users worldwide, including 224 million in India alone, areca nut consumption is deeply embedded in cultural traditions. [4]

7.2 Areca Nut

The term 'areca nut' is widely used in the literature. It is the seed of the fruit (berry) of the palm *Areca catechu*. This nut is chewed along with the leaf of a vine known as the betel vine (Piper betel L.). Betel quid typically consists of pieces of areca nut wrapped in a betel leaf and combined with slaked lime, spices and/or tobacco. While this practice is deeply rooted in cultural and social traditions, the health risks associated with its use, particularly its impact on oral health, are substantial and well-documented. [4]

K. Ranganathan (✉)
Department of Oral and Maxillofacial Pathology, Ragas Dental College, Chennai, Tamil Nadu, India

S. R. Prabhu et al. (eds.), *Lifestyle in Oral Health and Disease*,
https://doi.org/10.1007/978-3-032-05888-1_7

7.2.1 Areca Nut Types

Raw/Traditional Forms These can be soft, unripe nuts (green) or mature nuts (orange/red). They have a high moisture content and are used in certain regions of Taiwan, India and the Pacific islands (Fig. 7.1a).

Processed Raw Forms The nuts are sun-dried, boiled, fermented or roasted and used in whole or sliced preparations (Fig. 7.1b–d), as well as in dried areca husk [5]. Additionally, areca nuts are combined with Piper betel inflorescence. [6]

Basic Betel Quid (Paan) Whole or crushed areca nuts are wrapped in betel leaf (Piper betel), slaked lime (calcium hydroxide) and a variety of condiments/spices. Preparation varies regionally (Fig. 7.2a–c).

Pan Masala Commercial product without tobacco. They contain processed areca pieces, sweeteners, flavouring and aromatic substances.

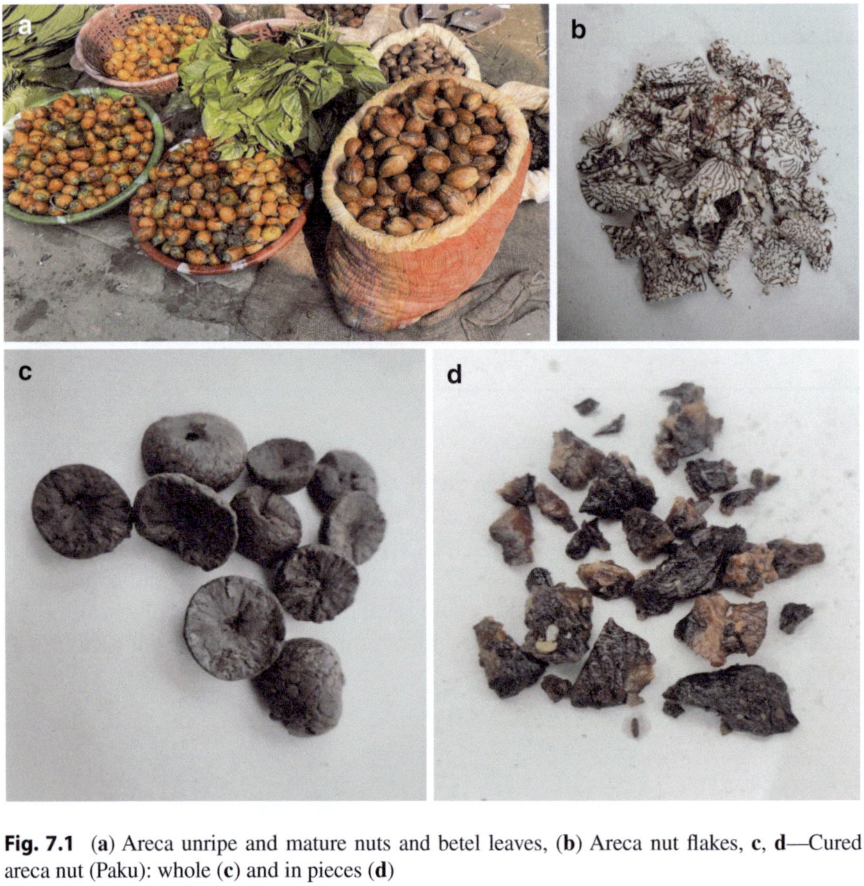

Fig. 7.1 (**a**) Areca unripe and mature nuts and betel leaves, (**b**) Areca nut flakes, **c**, **d**—Cured areca nut (Paku): whole (**c**) and in pieces (**d**)

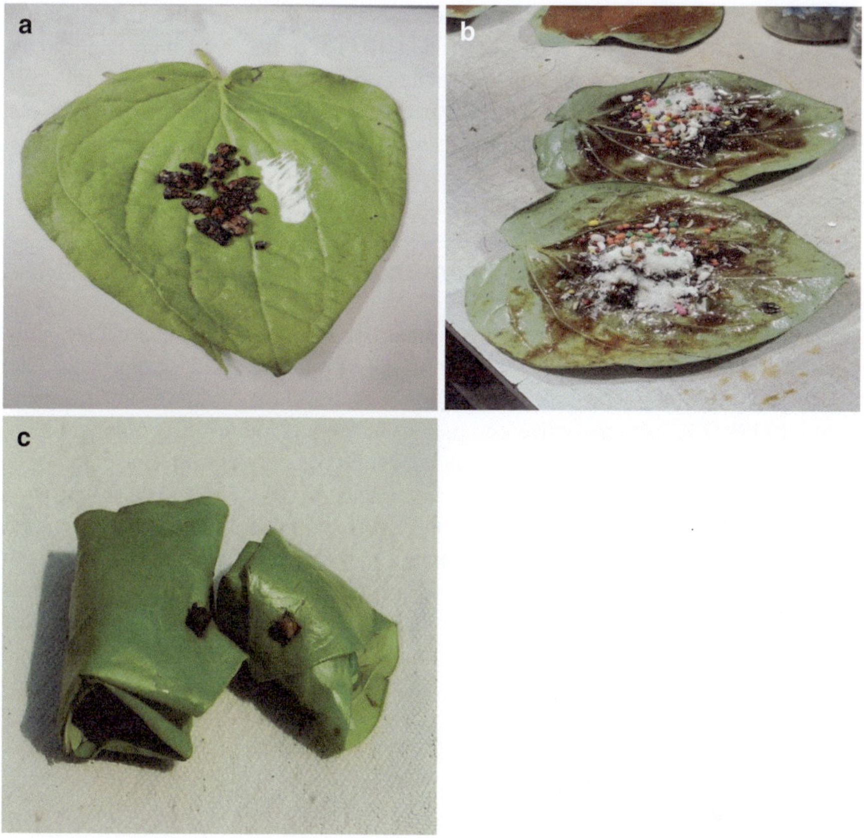

Fig. 7.2 (**a**) Areca nut pieces and (slaked lime (calcium hydroxide)) on betel leaves. The final betel quid, with all the ingredients (**b**), folded and held in place with a clove (**c**). Ready to chew

Gutka These are pan masala products that contain tobacco.

Other commercially available forms of areca nuts include scented supari, sweet supari, flavoured areca pieces, candy-coated varieties, silver-coated nuts and flavoured pastes.

7.3 Areca Nut Use Demographics

The highest prevalence is observed in South and Southeast Asian countries, particularly in India, Taiwan, Pakistan, Bangladesh, Sri Lanka, Myanmar and Southern regions of China [7, 8]. There has been a growing usage among Asian immigrant communities in Western countries. Globally, around 600 million people use areca nuts. Approximately 224 million people (24%) of India's adult population consume areca nuts. The majority (14%) combine it with tobacco, potentially amplifying its harmful effects [9]. Most users start in adolescence or early adulthood. Peak usage typically occurs between the ages of 20 and 40. There has been increasing prevalence among younger populations due to the easy availability of commercial packaged products. Gender distribution varies by region and cultural practices. Traditionally, it is more common among males; however, female usage is increasing. [7, 8]

7.4 Areca Nut/Betel Quid Contents

Areca nut contains alkaloids (arecoline, arecaidine, guvacine and guvacoline), polyphenols (catechin), flavonoids and tannins (gallotannic acid, gallic acid and d-catechol), as well as trace elements (copper, sodium, magnesium, vanadium and bromine) [9]. The primary active component of the areca nut is arecoline, an alkaloid with psychoactive properties. Areca nut is classified as a group-one carcinogen by the International Agency for Research on Cancer. [10]

Betel quid comprises betel leaf (safrole, hydroxychavicol, eugenol, isoeugenol, quercetin), slaked lime (Calcium hydroxide), catechu (a reddish-brown astringent from the heartwood of tropical acacia trees) and additional substances, such as tobacco, which significantly compounds its adverse health effects. The slaked lime used in the preparation raises the pH, enhancing the absorption of arecoline and other harmful substances [10].

7.5 Systemic Effects of Areca Nut

Cardiovascular and metabolic impacts include an increased risk of hypertension, a higher likelihood of metabolic syndrome, potential cardiovascular system damage, disrupted metabolic regulation and liver disease [11]. Arecoline acts as an agonist of muscarinic acetylcholine receptors, and neurochemical dependency occurs due to the modulation of acetylcholine and engagement of the dopaminergic system [3]. Cessation may be associated with mild cognitive disruptions, mood fluctuations, reduced concentration capacity, psychological cravings and difficulties in stress management.

7.6 Areca Nut and Oral Health

Chewing habits involving areca nuts are associated with several oral manifestations. These are briefly discussed below:

7.6.1 Erosive and Mechanical Damage of Teeth

The fibrous nature of the areca nut can cause mechanical wear and tear on teeth, resulting in enamel erosion and exposure of underlying dentin, which can lead to sensitivity. Severity depends on the hardness of the areca nut, chewing frequency and duration of the habit. Chronic chewing exacerbates this damage and can potentially lead to root fractures due to increased masticatory load.

7.6.2 Staining and Discolouration

Regular use of betel quid can cause dark, reddish-brown staining of the teeth and gums, resulting from the pigments in the betel quid. The oral mucosal changes are called betel chewer's mucosa. This presents as brownish-red discolouration of mucosa (Fig. 7.3). The discoloured mucosa may present with encrusted quid particles and a wrinkled appearance, which is localised to the quid placement site. It is more prominent when oral hygiene is poor. While primarily a cosmetic issue, these stains can also harbour bacteria, worsening oral hygiene. It is not considered potentially malignant but may coexist with precancerous lesions. [12, 13]

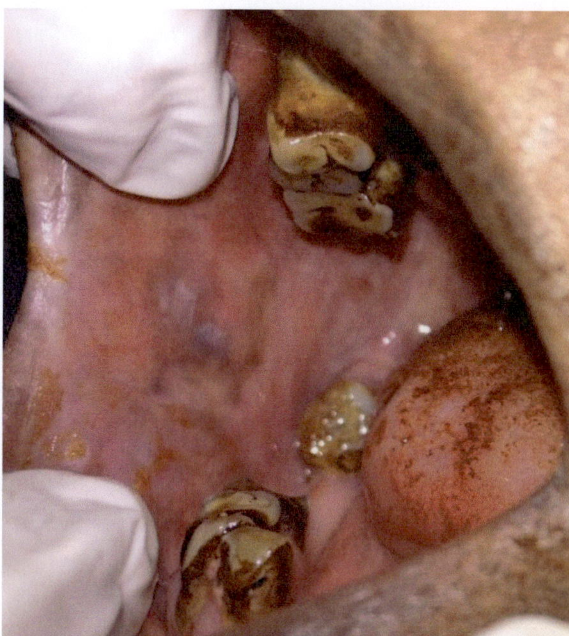

Fig. 7.3 Red discolouration of teeth and mucosa from chewing betel quid

7.6.3 Periodontal Disease and Tooth Loss

Chewing betel quid increases the risk of periodontal disease. The abrasive nature of the nut damages the gingiva and periodontium, creating an environment conducive to bacterial growth. In vitro studies have shown that arecoline inhibits the growth of periodontal fibroblasts, impairs epithelial cell attachment and reattachment and worsens existing periodontal disease [14]. Chronic inflammation and infection result in gingival recession, bone loss and eventual tooth loss.

7.6.4 Oral Submucous Fibrosis (OSF)

Oral submucous fibrosis (OSF) is a chronic, irreversible and progressive disease characterised by fibrosis that affects the lining mucosa of the upper digestive tract, including the oral cavity, oropharynx and upper third of the oesophagus. The fibrosis can extend into underlying musculature. This limits mouth opening, making speaking, eating and swallowing difficult. The prevalence rates of OSF are 0.07–3.2% in India and 0.5–3.4% in South Africa, with a rising trend noted in India due to increased areca consumption among the younger age group [15].

It can occur at any age, with an average age of diagnosis ranging from 20 to 30 years. The male-to-female ratio varies by region and local customs. Risk factors for OSF depend on the duration and frequency of areca nut use, the form of consumption (such as quid or commercial products), genetic susceptibility and nutritional deficiencies of the user, particularly iron and vitamin B complex deficiencies. The condition is irreversible and has a high potential to progress to oral cancer, with a transformation rate of 2–87–13% (References, please) [16].·

Clinical features of SMF include a range of symptoms and signs, which can be clinically divided into three stages: [17]

Early Stage At this stage, common symptoms include a burning sensation, mild blanching of the oral mucosa, mucosal petechiae, oral vesicles and ulceration, leathery mucosa and depapillation of the dorsum of the tongue. Mouth opening is normal at this stage.

Intermediate Stage Clinical features at this stage include sore mouth, discomfort to hot and spicy food, palpable fibrous bands, blanching of oral mucosa, mucosal depigmentation, limited mouth opening (20–40 mm) (Fig. 7.4a) and limitation of tongue mobility.

Advanced Stage In this stage, the mucosa appears 'marble-like'. Extensive fibrous bands, accompanied by trismus with significant limitation in mouth opening (<20 mm), is a consistent feature (Fig. 7.4b). Other features include sunken cheeks, flattening of the palate, a 'Hockey stick' shape or deformity of the uvula (Fig. 7.4c), severe limitation of tongue mobility, dysphagia and weight loss.

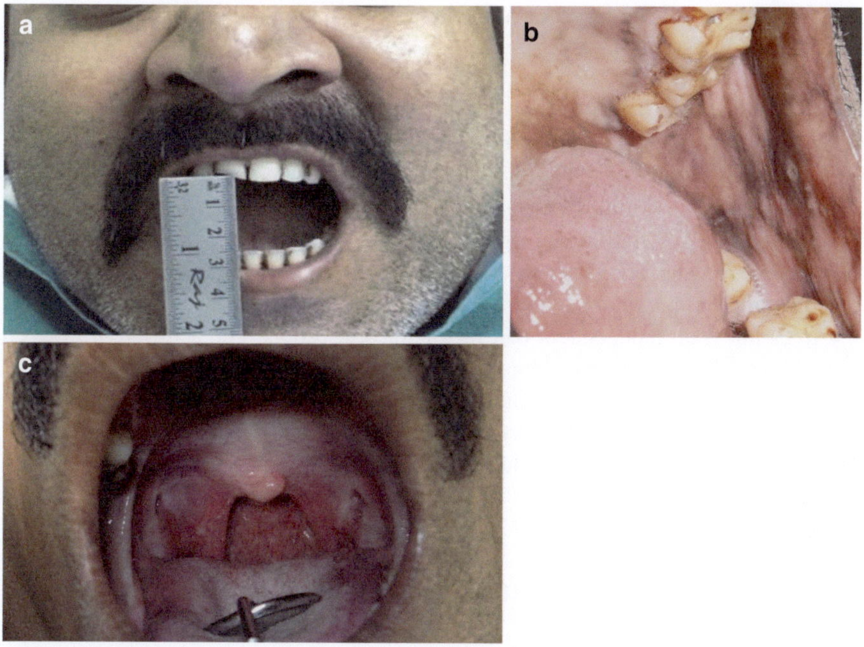

Fig. 7.4 (**a**) Limitation of mouth opening in the intermediate stage of SMF. (**b**) Vertical 'fibrous' bands in the buccal mucosa in the advanced stage of SMF. (**c**) Deformed uvula in the advanced stage of SMF. Also, note the marble-like appearance of the palatal mucosa

7.7 OSF Pathogenesis

The pathogenesis of OSF involves complex interactions between various molecular pathways [13]. Areca nut contents, mainly two alkaloids, arecoline and arecaidine, initiate the following three processes [18].

1. *Fibroblast Stimulation:* This process is characterised by enhanced proliferation of fibroblasts, increased collagen synthesis, reduced collagen degradation and altered collagen metabolism.
2. *Copper-Mediated Effects:* This process features upregulation of lysyl oxidase activity, enhanced collagen cross-linking, increased collagen stabilisation and resistance to degradation.
3. *Inflammatory Response:* The main events in this process include cytokine production alteration, enhanced inflammatory mediator release, chronic inflammatory state maintenance and tissue remodelling promotion.

Genetic susceptibility plays a crucial role in the development of OSF. HLA associations (DR, B76), genetic polymorphisms affecting collagen metabolism and gene variations related to inflammatory response contribute to individual susceptibility differences. The Major Histocompatibility Complex Class I Chain-Related Gene A

(MICA) polymorphism has been associated with an increased risk of OSF, particularly the allele A6 in MICA [19].

7.8 Areca Nut as a Risk Factor for Oral Cancer

Areca nut contains carcinogenic compounds, such as arecoline, which contribute to abnormal cell proliferation and malignant transformation by increasing the secretion of tumour-promoting cytokines, triggering DNA damage in oral keratinocytes and inducing inflammatory proteins like COX-2 and PGE2. [20]

Areca nut is an independent risk factor for oral cancer. The addition of tobacco in betel quid further escalates the risk. Around 68% of women with buccal cancer and 84% of women with tongue cancer who are non-smokers chew betel quid. Betel leaf with areca nut chewing accounts for 31% of oral cancers in South India. Eliminating chewing habits could reduce the risk of malignancy by up to 91% [21, 22].

7.9 Reduced Salivary Function and Dry Mouth

While initial saliva stimulation may occur, prolonged use can lead to long-term impairment of salivary gland function, resulting in dry mouth (xerostomia). This condition predisposes individuals to cavities, infections and discomfort.

7.10 Lichenoid Lesions

Lichenoid lesions appear at quid retention sites, usually on buccal mucosa or tongue. These lesions are usually unilateral and present as white keratotic lines (Fig. 7.5), often accompanied by red or atrophic areas [23]. They are hypersensitive reactions that usually resolve on cessation of the habit.

7.11 Conclusion

Areca nut consumption is a significant public health concern with far-reaching health implications, particularly the debilitating and life-threatening effects of OSF and oral cancer. Its adverse impacts on oral, systemic and mental health necessitate coordinated interventions. The problem of areca nut illustrates the complex challenges faced in public health when addressing substances deeply embedded in cultural traditions. Moving forward requires a balanced approach that acknowledges cultural sensitivity while actively working to protect public health through education, intervention and continued research. Comprehensive strategies that combine education, regulation, medical intervention and research are crucial for mitigating the harmful effects and enhancing public health outcomes. Success will require

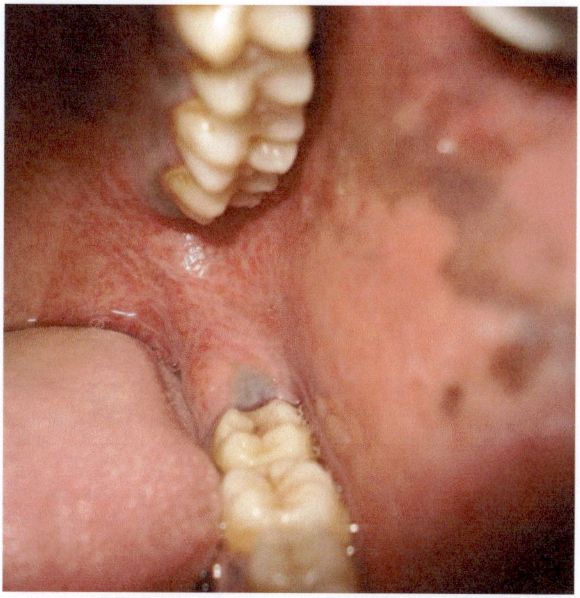

Fig. 7.5 Lichenoid changes in OSF. Lace-like lesions mimic reticular lichen planus

continued collaboration between healthcare providers, researchers, policymakers and community leaders to create sustainable solutions to this significant public health challenge.

References

1. Winstock AR, Trivedy CR, Warnakulasuriya KA, Peters TJ. A dependency syndrome related to areca nut use: some medical and psychological aspects among areca nut users in the Gujarat community in the UK. Addict Biol. 2000;5(2):173–9. https://doi.org/10.1080/13556210050003766. PMID: 20575832
2. Winstock A. Areca nut-abuse liability, dependence and public health. Addict Biol. 2002;7(1):133–8. https://doi.org/10.1080/13556210120091509. PMID: 11900633
3. Papke RL, Hatsukami DK, Herzog TA. Betel quid, health, and addiction. Subst Use Misuse. 2020;55(9):1528–32. https://doi.org/10.1080/10826084.2019.1666147. PMID: 32569542; PMCID: PMC7737392
4. Gupta PC, Ray CS, Papke RL, et al. Perspectives on areca nut with some global implications: symposium report. Transl Res Oral Oncol. 2018:3. https://doi.org/10.1177/2057178X18814068.
5. Zhang X, Li C, Liao Q, Reichart PA. Areca chewing in Xiangtan, Hunan province, China: interviews with chewers. J Oral Pathol Med. 2008;37(7):423–9. https://doi.org/10.1111/j.1600-0714.2008.00640.x. Epub 2008 Feb 19
6. Wu MT, Wu DC, Hsu HK, Kao EL, Lee JM. Constituents of areca chewing related to esophageal cancer risk in Taiwanese men. Dis Esophagus. 2004;17(3):257–9. https://doi.org/10.1111/j.1442-2050.2004.00419.x. PMID: 15361101
7. Gupta PC, Warnakulasuriya S. Global epidemiology of areca nut usage. Addict Biol. 2002 Jan;7(1):77–83. https://doi.org/10.1080/13556210020091437.

8. More CB, Patil DJ. Epidemiology of oral submucous fibrosis: prevalence and trends. In: Warnakulasuriya S, Ranganathan K, editors. Oral submucous fibrosis. A guide to diagnosis and management. Cham: Springer; 2023. p. 17–29. https://doi.org/10.1007/978-3-031-12855-4_2.
9. Singh PK, Yadav A, Singh L, Mazumdar S, Sinha DN, Straif K, Singh S. Areca nut consumption with and without tobacco among the adult population: a nationally representative study from India. BMJ Open. 2021;11(6):e043987. https://doi.org/10.1136/bmjopen-2020-043987. PMID: 34130957; PMCID: PMC8208015
10. Betel-quid and Areca-nut Chewing and Some Areca-nut-derived Nitrosamines. IARC monographs on the evaluation of carcinogenic risks to humans, No. 85.IARC Working group on the evaluation of carcinogenic risks to humans. Lyon (FR): International Agency for Research on Cancer; 2004.
11. Javed F, Al-Hezaimi K, Warnakulasuriya S. Areca-nut chewing habit is a significant risk factor for metabolic syndrome: a systematic review. J Nutr Health Aging. 2012 May;16(5):445–8. https://doi.org/10.1007/s12603-011-0353-5.
12. Zain RB, Ikeda N, Gupta PC, Warnakulasuriya S, van Wyk CW, Shrestha P, Axéll T. Oral mucosal lesions associated with betel quid, areca nut and tobacco chewing habits: consensus from a workshop held in Kuala Lumpur, Malaysia, November 25–27, 1996. J Oral Pathol Med. 1999 Jan;28(1):1–4. https://doi.org/10.1111/j.1600-0714.1999.tb01985.x.
13. Ramanathan A, Zain RB. Associated conditions of Oral submucous fibrosis. In: Warnakulasuriya S, Ranganathan K, editors. Oral Submucous Fibrosis. A guide to diagnosis and management. Cham: Springer; 2023. p. 17–29. https://doi.org/10.1007/978-3-031-12855-4_2.
14. Berniyanti T, Jamaludin MB, Eky YE, Bramantoro T, Palupi R. Duration and frequency of betel quid chewing affects periodontitis severity and life quality of people in Tanini Village, Kupang, Indonesia. Int J Dent Hyg. 2024;22(1):229–35. https://doi.org/10.1111/idh.12749. Epub 2023 Sep 18
15. Wang M, Duan C, Wei Y, Xu X. Prevalence of oral submucous fibrosis across diverse populations: a systematic review and meta-analysis. Peer J. 2024;12:e18385. https://doi.org/10.7717/peerj.18385. PMID: 39525471; PMCID: PMC11549909
16. Ray JG, Ranganathan K, Chattopadhyay A. Malignant transformation of oral submucous fibrosis: overview of histopathological aspects. Oral Surg Oral Med Oral Pathol Oral Radiol. 2016;122(2):200–9. https://doi.org/10.1016/j.oooo.2015.11.024. Epub 2016 Apr 19
17. Warnakulasurya S. Clinical features: Oral submucous fibrosis. In: Warnakulasuriya S, Ranganathan K, editors. Oral submucous fibrosis. A guide to diagnosis and management. Cham: Springer; 2023. p. 17–29. https://doi.org/10.1007/978-3-031-12855-4_2.
18. Tilakaratne WM, Klinikowski MF, Saku T, Peters TJ, Warnakulasuriya S. Oral submucous fibrosis: review on aetiology and pathogenesis. Oral Oncol. 2006;42(6):561–8. https://doi.org/10.1016/j.oraloncology.2005.08.005. Epub 2005 Nov 28
19. Liu CJ, Lee YJ, Chang KW, Shih YN, Liu HF, Dang CW. Polymorphism of the MICA gene and risk for oral submucous fibrosis. J Oral Pathol Med. 2004 Jan;33(1):1–6. https://doi.org/10.1111/j.1600-0714.2004.00047.x.
20. Senevirathna K, Pradeep R, Jayasinghe YA, Jayawickrama SM, Illeperuma R, Warnakulasuriya S, Jayasinghe RD. Carcinogenic effects of areca nut and its metabolites: a review of the experimental evidence. Clin Pract. 2023;13(2):326–46. https://doi.org/10.3390/clinpract13020030. PMID: 36961055; PMCID: PMC10037666
21. Warnakulasuriya S, Trivedy C, Peters T. Areca nut use: an independent risk factor for oral cancer. BMJ. 2002;324:799–800.
22. Jasim A, Li X, Octavia A, Gunardi I, Crocombe L, Sari EF. The association between betel quid use and oral potentially malignant and malignant disorders in southeast Asian and Pacific regions: a systematic review and meta-analysis with GRADE evidence profile. Front Oral Health. 2024;5:1397179. https://doi.org/10.3389/froh.2024.1397179. PMID: 38846318; PMCID: PMC11153687
23. Reichart PA, Warnakulasuriya S. Oral lichenoid contact lesions induced by areca nut and betel quid chewing: a mini-review. J Investig Clin Dent. 2012;3(3):163–6. https://doi.org/10.1111/j.2041-1626.2012.00130.x.

Khat (*Catha edulis*) Chewing and Oral Health

8

Sadeq Ali Al-Maweri and Esam Saleh Halboub

8.1 Introduction

Catha edulis, commonly known as khat (or qat or chat), is an evergreen plant native to the Arabian Peninsula (mainly Yemen) and East Africa (Fig. 8.1) [1]. Khat chewing is a widespread practice in these regions, primarily due to its stimulating, amphetamine-like effects [1–3]. With increased immigration and easier trade routes, this habit has spread to other parts of the world, and it is now practised by tens of millions globally [3, 4]. The primary chemical components of khat are *cathinone* and *cathine*, along with traces of other substances, including tannins, carbohydrates, alkaloids, flavonoids and terpenoids [3]. Cathinone, the most active compound, has sympathomimetic effects similar to those of amphetamines, albeit with less potency [3, 4].

People typically chew fresh khat leaves during social gatherings, such as weddings, celebrations or casual meetings [3]. It is also commonly used by students, labourers and night guards due to its stimulating properties [1, 3]. Khat sessions usually begin after lunchtime and last for several hours. The habit generally involves chewing fresh khat leaves on one side of the mouth and holding the chewed material in the mucobuccal fold for extended periods, often for several hours each day (Fig. 8.2) [1, 3, 5].

While khat plays a significant role in the economy of certain regions, its use has been reported to be associated with several systemic health issues, including liver disease, cardiovascular disorders, gastrointestinal problems and psychological conditions [6, 7]. Moreover, long-term khat chewing has been associated with

S. A. Al-Maweri (✉)
Department of Preclinical Oral Health Sciences, College of Dental Medicine, QU Health, Qatar University, Doha, Qatar

E. S. Halboub
Department of Maxillofacial Surgery and Diagnostic Sciences, College of Dentistry, Jazan University, Jazan, Saudi Arabia

S. R. Prabhu et al. (eds.), *Lifestyle in Oral Health and Disease*,
https://doi.org/10.1007/978-3-032-05888-1_8

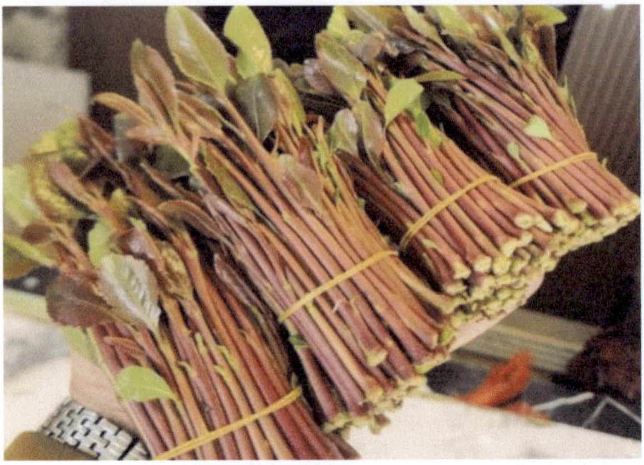

Fig. 8.1 Bunches of khat (*Catha edulis*) sold in the marketplace

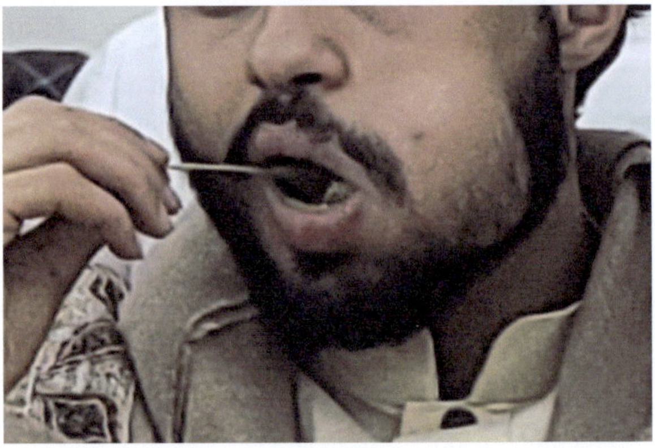

Fig. 8.2 The habitual khat user chews fresh khat leaves on one side of the mouth and holds the chewed material in the mesiobuccal fold for extended periods

numerous oral and dental health issues, including periodontal disease, mucosal lesions, tooth discolouration, tooth loss, xerostomia (dry mouth), taste changes and temporomandibular joint (TMJ) disorders [3, 8–14]. Although many studies have investigated the potential role of khat in the development of oral squamous cell carcinoma, the results remain inconclusive [15–17]. The oral and systemic health effects of khat are believed to result partly from its psychoactive components (particularly cathinone), which mimic the effects of amphetamines, as well as from the pesticides used in its cultivation [3, 6, 10]. The frictional effects of prolonged chewing also contribute to these oral health issues [18–20].

Another significant concern is the concurrent use of khat and tobacco products, including smoking, water pipe smoking (shisha) and smokeless tobacco (locally known as Shammah) [21, 22]. Research indicates that most khat chewers tend to smoke or use shisha more frequently during khat sessions, and some individuals only use tobacco while chewing khat [21]. The primary reason for combining these habits is to enhance the stimulant effects of khat [21]. Consequently, in addition to the health risks associated with khat, there is also an increased exposure to tobacco-related harms among khat chewers.

Due to the widespread use of khat, oral lesions induced by khat use are likely to be encountered worldwide. Therefore, dental practitioners, students and interns worldwide need to be aware of this habit and its potential impact on oral health. This chapter provides an overview of the epidemiology of khat chewing and its various oral and dental health consequences.

8.2 Epidemiology of Khat Chewing

The prevalence of the khat chewing habit has significantly increased over the past few decades, with an estimated tens of millions of people chewing khat daily [1–4]. This habit is prevalent in regions where khat is cultivated and/or marketed, either legally or illegally, such as East African countries (primarily Ethiopia, Eritrea, Djibouti, Somalia and Kenya) and the Arabian Peninsula, particularly Yemen and southern Saudi Arabia [1, 3]. However, due to immigration and improved transportation, khat chewing has spread rapidly beyond its countries of origin and is now practised by millions of people in various parts of the world [3, 4]. The prevalence of khat chewing varies widely between countries and even within different cities of the same country. In Yemen, khat chewing is deeply rooted in the culture, with 70% of men and 30% of women are estimated to chew khat daily [23]. Among Yemeni schoolchildren (13 to 19 years-old), the prevalence of khat chewing was estimated at 42.4% (51.4% of boys and 23.5% of girls) [2].

In Ethiopia, khat chewing is also a common practice. A recent meta-analysis reported a prevalence rate of 19.55% (95% confidence interval [CI]: 14.62–25.64%) of current khat use and a lifetime prevalence of 26.14% (95% CI: 17.66–36.87%) [1]. Khat chewing is similarly widespread in other countries, with varying reported lifetime prevalence rates: Somalia (18.3–55%) [24], South Saudi Arabia (33.2%) [25], Kenya (68%) [26] and Djibouti (90%) [3]. As mentioned earlier, the habit of khat chewing has spread beyond its traditional regions. It is now common in Europe, North America, Australia, East Asia and other African countries, primarily due to immigration from khat-producing nations [3, 4, 27].

8.3 Dental and Oral Effects of Khat Chewing

Long-term khat chewing has been linked to the development of several disorders affecting the oral and para-oral structures. These include periodontal diseases, oral mucosal alterations, defects of hard dental tissues (such as teeth discolouration and attrition), salivary dysfunction, taste impairment and masticatory system dysfunction [4] (Box 8.1).

Box 8.1: Oral Consequences of Khat

Hard tissue effects:

Dental attrition
Dental caries
Teeth discoloration
TMJ disorders

Soft tissue effects:

Keratotic white lesions
Plasma cell stomatitis
Periodontal defects
Fissured tongue
Hairy tongue
Chronic ulcers
Salivary gland disorders
Xerostomia
Taste changes

8.3.1 Dental Hard Tissues

8.3.1.1 Teeth Attrition and Discoloration

Teeth Attrition: Several studies have linked long-term khat chewing to significant damage to tooth structures [28, 29]. The continuous, repetitive chewing of khat can cause mechanical wear and tear on the teeth, potentially leading to enamel loss [28]. Numerous clinical and epidemiological studies have reported a notably high prevalence of tooth attrition among khat chewers, particularly on the side of the mouth used for chewing [28, 29]. In a study by Gibson and Hill, long-term khat chewers (those who had been chewing for more than 20 years) exhibited generalised tooth attrition on the chewing side [29]. A more recent study among Saudi khat chewers revealed a significantly higher prevalence and more severe tooth wear compared to non-chewers [28]. The attrition observed in khat chewers can be attributed to the repetitive chewing on one side of the mouth. The role of khat-induced low saliva production (hyposalivation) and the concurrent consumption of acidic beverages could be contributory as well [3, 28].

Teeth Discolouration: Khat chewing has been linked to tooth staining and discolouration of dental restorations [3]. Numerous studies have reported a significantly higher prevalence of tooth staining among khat chewers compared to non-chewers [29–31]. Additionally, a recent in vitro study found that khat extract caused the most significant colour change in composite fillings compared to other staining agents, such as Pepsi [32]. The discolouration caused by khat is attributed to tannin, a chemical compound found in khat leaves [32].

8.3.1.2 Dental Caries

The relationship between khat chewing and dental caries remains a topic of controversy. While some studies have found that khat chewing is associated with an increased prevalence of dental caries [8, 10, 12], others have found no such link [33], and one study even reported a lower prevalence of caries among khat chewers [29]. The inconsistencies in the literature regarding khat's potential role in the development of dental caries may be due to differences in methodologies, study populations, confounding factors and variations in khat chewing habits. However, it is essential to note that while khat in itself may not be cariogenic, the excessive consumption of sugary drinks (such as soda and energy drinks) along with the common practice of adding sugar to khat to mask its bitterness are significant contributing factors to dental caries, particularly cervical caries [3, 8].

8.3.1.3 TMJ and Muscles of Mastication Disorders

The connection between khat chewing and TMJ disorders, including disorders of the masticatory system, has attracted considerable attention in recent years. Numerous studies have reported long-term khat use as a risk factor for various TMJ disorders [10, 29]. The first study to document TMDs among khat chewers was conducted by Hill and Gibson, who found that 40% of khat chewers experienced TMJ pain [29]. More recent clinical and epidemiological studies have confirmed these findings, reporting a high prevalence of TMJ signs and symptoms such as pain and clicking among khat chewers [10, 29, 34]. More recent radiographic investigations, including CBCT studies, have also revealed significant radiographic changes in the TMJ of khat chewers, particularly on the chewing side, when compared to non-chewers [11, 35]. Additionally, some studies have identified a significant association between the severity of TMJ disorders and the frequency and duration of khat chewing [35]. These findings can be attributed to the continuous and repetitive chewing, which places excessive strain on the TMJ and masticatory system, resulting in macro- and microstructural changes to the TMJ tissues and its supporting structures [11, 34, 35].

8.3.2 Periodontal Diseases

The most investigated topic regarding the impact of khat chewing on oral tissues is its effects on periodontal health. Despite the controversy that covers this issue, most of the studies conducted so far confirm that khat chewing exerts deteriorative effects on the periodontium, presenting as clinical attachment loss and gingival recession confined mainly to the chewing side (Fig. 8.3), reflective of the mechanical effects of the khat bolus that is kept for long hours therein [12, 36–39].

One study employed the 'experimental gingivitis model', where khat chewers volunteered not to brush their teeth or use mouthwashes for 20 days [40]. The scores of the plaque index were lower on the chewing side compared to non-chewing side, and among chewers compared to non-chewers. The differences were significant at day 20. Although their baseline gingival inflammation indices were higher, the chewers and chewing sides showed significantly lower scores of gingival bleeding on the probing index at days 10 and 20. The claimed beneficial effect of khat chewing was evident on both the lingual and buccal aspects. The study concluded that the khat chewing habit has anti-plaque and anti-gingivitis properties rather than being detrimental to the periodontium [40]. Some observational studies support such findings [13, 30, 37].

Nevertheless, a systematic review and meta-analysis of 12 relevant studies revealed worse periodontal health among khat chewers compared to non-chewers, and in the chewing side compared to the non-chewing side in terms of periodontal pocket depth, attachment loss and gingival recession. [41]. Another systematic review (without meta-analysis) that included 10 relevant studies reported a higher risk of periodontal disease among khat chewers, as reflected by higher measurements of attachment loss and gingival recession [42]. The study concluded that such detrimental effects of khat chewing on the periodontium outweigh its beneficial antimicrobial properties [42].

It appears that the mechanical effect exerted by the khat bolus, which is kept in place on one side of the mouth against the buccal and alveolar mucosae and gingiva for prolonged periods, causes gingival recession, ultimately leading to attachment loss (Fig. 8.3) [42]. At the same time, this mechanical effect also has a cleansing effect, reducing plaque accumulation and making it less pathogenic. Many microbiological studies that harvested microbial samples from the gingival sulci of khat chewers and non-chewers, as well as from chewing and non-chewing sides, revealed a decrease in the colonisation of gingival plaque by periodontal pathogens, which are known as causative factors for periodontal disease [39, 43, 44]. Furthermore, these studies reported that khat promotes the presence of species compatible with periodontal health, similar to the effects of prebiotics on intestinal microflora [39, 43]. Other effects on periodontium associated with khat chewing have been documented, like periodontal pockets [36], plaque accumulation [38] and tooth loss [12, 33].

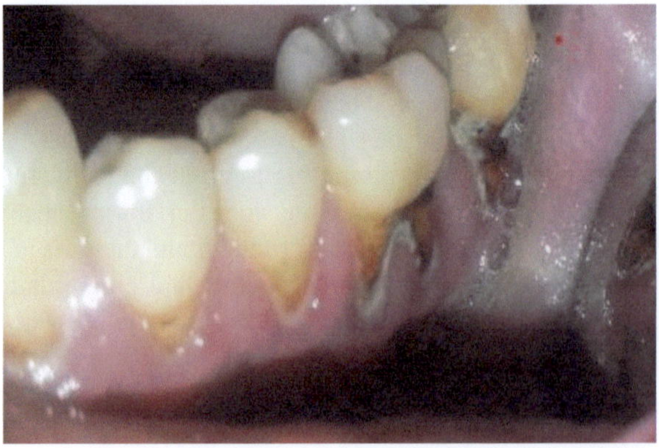

Fig. 8.3 Gingival recession in a khat chewer

8.3.3 Oral Mucosal Lesions

There is compelling evidence that khat chewing induces keratotic white lesions at the site of chewing (Fig. 8.4a, b). In a large cross-sectional study involving Yemeni adults, 343 cases of keratotic white lesions were identified among 1528 khat chewers, representing 22.4%, compared to only 6 cases (0.6%) among 978 non-khat chewers. The reported odds ratio was strikingly high (46.43), which strengthened their argument that khat chewing can provoke the development of oral keratotic white lesions at the site of chewing, whose prevalence and severity increase with duration and frequency of the habit [20]. Other research on Yemenis [18, 45, 46], Yemeni Jews [19, 30], Ethiopians [47] and the Kenyan people [48] supports such an association.

Clinically, these white lesions vary from merely homogeneous, transparent whitening to coarse, irregular and even corrugated lesions (Fig. 8.4a, b). This variability may reflect the maturity of the lesion, secondary to the frequency and duration of khat chewing. Mostly, these lesions are diffused and not well-demarcated. The most affected sites in ascending order of occurrence are the buccal mucosa, lower buccal vestibule, upper buccal vestibule and buccal gingiva of the chewing side [18–20, 30, 45].

The white appearance of these lesions is attributed to the production of keratin and thickening of the epithelium secondary to hyperplasia and acanthosis [48–50]. These changes are believed to be protective mechanisms. Hence, the diagnostic terms of 'frictional keratosis' or 'khat-induced white lesion' are used. Additionally, khat chewing was found to be associated with increased intracellular oedema [48–50], melanin pigment deposits and an increased number of thin and deep rete pegs [48].

Another oral lesion believed to be khat-induced is plasma cell mucositis/gingivitis, although it has been documented only in case reports. These patients reported a complaint of a burning sensation with recurrent bleeding of the affected site. Clinically, the lesions appear to be widespread, involving a large area on the chewing side, with a velvety texture and ranging from erythematous to ulcerative. Histopathologically, the lesions are characterised by a dense chronic inflammatory infiltrate dominated by plasma cells. Further evaluations excluded all other potential

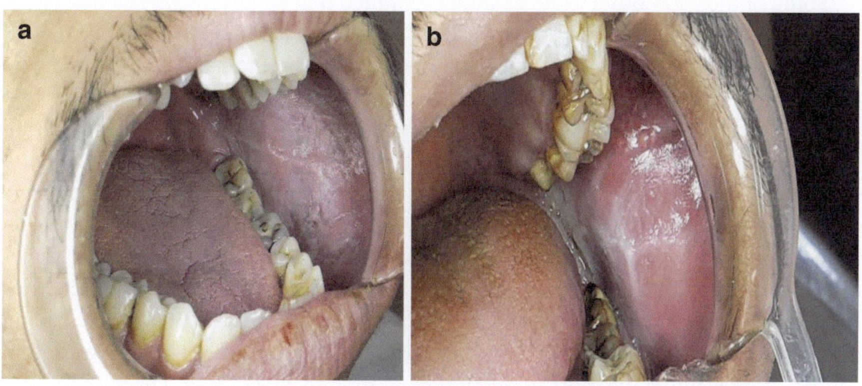

Fig. 8.4 (**a** and **b**) Keratotic white lesions on the buccal mucosa in habitual khat chewers

diseases, confirming the clinicopathological diagnosis of plasma cell mucositis/gingivitis [9, 51, 52]. Based on our experience with these lesions, no improvement can be achieved, even with a high dose of prednisolone (1–2 mg/kg body weight), unless the patient stops chewing khat. However, upon cessation of khat use, recovery is inevitable and typically occurs within two to several weeks, even without the need for topical or systemic corticosteroids. Recurrence has been observed in cases where patients resume chewing khat.

Another crucial soft tissue lesion associated with khat chewing, as noted recently, is deep ulceration at the site of chewing. Many young adults with a history of long-term khat chewing present with deep ulcers confined mainly to the posterior buccal mucosa, the retromolar pad area and the anterior tonsillar pillar. Although these ulcers may appear frightening to both patients and dentists, they are symptomless. However, we reported a case of deep ulcers associated with severe bleeding. The healing of these ulcers was not possible without quitting khat chewing [53].

Other, but less frequent, oral lesions or conditions associated with khat chewing included hairy tongue, fissured tongue, benign tumours and traumatic ulcers [5, 14, 54]. Although Yarom et al. found a higher prevalence of oral pigmented lesions among Yemeni Jewish khat chewers [30], and Lukandu OM et al. confirmed the presence of melanin deposits in biopsies taken from the chewing sides of Kenyan khat chewers [48], one recent large-scale study in Yemen failed to correlate khat chewing with the diagnosed cases of pigmentation [2].

8.3.4 Oral Potentially Malignant Lesions and Oral Cancer

The link between khat chewing and cancers, including oral cancer, remains controversial. A large fraction of the basic medical research in this respect supports the notion that khat is cytotoxic, teratogenic and hence carcinogenic. Numerous observational studies support this hypothesis, indicating a higher incidence of oral cancer among khat chewers, particularly long-term chewers. Further support comes from sporadic case reports. This controversy is detailed below.

Some of the early observational studies claimed that khat chewing is a risk factor for the development of oral cancer, while others didn't. Although Ibrahim E M et al. (1986) diagnosed 64 patients with squamous cell carcinoma, 52 of them were Shammah (a form of smokeless tobacco) users, in contrast to only 22 who were khat chewers. This matter may invalidate their conclusion [55]. Another study by Soufi HE et al. (1991), included 28 patients with squamous cell carcinoma, reached a similar conclusion. They based their conclusion solely on the presence of 10 patients with a history of khat chewing [56]. Nasr AH and Khatri ML (2000) reported 36 Yemeni patients with head and neck cancers, of whom 30 patients were khat chewers. Given that all patients with oral cancer were khat chewers, the authors considered it a significant contributing factor [57]. Upon reviewing hospital-based data on 649 primary cancers in Yemen, Sawair et al. (2004) found that 149 cases were oral cancers, representing the most frequent type of malignancy (23%). The authors suggested that khat may be a predisposing factor given that up to 60% of these patients were khat chewers [58]. In one study, 6 cases of cellular atypia and 24 cases of parakeratosis were identified in cytological smears collected from the khat chewing side of 150 khat chewers, with no single case of such changes identified in cytological smears collected from 150 non-khat chewers. The study concluded that khat chewing contributes to the development of cytological atypia that might develop to oral potentially malignant lesions or even malignant lesions [17]. A recent study recruited 83 khat chewers affected with oral squamous cell carcinoma (41 were short-term khat chewers, with a duration of less than 20 years, and 42 were long-term khat chewers, with a duration of more than 20 years), as well as 30 subjects as healthy controls. The DNA analyses of samples from the peripheral blood revealed seven somatic mutations in four out of nine cancer-related genes among short-term khat chewers and nine somatic mutations in five out of nine cancer-related genes among long-term khat chewers. Hence, the study concluded that khat is a mutagenic and carcinogenic plant provoking oral squamous cell carcinoma. However, it is worth mentioning that 42% of khat chewers reported being smokers [15].

In contrast, other studies claimed no role for khat chewing in the development of oral cancer. Furthermore, one study reported protective effect against the carcinogenicity induced by Shammah among dual users [16]. Hill CM and Gibson A (1987) failed to report any detrimental impact on the oral tissues as a consequence of khat chewing other than benign keratosis on the buccal mucosa [29]. In a study involving 803 Kenyan adults, leucoplakia was diagnosed in 85 patients (10.6%). In terms of predisposing factors, 8.3% of these leukoplakias were tobacco-induced, and 2.2% were idiopathic, indicating no role for khat chewing [59]. The authors of the previous study took this one step further in another case–control study, in which these 85 patients with leucoplakia were matched with 141 controls. The results confirmed the role of tobacco, but no any role for traditional beer, khat or chillies [60]. As mentioned earlier, a large cross-sectional study in Yemen involving 2500 adults, 1528 of whom were khat chewers, failed to report a single case of oral cancer or even an oral potentially malignant lesion [20].

Most of the evidence on the deleterious effects of khat came from basic research at the cellular level, where khat is considered carcinogenic/toxic. Research on the impact of khat extract on primary normal human oral keratinocytes and fibroblasts has shown that khat induces apoptotic cell death through its early effect on mechanisms that increase intracellular reactive oxygen species while depleting glutathione, a potent antioxidant molecule. It was postulated that khat induces stress in these cells, resulting in morphological changes and G1 phase arrest of the cell cycle, with increased concentrations of p53, p21 and p16, which are suggestive of senescence related to cellular differentiation, especially in the keratinocyte cycle. Further research on the topic revealed a novel, mitochondria-mediated mechanism associated with the loss of mitochondrial membrane potential upon exposure to khat extract for 0.5 to 1 h. This effect is claimed to be closely linked to the survival of the cells. In an attempt to take it one step further, research has focused on reconstructed human oral mucosa, with results indicating that khat induces toxic effects, including premature differentiation, senescence and abnormal keratinisation [61–64].

There is a case report linking khat chewing and oral cancer. A 42-year-old Kenyan female khat chewer presented with a speckled, red and white ulcerated lesion on the left floor of the mouth, measuring 1.5 cm in diameter, discoid in shape, with a slightly rolled border. The histopathology revealed squamous cell carcinoma. The authors debated that such a relatively early presentation of oral squamous cell carcinoma may be linked to the synergistic effect of khat chewing. However, the patient reported smoking (30–40 cigarettes a day for 15 years) and alcohol consumption of approximately 50 units (25 standard drinks) per week [65]. A recent case report linked khat with extensive erythroplakia involving the whole buccal mucosa and half of the tongue on the chewing side [66]. The histopathology report claimed the presence of dysplasia, although it was considered doubtful from our perspective. Instead, the lesion mimics the plasma cell mucositis, as mentioned above.

To sum up, the evidence for the notion that khat is a risk factor for oral cancer and potentially malignant oral lesions is very weak and further well-designed research is warranted [67].

8.3.5 Salivary and Taste Functions

The detrimental effects of khat chewing on saliva and salivary glands have been established in the literature [3, 10, 68]. Khat chewers have been found to have a higher prevalence of xerostomia compared to non-chewers [5, 10, 14, 30, 34]. Interestingly, some studies also found a significant association between the severity of mouth dryness and the frequency and duration of chewing [69]. Khat-induced xerostomia is attributed to the parasympathetic action of khat chemical components, mainly cathinone [68]. Additionally, the direct effect of khat's chemical elements on the salivary glands has also been suggested [68, 70]. For example, one experimental study on mice reported that khat extracts caused significant degeneration and alterations in the secretory cells of the submandibular glands [70].

Taste Functions: Studies on the effect of khat on taste functions are minimal. Two studies found a higher prevalence of self-reported taste impairment among khat chewers compared to control subjects [10, 34]. A recent study investigated the effects of khat chewing on the taste threshold using four primary tastes: sweet, salty, sour and bitter [69]. The results revealed significantly lower mean taste sensation scores for sweet, salty and bitter tastants among khat chewers as compared to non-chewers [69]. Additionally, 20% of chewers were found to have hypogeusia compared to only 4.5% of non-chewers [69]. The plausible explanation for the taste impairment among khat chewers is hyposalivation, a common adverse effect of khat chewing [68]. Saliva plays a vital role in taste perception by dissolving food and stimulating the taste buds, in addition to its chemical components, such as salivary growth factors (Gustin), which are crucial for the homeostasis and integrity of the taste buds [69]. Another possible explanation is the direct effect of khat's chemical components (mainly cathinone) and/or chemical pesticides on the taste buds [69].

Regarding the effect of khat on smell, the literature is scarce in this regard, and to date, no published studies have explored the effects of khat on the olfactory system.

8.4 Concurrent Use of Khat and Tobacco Products

One of the significant concerns regarding khat chewing is the concurrent use of tobacco. Khat users often tend to smoke or use other forms of tobacco, such as shisha or smokeless tobacco, during their chewing sessions. Research indicates that approximately 64% of khat chewers are also smokers, and they tend to consume more cigarettes while chewing khat [21]. Additionally, some chewers, particularly women, may use shisha or other tobacco products exclusively during khat chewing, which increases the associated health risks [21]. A recent systematic review and meta-analysis on the risk factors for smoking among Ethiopian adults found that khat chewers are 7.99 times more likely to smoke cigarettes compared to non-chewers [22]. This highlights the strong association between khat chewing and smoking, indicating that khat chewing may act as a gateway to tobacco consumption [21, 22]. The simultaneous use of khat and tobacco presents a significant public health challenge, as it synergises the adverse effects on both systemic and oral health [22]. While khat itself has harmful effects, it also encourages individuals to adopt other risky habits, such as tobacco use, which exacerbates the negative health outcomes of both behaviours [21, 22]. The combined impact of khat chewing and tobacco use increases the risk of severe health conditions, including cardiovascular diseases, respiratory issues and various cancers, including oral cancer [21].

References

1. Ayano G, Ayalew M, Bedaso A, Duko B. Epidemiology of Khat (Catha edulis) chewing in Ethiopia: a systematic review and meta-analysis. J Psychoactive Drugs. 2024;56(1):40–9.
2. Al-Maweri SA, Alhajj MN, Al-Soneidar WA, Shamala A, Alkadasi BA, Amran AG, Abu-Lohom F, Al-Sharani HM, Basalamah MA, Al-Muaalemi Z, et al. Tobacco use and khat chewing among adolescents in Yemen: a large-scale school-based cross-sectional study. BMC Public Health. 2024;24(1):2406.
3. Al-Maweri SA, Warnakulasuriya S. Samran A: Khat (Catha edulis) and its oral health effects: an updated review. J Investig Clin Dent. 2018;9(1)
4. Nakajima M, Molla K, Belachew B, Mohammed A, Hassan A, Kroll J, Al'Absi M. Khat use is associated with tobacco, alcohol, and illicit drug use: a cross-sectional examination in the United States. J Psychoactive Drugs. 2017;49(5):413–9.
5. Al-Maweri SA, Alaizari NA, Al-Sufyani GA. Oral mucosal lesions and their association with tobacco use and qat chewing among Yemeni dental patients. J Clin Exp Dent. 2014;6(5):e460–6.
6. Nigussie T, Gobena T, Mossie A. Association between khat chewing and gastrointestinal disorders: a cross sectional study. Ethiop J Health Sci. 2013;23(2):123–30.
7. Alsanosy R, Mahfouz MS, Arishi AM, Abdelwahab SI, Taha M, Albasheer O, Daghriri HM, Majrashi KA, Farasani A, Altraifi AAA, et al. Risk of acute coronary syndrome and relationship with the use of khat and tobacco products in the Jazan region, Saudi Arabia: a prospective case-control study. Tob Induc Dis. 2024:22.

8. Halboub E, Alamri AA, Kamili G, Alqahtani AS. Dental caries experience among qat chewers in dental college clinics, Jazan, Saudi Arabia. BMC Oral Health. 2023;23(1):114.
9. Tailor A, Pemberton MN, Murphy R, Hegarty AM. Plasma cell mucositis related to qat chewing: a report of 2 cases and review of the literature. Oral Surg Oral Med Oral Pathol Oral Radiol. 2021;131(3):e65–70.
10. Bennani A, Mohamed S. Effect of Khat consumption on oral health: study carried out in Djibouti City. Oral Health Dental Sci. 2021;5(1):1–8.
11. Almashraqi AA, Barngkgei I, Halboub ES, Al-Maweri SA, Al-Wesabi MA, Al-Kamel A, Alhammadi MS, Alamir AH. Cone beam computed tomography findings in the temporomandibular joints of chronic qat chewers: radiographic bone density and trabecular microstructural analyses. Oral Surg Oral Med Oral Pathol Oral Radiol. 2021;132(4):465–74.
12. Noman NA, Aladimi AA, Alkadasi BA, Alraawi MA, Al-Iryani GM, Shaabi FI, Khalid A, Moaleem MMA. Social habits and other risk factors that cause tooth loss: an associative study conducted in Taiz Governorate, Yemen. J Contemp Dent Pract. 2019;20(4):428–33.
13. Al-Alimi A, Halboub E, Al-Sharabi AK, Taiyeb-Ali T, Jaafar N, Al-Hebshi NN. Independent determinants of periodontitis in Yemeni adults: a case-control study. Int J Dent Hyg. 2018;16(4):503–11.
14. Al-Maweri SA, Al-Jamaei AA, Al-Sufyani GA, Tarakji B, Shugaa-Addin B. Oral mucosal lesions in elderly dental patients in Sana'a, Yemen. J Int Soc Prev Community Dent. 2015;5(Suppl 1):S12–9.
15. Alshahrani SA, Al-Qahtani WS, Almufareh NA, Domiaty DM, Albasher GI, Safhi FA, AlQassim FA, Alotaibi MA, Al-Hazani TM, Almutlaq BA. Oral cancer among Khat users: finding evidence from DNA analysis of nine cancer-related gene mutations. BMC Oral Health. 2021;21(1):626.
16. Quadri MF, Alharbi F, Bajonaid AM, Moafa IH, Sharwani AA, Alamir AH. Oral squamous cell carcinoma and associated risk factors in Jazan, Saudi Arabia: a hospital based case control study. Asian Pac J Cancer Prev. 2015;16(10):4335–8.
17. Ahmed HG, Omer AS, Abd Algaffar SA. Cytological study of exfoliative buccal mucosal cells of Qat chewers in Yemen. Diagn Cytopathol. 2011;39(11):796–800.
18. Al-Maweri SA, Al-Jamaei A, Saini R, Laronde DM, Sharhan A. White oral mucosal lesions among the Yemeni population and their relation to local oral habits. J Investig Clin Dent. 2018;9(2):e12305.
19. Gorsky M, Epstein JB, Levi H, Yarom N. Oral white lesions associated with chewing khat. Tob Induc Dis. 2004;2(3):145–50.
20. Ali AA, Al-Sharabi AK, Aguirre JM, Nahas R. A study of 342 oral keratotic white lesions induced by qat chewing among 2500 Yemeni. J Oral Pathol Med. 2004;33(6):368–72.
21. Kassim S, Jawad M, Croucher R, Akl EA. The epidemiology of tobacco use among Khat users: a systematic review. Biomed Res Int. 2015;2015:313692.
22. Tegegne KT. Khat chewing as a risk factor of cigarette smoking in Ethiopia Systemic review and meta-analysis. EC Psychology and Psychiatry. 2021;10:69–78.
23. Nakajima M, Al'Absi M, Dokam A, Alsoofi M, Khalil NS, Al Habori M. Gender differences in patterns and correlates of khat and tobacco use. Nicotine Tob Res. 2013;15(6):1130–5.
24. Elmi AS. The chewing of khat in Somalia. J Ethnopharmacol. 1983;8(2):163–76.
25. Mahfouz MS, Rahim BE, Solan YM, Makeen AM, Alsanosy RM. Khat chewing habits in the population of the Jazan Region, Saudi Arabia: prevalence and associated factors. PLoS One. 2015;10(8):e0134545.
26. Njuguna J, Olieva S, Muruka C, Owek C. Khat consumption in Masalani town, northeastern Kenya. J Psychoactive Drugs. 2013;45(4):355–9.
27. Young JT, Butt J, Hersi A, Tohow A, Mohamed DH. Khat dependence, use patterns, and health consequences in Australia: an exploratory study. J Stud Alcohol Drugs. 2016;77(2):343–8.
28. Sayed ME, Hamdi AD, Hakami BM, Mugri MH, Bhandi SH. Tooth wear patterns among Khat and Shammah users in Jazan City, Kingdom of Saudi Arabia: a cross-sectional survey. J Contemp Dent Pract. 2017;18(6):429–36.

29. Hill CM, Gibson A. The oral and dental effects of q'at chewing. Oral Surg Oral Med Oral Pathol. 1987;63(4):433–6.
30. Yarom N, Epstein J, Levi H, Porat D, Kaufman E, Gorsky M. Oral manifestations of habitual khat chewing: a case-control study. Oral Surg Oral Med Oral Pathol Oral Radiol Endod. 2010;109(6):e60–6.
31. Al-Kholani AI. Influence of Khat chewing on periodontal tissues and oral hygiene status among Yemenis. Dent Res J (Isfahan). 2010;7(1):1–6.
32. Al-Anesi WA, Madfa AA, Dubais MA, Albahari AA. Effects of khat extract and other staining media on color change of composite resins subjected to various polishing methods. Mater Sci. 2019;7(1):10.7243.
33. Halboub E, Dhaifullah E, Yasin R. Determinants of dental health status and dental health behavior among Sana'a University students, Yemen. J Investig Clin Dent. 2013;4(4):257–64.
34. Astatkie A, Demissie M, Berhane Y, Worku A. Oral symptoms significantly higher among long-term khat (Catha edulis) users in Ethiopia. Epidemiol Health. 2015;37:e2015009.
35. Almashraqi AA, Halboub ES, Al-Maweri SA, Barngkgei I, Al-Wesabi MA, Al-Kamel A, Alhammadi MS, Alamir AH. Cone beam computed tomography findings in temporomandibular joint of chronic qat chewers: dimensional and osteoarthritic changes. J Oral Rehabil. 2020;47(12):1538–49.
36. Dhaifullah E, Al-Maweri SA, Al-Motareb F, Halboub E, Elkhatat E, Baroudi K, Tarakji B. Periodontal health condition and associated factors among University Students, Yemen. J Clin Diagn Res. 2015;9(12):ZC30–33.
37. Al-Sharabi AK, Shuga-Aldin H, Ghandour I, Al-Hebshi NN. Qat chewing as an independent risk factor for periodontitis: a cross-sectional study. Int J Dent. 2013;2013:317640.
38. Al-Maweri SA, AlAkhali M. Oral hygiene and periodontal health status among khat chewers. A case-control study. J Clin Exp Dent. 2017;9(5):e629–34.
39. Al-Alimi A, Taiyeb-Ali T, Jaafar N, Al-hebshi NN. Qat chewing and periodontal pathogens in health and disease: further evidence for a prebiotic-like effect. Biomed Res Int. 2015;2015:291305.
40. Al-hebshi NN, Al-ak'hali MS. Experimental gingivitis in male khat (Catha edulis) chewers. J Int Acad Periodontol. 2010;12(2):56–62.
41. Al-Akhali MS, Al-Moraissi EA. Khat chewing habit produces a significant adverse effect on periodontal, oral health: a systematic review and meta-analysis. J Periodontal Res. 2017;52(6):937–45.
42. Kalakonda B, Al-Maweri SA, Al-Shamiri HM, Ijaz A, Gamal S, Dhaifullah E. Is Khat (Catha edulis) chewing a risk factor for periodontal diseases? A systematic review. J Clin Exp Dent. 2017;9(10):e1264–70.
43. Al-Hebshi NN, Al-Sharabi AK, Shuga-Aldin HM, Al-Haroni M, Ghandour I. Effect of khat chewing on periodontal pathogens in subgingival biofilm from chronic periodontitis patients. J Ethnopharmacol. 2010;132(3):564–9.
44. Al-Hebshi NN, Skaug N. Effect of khat chewing on 14 selected periodontal bacteria in sub- and supragingival plaque of a young male population. Oral Microbiol Immunol. 2005;20(3):141–6.
45. Halboub E, Dhaifullah E, Abdulhuq M. Khat chewing and smoking effect on oral mucosa: a clinical study. Acta Medica (Hradec Kralove). 2009;52(4):155–8.
46. Hijazi M, Jentsch H, Al-Sanabani J, Tawfik M, Remmerbach TW. Clinical and cytological study of the oral mucosa of smoking and non-smoking qat chewers in Yemen. Clin Oral Investig. 2016;20(4):771–9.
47. Demissie S, Mekonen S, Awoke T, Teshome B, Mengistie B. Prevalence of arsenic-induced skin lesions and associated factors in Ethiopia: community-based study. Toxicol Rep. 2023;11:153–61.
48. Lukandu OM, Koech LS, Kiarie PN. Oral lesions induced by chronic Khat use consist essentially of thickened hyperkeratinized epithelium. Int J Dent. 2015;2015:104812.
49. Ali AA. Histopathologic changes in oral mucosa of Yemenis addicted to water-pipe and cigarette smoking in addition to takhzeen al-qat. Oral Surg Oral Med Oral Pathol Oral Radiol Endod. 2007;103(3):e55–9.

50. Ali AA, Al-Sharabi AK, Aguirre JM. Histopathological changes in oral mucosa due to takhzeen al-qat: a study of 70 biopsies. J Oral Pathol Med. 2006;35(2):81–5.
51. Al-ak'hali MS, Al-haddad KA, Al-hebshi NN. Oral plasma-cell mucositis exacerbated by qat chewing – a case series. Saudi J Dent Res. 2015;6:60–6.
52. Marker P, Krogdahl A. Plasma cell gingivitis apparently related to the use of khat: report of a case. Br Dent J. 2002;192(6):311–3.
53. Halboub E, Alkadasi B, Saif E, Almurisi E, Abdulrab S. Extensive and deep oropharyngeal ulcerations induced by Qat chewing: a case report. Authorea. Authorea. 2025;
54. Gazal G. Surgical removal for khat inducible verruca vulgaris lesion of the oral mucosa. Niger J Clin Pract. 2019;22(3):439–41.
55. Ibrahim EM, Satti MB, Al Idrissi HY, Higazi MM, Magbool GM, Al Quorain A. Oral cancer in Saudi Arabia: the role of alqat and alshammah. Cancer Detect Prev. 1986;9(3-4):215–8.
56. Soufi HE, Kameswaran M, Malatani T. Khat and oral cancer. J Laryngol Otol. 1991;105(8):643–5.
57. Nasr AH, Khatri ML. Head and neck squamous cell carcinoma in Hajjah, Yemen. Saudi Med J. 2000;21(6):565–8.
58. Sawair FA, Al-Mutwakel A, Al-Eryani K, Al-Surhy A, Maruyama S, Cheng J, Al-Sharabi A, Saku T. High relative frequency of oral squamous cell carcinoma in Yemen: qat and tobacco chewing as its aetiological background. Int J Environ Health Res. 2007;17(3):185–95.
59. Macigo FG, Mwaniki DL, Guthua SW. Prevalence of oral mucosal lesions in a Kenyan population with special reference to oral leukoplakia. East Afr Med J. 1995;72(12):778–82.
60. Macigo FG, Mwaniki DL, Guthua SW. The association between oral leukoplakia and use of tobacco, alcohol and khat based on relative risks assessment in Kenya. Eur J Oral Sci. 1995;103(5):268–73.
61. Lukandu OM, Bredholt T, Neppelberg E, Gjertsen BT, Johannessen AC, Vintermyr OK, Costea DE. Early loss of mitochondrial inner transmembrane potential in khat-induced cell death of primary normal human oral cells. Toxicology. 2009;263(2-3):108–16.
62. Lukandu OM, Costea DE, Dimba EA, Neppelberg E, Bredholt T, Gjertsen BT, Vintermyr OK, Johannessen AC. Khat induces G1-phase arrest and increased expression of stress-sensitive p53 and p16 proteins in normal human oral keratinocytes and fibroblasts. Eur J Oral Sci. 2008;116(1):23–30.
63. Lukandu OM, Costea DE, Neppelberg E, Johannessen AC, Vintermyr OK. Khat (Catha edulis) induces reactive oxygen species and apoptosis in normal human oral keratinocytes and fibroblasts. Toxicol Sci. 2008;103(2):311–24.
64. Lukandu OM, Neppelberg E, Vintermyr OK, Johannessen AC, Costea DE. Khat alters the phenotype of in vitro-reconstructed human oral mucosa. J Dent Res. 2010;89(3):270–5.
65. Fasanmade A, Kwok E, Newman L. Oral squamous cell carcinoma associated with khat chewing. Oral Surg Oral Med Oral Pathol Oral Radiol Endod. 2007;104(1):e53–5.
66. Al-Jamaei AAH, Al-Kebsi K, Al-Qafaf E, Hanash MHM, Subramanyam RV, de Visscher JGAM. Habitual khat chewing induced oral erythroplakia: a case report. Oral Oncol Rep. 2024;9(March):100230.
67. El-Zaemey S, Schuz J, Leon ME. Qat chewing and risk of potentially malignant and malignant oral disorders: a systematic review. Int J Occup Environ Med. 2015;6(3):129–43.
68. Al-Alimi KR, Razak AAA, Saub R. Salivary caries parameters: comparative study among Yemeni khat chewers and nonchewers. J Dent Sci. 2014;9(4):328–31.
69. Al-Akwa'a OM, Al-Hajri MM, ALHowshabi AM, Al-Maweri SA, Halboub E. Effects of khat (Catha edulis) chewing on dry mouth and taste function: a comparative cross-sectional study. Oral Surg Oral Med Oral Pathol Oral Radiol. 2025;140(3):291–9. https://doi.org/10.1016/j.oooo.2025.03.016. Epub 2025 Apr 11. PMID: 40393882.
70. Al-Qadhi G, Mubarak R. Qualitative ultrastructural analysis of the submandibular salivary glands after administration of khat: in vivo study. BMC Res Notes. 2021;14(1):180.

9 Impact of Chewing Gum on Oral Health

Faiez Najeeb Hattab

9.1 Introduction

People worldwide have chewed on natural materials for hundreds of years. Some of these materials include thickened resin and latex from certain types of trees, as well as various sweet grasses, leaves, grains and waxes. Today, chewing gum is one of the most common candies globally, especially among teenagers. It is estimated that the global chewing gum market is approximately 560,000 tons per year, valued at around $5 billion, with international sales of approximately 374 billion chewing sticks per year [1]. Drug delivery vehicles with short treatment cycles and low side effects have always been an attractive target in medicine and pharmaceuticals. Among them, chewing gum has shown promise in delivering dental and oral health medications. Compared to other oral therapeutic products, its advantage is that individual compliance is higher [2, 3]. The water-soluble substances in chewing gum are released completely and rapidly, and methods for delaying their release can be employed to provide extended-release characteristics. Gum bases are often hydrophobic, which can alter the release rate of the loaded drug [2]. The basic ingredients of chewing gum are gum base (25–35%; polymers, plasticisers and resins); sweeteners (40–50%; sugar alcohols or polyols (sorbitol, xylitol or mannitol)); softeners (2–15%; glycerine or vegetable oil); flavours (1.5–3%; mint, fruit, spearmint, menthol); and colourants [3]. Softeners are used to blend ingredients and prevent the gum from becoming hard or stiff. Today, synthetic materials have replaced natural gum ingredients to provide chewing gum with better quality, texture and taste.

Chewing gum was initially sweetened with sugar, which can cause dental caries. Today, however, more than 50% of chewing gum sold in Europe is sweetened with sugar substitutes [1]. Clinical evidence shows that chewing gum containing sugar substitutes does not cause caries because plaque bacteria do not metabolise them to produce acid by-products. It is widely accepted that saliva plays a crucial protective

F. N. Hattab (✉)
Oskar-Maria-Graf-Ring, Munich, Germany

S. R. Prabhu et al. (eds.), *Lifestyle in Oral Health and Disease*,
https://doi.org/10.1007/978-3-032-05888-1_9

role in preventing the development of dental caries and periodontal disease [1, 4–6]. Chewing gums labelled 'Safe for teeth' or 'Tooth-friendly' are sweetened with sugar substitutes, mainly sorbitol, xylitol or mannitol. The American Dental Association (ADA) recommends brushing twice daily with fluoride toothpaste, interdental cleaning and chewing sugar-free gum to reduce the risk of tooth decay [4]. This chapter highlights and updates the use of chewing gum to promote oral and dental health based on research data from the past 40 years. Nicotine-containing chewing gum (Nicorette®) was the first medicated gum marketed in Switzerland (1976) to aid in smoking cessation.

9.2 Function of Chewing Gum

Chewing gum is a natural or synthetic resin that is typically sweetened and flavoured with various ingredients. There are four main types of chewing gum: (i) sugar-containing chewing gum, (ii) sugar-free chewing gum, (iii) coated chewing gum and (iv) medicated chewing gum. The primary benefit of chewing gum is its ability to enhance the function of the salivary glands. The mechanical action of chewing gum stimulates these glands, accelerating the flow of saliva and increasing its secretion by 10–12 times compared to unstimulated saliva. The flavours in the gum can activate taste receptors on the tongue, further boosting saliva production. Saliva plays a vital role in preventing dental caries by removing bacteria and food particles from the mouth, inhibiting plaque formation, neutralising plaque acidity, promoting the remineralisation of early enamel lesions, controlling enamel demineralisation, exhibiting antibacterial action and maintaining an environment saturated with calcium and phosphate, while providing a buffering system (bicarbonate, phosphate, and protein) [3–5]. Each time fermentable carbohydrates (primarily sugars) are consumed from food and beverages, the pH of dental plaque decreases due to acid production by bacteria. Following these cycles, chewing sugar-free gum significantly enhances saliva function [6–8]. Chewing gum is recommended for individuals with poor oral hygiene, those with physical and mental disabilities, patients at risk of dental caries and gingivitis and patients with low salivation due to radiation therapy for head and neck cancers and medications with antisialagogue effects, such as antipsychotics, antidepressants and antihistamines [9, 10].

Various therapeutic agents have been incorporated into chewing gum to promote oral and dental health. These include antiplaque/antibacterial agents (chlorhexidine [CHX], eucalyptus, mastic, sodium bicarbonate, zinc acetate), anticaries agents (fluoride (F), chlorhexidine (CHX), calcium phosphate), antigingivitis agents (CHX, hydrogen peroxide, sodium bicarbonate, vitamin C, eucalyptus and herbal extracts), anti-oral candidiasis agents (nystatin, clotrimazole, fluconazole), teeth whitening agents (hydrogen peroxide, carbamide peroxide, sodium bicarbonate, citric acid, malic acid, silica) and anti-hyposalivation agents (mint, methylcellulose). Adding CHX to chewing gum serves as an attractive supplement to conventional oral hygiene measures. The antiplaque properties of CHX are more effective than those of other antimicrobial agents used in mouthwashes due to a higher retention rate and greater sustainability. In a clinical trial involving elderly individuals living in residential homes, subjects who chewed two pieces of CHX/xylitol gum for 15 min per day showed a significant ($P < 0.001$) decrease in plaque and gingival indices after 12 months compared to the control group [11]. Most commercially available fluoridated chewing gums contain 0.25 mg of fluoride (as sodium fluoride, NaF) per gum stick. Almost all fluoride in the gum is released within the first 30 min of chewing, with peak fluoride release occurring after 5 min [8, 12]. Co-administration of CHX and fluoride resulted in higher diffusion rates in human tooth enamel compared to CHX alone [13]. This synergistic effect of CHX with fluoride in caries prevention has been demonstrated [14]. In situ studies have shown that chewing sugar-free gum after meals can reduce the development of dental caries. A 2-year study of 547 schoolchildren in Budapest found that children who chewed sorbitol gum for 20 min after meals had a 38.7. 7% reduction in dental caries increments compared to a control group without gum [15].

9.3 Sugar-Containing Chewing Gum

In contrast to beneficial sugar-free gum, clinical trials have shown that sugar-containing gum can increase the incidence of dental caries by promoting plaque growth, bacterial colonisation and a drop in plaque pH below the critical level of 5.5, where enamel minerals begin to demineralise. [16, 17]. Sucrose is readily metabolised by oral cariogenic bacteria, leading to a more significant decrease in plaque pH than any other carbohydrate. In a clinical trial conducted on schoolchildren aged 9 to 11, one group served as the control (no gum chewing), while the other groups chewed gum sticks containing sucrose, sorbitol or xylitol five times a day. At the end of the 40-month trial, children who chewed the sucrose-containing gum had an increased incidence of caries compared to those who received no chewing gum. Children who chewed sorbitol gum or xylitol gum showed a respective 20.8% decrease in caries incidence compared to the control group [18]. Clinical and experimental studies have demonstrated that chewing sugary gum has a cariogenic effect.

9.4 Sugar-Free Chewing Gum

According to the US Federal Regulations, 2022 [21 CFR 101], food and chewing gum can be labelled as 'sugar-free' if they contain less than 0.5 g of sugar per serving. Instead of sugar, gums are sweetened with sugar alcohols (polyols) such as sorbitol, xylitol or mannitol. Intense sweeteners such as acesulfame, aspartame, neotame, saccharin or sucralose are also used. Unlike sugar, these sweeteners are not metabolised by bacterial plaque, except for sorbitol and mannitol, which are slowly metabolised. Sorbitol was introduced into the diabetic diet as early as 1929 and is widely distributed in plants such as berries, apples, plums and pears.

Sugar-free chewing gum first appeared on the market in the early 1950s, and its quality, texture and taste have since improved. Sorbitol is commercially produced from sucrose or starch and is about half as sweet as sucrose, with one-third fewer calories. It serves as a sugar substitute in confections, chewing gums, chocolates, jams, jellies and other products labelled as a 'dentally safe' sweetener. Sorbitol is also used in formulating oral care products such as toothpaste and mouthwash. Xylitol is found in small amounts in fruits and vegetables, including bananas, strawberries, cauliflower and mushrooms, and is commercially produced from coconut shells, birch trees and xylan-containing wood. Its sweetness equals that of sucrose (table sugar), and it has 40% fewer calories than sucrose. Xylitol is 10 times more expensive than sucrose and is produced from corn cobs to reduce production costs. Sorbitol and xylitol are widely used in food, confectionerty, medicines, and health product. Oral microorganisms, especially *Streptococcus mutans*, do not possess the enzymes necessary to utilise xylitol to produce acid and synthesise extracellular polysaccharides involved in plaque formation.

Several clinical trials have evaluated the effectiveness of chewing gum for oral and dental health. A literature review showed that xylitol was least associated with caries compared to other polyols and had antimicrobial effects in some studies, including against *S. mutans* [19]. Burt [20] reported that chewing sorbitol gum three times a day was less cariogenic than sugar gum, while xylitol gum was not cariogenic in all tested products. In a 2-year study, using chewing gum containing xylitol, sorbitol or a mixture of both resulted in a significant decrease in caries incidence in primary teeth, with caries reduction in the xylitol and sorbitol gum groups of 35 and 44%, respectively, compared to the no-gum group [21]. Isogangas et al. [22] found that children who used xylitol chewing gum daily had significantly lower caries incidence than the control group (no chewing gum). A 2-year study of Danish schoolchildren aged 8–12 years who chewed gum containing sorbitol after each meal showed that caries increments were 5.6 compared to 6.2 in the control group with no gum chewing [23]. A systematic review (2021) showed that xylitol chewing gum significantly reduced the number of *S. mutans* compared with no gum chewing or F varnish [24]. One study on subjects with gingivitis showed that after chewing xylitol or maltitol gum for 10 min, five times a day for 3 weeks, marginal probing bleeding and plaque scores were significantly ($P < 0.001$) lower compared to chewing gum base in the absence of toothbrushing [25]. Clinical reports have shown that in the absence of toothbrushing, chewing xylitol or maltitol gum significantly inhibited gingivitis scores compared to chewing gum base [26]. It can be concluded that the regular use of xylitol chewing gum to aid toothbrushing effectively removes dental biofilm and reduces gingival inflammation. Chewing sugar-free gum for 5–10 min after meals is recommended three times daily.

9.5 Fluoride Chewing Gum

It is well known that the frequent use of low-concentration fluoride is an effective method to promote the remineralisation of early carious lesions and prevent dental caries. Fluoride-containing chewing gum (e.g. Fluomin, Fluorette, Fluogum) fits this concept. These chewing gums can rapidly and thoroughly deliver fluoride ions to the enamel-plaque-saliva biosystem through mechanical degradation. Bruun and Givskov [27] found that chewing gum containing 0.25 mg of fluoride released 11.7 and 15.3 ppm after 2 and 5 min, respectively, which decreased to 3.9 ppm after 10 min of chewing. The study also found that chewing gum releases significantly more fluoride than chewing fluoride tablets. In contrast, one study showed no significant difference in saliva fluoride concentration after chewing gum compared to chewing fluoride tablets, suggesting that fluoride gum could be an effective alternative to fluoride tablets for preventing dental caries [28].

Few publications provide information on the clinical effects of F-containing chewing gum on enamel remineralisation and caries prevention. In situ enamel sections with subsurface lesions were mounted in removable lower appliances, and subjects chewed five sticks/day of F gum (0.1 mg F/stick) for 3 days. The results showed a significantly higher microhardness value of the test group than those of the control group that did not chew gum [29]. Another *in situ* experiment, in which enamel sections with early caries lesions were mounted in removable lower appliances. The test group chewed five sticks of gum day (0.1 mg F/stick) daily for 21 days, while the control group used F-free dentifrice. Enamel remineralisation and F uptake were significantly higher in the test group compared to the control group [30]. Hattab et al. [12] first studied the effects of F-chewing gum on the remineralisation of white spot caries lesions, plaque F uptake and plasma F level. The following are the local and systemic effects of F-chewing gum [8, 12].

Salivary F Release: Healthy adults refrained from brushing with F toothpaste for three days and avoided consuming F-rich foods and drinks. Subjects chewed a stick of sugar-free Fluogum® (containing 0.113 mg F as NaF) for 15 min. Saliva samples were collected at intervals ranging from 2 to 180 min. On separate occasions, two sticks of Fluogum® (0.23 mg F) were chewed simultaneously. Fluoride analysis was performed using an F-ion electrode. After chewing a stick of Fluogum®, salivary F concentrations increased from a baseline value of 0.03 ppm to a peak of 1.2 ppm after 5 min of chewing. The corresponding peak F concentration after chewing two sticks was 2.73 ppm (Fig. 9.1). The area under the curve (AUC) of salivary F concentration versus time was 0.78 h × µg/mL for one stick and 1.89 h × µg/mL for two sticks, respectively. The mean saliva flow rates for one and two sticks were 2.1 and 2.8 mL/min, respectively.

Plaque F Content: Before chewing the gum, baseline plaque samples were collected from all accessible sites using a plastic spatula. The subjects then chewed two sticks of Fluogum for 15 min. Plaque was sampled after 1 and 3 h. The samples

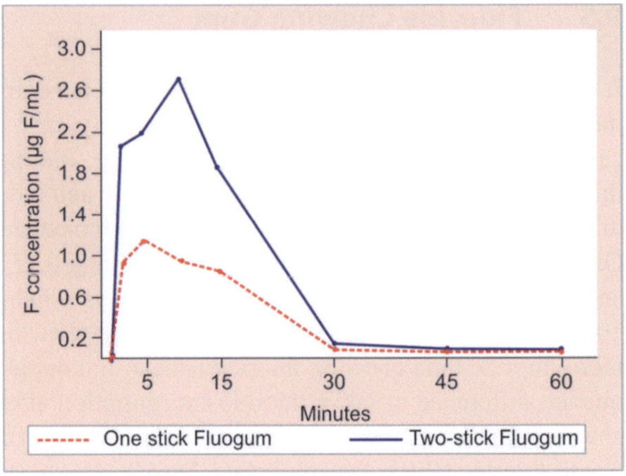

Fig. 9.1 Mean F concentrations (μg/mL) in whole saliva at time intervals during and after 15-minutes of chewing one or two gum containing 0.113 mg F and 0.23 mg F (as NaF), respectively. The peak salivary F level occurred 5 minutes after chewing one stick of Fluogum®, and 10 minutes after chewing two Fluogum sticks. Chewing two gum sticks resulted in significant increase in F concentration. Both concentration lines dropped rapidly after 15 minutes and stabilized after 30 minutes

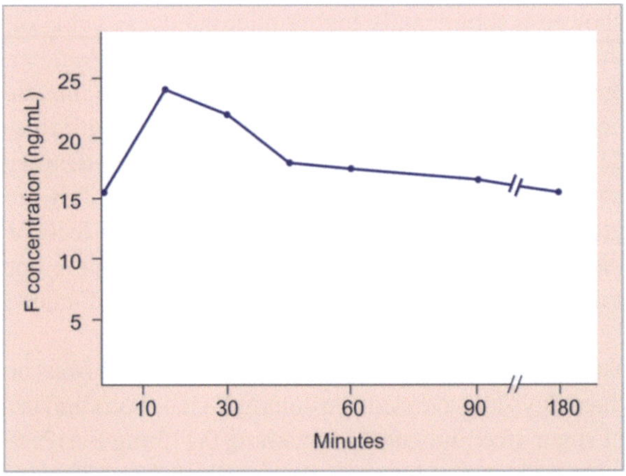

Fig. 9.2 Plasma F concentrations (ng/mL) in fasting subjects chewed two Fluogum sticks (0.23 mg F, in the form of NaF) for 15 minutes and swallow the pooled saliva. Peak F concentration was reached after 5 minutes

were suspended in 0.5 $HClO_4$ for 12 h, then F was determined. Gum chewing increased the F content in plaque from 2.94 to 4.87 μg/g. A positive correlation was found between F levels in saliva and dental plaque.

Plasma F Levels: After fasting overnight, the subject chewed two sticks of Fluogum for 15 min and swallowed the pooled saliva. Fingertip blood samples were collected before chewing gum and at 15, 30, 45, 60, 90, 120 and 180 min after chewing gum. The plasma F level increased slightly from 16 ng/mL (baseline value) to a peak of 24 ng/mL, returning to the baseline value after 20 min of chewing (Fig. 9.2). The AUC was 6.3 h × ng/mL, accounting for one-third of that for saliva AUC.

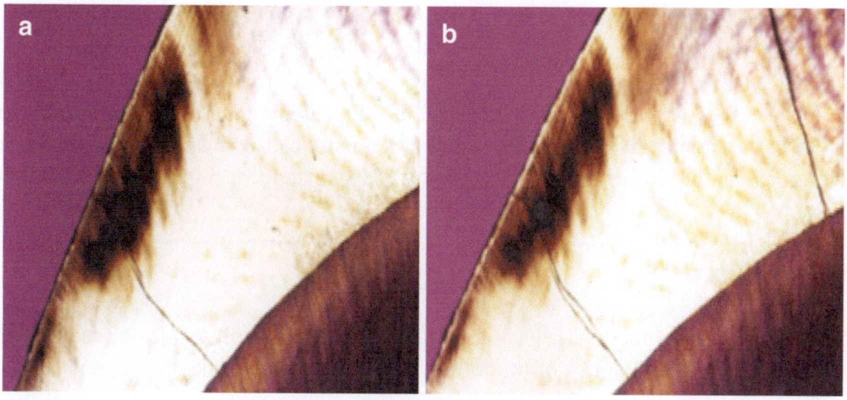

Fig. 9.3. Remineralising effects of chewing sugar-free F gum. (**a**) Enamel caries lesion observed in PLM after imbibition in water. The lesion exhibited positive birefringence, indicating demineralisation. (**b**) After three days of gum chewing, the outer surface of the lesion increased in thickness (remineralisation) exhibited negative birefringence, and the lesion body showed a tendency to remineralise

Remineralisation: Subjects wore maxillary acrylic appliances containing enamel sections with white spot caries lesions. They chewed 15 sticks (5 sticks a day) of Fluogum®. Birefringence values before and after chewing were assessed using polarised light microscopy (PLM). After 3 days of the test period, there was a significant reduction in both lesion depth and lesion body size ($P < 0.001$), with decreases of 10 and 28%, respectively (Fig. 9.3a, b). In a separate experiment involving F-free gum chewing, there was a significant reduction in the lesion body (5%) but not in the lesion depth.

9.6 Chlorhexidine Chewing Gum

Chlorhexidine (CHX; chlorhexidine gluconate) is a potent antiseptic widely used as an antimicrobial agent. CHX has high retention and greater sustainability in both hard and soft tissue effects, making it the material of choice for anti-plaque and anti-gingivitis applications. CHX, either alone or in combination with F, is used in mouthwashes, gels, lozenges, sprays, varnishes, toothpaste, dental floss and toothpicks. Although CHX is non-toxic, it has an unpleasant taste, alters taste perception and can cause brown stains on teeth, tongue and restorations with prolonged use [31]. Adding CHX to chewing gum is an attractive adjunct to conventional oral hygiene measures. During the 6-day trial, subjects chewed five pieces of CHX, xylitol and sorbitol gum for 20 min per day on different occasions. The results showed that chewing gum containing CHX significantly reduced the plaque value to 0.7 compared to 1.7 for the xylitol gum and 2.7 for the sorbitol gum, with the plaque value of xylitol considerably lower than that of sorbitol chewing gum [32]. In another trial, the effectiveness of CHX was tested in three groups: Group 1 chewed two pieces of CHX chewing gum for 10 min twice a day, Group 2 chewed placebo chewing gum and Group 3 rinsed with 10 mL of 0.2% CHX mouthwash for 1 minute twice a day. After 8 weeks, plaque and gingival bleeding scores in the CHX gum group were significantly lower than those in the placebo gum group and similar to those in the mouthwash group. The staining intensity caused by CHX chewing gum was considerably lower than that caused by CHX rinse [33].

9.7 Discussion

Saliva has several functions related to oral and systemic health. It play a crucial role in maintaining the integrity of the mouth and teeth, physiological functions (swallowing, chewing and speaking), and preventing dental caries and periodontal disease. Chewing gum increases salivary flow in response to mechanical (chewing) and gustatory (taste) stimuli, elevating resting values of 0. 0.4–0. 0.5 mL/min to approximately 5–6 mL/min, representing a tenfold increase. Hyposalivation is diagnosed when the stimulated salivary flow rate is ≤0. 0.5–0. 0.7 mL/min and the unstimulated salivary flow rate is ≤0. 0.1 mL/min. The key functions of saliva include removing oral bacteria and food debris, neutralising plaque pH after a sugar challenge through its buffering action, enhancing the remineralisation of early caries lesions by maintaining an environment saturated with calcium and phosphate and controlling demineralisation [6–9]. Increased levels of *S. mutans* and Lactobacilli are often associated with low salivary rates. Studies have shown that chewing gum and increasing saliva flow for five days can significantly reduce plaque buildup and allow for the removal of 50% of food particles. To date, the only gum approved by the ADA is sugar-free. These are sweetened with non-cariogenic substances such as sorbitol, xylitol, mannitol and aspartame. Research indicates that the peak F released from chewing gum occurs after 5 min of chewing and then declines sharply within the first 30 min, with the area under the curve (AUC) of salivary F concentration being two to three times higher than that of non-chewing individuals. The AUC of F concentration in saliva when chewing two sticks of gum is 2.4 times that of chewing one stick (Fig. 9.1). Chewing F-gum enhanced plaque pH recovery after rinsing with a 10% sucrose solution [34]. In situ tests have shown that chewing F gum significantly promotes the remineralisation of early enamel caries lesions, increases enamel microhardness, reduces plaque deposits and boosts F content in enamel and dental plaque. Subjects wearing intraoral appliances with demineralised enamel blocks were tested with chewing gum made from green tea extract and supplemented with 50 μg of F. After chewing two pieces of gum twice a day for 4 weeks, participants exhibited a fourfold higher F concentration in the demineralised area compared to those chewing placebo gum [35]. A 12-week trial in patients with gingivitis who chewed gum made from eucalyptus extract demonstrated a significant reduction in plaque accumulation, gingival index, bleeding on probing and periodontal probing depth [36].

The safety of using chewing gum in warrants discussion. Bijella et al. [37] reported that Brazilian Happydent chewing gum, which contains 3.38 mg F/piece (as Na_2PO_3F), can lead to dental fluorosis. It should be noted that Na_2PO_3F contains 13% F−, while NaF contains 45% F−; consequently, the impact of $Na_2PO_3F_2$ on increasing plasma F concentration is 3.5 times lower than that of Naf. Therefore, the amount of ingested F reported by Bijella et al. is 8.7 times lower than the recommended optimal daily F intake for children, which is 0.05–0.07 mg F/kg body weight. A study by Oliveby et al. [38] involving four subjects living in a non-fluoridated area demonstrated that the use of two pieces of chewing gum (Fluomin®) containing 0.5 mg F (as NaF) taken ten times a day resulted in slightly elevated plasma F levels from 1 to 3 µmol/L (0.019 to 0.057 ppm). Our findings indicate that chewing F gum only slightly increases plasma F levels, from 16 ng/mL to a peak of 24 ng/mL (Fig. 9.2). The highest plasma F level from chewing F gum falls within the range of 3–4 µmol/L (0.057–0.76 ppm). For individuals living in areas with fluoridated drinking water plasma F levels are in range of 1 to 4 µmol/L. This supports the safety of using F-chewing gum.

9.8 Conclusion

Chewing gum is an appealing delivery vehicle for low-concentration broad-spectrum therapeutic agents, providing ease of use, frequent topical application of low therapeutic doses and improved human compliance. Advantages of using chewing gum include the following:

1. Powerfully increases saliva flow and volume through its mechanical action and the flavours it contains.
2. Saliva and its various components play an essential role in maintaining dental and oral health by removing food particles, reducing the number of microorganisms, neutralising the pH of dental plaque after a sugar challenge, inhibiting plaque buildup, promoting the remineralisation of early caries lesions and controlling enamel demineralisation.
3. Chewing gum with F and CHX is an essential adjunct in preventing dental caries and periodontal disease.
4. Chewing sugar-free gum is a safe product with no side effects. Among its many benefits, chewing gum is particularly valuable for patients with hyposalivation or xerostomia, who may face functional problems due to dry mouth and a diminished quality of life.

References

1. Imfeld T. Chewing gum – facts and fiction: a review of gum-chewing and oral health. Crit Rev Oral Biol Med. 1999;10(3):405–19.
2. Rassing MR. Chewing gum as a drug delivery system. Adv Drug Deliv Rev. 1994;13(1–2):89–121.
3. Banakar M, Moayedi S, Shamsoddin E, et al. Chewing gums as a drug delivery approach for oral health. Int J Dent. 2022;20:9430988.

4. American Dental Association (ADA). Chewing gum, 2023.
5. Edgar M, Dawes C, O'Mullane D, editors. Saliva and oral health. 4th ed. Stephen Hancocks Ltd; 2012.
6. Edgar WM, Geddes DAM. Chewing gum and dental health. Br Dent J. 1990;169:173–7.
7. Dodds MW. The oral health benefits of chewing gum. J Ir Dent Assoc. 2012;58(5):253–61.
8. Hattab FN. Chewing gum for oral and dental health: a review. J Oral Health Comm Dent. 2023;17(1):12–9.
9. Newton JT, Awojobi O, Nasseripour M, et al. A systematic review and meta-analysis of the role of sugar-free chewing gum in dental caries. JDR Clin Trans Res. 2020;5(3):214–23.
10. Saheer PA, Parmar P, Majid SA, et al. Effect of sugar-free chewing gum on plaque and gingivitis among 14-15-year-old school children: a randomized controlled trial. Indian J Dent Res. 2019;30(1):61–6.
11. Simons D, Brailsford S, Kidd EA, et al. The effect of chlorhexidine acetate/xylitol chewing gum on the plaque and gingival indices of elderly occupants in residential homes. J Clin Periodontol. 2001;28(11):1010–5.
12. Hattab FN, Green RM, Pang KM, Mok YC. Effect of fluoride-containing chewing gum on remineralisation of carious lesions and on fluoride uptake in man. Clin Prevent Dent. 1989;11:6–11.
13. Linden L-A, Bjorkman S, Hattab F. The diffusion in vitro of fluoride and chlorhexidine in the enamel of human deciduous and permanent teeth. Arch Oral Biol. 1986;31:33–7.
14. Hattab F. Effect of topical application of alginate containing fluoride or fluoride and chlorhexidine on dental caries in rats. Caries Res. 1984;18:367–74.
15. Szöke J, Bánóczy J, Proskin HM. Effect of after-meal sucrose-free gum-chewing on clinical caries. J Dent Res. 2001;80(8):1725–9.
16. Addy M, Perriam E, Sterry A. Effects of sugared and sugar-free chewing gum on the accumulation of plaque and debris on the teeth. J Clin Periodontal. 1982;9:346–54.
17. Ainamo J, Sjoblom M, Ainamo A, Tiainen L, et al. Growth of plaque while chewing sucrose and sorbitol flavoured chewing gum. J Clin Periodontal. 1977;4:151–60.
18. Mäkinen KK, Bennett CA, Hujoel PP, et al. Xylitol chewing gums and caries rates: a 40-month cohort study. J Dent Res. 1995;74(12):1904–13.
19. Deshpande A, Jadad AR. The impact of polyol-containing chewing gums on dental caries: a systematic review of original randomised controlled trials and observational studies. J Am Dent Assoc. 2008;139(12):1602–14.
20. Burt BA. The use of sorbitol- and xylitol-sweetened chewing gum in caries control. J Am Dent Assoc. 2006;137(2):190–6.
21. Mäkinen KK, Hujoel PP, Bennett CA, et al. Polyol chewing gums and caries rates in primary dentition: a 24-month cohort study. Caries Res. 1996;30(6):408–17.
22. Isogangas P, Mäkinen KK, Tiekso J, Alanen P. Long-term effect of xylitol chewing gum in the prevention of dental caries: a follow-up 5 years after termination of a prevention program. Caries Res. 1993;27(6):495–8.
23. Möller IJ, Poulsen S. The effect of sorbitol-containing chewing gum on the incidence of dental caries; plaque and gingivitis in Danish schoolchildren. Community Dent Oral Epidemiol. 1973;1(2):58–67.
24. Nasseripour M, Newton JT, Warburton F, et al. A systematic review and meta-analysis of the role of sugar-free chewing gum on Streptococcus mutans. BMC Oral Health. 2021;21(1):217.
25. Söderling E, Pienihäkkinen K, Gursoy UK. Effects of sugar-free polyol chewing gums on gingival inflammation: a systematic review. Clin Oral Investig. 2022;26(12):6881–91.
26. Keukenmeester RS, Slot DE, Rosema NA, et al. Effects of sugar-free chewing gum sweetened with xylitol or maltitol on the development of gingivitis and plaque: a randomized clinical trial. Int J Dent Hyg. 2014;12(4):238–44.
27. Bruun C, Givskov H. Release of fluoride from fluoride-containing chewing gum. Community Dent Oral Epidemiol. 1978;6(1):27–9.

28. Cagetti MG, Brambilla E, Fadini L, Strohmenger L. Comparative study of salivary and urinary fluoride levels and clearance patterns between fluoridated chewing gum and fluoride tablets in children. Eur J Paediatr Dent. 2002;3(1):27–32.
29. Lamb WJ, Corpron RE, More FG, et al. In situ remineralisation of subsurface enamel lesion after the use of a fluoride chewing gum. Caries Res. 1993;27(2):111–6.
30. De Los SR, Lin YT, Corpron RE, et al. In situ remineralisation of root surface lesions using a fluoride chewing gum or fluoride-releasing device. Caries Res. 1994;28(6):441–6.
31. Hattab FN, Qudeimat MA, AL-Rimawi HS. Dental discoloration: an overview. J Esthet Dent. 1999;11:292–311.
32. Tellefsen G, Larsen G, Kaligithi R, Zimmerman GJ, et al. Use of chlorhexidine chewing gum significantly reduces dental plaque formation compared to use of similar xylitol and sorbitol products. J Periodontol. 1996;67(3):181–3.
33. Smith AJ, Moran J, Dangler LV, et al. The efficacy of an anti-gingivitis chewing gum. J Clin Periodontol. 1996;23(1):19–23.
34. Sjögren K, Lingström P, Lundberg AB, Birkhed D. Salivary fluoride concentration and plaque pH after using a fluoride-containing chewing gum. Caries Res. 1997;31:366–72.
35. Suyama E, Tamura T, Ozawa T, et al. Remineralisation and acid resistance of enamel lesions after chewing gum containing fluoride extracted from green tea. Aust Dent J. 2011;56(4):394–400.
36. Nagata H, Inagaki Y, Tanaka M, et al. Effect of eucalyptus extract chewing gum on periodontal health: a double-masked, randomised trial. J Periodontol. 2008;79(10):1378–85.
37. Bijella MFTB, Brighenti FL, Bijella MFB, et al. Fluoride kinetics in saliva after the use of a fluoride-containing chewing gum. Braz Oral Res. 2005;19(4):256–60.
38. Oliveby A, Ekstrand J, Lagerlöf F. Effect of salivary flow rate on salivary fluoride clearance after use of a fluoride-containing chewing gum. Caries Res. 1987;21(5):393–401.

Alcohol Abuse and Oral Health

10

Aruni Tilakaratne, Yet Ching Goh,
and Wanninayake Mudiyanselage Tilakaratne

10.1 Introduction

Alcohol consumption trends show variation across different geographical regions and cultural practices. The World Health Organization (WHO) data reveals alcohol consumption by more than half of the population in America, Europe and the Western Pacific region [1]. It has been estimated that 2.5 billion people aged over 15 years consume alcohol. The highest alcohol consumption was reported in Europe, North and South America and the Western Pacific region. The fact that the prevalence of alcohol consumption is notably higher across Europe in comparison to North Africa and the Middle East may signify a link between alcohol habits and social and cultural beliefs and practices. It is documented that more than a quarter of adolescents worldwide are current drinkers, with the highest rates among WHO European region. Further, the estimates for 2019 based on the WHO Global Health Status Report reveal that the overall per capita consumption of alcohol was 5.5 litres of pure alcohol, with higher consumption among men (8.2 litres) than women (2.2 litres). The types of alcohol consumed are spirits, beer and wine. Spirits are recorded as the most consumed alcohol worldwide. The alcohol consumption trend is declining or stabilising in many high-income countries, attributed to the health awareness and availability of non-alcoholic alternatives. Alcohol consumption, on the

A. Tilakaratne
Department of Restorative Dentistry, Faculty of Dentistry, Universiti Malaya, Kuala Lumpur, Malaysia
e-mail: aruniti@um.edu.my

Y. C. Goh · W. M. Tilakaratne (✉)
Department of Oral and Maxillofacial Clinical Sciences, Faculty of Dentistry, Universiti Malaya, Kuala Lumpur, Malaysia
e-mail: gohyetching@um.edu.my; wmtilak@um.edu.my

S. R. Prabhu et al. (eds.), *Lifestyle in Oral Health and Disease*,
https://doi.org/10.1007/978-3-032-05888-1_10

contrary, is increasing trend in some developing countries, most probably due to economic growth and urbanisation [2].

The harmful use of alcohol is a decisive risk factor for more than 200 diseases, including conditions related to injuries. Among the alcohol-related diseases, non-communicable diseases (NCDs) such as cardiovascular diseases, digestive diseases as well as oral diseases are of prime concern. However, out of all oral diseases, harmful alcohol habits largely influence the development of oral cavity cancer. The global and regional burden of lip and oral cavity cancer reveals an estimated 377,713 new cases and 177,757 deaths from lip and oral cavity cancers worldwide in 2020 [2, 3].

Additionally, harmful alcohol consumption is associated with a variety of family, social and economic issues, as well as mental and behavioural disorders. At a global scale, the harmful use of alcohol causes an estimated three million deaths per year, representing 5.3% of all deaths. Of the worldwide burden of disease and injury, 5.1% is attributable to alcohol [1]. Exposure to risk factors such as alcohol appears to pose a significant challenge, paving the way for persisting or even increasing inequalities [1].

10.2 Definition of Alcohol Abuse

Alcohol abuse is also termed as alcohol use disorder (AUD), referring to harmful or excessive consumption of alcohol causing adverse effects on an individual's physical, mental and social well-being. The World Health Organization classifies heavy episodic drinking (HED) as the consumption of 60 or more grams of pure alcohol on at least one occasion per month. The prevalence of HED has decreased globally from the year 2000 to 2016 but remains high, particularly in some parts of Eastern Europe. HED peaks between the ages of 20 and 24. The prevalence of HED is remarkably higher among men [1]. The fifth edition of the Diagnostic and Statistical Manual of Mental Disorders (DSM-5) defines AUD as the presence of behavioural and physical symptoms, such as withdrawal, tolerance and craving [4]. AUD may range from mild-to-severe depending on the symptoms present and the proposed diagnostic criteria. Biomarkers such as ethyl glucuronide (EtG), fatty acid ethyl esters, phosphatidyl ethanol, acetaldehyde adducts to protein and 5-hydroxytryptophan are used to support a diagnosis of alcohol consumption. However, no laboratory test is sufficiently reliable to support the diagnosis of AUD.

10.3 Pathophysiological Effects of Alcohol

Alcohol can permeate human organs and soft tissue, resulting in tissue injury and organ dysfunction following alcohol abuse. Chronic alcohol abuse could lead to medical consequences affecting the liver, lung, endocrine, immune system and brain. Alcohol-induced organ damage is usually a cumulative process as a result of long-term alcohol intake. Liver disease is a well-documented medical consequence of heavy drinking. Elevated liver enzymes, specifically alanine aminotransferase (ALT) and gamma-glutamyl transferase (GGT), are associated with excessive alcohol intake [5]. The level of these enzymes is medically used as an indicator of liver damage.

The endocrine system serves as a communicator between organs, maintaining constant internal homeostasis. Alcohol abuse can disrupt the endocrine system, causing hormonal disturbances and functional disorders. The studies show alcohol can affect the essential hormonal regulating pathways, namely, the hypothalamic–pituitary–adrenal (HPA) axis, hypothalamic–pituitary–gonadal (HPG) axis, hypothalamic–pituitary–thyroid (HPT) axis, hypothalamic–pituitary–growth hormone/insulin-like growth factor-1 (GH/IGF-1) axis and hypothalamic–posterior-pituitary (HPP) axis [5, 6]. The hormonal disturbances can lead to cardiovascular disorders, reproductive deficits, immune dysfunction, psychological and behavioural disorders and other hormonal-influencing disorders.

Alcohol-induced immune activation or suppression can increase susceptibility to a wide range of health problems and weaken the host's defences against infection. Alcohol can affect the structure and integrity of the gastrointestinal (GI) system significantly as it is the first system in contact with alcohol [6, 7]. The microbiome of the GI system plays an essential role in the maturation and function of the immune system. Extensive alcohol consumption is also linked to respiratory diseases, attributing to the disturbances to ciliary function and immune cells, jeopardising the barrier function of the respiratory epithelium [7].

10.4 Economic Impact of Alcohol Abuse on the Healthcare System (Health Economics Burden)

Alcohol abuse causes a substantial and broad economic impact on the healthcare system, as illustrated by various statistics conducted regionally and globally. The financial implications of healthcare abuse involve direct healthcare costs and indirect costs from productivity losses, alcohol-related accidents and injuries, social services costs and disability burdens. It is estimated that alcohol contributes to 5.1% of global deaths each year, impacting economic development and progress worldwide. The global economic burden of alcohol-related issues is estimated at $1.4 trillion annually [1, 8]. This figure is definitely a significant burden on the healthcare system and represents a large component of global expenditures.

10.5 Oral Conditions Linked to Alcohol Abuse

10.5.1 Xerostomia

Xerostomia in alcohol abuse is primarily attributed to the effects of alcohol on salivary glands and the nervous system. Alcohol acts as a diuretic by increasing urine production and causing dehydration. This, in turn, reduces the volume of fluids channel for saliva production. As the major component of saliva is water, alcohol-induced dehydration leads to reduced saliva production and subsequently causes xerostomia. Alcohol diffuses into the salivary glands and damages salivary glandular tissue through inflammation, fibrosis and direct toxic effects on glandular cells [9, 10]. The ability to produce saliva is compromised in impaired glandular tissues.

Alcohol abuse can interfere with the nervous system, particularly the parasympathetic system that is responsible for saliva production. Chronic alcohol intake disrupts the signalling required for saliva secretion and results in disturbances of salivary glands metabolism process [11]. Chronic alcohol intake causes elevation of tumour necrosis factor-alpha (TNF-α) leading to induction of acinar cell apoptosis. Other reported changes to the salivary glands following chronic alcohol abuse include accumulation of fat tissue in the salivary glands and acinar cell atrophy [12]. Although studies directly linking xerostomia to alcohol abuse differ, it is widely recognised that alcohol consumption significantly raises the risk of developing dry mouth. Many studies demonstrate the reduction in salivary flow in alcoholic patients and the correlation between xerostomia and other oral health conditions [13, 14].

10.5.2 Periodontal Disease

Periodontal disease is a multifactorial, chronic inflammatory disease of the tooth-supporting tissues, which comprise the gingiva, alveolar bone, cementum and periodontal ligament. The mildest form of periodontal disease is gingivitis, characterised by inflammation of the gingiva. The more severe form is referred to as periodontitis, characterised by loss of periodontal support due to the periodontal ligament, cementum and alveolar bone.

While gingivitis is the most prevalent periodontal disease affecting about 90% of the world's population, more than 50% of adults in the global population suffer from some form of periodontitis, with severe periodontitis reported as about 19% of people aged over 15 years. This prevalence corresponds to more than one billion cases of severe periodontal disease worldwide [2].

Dental plaque biofilm is established as the aetiology of periodontal disease. However, the current understanding of periodontal disease is that it is a risk-factor-driven non-communicable disease (NCD). Therefore, similar to other non-oral NCDS, there is a strong influence of both modifiable and non-modifiable risk factors for periodontal disease.

Although tobacco use and systemic diseases like diabetes are well established as risk factors of periodontal disease, the synergistic effects of alcohol have been discussed in understanding the pathogenic process and progression of periodontal disease in alcohol consumers, especially with harmful levels of alcohol use or abuse. More recently, a 'common-risk-factor model' and control of shared risk factors have been proposed to tackle oral and non-oral NCDs. This is because both tobacco and alcohol habits are modifiable risk factors, common for both oral and non-oral NCDs, as they predispose individuals to cardiovascular diseases, respiratory diseases, cancers including lip and oral cavity cancer and severe periodontal disease [2]. It is also known that harmful tobacco and alcohol habits may work in synergy, which could impact the immune responses, lowering the immune protective mechanisms in the body and heightening the susceptibility of the individual towards disease. Therefore, the approach for tackling shared risk factors is the basis for oral and non-oral disease prevention in the broader scope of the NCD agenda recommended in the WHO health reports.

10.5.3 Dental Erosion

Alcohol abuse can contribute to erosion of teeth through several mechanisms, including the acidic nature of alcohol, reduced salivation and development of gastroesophageal reflux disease (GERD). The majority of alcoholic beverages are acidic, especially wine. Prolonged exposure to acidic alcoholic drinks increases the susceptibility of enamel to demineralisation, leading to erosion of non-carious tooth surface wear [15].

Saliva plays a crucial role in buffering the oral environment and protecting teeth by neutralising the acidic condition. The protective effect is diminished following reduced saliva flow, increasing the vulnerability to the damaging effects of acid from alcoholic beverages. It is reported that the incidence of erosion of teeth is significantly higher in alcohol addicts, up to three times higher than in those who abstain from alcoholic beverages. Research evidence reveals that between 49% and 92% of teeth in individuals with alcoholism show signs of erosion.

Alcohol consumption likely triggers GERD, as it can directly damage the mucous membranes of the oesophagus and stomach, leading to irritation. This condition leads to regurgitation of stomach acids into the oesophagus and oral cavity, further contributing to dental erosion [16, 17].

10.5.4 Oral Potentially Malignant Disorders (OPMDs)

OPMDs refer to a heterogeneous group of clinical conditions associated with a risk of progressing to oral malignancy [18]. OPMDs can clinically manifest in any intra-oral site. Alcohol abuse is globally recognised as one of the main aetiological factors associated with the development of these disorders. Alcohol can alter the normal oral mucosal integrity by destroying the lipid composition of the oral mucosa and disrupting the order of normal epithelial lipid molecules. This leads to a gap between epithelial cells, increasing mucosal permeability.

Alcohol is primarily metabolised through alcohol dehydrogenase (ADH) pathway in the liver. The ethanol is first converted into acetaldehyde by alcohol dehydrogenase, then metabolised by acetaldehyde dehydrogenase (ALDH) into acetate. Microsomal Ethanol-Oxidizing System (MEOS) is activated in chronic alcohol consumption, leading to slower alcohol metabolism and higher tolerance to alcohol [19]. This system produces reactive oxygen species (ROS) that can harm liver health. Acetaldehyde is a highly reactive compound and potent carcinogen that can promote precancerous transformation in the oral epithelium.

Repeated exposure to alcohol induces the interaction between acetaldehyde with epithelial cells, causing cellular DNA changes and potential genetic damage, making the oral mucosa more prone to develop OPMDs. Leukoplakia and erythroplakia are two most commonly reported OPMDs related to alcohol consumption. The altered inflammatory response is also observed in chronic alcohol consumption. The prolonged inflammatory response could lead to changes in epithelial integrity and induce dysplastic changes in the oral epithelium.

10.5.5 Oral Cancer

Globally, head and neck cancer is responsible for over 890,000 cases and approximately 450,000 deaths each year. Oral cancer is the 16th most common cancer worldwide, and oral squamous cell carcinoma (OSCC) accounts for approximately 90% of all oral cancers and often presents with advanced stage and lower mean 5-year survival. Two of the main aetiological factors for oral cancer are tobacco and alcohol, contributing to more than 70% of attributable risk in European oral cancer cases. Recent research documents a 1.8-fold higher risk in moderate alcohol drinkers and 5.5-fold higher risk in heavy alcohol drinkers for the occurrence of oral cavity cancers [1]. The International Agency for Research on Cancer (IARC) classifies alcohol as a Group 1 carcinogen, acknowledging its harmful carcinogenic properties [20]. Up to 26.4% of all oral cavity and lip cancers worldwide are linked to heavy alcohol drinking [21].

In general, several molecular mechanisms of alcohol-associated carcinogenesis have been proposed. Three major alcohol-associated processes in relation to carcinogenesis involve disturbances of metabolism in squamous epithelial cells, disruption of systemic nutrient metabolism and alteration of signalling pathways in squamous epithelial cells [22]. Interaction of acetaldehyde with oral cells induces genetic alteration, which further alters cell cycle regulation and DNA repair, amplifying the tumorigenesis and development of oral cancer. The link between OPMDs and the development of oral cancer is well established. Untreated OPMDs may progress into oral squamous cell carcinoma, with an increased malignant transformation rate associated with risk factors such as alcohol consumption [23, 24].

A study investigating the effects of tobacco and alcohol on cancer location of OSCC revealed that OSCC shows notably different sites about the aetiology. The study reported that smoking and alcohol exposure were 25.8-fold more likely to have OSCC on the floor of the mouth [25]. Floor of the mouth is structurally more sensitive to carcinogen exposure due to the difference in tissue composition, molecular marker expression and epithelium turnover rates. Having composed of thin, non-keratinised stratified squamous epithelium, carcinogens that mixed with saliva would pool at the floor of the mouth, allowing longer contact time. The keratin surface of keratinised stratified squamous epithelium in some parts of the oral cavity could be a barrier against harmful exposure.

10.6 Correlation Between Alcohol Consumption and Increased Oral Potentially Malignant Disorders and Oral Cancer Risk

Chronic alcohol consumption is reportedly contributing to 3.6% of all cancers worldwide, affecting the upper aerodigestive tract, liver, colorectal and breast [22, 24]. The alcohol-associated carcinogenesis is primarily linked to alcohol metabolite, acetaldehyde as well as the frequency and amount of alcohol consumption. The combination of alcohol and tobacco can synergistically promote the occurrence of oral squamous cell carcinoma by two to three times higher than with smoking alone [26]. Alcohol consumption increases susceptibility for OPMDs and oral cancer through several mechanisms: (i) induce DNA damage and mutagenesis, (ii) generation of reactive oxygen species (ROS) and (iii) alteration of host immune system.

The adverse effects of alcohol are associated with pro-inflammatory effects. Prolonged alcohol exposure was reported to elevate serum interleukin-6 (IL-6) and IL-1β levels [26]. IL-6 has been linked to tumourigenesis by altering long interspersed nuclear element-1 (LINE-1) hypermethylation. Acetaldehyde, a metabolic product of alcohol, is a potent mutagen that can cause damage to cellular genetic pathways and result in tumour growth. Acetaldehyde binds to protein molecules and alters the integrity functions, particularly the enzymes involved in cellular genetic repair and glutathione. Additionally, acetaldehyde can bind to DNA and form DNA adducts, resulting in tumoural cell immortalisation and clonal expansion, which eventually progress to cancer [27]. Researchers suggest measuring aldehyde-induced DNA and protein adducts as indicators for AUD detection while establishing its exact relationship with oral cancer initiation.

Chronic alcohol consumption could activate the Microsomal Ethanol-Oxidizing System (MEOS) involving the cytochrome P450 (CYP) family that generates reactive oxygen species (ROS) and results in oxidative damage of normal cells. It is noteworthy to highlight that ethanol metabolism by MEOS typically occurs at high levels of alcohol in the body, such as alcohol abuse [22]. This pathway accounts for about 10% of the body's alcohol metabolism [27]. Oxidative stress impacts the balance between the production of ROS and the body's antioxidant defence system. This, in turn, creates a hypoxic environment and activates cancer development in humans. Prolonged alcohol exposure also weakens the host's immune system and impairs the body's ability to suppress tumour growth.

Recent research has highlighted the somatic alteration of oncogenes and tumour suppressors linked to heavy alcohol intake. The mutations that were triggered include CDKN2A, FHIT, 11q13region, HER2, 3q25-qter and CSMD 1 [26]. Aldehyde dehydrogenase 1 (ALDH1), which is one of the components of the alcohol metabolism pathway located at chromosome 9q21.13, is regarded as a prognostic marker in head and neck cancer.

As ADH1B polymorphisms are of concern, moderate or heavy Asian drinkers carrying the ADH1B*1/*1 genotype are found more likely to develop cancers of the upper aerodigestive tract than those carrying the ADH1B*2 allele [26, 27]. It is postulated that ADH1B*2 exhibits protective effects compared to ADH1B*1/*1.

This finding, however, is contrary to laryngeal cancer in white populations, where no association was found between ADH1B genotype and alcohol consumption [27].

10.7 Correlation Between Alcohol Consumption and Periodontal Disease

The detrimental effects of alcohol on systemic health have been substantially validated with established research evidence for the past few decades. Correspondingly, the potential negative effects of harmful alcohol habits on the oral cavity have also been reported. However, the effects and the exact link between alcohol consumption and periodontal disease have not been studied extensively. The available studies from the recent past have focused on the potential synergy between alcohol consumption and periodontal disease, and the impact of alcohol in escalating the periodontal disease status of an individual. Accordingly, a few studies reveal the existence of a positive association between alcohol consumption and periodontitis, although the potential mechanisms behind this association are yet to be elucidated. The severity of periodontitis is reported to be higher among alcohol consumers, with a proportionate increase in the occurrence of periodontitis, along with the frequency of alcohol consumption [28, 29].

Pitiphat et al. in 2003 investigated the risk of periodontitis with alcohol consumption, and reported that alcohol consumption is an independent risk factor for periodontitis, although the different types of alcohols had no distinct effect on periodontitis [29]. Additionally, the alcohol consumers have been identified as having higher periodontal treatment needs. A higher level of loss of periodontal attachment has also been associated with alcohol consumption, even among the individuals without active periodontitis [28, 30]. As pointed out in another study by Lages et al., in 2015, the individuals with alcohol dependence had higher plaque index and higher severity of periodontitis [31]. According to Khocht et al., in 2009, alcohol dependence appeared to be related to higher dental plaque biofilm formation [32]. It is plausible that excessive intake of alcohol could contribute towards an increase in the rate of biofilm formation and accumulation, since alcohol can cause oral dryness reducing the salivary flow [33].

Additionally, it has been reported that periodontitis patients who were also alcohol-dependent demonstrated worse periodontal status with a higher frequency of harbouring periodontal pathogens such as *Prevotella intermedia*, *Eikenella corrodens* and *Fusobacterium nucleatum* [31]. The microbial analysis revealed a significant increase in the bacterial counts of those with periodontitis who were also alcohol consumers when compared with those with periodontitis but without alcohol habits. According to Szabo in 1999, alcohol intake appears to decrease the primary defence mechanisms, predisposing to a heightened level of bacterial growth [34].

While the etiopathogenesis of periodontal disease is multifaceted, there is well-established evidence supporting the importance of certain bacterial species and the host's immune-inflammatory response in the initiation, pathogenesis and progression of periodontal disease. At the same time, it is known that lifestyle risk factors such as harmful alcohol habits may alter the host–immunoinflammatory response and the host susceptibility, escalating the risk of severe periodontal destruction [34].

Although there is a scarcity of findings related to microbiological and immunological profiles associated with the periodontal disease of alcohol consumers, it is reported that alcohol may impair neutrophil, macrophage and T-cell functions, increasing the susceptibility of the individual to develop infections [34]. The same risk of infection applies to a heightened level of oral infections, including periodontal disease, which is primarily a disease of microbial aetiology.

Additionally, longstanding alcohol habits have also been associated with pathologies relating to altered inflammatory cells and adaptive immune responses, with an increase in the incidence of infections [35]. Therefore, it can be hypothesised that excessive and frequent alcohol consumption could affect the host response against bacterial infections, thus predisposing an individual to be a susceptible host [36]. Some studies have demonstrated that metabolic products of bacterial origin are capable of increasing the production of proinflammatory cytokines, and this increase is associated with the severity of periodontitis [37, 38]. According to Irie et al. (2006), chronic exposure to ethanol in an experimental rat model resulted in increased production of TNF-α , indicating a higher severity of inflammation in ligature-induced periodontitis in rats [39]. Therefore, alcohol is known for its ability to alter cytokine levels in both plasma and tissues and organs throughout the body.

Some studies have established the fact that individuals with intense alcohol consumption experience a higher severity of periodontitis, which was attributed to an exacerbation in the production of TNF-α [40–42]. As reported by Gonzalez-Quintela et al. in 2008, serum levels of TNF-α were much higher among intense alcohol consumers, although the same was null when the alcohol consumption was slight or moderate [43].

When considering the overall research findings reported thus far, it is envisaged that harmful alcohol habits could be considered as an independent risk factor for periodontal disease. However, the toxic threshold, intensity and other synergic effects are yet to be explained. This may warrant further research evidence in understanding the association, the mechanisms and the risk of developing periodontal disease attributable to alcohol consumption.

10.8 The Role of Alcohol in Social Settings and Its Impact on Oral Health

The destructive effects of alcohol misuse reach far beyond the individual health risks, with its consequences related to the impact on one's family, close social circle with friends and society at large. The cultural and social factors may be influential for an individual to resort to alcohol habits. Currently, most societies worldwide are exposed to a plethora of information flowing through various media. The excessive influx of information from multiple sources can be viewed as a double-edged sword.

Media advertising, product placements and other sources such as movies, television, social media and other forms of entertainment are some examples of direct or indirect promotion towards harmful alcohol habits. Media exposure significantly influences the people in a society, particularly in shaping their own choices of habits or behaviours, which, in the true sense, may have harmful consequences, yet are often viewed as societal norms.

Some studies have reported that alcohol commercials particularly affect younger adolescents to start alcohol habits. However, it is possible that the effects of advertisement differ across age groups and races. In general, the alcohol industry uses complex, targeted marketing strategies that focus certain age groups and demographic categories [44, 45]. Experimental studies also show that these targeted alcohol marketing results in individuals developing positive beliefs about drinking and creating an environment where alcohol use is socially-acceptable and encouraged [45, 46]. Emergence of flavoured alcoholic beverages is also another targeted marketing strategy by the alcohol industry in influencing the youth in general, especially the young women. Products with sweet, fruity flavours, colours and attractive packaging, particularly those aimed at young women, have a strong appeal. Although the alcohol industry claims that its marketing strategies target adults with age limits of over 21 or 29 years, flavoured alcoholic beverages are largely attractive to more younger individuals [44]. Furthermore, youth exposed to alcohol advertisements tend to drink more, on average, than their peers who were exposed to intense alcohol-related marketing [45]. According to the available research evidence for the last decade, social media platforms are most widely used by the youth, with 92% of teens reported to be online every day and 24% almost constantly [47].

There is also evidence that certain racial and ethnic minorities are exposed to targeted alcohol beverage advertising and their inclination to test these products at a younger age. For example, malt liquor typically has a higher alcohol content, but it is less expensive and sold in larger quantities [44]. This may attract some social groups with low income to consume highly concentrated alcohol products in excessive amounts, which may lead to a level of addiction.

As for the above information, the prevailing alcohol habits in some societies, especially at a harmful level, are currently viewed by oral healthcare professionals as a significant health and economic burden in combatting common oral diseases such as oral malignancies and periodontal disease.

10.9 Strategies for Maintaining Oral Health for Those Who Consume Alcohol

Maintaining good oral health for those who consume alcohol is ultimately crucial as alcohol can have a negative impact on oral health by resulting in xerostomia, erosion of teeth, periodontal diseases and development of oral cancer and potentially malignant disorders (Fig. 10.1).

Alcohol acts as a diuretic, which can lead to dehydration and xerostomia. Increased water intake helps to hydrate the mouth and reduce the severity of dry

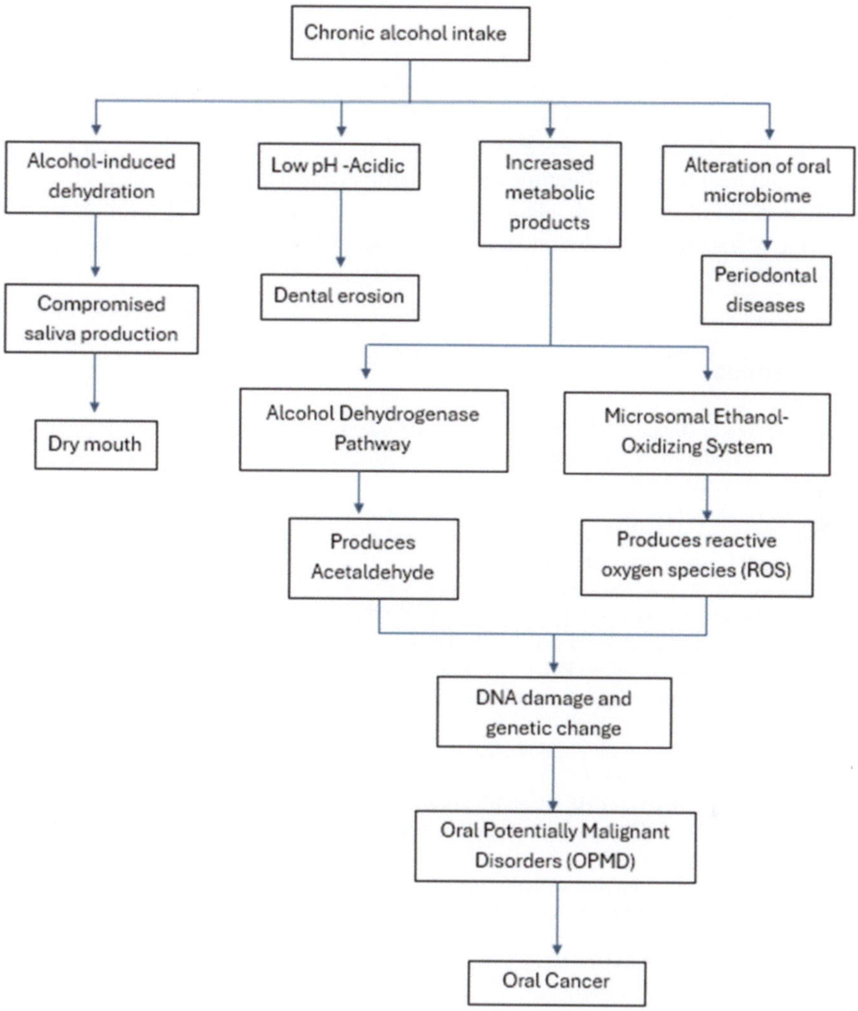

Fig. 10.1 Effects of alcohol abuse on oral health

mouth. Good oral hygiene practices help prevent dental caries and maintain an optimal environment for a balanced oral microbiome. As most alcoholic beverages are acidic and contain high amounts of sugar, the susceptibility to developing dental caries and enamel erosion is increased. A mindful selection of alcoholic drinks with low sugar content or low acidity is more likely to reduce the potential negative impacts. Regular dental checkups are essential for the early detection of dental caries, periodontal diseases or potentially malignant oral disorders. After all, either cessation or drinking in moderation is the most effective way to minimise the negative impact of alcohol on oral health.

10.10 Conclusion

The consumption of alcohol varies across different geographical regions and cultural practices. Moderate drinking can be part of a balanced recreational, social or artistic lifestyle. However, excessive alcohol intake or alcohol abuse can lead to significant health issues affecting various bodily systems, including the oral cavity. In the context of oral health, alcohol abuse increases the risk of xerostomia, dental erosion, periodontal diseases and the development of potentially malignant oral disorders, which can eventually progress into oral cancers.

References

1. World Health Organization. Global status report on alcohol and health and treatment of substance use disorders [Internet]. wwwwhoint. 2024. Available from: https://www.who.int/publications/i/item/9789240096745.
2. World Health Organisation. Global oral health status report: towards universal health coverage for oral health by 2030 [Internet]. www.who.int. 2022. Available from: https://www.who.int/publications/i/item/9789240061484.
3. Ghanem AS, Tóth Á, Nagy AC. Socio-demographic disparities in global trends of lip and oral cavity neoplasms from 1990 to 2021. Sci Rep. 2025;15(1):4230.
4. American Psychiatric Association. Diagnostic and statistical manual of mental disorders (DSM-5). 5th ed. American Psychiatric Publishing; 2013.
5. Rachdaoui N, Sarkar DK. Pathophysiology of the effects of alcohol abuse on the endocrine system. Alcohol Res. 2017;38(2):255–76.
6. The effects of alcohol on physiological processes and biological development. Alcohol Res Health. 2004;28(3):125–31.
7. Sarkar D, Jung MK, Wang HJ. Alcohol and the immune system. Alcohol Res. 2015;37(2):153–5.
8. Centres for Disease Control and Prevention. Addressing excessive alcohol use: state fact sheets [Internet]. www.cdc.gov. 2023. Available from: https://www.cdc.gov/alcohol/fact-sheets/states/excessive-alcohol-use-united-states.html.
9. Waszkiewicz N, Zalewska A, Szulc A, Kepka A, Konarzewska B, Zalewska-Szajda B, Chojnowska S, Waszkiel D, Zwierz K. The influence of alcohol on the oral cavity, salivary glands and saliva. Pol Merkur Lekarski. 2011;30(175):69–74.
10. Porter SR, Scully C, Hegarty AM. An update of the etiology and management of xerostomia. Oral Surg Oral Med Oral Pathol Oral Radiol Endod. 2004;97(1):28–46.
11. Aps JKM, Martens LC. Review: the physiology of saliva and transfer of drugs into saliva. Forensic Sci Int. 2005;150(2–3):119–31.
12. Inenaga K, Ono K, Hitomi S, Kuroki A, Ujihara I. Thirst sensation and oral dryness following alcohol intake. Jpn Dent Sci Rev. 2017;53(3):78–85.
13. Waszkiewicz N, Jelski W, Zalewska A, Szulc A, Szmitkowski M, Zwierz K, Szajda SD. Salivary alcohol dehydrogenase in non-smoking and smoking alcohol-dependent persons. Alcohol. 2014;48(6):611–6.
14. Dutta SK, Orestes M, Vengulekur S, Kwo P. Ethanol and human saliva: effect of chronic alcoholism on flow rate, composition, and epidermal growth factor. Am J Gastroenterol. 1992;87(3):350–4.
15. Schlueter N, Amaechi BT, Bartlett D, Buzalaf MAR, Carvalho TS, Ganss C, Hara AT, Huysmans MDNJM, Lussi A, Moazzez R, Vieira AR, West NX, Wiegand A, Young A, Lippert F. Terminology of erosive tooth wear: consensus report of a workshop organized by the ORCA and the Cariology Research Group of the IADR. Caries Res. 2020;54(1):2–6.

16. Chen SH, Wang JW, Li YM. Is alcohol consumption associated with gastroesophageal reflux disease? J Zhejiang Univ Sci B. 2010;11(6):423–8.
17. Ranjitkar S, Kaidonis JA, Smales RJ. Gastroesophageal reflux disease and tooth erosion. Int J Dent. 2011;2012:479850.
18. Muller S, Tilakaratne WM. Update from the 5th edition of the World Health Organization classification of head and neck tumors: tumours of the oral cavity and mobile tongue. Head Neck Pathol. 2022;16(1):54–62.
19. Ratna A, Mandrekar P. Alcohol and cancer: mechanisms and therapies. Biomolecules. 2017;7(3):61.
20. International Agency for Research on Cancer (IARC). Personal Habits and Indoor Combustions [Internet]. publications.iarc.fr. Available from: https://publications.iarc.fr/Book-And-Report-Series/Iarc-Monographs-On-The-Identification-Of-Carcinogenic-Hazards-To-Humans/Personal-Habits-And-Indoor-Combustions-2012.
21. Hoes L, Dok R, Verstrepen KJ, Nuyts S. Ethanol-induced cell damage can result in the development of oral tumors. Cancers (Basel). 2021;13(15):3846.
22. Liu Y, Chen H, Sun Z, Chen X. Molecular mechanisms of ethanol-associated oro-esophageal squamous cell carcinoma. Cancer Lett. 2015;361(2):164–73.
23. Le Dare B, Lagente V, Gicquel T. Ethanol and its metabolites: update on toxicity, benefits, and focus on immunomodulatory effects. Drug Metab Rev. 2019;51(4):545–61.
24. Pelucchi C, Gallus S, Garavello W, Bosetti C, La Vecchia C. Cancer risk associated with alcohol and tobacco use: focus on upper aero-digestive tract and liver. Alcohol Res Health. 2006;29(3):193–8.
25. Eloranta R, Vilén ST, Keinänen A, Salo T, Qannam A, Bello IO, Snäll J. Oral squamous cell carcinoma: effect of tobacco and alcohol on cancer location. Tob Induc Dis. 2024;22:1–9.
26. Ferraguti G, Terracina S, Petrella C, Greco A, Minni A, Lucarelli M, Agostinelli E, Ralli M, de Vincentiis M, Raponi G, Polimeni A, Ceccanti M, Caronti B, Di Certo MG, Barbato C, Mattia A, Tarani L, Fiore M. Alcohol and head and neck cancer: updates on the role of oxidative stress, genetic, epigenetics, oral microbiota, antioxidants, and alkylating agents. Antioxidants (Basel). 2022;11(1):145.
27. Zygogianni AG, Kyrgias G, Karakitsos P, Psyrri A, Kouvaris J, Kelekis N, Kouloulias V. Oral squamous cell cancer: early detection and the role of alcohol and smoking. Head Neck Oncol. 2011;3:2.
28. Lages EJ, Costa FO, Lages EM, Cota LO, Cortelli SC, Nobre-Franco GC, Cyrino RM, Cortelli JR. Risk variables in the association between frequency of alcohol consumption and periodontitis. J Clin Periodontol. 2012;39(2):115–22.
29. Pitiphat W, Merchant AT, Rimm EB, Joshipura KJ. Alcohol consumption increases periodontitis risk. J Dent Res. 2003;82(7):509–13.
30. Park JB, Han K, Park YG, Ko Y. Association between alcohol consumption and periodontal disease: the 2008 to 2010 Korea National Health and nutrition examination survey. J Periodontol. 2014;85(11):1521–8.
31. Lages EJ, Costa FO, Cortelli SC, Cortelli JR, Cota LO, Cyrino RM, Lages EM, Nobre-Franco GC, Brito JA, Gomez RS. Alcohol consumption and periodontitis: quantification of periodontal pathogens and cytokines. J Periodontol. 2015;86(9):1058–68.
32. Khocht A, Schleifer SJ, Janal MN, Keller S. Dental care and oral disease in alcohol-dependent persons. J Subst Abus Treat. 2009;37(2):214–8.
33. Enberg N, Alho H, Loimaranta V, Lenander-Lumikari M. Saliva flow rate, amylase activity, and protein and electrolyte concentrations in saliva after acute alcohol consumption. Oral Surg Oral Med Oral Pathol Oral Radiol Endod. 2001;92(3):292–8.
34. Szabo G. Consequences of alcohol consumption on host defence. Alcohol. 1999;34:830–41.
35. Achur RN, Freeman WM, Vrana KE. Circulating cytokines as biomarkers of alcohol abuse and alcoholism. J Neuroimmune Pharmacol. 2010;5:83–91.
36. Amaral CS, Luiz RR, Lea˜o AT. The relationship between alcohol dependence and periodontal disease. J Periodontol. 2008;79:993–8.

37. Schenkein HA, Barbour SE, Tew JG. Cytokines and inflammatory factors regulating immunoglobulin production in aggressive periodontitis. Periodontol. 2000;2007(45):113–27.
38. Tanaka S, Fakher M, Barbour SE, Schenkein HA, Tew JG. Influence of proinflammatory cytokines on Actinobacillus actinomycetemcomitans specific IgG responses. J Periodontal Res. 2006;41:1–9.
39. Irie K, Tomofuji T, Tamaki N, Sanbe T, Ekuni D, Azuma T, Maruyama T, Yamamoto T. Effects of ethanol consumption on periodontal inflammation in rats. J Dent Res. 2008;87(5):456–60.
40. Felver ME, Mezey E, McGuire M, Mitchell MC, Herlong HF, Veech GA, Veech RL. Plasma tumor necrosis factor alpha predicts decreased long-term survival in severe alcoholic hepatitis. Alcohol Clin Exp Res. 1990;14(2):255–9.
41. Bird GL, Sheron N, Goka AK, Alexander GJ, Williams RS. Increased plasma tumor necrosis factor in severe alcoholic hepatitis. Ann Intern Med. 1990;112:917–20.
42. Schafer C, Schips I, Landig J, Bode JC, Bode C. Tumor necrosis-factor and interleukin-6 response of peripheral blood monocytes to low concentrations of lipopolysaccharide in patients with alcoholic liver disease. Z Gastroenterol. 1995;33:503–8.
43. Gonzalez-Quintela A, Campos J, Loidi L, Quinteiro C, Perez LF, Gude F. Serum TNF-alpha levels in relation to alcohol consumption and common TNF gene polymorphisms. Alcohol. 2008;42:513–8.
44. Sudhinaraset M, Wigglesworth C, Takeuchi DT. Social and cultural contexts of alcohol use: influences in a social-ecological framework. Alcohol Res. 2016;38(1):35–45.
45. Snyder LB, Milici FF, Slater M, Sun H, Strizhakova Y. Effects of alcohol advertising exposure on drinking among youth. Arch Pediatr Adolesc Med. 2006;160(1):18–24.
46. Kann L, Kinchen S, Shanklin SL, Flint KH, Kawkins J, Harris WA, Lowry R, Olsen EO, McManus T, Chyen D, Whittle L, Taylor E, Demissie Z, Brener N, Thornton J, Moore J. Zaza S; Centers for Disease Control and Prevention (CDC). Youth risk behavior surveillance—United States, 2013. MMWR Suppl. 2014;63(4):1–168.
47. Teens LA. Social Media & Technology Overview 2015 [Internet]. Pew Research Center; 2015.

Illicit and Recreational Drug Abuse and Oral Health

11

Shankargouda Patil, Shilpa Bhandi, and Frank W. Licari

11.1 Introduction

Illicit drugs are substances whose non-medical use is prohibited under international drug control conventions and global drug control laws due to their significant potential for dependency and abuse [1, 2]. These substances pose substantial risks to individual health and societal well-being. Recreational drugs, on the other hand, refer to psychoactive substances consumed without medical supervision, primarily to alter consciousness for purposes of pleasure or relaxation [3]. Users often mistakenly assume that infrequent or sporadic consumption of these substances is non-addictive despite evidence to the contrary [4]. Recreational drugs can encompass both legal and illegal substances [5], with their primary use aimed at achieving an elevated or altered state of consciousness for non-medical reasons [6].

Common illicit drugs used recreationally include cannabis, amphetamines, cocaine and marijuana, among many others [7]. The effects of these substances on the human body vary widely, depending on the specific drug and its mechanism of action [8, 9].

11.2 Global and National Prevalence of Drug Abuse

The production and consumption of illicit drugs have escalated significantly over recent decades, with global drug use surpassing the rate of natural population growth [10]. The prevalence of substance use disorders has also increased over time for both men and women worldwide. In 2016, the Global Burden of Disease study, which examined alcohol and drug use across 195 countries and territories, identified cannabis dependence as the most prevalent drug use disorder, affecting 22.1 million

S. Patil (✉) · S. Bhandi · F. W. Licari
College of Dental Medicine, Roseman University of Health Sciences, South Jordan, UT, USA
e-mail: spatil@roseman.edu; sbhandi@roseman.edu; flicari@roseman.edu

S. R. Prabhu et al. (eds.), *Lifestyle in Oral Health and Disease*,
https://doi.org/10.1007/978-3-032-05888-1_11

individuals. This was followed by opioid dependence, with 26.8 million cases [11]. Amphetamine dependence was comparatively less common, and cocaine dependence was the least prevalent. The 2019 *World Drug Report* by the United Nations Office on Drugs and Crime (UNODC) estimated that in 2017, 5.5% of the global population—approximately 271 million individuals—had consumed drugs in the preceding year [12]. By 2018, around 53 million people worldwide were reported to have used opioids, with nearly 29 million consuming opiates such as heroin. In total, approximately 270 million individuals had used illicit drugs at least once in 2018 [13]. In 2020, the UNODC reported that over 250 million individuals globally used drugs, with more than 35 million people affected by drug use disorders [14]. By 2021, the global prevalence of illicit drug use had risen to 5.8% of the population, equating to approximately 296 million individuals. Within the European Union, 29% of adults aged 15–64 years reported using illicit drugs at least once in their lifetime [15].

Among illicit drugs, cannabis remains the most widely consumed, with 192.2 million users globally, followed by amphetamines, with an estimated 34.2 million users [16]. Cocaine and opiates also rank highly in terms of consumption. The overall consumption rates, measured in milligrams per day per 1000 people, reveal cannabis as the most consumed (7417.9 mg/day/1000 people), followed by cocaine (655.7 mg/day/1000 people) and morphine (384.9 mg/day/1000 people). Other substances include methamphetamine (296.2 mg/day/1000 people), codeine (222.7 mg/day/1000 people), methadone (200.2 mg/day/1000 people), methylene-dioxy-methamphetamine (MDMA) (126.3 mg/day/1000 people), amphetamine (118.2 mg/day/1000 people) and 2-ethylidene-1,5-dimethyl-3,3-diphenylpyrrolidine (33.7 mg/day/1000 people) [10].

Demographic patterns and behavioural factors Young adults aged 18–25 are particularly vulnerable to initiating or increasing substance use compared to other age groups [17]. This demographic is also less likely to perceive significant risks associated with drug use than adults aged 26 years or older [18]. Substance use is notably prevalent in social settings such as music festivals, raves, clubs, night parties and concerts [19]. Additionally, males exhibit a higher propensity for drug use compared to females [20].

Geographical variations in drug use Substantial geographical differences exist in the prevalence and patterns of substance use and dependence. Amphetamine dependence is most prevalent in Australasia, whereas cannabis, cocaine and opioid dependence are more commonly observed in North America [11]. Countries like New Zealand and the United States report higher cannabis use than other nations, with the United States also being an outlier in cocaine consumption. In Europe, cannabis is the most frequently used drug, followed by stimulants like cocaine and amphetamines [21]. However, opioid use in Europe remains comparatively low [22].

11.3 The Pharmacological Impact of Illicit Drugs on Oral Health

Drugs of abuse exert a wide range of effects on the human body, encompassing biochemical, behavioural and toxicological consequences, with a predominant impact on the brain and central nervous system (CNS) [22]. When individuals are under the influence of drugs, their neural responses undergo significant alterations, disrupting normal brain function [23]. At the biochemical level, drugs interfere with the natural process of neurotransmission. According to the National Institute on Drug Abuse (NIDA), substances like heroin and marijuana mimic endogenous neurotransmitters, leading to abnormal activation of neurons and improper impulse transmission. On the other hand, stimulants such as amphetamines and cocaine cause excessive release of neurotransmitters or inhibit their reuptake, thereby amplifying or disrupting normal signal transmission within the CNS [24].

Behaviourally, drug misuse impairs judgment and cognitive functions, induces euphoria or dysphoria and alters mood and emotional stability. Additionally, drug use is associated with various physiological and neurological complications, including vascular headaches, acute hypertension, cardiac dysrhythmias, haemorrhagic or ischaemic strokes, cerebral atrophy and peripheral neuropathy [25]. Drugs of abuse target specific brain regions, including the basal ganglia, prefrontal cortex and amygdala. The basal ganglia, which are involved in reward and motivation, are disrupted by repeated drug use, thereby altering the brain's reward system. The prefrontal cortex, which is responsible for decision-making and impulse control, is compromised, resulting in impaired regulatory functions. The amygdala, which governs emotional processing, is also affected, contributing to heightened stress and emotional dysregulation in individuals who misuse drugs. Opioids notably affect the brainstem, which controls vital autonomic functions, including heart rate, breathing and sleep cycles. An opioid overdose can suppress respiratory function, potentially resulting in fatal outcomes such as respiratory depression and death [25].

11.4 Drug-Induced Oral Manifestations

Drug abuse impacts oral health through both direct and indirect mechanisms [26]. Direct effects occur when drugs interact with oral tissues during ingestion or inhalation, while indirect effects arise from the systemic consequences of drug use. However, isolating the specific causes of oral conditions in individuals who misuse drugs can be challenging, as these individuals often exhibit multiple unhealthy behaviours [27].

Oral manifestations associated with drug use Drug users frequently present with various oral health issues, including xerostomia (dry mouth), increased risk of dental caries and periodontal diseases such as attachment loss and periodontitis [28]. Other common manifestations include mucosal lesions, halitosis, stomatitis, oral keratosis and an increased susceptibility to infections, such as oral candidiasis

[29, 30]. Dental erosion, tooth wear, bruxism and dry mouth are particularly prevalent in young individuals using recreational substances, often referred to as 'club drugs' [31].

Trauma and orofacial injuries In addition to pathological conditions, drug users experience a higher incidence of traumatic orofacial injuries, tooth loss and fractures. These injuries are often linked to accidents or physical altercations, which are more common in populations with substance use disorders.

11.4.1 Oral Health Complications Arising from Specific Drugs

- *Methamphetamine*

Methamphetamine, a synthetic derivative of amphetamine, was first synthesised in Japan in 1893 [32]. Initially utilised as a nasal decongestant and bronchial inhaler [33]. It stimulates the release and inhibits the reuptake of norepinephrine, dopamine and serotonin, leading to heightened alertness and euphoria [34]. However, this neurotransmitter imbalance contributes to neurodegeneration and eventual neurotoxicity [35]. Methamphetamine is a highly potent and long-lasting drug, classified by the FDA as a Schedule II substance due to its significant potential for misuse and dependence. Commonly referred to as 'meth', 'LA glass', 'super ice' or 'crank', it is notorious for its severe systemic and oral health consequences.

A hallmark of methamphetamine use is 'meth mouth', characterised by blackened, stained and severely decayed teeth that appear crumbled or rotten [36]. These dental lesions often resemble early childhood caries [37], with affected areas undergoing cycles of arrest and progression [34]. Lesions predominantly occur on the buccal, cervical and proximal surfaces of anterior teeth. Chronic methamphetamine users are twice as likely to have untreated caries and multiple missing or filled teeth compared to the general population [38]. These carious lesions are frequently irreparable, necessitating extractions.

Methamphetamine use is associated with severe xerostomia (dry mouth), gingivitis, periodontitis and fractured teeth [39, 40]. The acidic nature of the drug exacerbates these effects, particularly when smoked or inhaled, causing corrosive damage to oral tissues [36]. Bruxism and jaw clenching, resulting from increased neuromuscular activity, further contribute to dental attrition and temporomandibular joint (TMJ) complications [41].

- *Opioids (oxycodone)*

Opioids, derived from the opium poppy plant, have been used as potent analgesics for centuries [42, 43]. This class includes synthetic drugs such as fentanyl, prescription medications like oxycodone and hydrocodone, and illicit substances like heroin [44]. Opioids exert their effects by acting as agonists on delta, mu and kappa receptors within the central and peripheral nervous systems, inducing analgesia, euphoria, respiratory depression and other systemic effects [45].

Among opioid users, oral health is often severely compromised [46]. High rates of dental caries, particularly on smooth surfaces and in cervical areas, are common. Chronic periodontitis and acute necrotising gingivitis are also prevalent in this population [47, 48]. These conditions are exacerbated by xerostomia caused by opioid-induced salivary gland hypofunction.

Oral health implications of opioid abuse Opioid use impairs the immune response, with morphine known to inhibit macrophage phagocytosis of *Candida albicans*. Combined with reduced salivary flow, this can increase susceptibility to oral candidiasis [49]. While no direct link has been established between opioid use and oral carcinoma, concurrent use of other substances, such as cannabis or cocaine, may predispose individuals to mucosal dysplasia [50, 51].

Bruxism, characterised by heightened neuromuscular activity, is another significant complication, resulting in dental attrition and temporomandibular joint dysfunction [52]. Additionally, opioid users are at increased risk for systemic infections, including HIV and hepatitis, which often present with oral manifestations such as oral ulcers, xerostomia and periodontal infections [53, 54].

- *Cocaine*

Cocaine, a naturally occurring alkaloid derived from the *Erythroxylon coca* bush, possesses both psychoactive and local anaesthetic properties [55]. It primarily acts on the brain's limbic system, inducing psychoactive effects and promoting addiction by inhibiting dopamine reuptake. This dopamine accumulation produces euphoria and reinforces the desire for repeated drug use [56].

Oral health implications of cocaine use Cocaine use is associated with various oral health complications:

Gingival lesions Oral administration of cocaine can cause ulcerated and erythematous gingival lesions. Its vasoconstrictive properties and direct caustic effects contribute to gingival erosion and recession. Addicts often apply cocaine to the gingiva as a 'quality check', exacerbating gingival recession [57].

Tooth erosion and decay The use of pure cocaine lowers salivary pH, thereby enhancing the disintegration of tooth structure and increasing susceptibility to dental erosion [57].

Orofacial tissue necrosis The vasoconstrictive action of cocaine can lead to ischaemia and necrosis of orofacial tissues, manifesting as palatal or nasal septum perforation and chronic sinusitis. These perforations can severely impair speech [55, 58].

Oral cellular damage The use of cocaine stimulates cellular proliferation in the buccal mucosa, induces chromosomal breakage and promotes cellular death, thereby increasing the risk of oral mucosal damage [59, 60].

Bruxism and temporomandibular joint (TMJ) issues Bruxism and TMJ discomfort are commonly reported among cocaine users due to increased neuromuscular activity [57].

Crack cocaine complications The use of crack cocaine can cause sores and burns on the lips and oral mucosa, increasing the risk of HIV transmission [61].

- *Heroin*

Heroin, also known as diacetylmorphine, is a highly potent opioid synthesised from morphine [62]. It is available as a white or brown powder or a sticky black substance known as 'black tar heroin'. Widely abused for its euphoric effects, heroin is associated with severe systemic and oral health consequences, including respiratory depression and, in some cases, fatal outcomes [63, 64].

Oral health implications of heroin use Heroin abuse directly contributes to poor oral health due to a combination of personal neglect, systemic effects and addiction-related behaviours [51]:

Neglect of oral hygiene Heroin users often exhibit poor oral care due to their emotional and physical dependence on the drug, which leads to disinterest in personal hygiene. The analgesic and mental detachment effects of heroin mask dental pain, delaying or preventing treatment [65].

Dental caries Heroin use is linked to rampant caries, often presenting as pathognomonic lesions. These caries are darker in appearance, predominantly affecting the buccal and labial surfaces and covering broader areas than typical cervical lesions [66].

Periodontal disease Chronic heroin use is strongly associated with periodontal disease, including attachment loss and gingival inflammation [67].

Xerostomia and salivary gland disorders Hyposalivation caused by heroin use leads to xerostomia, which contributes to the development of dental caries, sialosis, sialadenitis and burning mouth syndrome [65].

Diet and malnutrition Poor dietary habits and malnutrition commonly seen in heroin users exacerbate oral health deterioration, as insufficient nutrients impair immune response and tissue repair [51].

Increased DMF scores Former heroin addicts exhibit significantly higher decayed, missing and filled (DMF) scores, with more missing and untreated decayed teeth compared to non-users [68]. These findings highlight the multifactorial aetiology of heroin-related oral health issues, encompassing poor hygiene, malnutrition, anxiety and lack of motivation toward dental care.

- *Cannabis*

Cannabis, also known as marijuana, weed, or pot, is a complex plant containing over 60 cannabinoid compounds, with delta-9-tetrahydrocannabinol (Δ-9-THC) identified as its primary psychoactive component [69]. Δ-9-THC was first isolated in 1964 and acts as a partial agonist at CB1 receptors (CB1R). It modulates neurotransmitter release, often by interfering with the natural regulatory effects of endogenous cannabinoids such as anandamide (AEA) and 2-arachidonoylglycerol (2-AG). Cannabis use also enhances the release of dopamine, glutamate and acetylcholine in specific brain regions, possibly by inhibiting the activity of gamma-aminobutyric acid (GABA) [70]. This mechanism underlies the desired psychoactive effects of cannabis but also contributes to significant oral health risks [71].

Oral health implications of cannabis use Inadequate oral hygiene practices, infrequent dental visits and concurrent use of substances such as tobacco and alcohol often compound poor oral health among cannabis users [72]. Common oral manifestations include:

Xerostomia (dry mouth) Δ-9-THC reduces salivary flow, leading to xerostomia, which increases the risk of dental caries and periodontal diseases in users [73].

Dietary habits As an appetite stimulant, THC encourages the consumption of sugary, cariogenic snacks, increasing the prevalence of smooth-surface caries among users compared to non-users [74].

Soft tissue changes Marijuana smoking is associated with leukoedema, gingival enlargement and erythroplakia (collectively referred to as cannabis stomatitis). These conditions carry a potential for malignant transformation [74–76].

Periodontal disease Cannabis use is linked to an elevated risk of periodontal disease, often manifesting at an earlier age compared to the general population. Confounding factors such as tobacco and alcohol use may exacerbate the severity of periodontitis [77]. Furthermore, a synergistic effect between cannabis and tobacco smoke increases the risk of oral and oropharyngeal cancers [78]. Studies suggest that younger cannabis users are at a greater risk of developing aggressive and malignant forms of these cancers [72].

Immunosuppression and oral candidiasis The immunosuppressive effects of cannabis contribute to a higher prevalence of oral infections such as candidiasis. This occurs as a result of impaired immune defences in the oral mucosa.

- *Ecstasy (MDMA)*

Methylene-dioxy-methamphetamine (MDMA), commonly referred to as ecstasy, is a synthetic psychoactive substance predominantly used in recreational settings such as rave parties and dance clubs [28] MDMA is categorised as a 'club drug' and is associated with multiple oral complications [27].

Oral health implications of MDMA Xerostomia and dental erosion: MDMA induces xerostomia, which increases the risk of dental caries and tooth wear. Users often consume large quantities of acidic beverages to alleviate dehydration and dry mouth, which can further exacerbate dental erosion. Erosive wear is typically observed on the occlusal surfaces of posterior teeth rather than the incisal edges [79].

Bruxism MDMA use leads to bruxism due to heightened neuromuscular activity. This habit accelerates tooth wear and can contribute to discomfort in the temporomandibular joint.

Soft tissue lesions Ulcers, vestibular oedema and mucosal necrosis have been reported in MDMA users, likely due to the combined effects of dehydration, mechanical trauma and local irritants [80].

- *Others (e.g. LSD, ketamine and inhalants)*

Lysergic acid diethylamide (LSD) is a potent hallucinogenic drug that exerts its effects by binding to serotonin, dopamine and adrenergic receptors in the central nervous system (CNS). This interaction results in a range of physiological and psychological effects, including hypertension, arrhythmias, mood disturbances, disorientation and convulsions [81].

Oral health implications of LSD

Bruxism LSD users frequently exhibit bruxism due to heightened neuromuscular activity, which can lead to tooth wear and temporomandibular joint discomfort [46].

Xerostomia Drug-induced dry mouth increases the risk of dental caries and periodontal diseases.

Nutritional deficiencies LSD-induced anorexia contributes to nutritional deficiencies, which can impair oral and systemic health.

Ketamine, derived from phencyclidine, is a dissociative anaesthetic commonly used recreationally as a 'club drug' [82]. It is known by various names, including 'Special K', 'Kit-Kat', 'Super K' and 'Keets' [83].

Oral health implications of ketamine The oral effects of ketamine use closely resemble those of MDMA (ecstasy) [27]:

Xerostomia A dry mouth associated with ketamine use exacerbates caries and periodontal issues [84].

Bruxism and dental erosion Consuming acidic beverages during or after bruxism can contribute to tooth wear and dental erosion.

Soft tissue complications Mucosal ulcers, vestibular oedema and necrosis have also been reported.

Inhalants encompass a broad group of volatile substances, including nitrites, anaesthetic gases and organic solvents that are deliberately inhaled for their psychoactive effects. Common methods of use include sniffing, huffing, or inhaling from a bag. These substances disrupt CNS function and interfere with emotional, physiological and neurological development [85].

Oral health implications of inhalant abuse

Chemical and thermal burns Inhalation of volatile substances can cause oral mucosa and perioral tissue burns [86].

Huffer's rash Chronic inhalant abuse may result in perioral dryness or pyoderma, commonly called 'Huffer's rash' [87].

Oedema and irritation Oedema of the lips and oropharynx is frequently observed in individuals who use inhalants [88].

Systemic associations with oral manifestations Conditions such as sinusitis, anxiety disorders and tuberculosis, which are associated with inhalant abuse, may present oral signs or symptoms.

11.5 Oral Manifestations Linked to Drug Abuse

11.5.1 Xerostomia

Xerostomia, or dry mouth, is a prevalent oral health complication associated with the use of various substances, significantly affecting oral health and overall quality of life. It results from reduced salivary flow and diminished buffering capacity, which predispose individuals to dental caries and oral infections [89]. Among substance users, methamphetamine is a prominent cause of xerostomia due to its sympathomimetic properties. By stimulating the sympathetic nervous system and acting on adrenergic receptors, methamphetamine reduces salivary gland activity, leading to the characteristic 'cotton mouth' sensation reported by approximately one-third of users [90]. This sensation often necessitates drinking water during meals to aid swallowing. Chronic users report a worsening of symptoms over time, with the prevalence of xerostomia increasing by 3% annually [91]. The lack of adequate saliva significantly reduces the oral cavity's natural ability to buffer acids, thereby drastically increasing the risk of tooth decay and other oral health problems.

Cannabis use is another significant contributor to xerostomia, primarily through the activation of CB1 receptors in the submandibular glands by endocannabinoids and THC, the psychoactive compound in cannabis. This interaction inhibits salivary secretion, further exacerbating dry mouth symptoms. Opioid use, while better known for its effects on pancreatic and gastric secretions, also contributes to xerostomia. Although opioid-induced dry mouth is not universally severe, it can become pronounced when opioids are used in conjunction with medications like antidepressants, which have drying effects on the oral mucosa [92]. Additionally, alcohol consumption and tobacco smoking, commonly concurrent with drug use, impair salivary gland function, compounding the severity of xerostomia [93].

The long-term effects of xerostomia extend beyond mere discomfort. The lack of sufficient salivary flow compromises essential protective functions, such as acid buffering, antimicrobial activity and enamel remineralisation, leaving individuals significantly more susceptible to dental caries and oral infections, including candidiasis and periodontal disease. Chronic xerostomia also contributes to difficulties in speaking, eating and swallowing, leading to a substantial decline in quality of life. Affected individuals often experience taste impairment, burning mouth syndrome and halitosis, which can further impact their psychological well-being and social interactions.

11.5.2 Periodontal Disease

Drug use is frequently associated with periodontal destruction. Various substances exert specific effects on periodontal health [75, 94, 95]. The immunosuppressive properties of opioids exacerbate periodontal disease by impairing immune defences and promoting microbial dysbiosis. Neglect, xerostomia and plaque accumulation further contribute to the progression of periodontal conditions in opioid users [51].

Recreational cannabis use is strongly linked to periodontitis, with frequent users exhibiting significantly more sites with deep pockets and attachment loss compared to non-users [96]. The mechanisms underlying this association include deeper inhalation, extended absorption time and prolonged tissue contact during cannabis smoking [97]. These factors, combined with the combustion of harmful by-products, negatively affect periodontal tissues more than cannabinoids themselves. Additionally, cannabinoids suppress key inflammatory pathways [98], although concurrent tobacco use often confounds studies on this subject [99]. Despite these associations, there is no evidence suggesting genetic susceptibility between cannabis use and periodontitis [100].

Crack cocaine use is also associated with a significantly higher prevalence of periodontitis [101]. Although the evidence linking methamphetamine use to periodontal conditions is limited, studies suggest that it may promote gingival inflammation and destruction by increasing interleukin-1 beta production in response to bacterial lipopolysaccharides in plaque [102].

11.5.3 Tooth Decay and Enamel Erosion

Tooth decay and enamel erosion are common findings among drug users, arising from behavioural, physiological and chemical factors. Opioid users are particularly prone to caries due to a preference for high-sugar diets, driven by the modulation of central opioid receptors, which enhance the palatability and reward of sweet substances [103]. Financial constraints and neglect often exacerbate poor dietary habits, increasing caries risk.

Methamphetamine users exhibit accelerated decay due to multiple mechanisms. The consumption of sugared sodas to alleviate xerostomia and sweet cravings contributes to caries formation [104]. Methamphetamine's acidic nature directly corrodes oral tissues, while its excretion through crevicular fluid during inhalation creates a caustic environment for teeth [105, 106]. Hyposalivation from adrenergic receptor stimulation, dehydration and poor hygiene amplifies susceptibility to decay [107].

Cocaine also promotes enamel and dentin disintegration due to its acidic pH (4.5) when in contact with oral tissues [108]. Crack cocaine users demonstrate an increased caries experience, although they report lower filled and missing teeth indices, particularly among men, likely reflecting barriers to dental care [109].

11.5.4 Oral Ulcers and Mucosal Damage

Drug use is associated with various mucosal changes, including chronic ulcers, frictional keratosis, extraction scars, aphthous stomatitis, tongue depapillation and candidiasis [110, 111]. Smoking or the direct application of drugs in the mouth frequently leads to ulceration and burns. For instance, cocaine use is linked to ulcerated erythematous lesions, increased cell proliferation, chromosomal damage and cell death in buccal mucosal cells [59, 111]. Clinical manifestations include mucosal erythema on the palate, painful, well-circumscribed palatal ulcers and bilateral leukoplakia [112, 113]. Users of crack cocaine often exhibit traumatic ulcers, actinic cheilitis and fistulae, while methamphetamine users demonstrate mucosal fenestrations of the attached gingiva [114].

Ecstasy (MDMA) users frequently display widespread oedema involving the labial and buccal mucosa and tongue [115]. Multifocal oral erosions with a painful yellow-white pseudo membrane surrounded by an erythematous halo have also been reported. Histopathological examination of these ulcers reveals acanthotic squamous epithelium with spongiosis, interstitial oedema and perivascular lymphoid infiltrate [116].

11.5.5 Bruxism and TMJ Disorders

Psychoactive substance use is strongly associated with temporomandibular joint disorders (TMDs), which affect both the skeletal structures and the musculature of the masticatory system [117]. Bruxism, temporomandibular joint discomfort and pain in the surrounding muscles are common orofacial manifestations in substance users, particularly among those using cocaine [118]. These symptoms are thought to arise from alterations in dopaminergic neurotransmission [56]. Bruxism and jaw clenching, often seen in drug users, can either cause or exacerbate existing TMDs.

The clinical presentation of TMDs in substance users includes a spectrum of signs and symptoms, such as myofascial pain, difficulty in jaw movement, chipping or fracturing of teeth, clicking or popping sounds in the temporomandibular joint and localised inflammation [119]. These symptoms not only create physical discomfort but also intensify the psychological challenges faced by individuals with substance use disorders, including heightened stress, anxiety and depression [120]. The poor nutritional status associated with substance abuse further compromises the health of masticatory muscles and joints. At the same time, trauma or physical injuries can lead to joint dislocations or exacerbation of TMDs [121].

The relationship between substance abuse and TMDs is complex and bidirectional. On one hand, individuals with TMDs may use substances as a coping mechanism for chronic pain. On the other, substance abuse can worsen or initiate symptoms of TMDs. Amphetamine users, for example, often report sensitivity in the masticatory muscles, restricted jaw opening and joint clicking during movement, with the latter being the most prevalent sign of TMDs. Similarly, bruxism is more frequently reported among individuals using heroin, cocaine and MDMA compared to non-users, underscoring the multifaceted impact of substance abuse on the temporomandibular joint and masticatory system [122].

11.6 Substance Abuse and Dental Health

Individuals with substance use disorders often exhibit reluctance to seek dental care, driven by a combination of psychological, financial and systemic barriers [123–125]. Anxiety about dental procedures, fear of pain and embarrassment over the condition of their oral health frequently deter drug users from accessing dental services [126]. Financial constraints further compound this issue, as individuals with unstable incomes or limited access to dental insurance often struggle to afford dental treatments [31]. Among socioeconomically marginalised populations, policymakers' concerns about the cost-effectiveness of providing dental care to drug users also limit access to oral healthcare services.

Studies show that 52% of individuals with substance use disorders had not visited a dentist in over a year, reflecting a significant gap in care [127]. Social stigma and structural discrimination also act as important barriers. Drug users often report feeling judged or excluded from healthcare decision-making, primarily due to a lack of understanding of their circumstances by dental professionals [128]. Concerns over confidentiality and legal implications further deter these individuals. For instance, patients may fear that disclosing their drug use could lead to legal repercussions or harm their dignity and self-esteem [129]. Dentists, on the other hand, may hesitate to treat drug users due to concerns about maintaining their practice's reputation or the potential for legal challenges [130].

Despite ethical obligations to protect patient confidentiality regarding substance abuse, there remains a pervasive mistrust among individuals with substance use disorders. This mistrust, combined with their greater susceptibility to oral health problems, leads to fewer dental restorations and other indicators of suboptimal dental care, highlighting the urgent need for better integration of dental and addiction treatment services [131].

11.7 Substance Use Disorder (SUD) and Oral Neglect

The relationship between substance use disorders (SUDs) and oral neglect is deeply intertwined with mental health. Individuals with mental health disorders are 80% more likely to have acute dental needs [132]. Approximately half of Americans with substance use disorders also have co-occurring mental illnesses [133]. For example, studies indicate that 84% of cocaine users have been diagnosed with a lifetime mental health disorder and one-third of individuals with bipolar disorder meet the criteria for SUD [134, 135].

Psychotropic medications used to manage mental health disorders often exacerbate oral health issues, primarily through side effects like xerostomia, which may be intensified by concurrent use of tobacco and psychostimulants. Conversely, the oral health complications seen in SUDs—such as severe caries, periodontal disease and tooth loss—can negatively affect mental well-being. Poor oral health impacts self-esteem, body image and social acceptance, creating a cyclical relationship where diminished mental health exacerbates oral neglect and vice versa.

This bidirectional relationship emphasises the need for integrated healthcare approaches that address both the psychological and physical aspects of substance use disorders. Tackling oral neglect in this population requires addressing the broader mental health challenges that fuel the neglect, ensuring a holistic approach to care.

11.8 Clinical Management of Oral Health in Drug-Dependent Patients

Dental clinicians play a pivotal role in identifying early signs of substance abuse through vigilant observation and sensitive questioning during medical history assessments [136]. Indicators of drug abuse include changes in appetite, lethargy, poor hygiene, unusual body odours, needle marks and a deteriorated appearance [76]. Many patients seek aesthetic dental treatments such as veneers or whitening to counteract the social stigma associated with these effects [137]. Employing validated screening tools like the Drug Abuse Screening Test (DAST-20), the Tobacco, Alcohol, Prescription Medication and Other Substance Use (TAPS) tool, or the Alcohol, Smoking and Substance Involvement Screening Test (ASSIST) can facilitate the discussion of substance use and guide appropriate referrals for cessation and recovery therapy. Addressing substance use before initiating dental treatment minimises risks such as adverse drug interactions and ensures the long-term success of aesthetic and restorative procedures [138].

11.9 Comprehensive Oral Health Examination

Comprehensive oral health assessments for drug-dependent patients require a detailed examination of hard and soft tissues [139]. Dentists should prioritise personalised treatment plans and consider the unique challenges of substance users, such as limited motivation and heightened anxiety. Radiographic evaluations often reveal severe bone loss, angular intra-bony defects and other structural damage associated with substance use [140]. Short, patient-centred appointments with frequent breaks can help alleviate anxiety and facilitate effective treatment delivery.

11.9.1 Preventive Measures

Preventive care is crucial for patients in recovery to prevent further deterioration in their oral health. Education on basic oral hygiene practices, including proper brushing techniques, should be emphasised and routinely reviewed. Preventive measures, such as fluoride treatments, alcohol-free chlorhexidine rinses, xylitol gum and candies, are recommended to combat caries and regulate salivary pH. For patients unable to tolerate traditional restorative care, silver diamine fluoride offers an alternative for caries management [141].

Dietary counselling should focus on reducing sugar intake, increasing water consumption and avoiding caffeine and alcohol to mitigate xerostomia. In cases of salivary gland dysfunction, sialagogues such as pilocarpine may be prescribed, provided there are no contraindications or interactions with other medications. For patients undergoing medication-assisted therapy with buprenorphine, naloxone, or methadone, rinsing the mouth immediately after consumption can reduce the risk of oral health complications. A proactive and patient-centred approach is essential to managing oral health in drug-dependent patients, ensuring both immediate relief and long-term care [141].

11.9.2 Restorative and Rehabilitative Approaches

Restorative and rehabilitative dental treatments play a key role in improving the oral health and quality of life of drug-dependent patients, especially those with extensive dental damage or edentulism. Before initiating restorative care, conducting a comprehensive risk assessment, stabilising oral health through preventive measures and addressing active caries is essential.

Removable prostheses, either full or partial, offer a practical and cost-effective solution for patients with partial or complete edentulism. These prostheses are especially advantageous for patients with challenging medical or behavioural management issues. Fixed prosthodontic solutions, such as dental crowns, bridges and implants, may also be considered. However, dental implants require meticulous evaluation and planning, particularly in individuals with systemic complications or poor oral hygiene habits related to substance use disorders. Adequate pre-implant therapy and commitment to maintenance are critical for achieving long-term success [142].

11.9.3 Pain Management Considerations

Pain management in drug-dependent patients presents unique challenges, as their history of substance use may complicate analgesic efficacy and increase the risk of relapse [143, 144]. Many individuals with substance use disorders rely on illicit drugs to self-manage pain and withdrawal during dental therapy can exacerbate discomfort and hinder successful treatment [144]. Additionally, comorbid psychiatric and medical conditions may obscure pain perception and reduce the effectiveness of conventional analgesics [143].

Non-opioid analgesics, such as acetaminophen or ibuprofen, are recommended as first-line pain management options [145]. These medications are effective in controlling mild to moderate pain without posing the risk of addiction. Care must be exercised when using local anaesthetics containing adrenaline, as these can worsen tachycardia in patients consuming cannabis or methamphetamine [146]. For methamphetamine users, dental treatment should be postponed for at least 6 hours after the last dose. If treatment cannot be delayed, anaesthetics without vasoconstrictors should be employed [34]. In cocaine users, the administration of lignocaine is contraindicated due to its synergistic vasoconstrictive effects, which can lead to serious complications such as cerebrovascular accidents or myocardial infarction. Dental treatment in these patients should be deferred for 6–12 hours after cocaine use to minimise risks [57].

Drug-dependent patients often exhibit reduced responsiveness to local anaesthesia, necessitating higher doses or alternative methods for adequate pain control. However, conscious sedation using nitrous oxide or intravenous benzodiazepines should be avoided due to the potential for abuse or adverse interactions [147]. For patients requiring sedation, non-pharmacologic techniques or general anaesthesia under close supervision may be considered safer alternatives. Effective pain management in drug-dependent patients requires a personalised approach that balances the need for adequate analgesia with the risks associated with their substance use history. Close collaboration with medical professionals and addiction specialists is essential to optimise outcomes while minimising risks.

11.10 Legal and Ethical Considerations for Practitioners

Legal obligations for reporting drug abuse vary across regions, requiring dental practitioners to navigate complex regulations. Practitioners must ensure compliance with local laws while safeguarding patient welfare. Balancing patient confidentiality with mandatory reporting obligations poses ethical challenges. Practitioners must carefully document substance use, providing only essential and accurate information after obtaining informed consent from the patient. Confidentiality concerns often deter full disclosure in medical records, especially when state-mandated disclosures can negatively impact patients. Sensitivity in addressing substance use during patient interactions, alongside adherence to ethical principles, ensures trust while mitigating risks of harm from breaches in confidentiality. Accurate and informed documentation prevents malpractice and supports the delivery of optimal patient care [148].

11.11 Conclusions

Illicit drug use is a pervasive global public health issue. Such disorders manifest through systemic and orofacial complications, compounded by poly-drug use, tobacco, alcohol consumption and associated behavioural and psychological challenges. This multifaceted impact complicates oral health management and emphasises the need for an integrative care approach.

Dental clinicians play a crucial role in identifying early signs of substance abuse, enabling timely referrals for rehabilitation. This proactive approach can prevent addiction-related complications, enhance the cost-effectiveness of drug control interventions and restore patients' oral health, general well-being and psychosocial recovery, achieving comprehensive care objectives.

References

1. Babor T. Drug policy and the public good. Published online 2010.
2. McAllister WB. Drug diplomacy in the twentieth century. Routledge; 2002.
3. Crocq M-A. Historical and cultural aspects of man's relationship with addictive drugs. Dialogues Clin Neurosci. 2007;9(4):355–61.
4. Starobin B, Jablonski S, Andrle AM, Powers JB. Recreational drugs: effects on the heart and cardiovascular system. Published online 2018.
5. Gossop M. Classification of illegal and harmful drugs. BMJ. 2006;333(7562):272–3. https://doi.org/10.1136/bmj.38929.578414.80.
6. Gabay M. The federal controlled substances act: schedules and pharmacy registration. Hosp Pharm. 2013;48(6):473.
7. Lopez MJ, Preuss CV, Tadi P. Drug enforcement administration drug scheduling. In: StatPearls [Internet]. StatPearls Publishing; 2023.
8. Larrat EP, Marcoux RM, Vogenberg FR. Implications of recent controlled substance policy initiatives. Pharm Ther. 2014;39(2):126.

9. Gabay M. Federal controlled substances act: controlled substances prescriptions. Hosp Pharm. 2013;48(8):644.
10. Zarei S, Salimi Y, Repo E, et al. A global systematic review and meta-analysis on illicit drug consumption rate through wastewater-based epidemiology. Environ Sci Pollut Res. 2020;27:36037–51.
11. Degenhardt L, Charlson F, Ferrari A, et al. The global burden of disease attributable to alcohol and drug use in 195 countries and territories, 1990–2016: a systematic analysis for the Global Burden of Disease Study 2016. Lancet Psychiatry. 2018;5(12):987–1012. https://doi.org/10.1016/S2215-0366(18)30337-7.
12. UNODC. World Drug Report 2019 methodology report. Word Drug Rep – 2019 Stimul. 2019;(June 2019):56.
13. Mercan S, Kuloglu M, Tekin T, et al. Wastewater-based monitoring of illicit drug consumption in Istanbul: preliminary results from two districts. Sci Total Environ. 2019;656:231–8.
14. Shen J, Hua G, Li C, Liu S, Liu L, Jiao J. Prevalence, incidence, deaths, and disability-adjusted life-years of drug use disorders for 204 countries and territories during the past 30 years. Asian J Psychiatr. 2023;86:103677. https://doi.org/10.1016/j.ajp.2023.103677.
15. Lojszczyk A, Wilson R, Wood J, Hutton A. Motivational characteristics of recreational drug use among emerging adults in social settings: an integrative literature review. Front Public Health. 2023;11:1235387.
16. Cossa F, Piastra A, Sarrion-Pérez MG, Bagán L. Oral manifestations in drug users: a review. J Clin Exp Dent. 2020;12(2):e193–200. https://doi.org/10.4317/jced.55928.
17. Lu W, Lopez-Castro T, Vu T. Population-based examination of substance use disorders and treatment use among US young adults in the National Survey on Drug Use and Health, 2011–2019. Drug Alcohol Depend Rep. 2023;8:100181. https://doi.org/10.1016/j.dadr.2023.100181.
18. Lipari R, Jean-Francois B. Trends in perception of risk and availability of substance use among full-time college students. Published online 2016.
19. Arnett JJ. The developmental context of substance use in emerging adulthood. J Drug Issues. 2005;35(2):235–54.
20. Degenhardt L, Chiu W-T, Sampson N, et al. Toward a global view of alcohol, tobacco, cannabis, and cocaine use: findings from the WHO World Mental Health Surveys. PLoS Med. 2008;5(7):e141.
21. Eurosurveillance Editorial Team C. The European Monitoring Centre for Drugs and Drug Addiction publishes the 'European Drug Report 2013: trends and developments.' Published online 2013.
22. Ciucă Anghel D-M, Nițescu GV, Tiron A-T, Guțu CM, Baconi DL. Understanding the mechanisms of action and effects of drugs of abuse. Molecules. 2023;28(13) https://doi.org/10.3390/molecules28134969.
23. Cunha-Oliveira T, Rego AC, Carvalho F, Oliveira CR. Medical toxicology of drugs of abuse. Princ Addict Addict Behav Disord. 2013;1:159–75.
24. Neiman J, Haapaniemi HM, Hillbom M. Neurological complications of drug abuse: pathophysiological mechanisms. Eur J Neurol. 2000;7(6):595–606. https://doi.org/10.1046/j.1468-1331.2000.00045.x.
25. Chen A, Ashburn MA. Cardiac effects of opioid therapy. Pain Med. 2015;16(Suppl 1):S27–31. https://doi.org/10.1111/pme.12915.
26. Reece AS. Dentition of addiction in Queensland: poor dental status and major contributing drugs. Aust Dent J. 2007;52(2):144–9.
27. Shekarchizadeh H, Khami MR, Mohebbi SZ, Ekhtiari H, Virtanen JI. Oral health of drug abusers: a review of health effects and care. Iran J Public Health. 2013;42(9):929.
28. Gahlinger PM. Club drugs: MDMA, gamma-hydroxybutyrate (GHB), Rohypnol, and ketamine. Am Fam Physician. 2004;69(11):2619–27.
29. Andreis K, Billingsley J, Naimi Shirazi K, et al. Cannabinoid CB1 receptors regulate salivation. Sci Rep. 2022;12(1):14182. https://doi.org/10.1038/s41598-022-17987-2.

30. Mateos-Moreno MV, del-Río-Highsmith J, Riobóo-García R, Solá-Ruiz MF, Celemín-Viñuela A. Dental profile of a community of recovering drug addicts: biomedical aspects. Retrospective cohort study. Med Oral Patol Oral Cir Bucal. 2013;18(4):e671.
31. Robinson PG, Acquah S, Gibson B. Drug users: oral health-related attitudes and behaviours. Br Dent J. 2005;198(4):219–24.
32. Lineberry TW, Bostwick JM. Methamphetamine abuse: a perfect storm of complications. In: Mayo clinic proceedings, vol. 81. Elsevier; 2006. p. 77–84.
33. Mukherjee A, Dye BA, Clague J, Belin TR, Shetty V. Methamphetamine use and oral health-related quality of life. Qual Life Res. 2018;27:3179–90.
34. Hamamoto DT, Rhodus NL. Methamphetamine abuse and dentistry. Oral Dis. 2009;15(1):27–37.
35. Cadet JL, Jayanthi S, Deng X. Speed kills: cellular and molecular bases of methamphetamine-induced nerve terminal degeneration and neuronal apoptosis. FASEB J. 2003;17(13):1775–88.
36. Shetty V, Mooney LJ, Zigler CM, Belin TR, Murphy D, Rawson R. The relationship between methamphetamine use and increased dental disease. J Am Dent Assoc. 2010;141(3):307–18.
37. Shaner JW. Caries associated with methamphetamine abuse. N Y State Dent J. 2002;68(10):20.
38. Shetty V, Harrell L, Clague J, Murphy DA, Dye BA, Belin TR. Methamphetamine users have increased dental disease: a propensity score analysis. J Dent Res. 2016;95(7):814–21.
39. Spolsky VW, Clague J, Murphy DA, et al. Periodontal status of current methamphetamine users. J Am Dent Assoc. 2018;149(3):174–83.
40. Yazdanian M, Armoon B, Noroozi A, et al. Dental caries and periodontal disease among people who use drugs: a systematic review and meta-analysis. BMC Oral Health. 2020;20:1–18.
41. Donaldson M, Goodchild JH. Oral health of the methamphetamine abuser. Am J Health Pharm. 2006;63(21):2078–82.
42. Goodrich JT. History of spine surgery in the ancient and medieval worlds. Neurosurg Focus. 2004;16(1):1–13.
43. Benyamin R, Trescot AM, Datta S, et al. Opioid complications and side effects. Pain Physician. 2008;11(2 Suppl):S105–20.
44. Teesson M, Ross J, Darke S, et al. One year outcomes for heroin dependence: findings from the Australian Treatment Outcome Study (ATOS). Drug Alcohol Depend. 2006;83(2):174–80.
45. Vanderah TW. Delta and kappa opioid receptors as suitable drug targets for pain. Clin J Pain. 2010;26(Suppl 1):S10–5. https://doi.org/10.1097/AJP.0b013e3181c49e3a.
46. Fazzi M, Vescovi P, Savi A, Manfredi M, Peracchia M. The effects of drugs on the oral cavity. Minerva Stomatol. 1999;48(10):485–92.
47. Davis RK, Baer PN. Necrotizing ulcerative gingivitis in drug addict patients being withdrawn from drugs. Report of two cases. Oral Surg Oral Med Oral Pathol. 1971;31(2):200–4. https://doi.org/10.1016/0030-4220(71)90074-0.
48. Shekarchizadeh H, Khami MR, Mohebbi SZ, Ekhtiari H, Virtanen JI. Oral health status and its determinants among opiate dependents: a cross-sectional study. BMC Oral Health. 2019;19(1):5. https://doi.org/10.1186/s12903-018-0691-3.
49. Szabo I, Rojavin M, Bussiere JL, Eisenstein TK, Adler MW, Rogers TJ. Suppression of peritoneal macrophage phagocytosis of Candida albicans by opioids. J Pharmacol Exp Ther. 1993;267(2):703–6.
50. Llewelyn J, Mitchell R. Smoking, alcohol and oral cancer in south east Scotland: a 10-year experience. Br J Oral Maxillofac Surg. 1994;32(3):146–52. https://doi.org/10.1016/0266-4356(94)90098-1.
51. Titsas A, Ferguson MM. Impact of opioid use on dentistry. Aust Dent J. 2002;47(2):94–8.
52. Colon PG Jr. Dental disease in the narcotic addict. Oral Surg Oral Med Oral Pathol. 1972;33(6):905–10.
53. Liang TJ, Ward JW. Hepatitis C in injection-drug users – a hidden danger of the opioid epidemic. N Engl J Med. 2018;378(13):1169–71. https://doi.org/10.1056/NEJMp1716871.
54. Ribera E, Miró JM, Cortés E, et al. Influence of human immunodeficiency virus 1 infection and degree of immunosuppression in the clinical characteristics and outcome of infective

endocarditis in intravenous drug users. Arch Intern Med. 1998;158(18):2043–50. https://doi.org/10.1001/archinte.158.18.2043.
55. Brand HS, Gonggrijp S, Blanksma CJ. Cocaine and oral health. Br Dent J. 2008;204(7):365–9.
56. Hyman SE, Malenka RC. Addiction and the brain: the neurobiology of compulsion and its persistence. Nat Rev Neurosci. 2001;2(10):695–703.
57. Blanksma CJ, Brand HS. Cocaine abuse: orofacial manifestations and implications for dental treatment. Int Dent J. 2005;55(6):365–9.
58. Gandara-Rey JM, Diniz-Freitas M, Gandara-Vila P, Blanco-Carrion A, Garcia-Garcia A. Lesions of the oral mucosa in cocaine users who apply the drug topically. Med Oral Organo Of la Soc Esp Med Oral y la Acad Iberoam Patol y Med Bucal. 2002;7(2):103–7.
59. das Graças Alonso de Oliveira M, Dos Santos JN, Cury PR, et al. Cytogenetic biomonitoring of oral mucosa cells of crack cocaine users. Environ Sci Pollut Res. 2014;21:5760–4.
60. Kapila YL, Kashani H. Cocaine-associated rapid gingival recession and dental erosion. A case report. J Periodontol. 1997;68(5):485–8.
61. Faruque S, Edlin BR, McCoy CB, et al. Crack cocaine smoking and oral sores in three inner-city neighborhoods. JAIDS: J Acquir Immune Defic Syndr. 1996;13(1):87–92.
62. Milella MS, D'Ottavio G, De Pirro S, Barra M, Caprioli D, Badiani A. Heroin and its metabolites: relevance to heroin use disorder. Transl Psychiatry. 2023;13(1):120. https://doi.org/10.1038/s41398-023-02406-5.
63. Oppenheimer E, Tobutt C, Taylor C, Andrew T. Death and survival in a cohort of heroin addicts from London clinics: a 22-year follow-up study. Addiction. 1994;89(10):1299–308. https://doi.org/10.1111/j.1360-0443.1994.tb03309.x.
64. Sporer KA. Acute heroin overdose. Ann Intern Med. 1999;130(7):584–90. https://doi.org/10.7326/0003-4819-130-7-199904060-00019.
65. Abed H, Hassona Y. Oral healthcare management in heroin and methadone users. Br Dent J. 2019;226(8):563–7. https://doi.org/10.1038/s41415-019-0206-x.
66. Madinier I, Harrosch J, Dugourd M, Giraud-Morin C, Fosse T. The buccal-dental health of drug addicts treated in the University Hospital Centre in Nice. Press Med (Paris, Fr 1983). 2003;32(20):919–23.
67. Picozzi A, Dworkin SF, Leeds JG, Nash J. Dental and associated attitudinal aspects of heroin addiction: a pilot study. J Dent Res. 1972;51(3):869.
68. Rosenstein DI. Effect of long-term addiction to heroin on oral tissues. J Public Health Dent. 1975;35(2):118–22. https://doi.org/10.1111/j.1752-7325.1975.tb04035.x.
69. Gaoni Y, Mechoulam R. Isolation, structure, and partial synthesis of an active constituent of hashish. J Am Chem Soc. 1964;86(8):1646–7.
70. Bhattacharyya S, Crippa JA, Martin-Santos R, Winton-Brown T, Fusar-Poli P. Imaging the neural effects of cannabinoids: current status and future opportunities for psychopharmacology. Curr Pharm Des. 2009;15(22):2603–14.
71. Atakan Z. Cannabis, a complex plant: different compounds and different effects on individuals. Ther Adv Psychopharmacol. 2012;2(6):241–54. https://doi.org/10.1177/2045125312457586.
72. Cho CM, Hirsch R, Johnstone S. General and oral health implications of cannabis use. Aust Dent J. 2005;50(2):70–4.
73. Rechthand MM, Bashirelahi N. What every dentist needs to know about cannabis. Gen Dent. 2016;64(1):40–3.
74. Joshi S, Ashley M. Cannabis: A joint problem for patients and the dental profession. Br Dent J. 2016;220(11):597–601.
75. Rawal SY, Tatakis DN, Tipton D. Periodontal and oral manifestations of marijuana use. J Tenn Dent Assoc. 2012;92(2):26.
76. Maloney WJ, Raymond GF. Common substances and medications of abuse. In: The ADA practical guide to substance use disorders and safe prescribing. Wiley Blackwell. Published online 2015. p. 83–118.
77. Thomson WM, Poulton R, Broadbent JM, et al. Cannabis smoking and periodontal disease among young adults. JAMA. 2008;299(5):525–31.

78. Thompson GR, Tuscano JM, Dennis M, et al. A microbiome assessment of medical marijuana. Clin Microbiol Infect. 2017;23(4):269–70.
79. Redfearn PJ, Agrawal N, Mair LH. An association between the regular use of 3, 4 methylenedioxy-methamphetamine (Ecstasy) and excessive wear of the teeth. Addiction. 1998;93(5):745–8.
80. Brand HS, Dun SN, Nieuw Amerongen AV. Ecstasy (MDMA) and oral health. Br Dent J. 2008;204(2):77–81.
81. Nichols DE. Hallucinogens. Pharmacol Ther. 2004;101(2):131–81.
82. Kohrs R, Durieux ME. Ketamine: teaching an old drug new tricks. Anesth Analg. 1998;87(5):1186–93.
83. Gahlinger P. Illegal drugs: a complete guide to their history, chemistry, use, and abuse. Penguin; 2003.
84. Edition F. Diagnostic and statistical manual of mental disorders. Am Psychiatry Assoc. 2013;21(21):591–643.
85. Howard MO, Bowen SE, Garland EL, Perron BE, Vaughn MG. Inhalant use and inhalant use disorders in the United States. Addict Sci Clin Pract. 2011;6(1):18–31.
86. Lubman DI, Yücel M, Lawrence AJ. Inhalant abuse among adolescents: neurobiological considerations. Br J Pharmacol. 2008;154(2):316–26. https://doi.org/10.1038/bjp.2008.76.
87. Baydala L. Inhalant abuse. Paediatr Child Health. 2010;15(7):443–54.
88. Brouette T, Anton R. Clinical review of inhalants. Am J Addict. 2001;10(1):79–94.
89. Klasser GD, Epstein J. Methamphetamine and its impact on dental care. J Can Dent Assoc (Tor). 2005;71(10):759–62.
90. Brown C, Krishnan S, Hursh K, et al. Dental disease prevalence among methamphetamine and heroin users in an urban setting: a pilot study. J Am Dent Assoc. 2012;143(9):992–1001.
91. Murphy DA, Harrell L, Fintzy R, Vitero S, Gutierrez A, Shetty V. Soda consumption among methamphetamine users in the US: impact on Oral health. Oral Health Prev Dent. 2016;14(3):227.
92. Odeh M, Oliven A, Bassan H. Morphine and severe dryness of the lips. Postgrad Med J. 1992;68(798):303.
93. Hopcraft MS, Tan C. Xerostomia: an update for clinicians. Aust Dent J. 2010;55(3):238–44.
94. Yukna RA. Cocaine periodontitis. Int J Periodontics Restorative Dent. 1991;11(1):72–9.
95. Brazier WJ, Dhariwal DK, Patton DW, Bishop K. Ecstasy related periodontitis and mucosal ulceration–a case report. Br Dent J. 2003;194(4):197–9.
96. Shariff JA, Ahluwalia KP, Papapanou PN. Relationship between frequent recreational cannabis (marijuana and hashish) use and periodontitis in adults in the United States: National Health and Nutrition Examination Survey 2011 to 2012. J Periodontol. 2017;88(3):273–80.
97. López R, Baelum V. Cannabis use and destructive periodontal diseases among adolescents. J Clin Periodontol. 2009;36(3):185–9.
98. Melamede R. Harm reduction-the cannabis paradox. Harm Reduct J. 2005;2:1–13.
99. Johnson GK, Slach NA. Impact of tobacco use on periodontal status. J Dent Educ. 2001;65(4):313–21. https://doi.org/10.1002/j.0022-0337.2001.65.4.tb03401.x.
100. Baumeister S, Alayash Z, Baurecht H, et al. Cannabis use and the risk of periodontitis: a two-sample Mendelian randomization study. J Clin Periodontol. Published online 2022:0–2. https://doi.org/10.1111/jcpe.13632.
101. Antoniazzi RP, Zanatta FB, Rösing CK, Feldens CA. Association among periodontitis and the use of crack cocaine and other illicit drugs. J Periodontol. 2016;87(12):1396–405.
102. Tipton DA, Legan ZT, Dabbous MK. Methamphetamine cytotoxicity and effect on LPS-stimulated IL-1β production by human monocytes. Toxicol Vitr. 2010;24(3):921–7.
103. Badiani A, Leone P, Noel MB, Stewart J. Ventral tegmental area opioid mechanisms and modulation of ingestive behavior. Brain Res. 1995;670(2):264–76.
104. Clague J, Belin TR, Shetty V. Mechanisms underlying methamphetamine-related dental disease. J Am Dent Assoc. 2017;148(6):377–86.

105. ADA Division of Communications, Journal of the American Dental Association, ADA Division of Scientific Affairs. For the dental patient... methamphetamine use and oral health. J Am Dent Assoc. 2005;136(10):1491.
106. De-Carolis C, Boyd G-A, Mancinelli L, Pagano S, Eramo S. Methamphetamine abuse and "meth mouth" in Europe. Med Oral Patol Oral Cir Bucal. 2015;20(2):e205.
107. Heng CK, Badner VM, Schiop LA. Meth mouth. N Y State Dent J. 2008;74(5):50.
108. Krutchkoff DJ, Eisenberg E, O'Brien JE, Ponzillo JJ. Cocaine-induced dental erosions. N Engl J Med. 1990;322(6):408.
109. Cury PR, Oliveira MGA, de Andrade KM, de Freitas MDS, Dos Santos JN. Dental health status in crack/cocaine-addicted men: a cross-sectional study. Environ Sci Pollut Res. 2017;24:7585–90.
110. Sordi MB, Massochin RC, de Camargo AR, Lemos T, Munhoz EDA. Oral health assessment for users of marijuana and cocaine/crack substances. Braz Oral Res. 2017;31:e102.
111. Parry J, Porter S, Scully C, Flint S, Parry MG. Mucosal lesions due to oral cocaine use. Br Dent J. 1996;180(12):462–4.
112. Mitchell-Lewis DA, Phelan JA, Kelly RB, Bradley JJ, Lamster IB. Identifying oral lesions associated with crack cocaine use. J Am Dent Assoc. 1994;125(8):1104–8. https://doi.org/10.14219/jada.archive.1994.0122.
113. Cury PR, Araujo NS, das Graças Alonso Oliveira M, Dos Santos JN. Association between oral mucosal lesions and crack and cocaine addiction in men: a cross-sectional study. Environ Sci Pollut Res Int. 2018;25(20):19801–7. https://doi.org/10.1007/s11356-018-2120-1.
114. Verheyden SL, Henry JA, Curran HV. Acute, sub-acute and long-term subjective consequences of 'ecstasy' (MDMA) consumption in 430 regular users. Hum Psychopharmacol Clin Exp. 2003;18(7):507–17.
115. Ahmed M, Islam S, Hoffman GR. Widespread oral and oropharyngeal mucosal oedema induced by ecstasy (MDMA): a case for concern. Br J Oral Maxillofac Surg. 2007;45(6):496–8.
116. Biancardi MR, da Silveira HA, Fernandes D, et al. Ecstasy abuse and its effects on the oral mucosa. J Craniofac Surg. 2019;30(3):e189–91. https://doi.org/10.1097/SCS.0000000000005033.
117. Aldosari LIN, Hassan SAB, Alshahrani AA, et al. Prevalence of temporomandibular disorders among psychoactive substances abusers: A systematic review and meta-analysis. J Oral Rehabil. 2023;50(9):894–901.
118. Giannakopoulos HE, Quinn PD, Granquist E, Chou JC. Posttraumatic temporomandibular joint disorders. Craniomaxillofac Trauma Reconstr. 2009;2(2):91–101.
119. Enguelberg-Gabbay JV, Schapir L, Israeli Y, Hermesh H, Weizman A, Winocur E. Methadone treatment, bruxism, and temporomandibular disorders among male prisoners. Eur J Oral Sci. 2016;124(3):266–71.
120. Rasinski KA, Woll P, Cooke A. Stigma and substance use disorders. Published online 2005.
121. Smit DA, Naidoo S. Oral health effects, brushing habits and management of methamphetamine users for the general dental practitioner. Br Dent J. 2015;218(9):531–6.
122. White R. Drugs and nutrition: how side effects can influence nutritional intake. Proc Nutr Soc. 2010;69(4):558–64.
123. Saeland M, Haugen M, Eriksen F-L, et al. High sugar consumption and poor nutrient intake among drug addicts in Oslo, Norway. Br J Nutr. 2011;105(4):618–24.
124. Kane SF. The effects of oral health on systemic health. Gen Dent. 2017;65(6):30–4.
125. Scheutz F. Anxiety and dental fear in a group of parenteral drug addicts. Eur J Oral Sci. 1986;94(3):241–7.
126. Jaffe K, Choi J, Hayashi K, Milloy M-J, Richardson L. A paradox of need: gaps in access to dental care among people who use drugs in Canada's publicly funded healthcare system. Health Soc Care Community. 2021;29(6):1799–806. https://doi.org/10.1111/hsc.13289.
127. D'Amore MM, Cheng DM, Kressin NR, et al. Oral health of substance-dependent individuals: impact of specific substances. J Subst Abus Treat. 2011;41(2):179–85.
128. Brondani MA, Alan R, Donnelly L. Stigma of addiction and mental illness in healthcare: the case of patients' experiences in dental settings. PLoS One. 2017;12(5):e0177388.

129. Peltier B, Giusti L, Hoover T, Fountain J, Persinger J, Sutter S. The dental patient who is "high:" ethical and scientific recommendations for the standard of care. J Am Coll Dent. 2010;77(1):21–34.
130. Wentworth RB. What should I Do when I suspect a patient may be abusing prescription drugs? J Am Dent Assoc. 2008;139(5):623–4. https://doi.org/10.14219/jada.archive.2008.0226.
131. Baghaie H, Kisely S, Forbes M, Sawyer E, Siskind DJ. A systematic review and meta-analysis of the association between poor oral health and substance abuse. Addiction. 2017;112(5):765–79.
132. Nguyen VH, Lin SC, Cappelli DP, Nair S. The association between dental, general, and mental health status among underserved and vulnerable populations served at health centers in the US. J Public Health Dent. 2018;78(1):41–8.
133. Fellows JL, Atchison KA, Chaffin J, Chávez EM, Tinanoff N. Oral health in America. J Am Dent Assoc. 2022;153(7):601–9. https://doi.org/10.1016/j.adaj.2022.04.002.
134. Hunt GE, Malhi GS, Cleary M, Lai HMX, Sitharthan T. Comorbidity of bipolar and substance use disorders in national surveys of general populations, 1990–2015: systematic review and meta-analysis. J Affect Disord. 2016;206:321–30.
135. Saffer H, Dave D. Mental illness and the demand for alcohol, cocaine, and cigarettes. Econ Inq. 2005;43(2):229–46.
136. Parish CL, Pereyra MR, Pollack HA, et al. Screening for substance misuse in the dental care setting: findings from a nationally representative survey of dentists. Addiction. 2015;110(9):1516–23. https://doi.org/10.1111/add.13004.
137. Denisco RC, Kenna GA, O'Neil MG, et al. Prevention of prescription opioid abuse: the role of the dentist. J Am Dent Assoc. 2011;142(7):800–10.
138. McNeely J, Wright S, Matthews AG, et al. Substance-use screening and interventions in dental practices: survey of practice-based research network dentists regarding current practices, policies and barriers. J Am Dent Assoc. 2013;144(6):627–38.
139. Lee CYS, Mohammadi H, Dixon RA. Medical and dental implications of cocaine abuse. J Oral Maxillofac Surg. 1991;49(3):290–3.
140. Laslett A, Dietze P, Dwyer R. The oral health of street-recruited injecting drug users: prevalence and correlates of problems. Addiction. 2008;103(11):1821–5.
141. Cuberos M, Chatah EM, Baquerizo HZ, Weinstein G. Dental management of patients with substance use disorder. Clin Dent Rev. 2020;4(1):14. https://doi.org/10.1007/s41894-020-00078-8.
142. Alqarni H, Alsaloum M, Alzaid A. Prosthetic rehabilitation of meth mouth with implant-supported fixed dental prostheses: A clinical report. J Prosthet Dent. 2022;128(6):1140–4. https://doi.org/10.1016/j.prosdent.2021.02.036.
143. Koenig TW, Clark MR. Advances in comprehensive pain management. Psychiatr Clin North Am. 1996;19(3):589–611.
144. Portenoy RK, Dole V, Joseph H, et al. Pain management and chemical dependency: evolving perspectives. JAMA. 1997;278(7):592–3.
145. Charnock S, Owen S, Brookes V, Williams M. A community based programme to improve access to dental services for drug users. Br Dent J. 2004;196(7):385–8.
146. Maloney WJ. Significance of cannabis use to dental practice. N Y State Dent J. 2011;77(3):36.
147. Rees TD. Oral effects of drug abuse. Crit Rev Oral Biol Med. 1992;3(3):163–84.
148. McCuistian C, Fokuo JK, Dumoit Smith J, Sorensen JL, Arnold EA. Ethical dilemmas facing substance use counselors during the COVID-19 pandemic. Subst Abus Res Treat. 2023;17:11782218231158338. https://doi.org/10.1177/11782218231158338.

Unbalanced Nutrition and Oral Health

12

Sachin Sarode, Gargi Sarode, and Abhirami Premarajan

12.1 Introduction

Oral health refers to the condition of the mouth, teeth and orofacial structures that enable individuals to perform essential functions such as eating, breathing and speaking. It encompasses psychosocial dimensions, including self-confidence, well-being and the ability to socialise and work without pain, discomfort, or embarrassment [1]. Oral health varies throughout life and is integral to overall health, supporting individuals in participating in society and reaching their full potential [1]. As oral health is subjective and dynamic in nature [2], it encompasses multiple facets that contribute to its complexity, comprising physical, psychological, emotional and social spheres, all of which are essential for overall well-being.

Oral health is a principal aspect of general health, and a bi-directional effect is evident [3]. Due to the high prevalence and significant social implications, oral diseases are regarded as an important public health problem [4]. An individual's oral health is maintained by structures such as teeth, the tongue and salivary glands [5]. To prevent dental diseases, it is essential to maintain good oral hygiene. Oral health encompasses various factors, including awareness and habits related to oral hygiene, nutrition, genetics and systemic diseases. Achieving excellent oral health requires a balance of all the elements responsible for good oral hygiene and habits and it is crucial to promote global awareness about it. The World Health Organization (WHO) has reported that 60–90% of school-aged children have at least one dental cavity, and nearly 100% of adults have at least one dental cavity. Severe gum disease has been observed in 15–20% of adults aged between 35 and 44 years, and 30% of individuals aged 65–74 years have no natural teeth [6]. Other oral diseases, such as oral potentially malignant disorders (OPMDs), oral manifestations of blood and

S. Sarode (✉) · G. Sarode · A. Premarajan
Department of Oral and Maxillofacial Pathology and Oral Microbiology, Dr. D. Y. Patil Dental College and Hospital, Dr. D. Y. Patil Vidyapeeth, Pune, Maharashtra, India
e-mail: sachin.sarode@dpu.edu.in; gargi.sarode@dpu.edu.in

S. R. Prabhu et al. (eds.), *Lifestyle in Oral Health and Disease*,
https://doi.org/10.1007/978-3-032-05888-1_12

metabolic disorders, and bacterial, viral and fungal infections, are also quite common. For the maintenance of oral health, various parts of the oral cavity play specific roles. The breakdown of food is facilitated by the teeth. The tongue is predominantly made up of muscles, which not only regulate taste perception but also assist in chewing and swallowing [5]. Daily, the salivary glands produce 0.5–1.5 l of saliva. Antimicrobial proteins such as lysozyme, lactoferrin, peroxidase enzymes and other substances that clump bacteria, like mucins, glycoproteins and fibronectin, are present in the saliva [5]. Additionally, saliva also protects the oral and peri-oral tissues through lubrication, antimicrobial and buffering activity, thereby improving chewing, swallowing and digestion [5]. There is a negative impact of oral diseases on mastication, which is the first step of digestion. Essential determinants of overall health status are mastication and the subsequent acquisition of nutrition. As the oral cavity is exposed to everything an individual consumes, this can lead to oral diseases that give rise to a majority of health problems.

12.2 The Connection Between Nutrition and Oral Health

The mouth is where the journey to good health commences. A definite correlation is observed between oral health and nutrition in health and disease. The normal health and function of the oral cavity are maintained with the help of balanced nutrition [7]. For healthy oral tissues, along with their growth and development, proper nutrients are essential for maintenance and healing [8]. Nearly every structure of the oral cavity is affected by various nutritional deficiencies [8]. The occurrence and development of various oral diseases, such as dental caries, periodontal diseases and OPMDs, are significantly impacted by diet and nutrition [9].

The oral health of an individual is determined by the consumption and utilisation of nutrients, and the state of oral health is influenced by the nutrients an individual consumes [10]. Masticatory modifications are enabled by the specialised structures of the oral cavity, which help nourish the body and facilitate comprehension and interaction with our immediate surroundings [10]. Maintenance of proper nutritional status is greatly influenced by the condition of the teeth and the supporting tissues, which also contribute to overall health [3]. Patients who experience significant tooth loss may be more likely to consume less food, which is an essential source of vitamins, minerals, fibre and protein. Various ailments, such as infections, oral mucosal lesions like OPMDs and mucocutaneous lesions, can lead to swallowing dysfunctions that impact nutrition. Since the oral cavity reflects systemic health, it is crucial to aid in the early diagnosis, intervention and prevention of various disorders, as the disease manifestation of these nutritional disorders is evident in the oral cavity [7].

12.3 Definitions of Diet, Nutrition and Malnutrition

Diet A diet is the sum of food consumed by an individual. A healthy diet is one in which macronutrients are consumed in appropriate proportions to support energetic and physiological needs without exceeding intake while also providing sufficient micronutrients and hydration to meet the body's needs and physiological requirements [11].

Nutrition Generally encompasses macronutrients and micronutrients that are essential for an individual's growth, development, well-being and survival. Nutrients are categorised into macronutrients and micronutrients: macronutrients are required in large quantities and include proteins, carbohydrates, fats, oxygen and water. Micronutrients are necessary in smaller amounts or traces and include calcium, vitamin D, vitamin C, phosphorus, fluoride, folate and vitamin A.

Malnutrition Malnutrition is a subacute or chronic state of nutrition in which a combination of varying degrees of under or overnutrition and inflammatory activity has led to changes in body composition and diminished function. This definition not only assesses undernutrition or overnutrition but also considers the changes in body composition and function that they have led to, as well as the body's inflammatory status [12]. Malnutrition can be presented in the form of acute, sub-acute, or chronic and may or may not be related to underlying inflammation.

Malnutrition encompasses three categories according to the WHO guidelines [13].

1. *Undernutrition*
   - Low weight-for-height
   - Low height-for-age
   - Low weight-for-age
2. *Micronutrient*
   - Deficient/ excess vitamins and minerals
3. *Overnutrition*
   - Overweight, obesity and other diet-related health conditions

Healthy individuals require adequate amounts of various nutrients and micronutrients to support life and normal body functioning [14]. Excess or deficiency of a dietary part in terms of the seven main nutrients is referred to as unbalanced nutrition.

Malnutrition develops when the diet fails to meet the necessary daily requirements for healthy tissue [14]. This imbalance between need and intake can affect an individual's oral health status by either reducing the structural integrity of the dentition, making it more susceptible to dental caries, or by diminishing resistance to oral pathogens, as observed in cases of protein malnutrition [15]. Dietary habits, along with any detrimental behaviours, can act synergistically with the prevailing malnutrition, leading to various systemic diseases, including oral cancer [10]. Thus, oral health and nutrition are interlinked.

12.4 Global Dietary Pattern

The healthy dietary pattern generally comprises foods that are health-promoting, including fresh fruits and vegetables, soy, nuts, sources of omega-3 fatty acids, animal-derived proteins and foods that contain low saturated fats and trans fats [11]. Global dietary patterns are diverse and are influenced by cultural traditions, economic factors and changing lifestyles.

A brief overview of the Mediterranean, Nordic and Asian dietary patterns discussed is provided below:

Mediterranean Diet: The Mediterranean diet is well-known for its preventive effects on cardiovascular diseases and effective strategies are being developed to promote and adopt this dietary pattern. This dietary approach is not the only speciality; their eating habits and lifestyle considerations also contribute to the overall benefits. Their primary diet includes cereals, fruits and vegetables that are rich in micronutrients and phytochemicals (which help in reducing the risk of hypertension), as well as fibre, olive oil as a source of lipids, white meat, fish and eggs as sources of animal protein, and legumes as plant protein [11, 16].

Okinawan-Based Nordic Diet: It is characterised by a low-carbohydrate and calorie-count diet, rich in vitamins and minerals, also including restrictions on sugar, salt, processed meat and saturated fats. Studies have suggested that their diet is known to improve blood lipids, improve metabolic status and reduce body weight and glucose levels [17].

Traditional Asian Diet: There is less published detail on the impact of traditional Asian diets on health outcomes. The traditional Korean diet typically contains multiple small portions and excludes fried foods, in contrast to Western culture, which suggests that this dietary pattern is associated with a reduced risk of metabolic syndrome. The traditional Chinese diet, on the other hand, is higher in carbohydrates and lower in fats. The traditional Japanese diet, also known as Washoku, includes rice, fish, fermented soybean paste (as the base of the soup) and soups. The use of chopsticks and alternating small portion sizes improves satiety and prevents overeating. Adherence to the Japanese dietary pattern is known to be linked to a lower prevalence of hypertension in men, but it is associated with higher diastolic blood pressure in women, as well as an increase in waist circumference and body mass index (BMI) in men [11].

12.5 Lifestyle-Related Dietary Patterns and Their Impact on Health: An Overview

A key part in maintaining the health of an individual is through nutrition, which is a basic need of humans. As the nutritional status of individuals influences the clinical outcome, it serves as a necessary component of the healthcare system. Carbohydrates, proteins, lipids, minerals, vitamins and water, along with fibres and micronutrients, are the essential nutrients which are classified into these six groups [13]. Nutritional needs of healthy individuals depend on numerous aspects, such as age, sex and level of activity. Malnutrition can cause an imbalance in nutritional intake [18]. An inadequate or surplus consumption of macronutrients and micronutrients can lead to malnutrition [19].

The most important foundation of normal living, that is, health, is being neglected in the fast-paced, technologically driven world [7]. The ubiquitousness of fast food has increased, urging a critical evaluation of its effect on oral health. Diet and nutrition may have additive and multiple effects leading to chronic diseases when combined with factors such as habits or physical activities. Nutritional intake is severely affected by social influences such as poverty, catastrophe, war and even crash diets, leading to inadequate nutritional consumption. Nutritional conditions such as vitamin and iodine deficiency, anaemia, underweight and stunted growth, low birth weight and protein-energy malnutrition are all caused due to insufficient food intake. Various lifestyle disorders might arise due to excessive food intake, leading to nutritional health problems [20]. Thus, an effect of nutritional health is not only seen on the physical health but also on the psychological, developmental and sociocultural impact [21].

12.6 Role of Essential Nutrients

Nutritional Needs for Oral Health Proper, balanced nutrition influences the health of the oral cavity in both the pre-eruptive and post-eruptive phases of life, which also has specific effects on systemic health. The balance of nutrients in the diet affects caries prevalence, periodontal health and other inflammatory and ulcerative lesions of the body. Incorporating these nutrients into the daily diet has a positive impact on maintaining gum and tooth health [5]. Vitamins A, C and D, proteins and minerals, including calcium, phosphorus and fluoride, are necessary for teeth, among which vitamin C is required for normal synthesis and vitamin A is essential for keratin in the enamel [5].

12.7 Essential Macronutrients: Proteins, Carbohydrates and Fats

Proteins A vital macronutrient, are essential for the overall functioning of the body. Various amino acids, including non-essential, essential and branched-chain amino acids, form the building blocks of proteins, which are necessary for the formation of body tissues, making them an elementary nutritional requirement for any living organism [8]. In addition to this, it plays an essential role in maintaining and repairing oral health. Collagen is implicated in the formation of dentin, cementum, periodontal ligaments, gingiva, oral mucosa and bones [8].

Carbohydrates The primary source of energy found in various fruits, vegetables, grains and legumes, are categorised into sugars, starches and fibres based on their chemical bonding and the quantity of sugar units [22]. The texture of carbohydrates, their frequency of intake and exposure to the tooth structure are some of the parameters that affect oral health [23].

Lipids Are an essential component of balanced nutrition, vital for many biological functions of the human body. Sources include meat, nuts and oils such as vegetable or fish oil. Lipids are important as they serve as the building blocks of biological membranes, playing a pivotal role in determining membrane properties such as elasticity, fluidity and permeability, while modulating the immune response, which affects the differentiation and activation of immune cells [23].

12.8 Essential Micronutrients: Vitamins and Minerals

Vitamins Based on their solubility, McCollum and Davis (1915) classified vitamins into water-soluble and fat-soluble vitamins [24]. Fat-soluble vitamins include vitamins A, D, E and K, which are essential for the fluidity of cell membranes; however, there is an increased risk of hypervitaminosis due to their delayed elimination rate. Water-soluble vitamins include vitamins B and C, which play an important role in enzyme activation; furthermore, there is a reduced risk of hypervitaminosis associated with them compared to fat-soluble vitamins, as they dissolve in water instantaneously.

Vitamins A, D, E and K are categorised as fat-soluble vitamins, which exhibit lipophilicity, characterised by fat solubility rather than water solubility. The sources of these vitamins include a variety of fruits, vegetables, nuts and animal products. These lipophilic vitamins help improve cell membrane fluidity, facilitate transport and engage in redox reactions. Once consumed and metabolised, these vitamins are retained as reserves in the body for future use [25]. Water-soluble vitamins include the Vitamin B complex and C, which dissolve in water upon entering the body and are thus termed water-soluble vitamins. The occurrence of deficiency is rare, but it can occur in alcoholics, individuals following a vegan diet without supplementation, or those with malabsorption syndrome [25].

Minerals Calcium is associated with the formation of bones and teeth and is present in the form of hydroxyapatite crystals (Ca10[PO4]6[OH]2) [26]. Calcium metabolism is regulated by the parathyroid hormone-vitamin D endocrine system, and its absorption depends on the level of vitamin D [26]. Fluoride is a mineral that strengthens teeth and makes them less susceptible to demineralisation. Fluoride can be obtained through food, topical treatments via salivary secretions, or by gingival crevicular fluids. An increase from 1 μmol/L to approximately 2–5 μmol/L is crucial for preventing dental caries. Among the essential micronutrients, iron is the most abundant mineral and plays a crucial role in human health. A diet rich in iron has demonstrated a reduction in caries.

12.9 Health Consequences of Malnutrition

12.9.1 Protein Deficiency

Protein deficiency can affect oral health in various ways. Saliva contains several antimicrobial properties and other components that mediate buffering and antimicrobial action [27]. Additionally, it contains certain defensive proteins involved in providing both innate and acquired immunity. Therefore, protein deficiency can alter the salivary composition, thereby affecting homeostasis and its ability to neutralise toxins [28]. However, more research is necessary to gain a deeper understanding of the impact on oral health. Protein is essential for the structural integrity of dentition. A diet deficient in protein and fats can lead to increased intake of carbohydrates and sugars, making the oral cavity more susceptible and less resistant to demineralisation. Studies have shown that higher protein intake reduces periodontitis [29]. As one ages, the condition and number of teeth decline, resulting in poor nutritional intake. Thus, with ongoing inadequate protein intake and poor-quality diet, the health of the periodontium deteriorates, leading to tooth loss. The prevalence of oral mucosal lesions increases with age, particularly among geriatric patients [30]. Alongside systemic diseases, medications, ill-fitting dentures and nutritional disorders, particularly those related to proteins, contribute to this issue. Consequently, protein deficiency, combined with other factors, renders the oral mucosa less resistant to bacteria and delayed wound healing, increasing the risk of mucosal lesions, potentially including oral cancer in later stages.

12.9.2 Excess Protein Intake

Protein is considered an essential nutrient needed for the growth, repair and functioning of the body, but excess protein leads to low-grade metabolic acidosis

(LGMA), which lowers blood pH. When this occurs chronically, it negatively impacts the bones, resulting in bone resorption and decreased bone mineral levels [5].

12.10 Carbohydrate Deficiency

Carbohydrate Deficiency The functional deficiency, or absence, of one of the enzymes that regulate glycogen metabolism causes a rare metabolic disorder known as glycogen storage disorder (GSD). Patients with this metabolic disorder, alongside hepatic involvement, have exhibited symptoms of inflammation and infection in the oral cavity; however, no alterations to the mucosa or dentition have been recorded [31].

Excess Carbohydrate Intake The more these carbohydrates are retained in the oral cavity, the more chances of demineralisation of the tooth are observed. Frequent consumption, higher intake and intake of these simple carbohydrates between meals increase the probability of dental caries [23].

12.11 Fat Intake Deficiency and Excess

Lipid deficiency occurs when the body does not receive sufficient dietary fats. These fats are vital nutrients, providing energy, aiding the absorption of vitamins and supporting various essential bodily functions. A deficiency of essential fatty acids can result in dry skin, stunted growth and weakened immune function. In rare cases, genetic disorders may also lead to lower lipid levels in the body. Understanding the mechanism of lipid interaction is essential, as imbalances in their levels can be both beneficial and harmful. They are associated with acute or chronic inflammation, as well as a range of heart, neurological, metabolic and cancer-related diseases [23]. Lipids in the saliva might have a role in mineralising the plaque deposited, that is, for calculus formation. Low salivary lipid levels are better for a healthy oral cavity; excess may be harmful [32].

Excess lipid intake can lead to hyperlipidaemia. High lipid levels are not only a risk factor for the cardiovascular system; it has also been noted that chronic and acute systemic diseases induce cytokine changes that result in increased lipid levels. This suggests that oral infections (periodontitis) cause alterations in lipid levels [33].

12.12 Vitamin Deficiency

Vitamin A Deficiency Vitamin A is essential for vision, cellular differentiation, functioning as an epithelial barrier and related immune functions. There are various oral manifestations, such as amelogenesis imperfecta, which carries a high risk for dental caries and compromised enamel integrity [34], abnormal calcification and alterations in pulp structure, affecting the dentin, alongside oral mucosal fungal infections presenting white, soft plaques that complicate feeding and swallowing. Vitamin A has a vital role in the phases of wound healing, angiogenesis, collagen synthesis and more, which suggests that when there is a deficiency of this vitamin, it can lead to problems with the above-mentioned functions [34]. Other oral complications from vitamin A deficiency include oral keratosis, disorders of mucosal keratinisation [25] and periodontitis.

Vitamin D Deficiency Vitamin D is necessary to carry out basic functions in the body as it enhances mineral absorption (calcium, magnesium, iron, phosphate, zinc) in the intestine [10], reduces the periodontitis risk by promoting antimicrobial peptide production to reduce oral inflammation [35], reduces the risk of dental caries and also is immunosuppressive and prevents infections of oral cavity.

Vitamin D deficiency occurs when the serum level of 25(OH)D falls below 20 ng/dL for several reasons, such as low intake, decreased cutaneous synthesis and a high rate of exclusive breastfeeding. The oral impacts of this deficiency include various developmental disorders, such as amelogenesis imperfecta, where enamel is not properly formed, resulting in discolouration and structural alterations; dentinogenesis imperfecta, characterised by discoloured, translucent, weak and short teeth, bulbous crowns and small pulp chambers; and ectodermal dysplasia, which is characterised by oligodontia, hypoplastic teeth and irregularly shaped teeth (cone-shaped). Severe vitamin D deficiency occurs when the serum level drops to less than 10 ng/mL, causing hypocalcaemia, hypophosphatemia, secondary hyperparathyroidism, increased intestinal absorption of calcium, renal production of 1 α,25-dihydroxyvitamin D, enhanced bone turnover, high serum calcium levels, low serum inorganic phosphate levels, loss of vitamin D signalling pathways in odontogenic cells, inhibited teeth mineralisation and an increased risk of oral squamous cell carcinoma.

Vitamin E Deficiency Premature infants, children and pregnant women are at greater risk due to limited fat absorption or metabolic issues. Alpha-tocopherol, a chemical variant of vitamin E, is crucial for health. It functions as an antioxidant and also displays anti-inflammatory properties through T cell differentiation, thereby strengthening the immune system [37]. Furthermore, it has the ability to modulate inflammation, making it advantageous for managing oral conditions [38]. Signs of vitamin E deficiency include weakened immunity, haemolytic anaemia [39] and oral mucositis.

Vitamin K Deficiency The synthesis of blood coagulation depends on vitamin K, with K1 (phylloquinone) and K2 (menaquinone) playing a key role in human health. Vitamin K1 is obtained from the diet, whereas vitamin K2 is synthesised by bacteria

[40]. The irrational use of antimicrobial drugs can disrupt the balance of these bacteria, thus leading to a deficiency of this vitamin. Its deficiency can cause haemorrhagic diseases, manifested by sudden and possibly life-threatening haemorrhages from various body parts, which can also lead to fatal neurological consequences.

Vitamin B Complex Deficiency In the oral cavity, deficiencies in the vitamin B complex typically present as oral ulcers, glossitis and stomatitis. Risk factors for vitamin B deficiencies include age, medication, long-term alcohol misuse, malabsorptive syndromes and vegetarian and vegan diets. Atrophic gastritis, characterised by chronic inflammation of the stomach wall, results in the atrophy of gastric mucosa, leading to reduced gastric acid secretion and malabsorption; this condition is highly prevalent within the elderly population. Medications such as proton pump inhibitors, prescribed for gastritis and metformin both have adverse effects. Proton pump inhibitors tend to inhibit gastric acid secretion [41], while metformin (a drug used for type 2 diabetes) inhibits gluconeogenesis by reducing glucose output, thereby increasing insulin sensitivity [42]. Due to fundamental alterations in the metabolism of oral epithelial cells, vitamin deficiencies, particularly those of the B group, can affect various oral structures. Consequently, disorders such as angular cheilosis, ulceration and inflammation of the oral mucosa, cracked lips and ulcerative or erosive lesions in the head, neck, face and limbs are more likely to arise [15].

Thiamine (B1) Deficiency Thiamine (B1) serves as a cofactor for several enzymes involved in glucose breakdown. A deficiency can result in adenosine triphosphate (ATP) exhaustion, substantially disturbing aerobic tissues such as the brain, nerves and heart. When the heart is affected, it is termed wet beriberi, characterised by high-output heart failure, oedema and dyspnoea on exertion [43]. The deficiency is frequently part of the manifestations observed in individuals suffering from malnutrition or alcohol use disorder related to malnutrition and malabsorption. The deficiency may present in the oral cavity with various symptoms, including cracked lips, angular cheilitis and a burning sensation on the tongue. It may also be associated with recurrent aphthous stomatitis and can hinder the development of tooth enamel, particularly in children [25, 43].

Riboflavin (B2) Deficiency Riboflavin (B2) serves as a cofactor in redox reactions. Its deficiency may lead to corneal vascularisation [26]. Riboflavin deficiency can adversely affect oral health, resulting in various symptoms in the mouth and lips. These symptoms include angular cheilitis, glossitis and recurrent aphthous stomatitis. B2 deficiency may also result in enamel hypocalcification.

Niacin (B3) Deficiency Niacin (B3) is also involved in redox reactions derived from tryptophan. Its deficiency can manifest as pellagra, known by the three Ds:

diarrhoea, dermatitis and dementia. It may occur in alcoholics and those who are malnourished. Before the onset of pellagra, a prodromal burning sensation in the mouth is observed. A thick, grey discharge of degenerating cells forms a pseudo membrane on the dorsal surface of the tongue. Other oral manifestations of niacin deficiency include recurrent aphthous ulceration (RAU), angular cheilitis and gingivitis. In these individuals, intense halitosis is present [44].

Pantothenic Acid (B5) Deficiency Pantothenic acid (B5) is a component of coenzyme A and fatty acid synthase, both of which are necessary for energy production and hormone formation. Deficiency is characterised by dermatitis, enteritis, alopecia and adrenal insufficiency. Pantothenic acid deficiency leads to xerosis (dry skin) and cheilitis, resulting in similar oral complications to those observed with other B vitamins [45].

Pyridoxine (B6) Deficiency Pyridoxine (B6) is involved in transamination, decarboxylation and glycogen phosphorylase activity reactions. It is essential for erythropoiesis. Deficiency can result in sideroblastic anaemia, hyperirritability, convulsions, peripheral neuropathy and mental confusion. Pyridoxine deficiency leads to atrophic glossitis, gingivitis, angular stomatitis and minor mucosal aphthous ulcerations. A burning sensation in the tongue, resembling that associated with pellagra, along with severe redness and flattening of the filiform papillae, contributes to glossitis. Furthermore, pyridoxine deficiency also promotes oral fungal infections [46].

Biotin (B7) Deficiency Biotin (B7) metabolises proteins, fats and carbohydrates. A deficiency can lead to muscle pain, heart problems, anaemia and depression. Biotin contributes to keratin, enhancing the quality of hair, skin and nails. A deficiency in biotin can cause perioral dermatitis, sometimes accompanied by generalised oral erythema, dry, crusted lips and sparse atrophy of the tongue papillae [47].

Folate (B9) Deficiency Folate (B9) is essential for the synthesis of DNA and RNA. A deficiency can lead to neural tube defects and macrocytic megaloblastic anaemia. This deficiency is also linked to alcohol use disorder. Folate is necessary for the turnover of oral epithelial cells. Its deficiency can result in inadequate keratinisation of the gingival surface, decreased resistance to infection, gingival necrosis and damage to the periodontium. In individuals with severe folic acid deficiency, a higher incidence of orofacial clefts and oral cancer has been reported due to folate's crucial role in preserving DNA integrity [48].

Cobalamin (B12) Deficiency Cobalamin (B12) is critical for erythropoiesis and the development of the nervous system. A deficiency can cause pernicious anaemia and subacute combined spinal cord degeneration. The macrocytic megaloblastic anaemia appears similar to folate deficiency. However, B12 deficiency may manifest with neurological indications, whereas folate deficiency does not. Cobalamin deficiency can present oral symptoms such as glossitis, glossodynia, recurrent ulcers, cheilitis, dysgeusia, lingual paraesthesia and a burning sensation. The red, atrophic, meaty tongue exhibits a loss of filiform papillae, along with generalised stomatitis and taste disturbances. Fissuring and loss of circumvallate papillae lead to reduced taste sensitivity [45, 46]. Occasionally, Hunter's glossitis- a painful, atrophic, red tongue resulting from vitamin B12 deficiency- can be mistaken for primary burning mouth syndrome [49, 50].

Vitamin C Deficiency Vitamin C, an essential water-soluble antioxidant, is found in citrus fruits, tomatoes, potatoes and green vegetables [21]. It is essential for collagen, which constitutes about one-third of the total proteins that make up the oral hard and soft tissues, such as bones, cartilage, ligaments, tendons and teeth [51]. It induces calcium deposition and mineralisation, thereby providing support, structure and maintenance for the teeth [51]. It prevents the development of dental caries by exerting a concentration-dependent repressive influence between vitamin C and *Streptococcus mutans* [51]. It acts as an antioxidant, inhibiting carcinogenesis.

The deficiency of vitamin C occurs among populations with limited dietary diversity, the elderly and alcoholics [52]. In addition to these, smokers and individuals exposed to passive smoking include those with chronic conditions like renal diseases and malabsorption syndromes. A deficiency of vitamin C can cause scurvy, which includes inflamed, bleeding gums (gingivitis) and tooth mobility (periodontitis) [38], increased oxidative stress [53], atrophy of ameloblasts and odontoblasts [54] and an increased risk of oral premalignant disorders as well as head and neck cancers [51].

12.13 Hypervitaminosis

As the insufficient intake of nutrients influences an individual's health status, excessive intake can also be toxic. Excessive intake of vitamins causes hypervitaminosis or vitamin toxicity. The hypervitaminosis caused by fat-soluble vitamins has more serious consequences compared to water-soluble ones, leading to severe intoxication of the vitamins in tissues. Hypervitaminosis D causes dental enamel hypoplasia and focal pulp calcification [55]. The increase in iron absorption and transportation functions of vitamin C presents a risk to patients with sickle cell anaemia, haemochromatosis, beta-thalassemia major, or sideroblastic anaemia with iron overload [56]. Despite the role of vitamin C in the formation of collagen and other beneficial effects, foods containing vitamin C, such as citrus fruits, juices and chewable vitamin C, have low pH levels, which cause significant tooth wear as well as erosion [57].

12.14 Mineral Deficiency and Excess

Calcium Deficiency During odontogenesis, a proper supply of nutrients for the mineralisation of enamel, dentine and cementum is required. However, if there is an impairment in the supply of nutrients, especially calcium, during gestation and childhood, it can adversely affect tooth structure [58]. An aggravation of the reduction in bone mineralisation can result in pathological periodontal changes, leading to tooth mobility [21]. A decrease in calcium and the calcium-phosphorus ratio increases the rate of bone resorption [35]. The jawbone (mainly the alveolar bone) is initially affected and may be severely compromised over a long period, followed by the cranial bone, ribs, vertebrae and long bones.

Excess Calcium Intake An excessive intake of calcium can lead to hypercalcaemia. Thinning of bones, mobile and/or floating teeth, jaw pain, sensitivity in teeth during occlusion or percussion, soft tissue calcifications and various developmental disturbances related to teeth, particularly during eruption, may be observed. Furthermore, a brown tumour of the jaw may arise due to hypercalcaemia resulting from hyperparathyroidism [59].

Fluoride Deficiency A deficiency of fluoride does not affect the oral mucosa, but it makes the dentition more susceptible to caries. However, if consumed in excess, fluoride can lead to mild white flecks, brown discolouration and pitting of enamel, known as mottling of enamel, as well as skeletal abnormalities [60].

Excess Fluoride Consumption Excessive fluoride intake occurs due to the consumption of groundwater that is naturally rich in fluoride or when high-fluoride water is utilised in cooking or crop irrigation. This can lead to dental or skeletal fluorosis, osteosclerosis, tendon and ligament calcification and various bone deformities [61].

Iron deficiency is the most common cause of anaemia. In this condition, red blood cells are usually microcytic and hypochromic and iron stores are depleted. When the body does not have enough iron, the production of haemoglobin decreases. Haemoglobin binds to oxygen, allowing red blood cells to deliver oxygenated blood throughout the body. Symptoms of iron deficiency anaemia include fatigue, decreased stamina, shortness of breath, weakness, dizziness and pallor. Oral manifestations of iron-deficiency anaemia include papillary atrophy of the tongue, erythema and a burning sensation on the tongue, angular cheilitis, dysphagia, pallor and recurrent aphthous ulceration (RAU) [60].

Excess Iron Intake Excess iron intake can lead to hemochromatosis, which results in various adverse effects such as decreased growth (both linear growth and weight), diarrhoea, interactions with other trace elements such as copper and zinc, altered gut microbiota (to pathogenic bacteria), enhanced inflammatory markers and impaired cognitive and motor development [62].

12.15 Oral Health-Friendly Dietary Recommendations

To develop a systematic and comprehensive healthcare plan, the healthcare model should encompass an interdisciplinary and holistic approach involving physicians, dentists and registered dietitians [7]. Patients must receive education on how to maintain healthy eating habits, alongside knowledge regarding the cessation of harmful practices such as tobacco use and alcoholism [43]. It is vital to have nutritional counselling with a nutritionist/dietitian. Regular intraoral examinations facilitate the timely identification of various deficiencies and a range of pathological conditions, thus aiding in their prompt correction. Patient education and awareness are crucial in detecting the nature of deficiencies, their implications, treatment planning and the implementation of preventative measures, as well as post-treatment care [36].

12.16 Conclusion

Nutrition is a crucial factor in maintaining good oral health. The key to excellent oral health is a balanced diet that includes all the necessary nutrients. A holistic approach that integrates nutritional education and oral healthcare is essential for maintaining overall wellness and preventing oral and systemic complications.

References

1. https://www.who.int/health-topics/oral-health/#tab=tab_1
2. Barranca-Enríquez A, Romo-González T. Your health is in your mouth: a comprehensive view to promote general wellness. Front Oral Health. 2022;3:971223.
3. Valdivia A, Sánchez M, Cortés D, Cortes E. Oral health: fundamentals, importance, and perspectives. In: Human teeth – from function to esthetics. IntechOpen; 2023.
4. Kaushal N, Adhikari B, Negi M, Pant N, Panwar P, Gusain S. Oral Hygiene. Int J Adv Res. 2023;11:465–75.
5. Jayasinghe TN, Harrass S, Erdrich S, King S, Eberhard J. Protein intake and oral health in older adults-a narrative review. Nutrients. 2022;14(21):4478.
6. Jain N, Dutt U, Radenkov I, Jain S. WHO's global oral health status report 2022: actions, discussion and implementation. Oral Dis. 2023;30(2):73–9.

7. Bhatnagar P. Nutrition and dental caries: strong teeth for good eat. Int J Creat Res Thoughts. 2023;11(3):954–63.
8. Pflipsen M, Zenchenko Y. Nutrition for oral health and oral manifestations of poor nutrition and unhealthy habits. Gen Dent. 2017;65(6):36–43.
9. https://www.ada.org/resources/ada-library/oral-health-topics/nutrition-and-oral-health
10. Ahn-Jarvis JH, Piancino MG. Chapter 14: impact of oral health on diet/nutrition. Monogr Oral Sci. 2020;28:134–47.
11. Cena H, Calder PC. Defining a healthy diet: evidence for the role of contemporary dietary patterns in health and disease. Nutrients. 2020;12(2):334.
12. Soeters P, Bozzetti F, Cynober L, Forbes A, Shenkin A, Sobotka L. Defining malnutrition: a plea to rethink. Clin Nutr. 2017;36(3):896–901.
13. Kesari A, Noel JY. Nutritional assessment. 2023. In: StatPearls. Treasure Island: StatPearls Publishing. p. 2025.
14. Gondivkar SM, Gadbail AR, Gondivkar RS, Sarode SC, Sarode GS, Patil S, Awan KH. Nutrition and oral health. Dis Mon. 2019;65(6):147–54.
15. Jadhav H, Khairnar M, Naik R, Vishwakarma P, Deshmukh M, Chandra A. Assessment of oral health status and nutritional status of tribal children residing in tribal area of Maharashtra state, India. RUHS J of Health Sci. 2022;7(4):198–203.
16. Popovac A, Jaćimović J, Trichopoulou A, Peppa E, Kotrokois K, Stančić I, Milić-Lemić A, Kossioni A. Mediterranean diet and oral health: is there an association? A scoping review. Nutr Res Rev. 2024;18:1–15.
17. Persson GR, Widén C, Wohlfart B, Sjöberg K, Steen S, Coleman MD, Holmer H. Impact of an Okinawa/Nordic based diet on endocrinological and periodontal conditions in individuals with type 2 diabetes. A randomized case-control study. BMC Oral Health. 2023;23(1):544.
18. Elia M. Defining, recognizing, and reporting malnutrition. Int J Low Extrem Wounds. 2017;16(4):230–7.
19. Mueller C, Compher C, Ellen DM. American Society for Parenteral and Enteral Nutrition (A.S.P.E.N.) Board of Directors. A.S.P.E.N. Clinical guidelines: nutrition screening, assessment, and intervention in adults. JPEN J Parenter Enteral Nutr. 2011;35(1):16–24.
20. Sarıkaya B. Unbalanced distribution of food. Soc Regist. 2017;1:199–208.
21. Tolkachjov SN, Bruce AJ. Oral manifestations of nutritional disorders. Clin Dermatol. 2017;35(5):441–52.
22. Slavin J, Carlson J. Carbohydrates. Adv Nutr. 2014;5(6):760–1.
23. Frydrych A, Kulita K, Jurowski K, Piekoszewski W. Lipids in clinical nutrition and health: narrative review and dietary recommendations. Foods. 2025;14(3):473.
24. Panchumarth A, Sankar R. The comprehensive review on fat soluble vitamins. IOSR J Pharm. 2015;5(11):12–28.
25. Lešić S, Ivanišević Z, Špiljak B, Tomas M, Šoštarić M, Včev A. The impact of vitamin deficiencies on oral manifestations in children. Dent J (Basel). 2024;12(4):109.
26. Balasubramaniam S, Christodoulou J, Rahman S. Disorders of riboflavin metabolism. J Inherit Metab Dis. 2019;42(4):608–19.
27. Psoter W, Reid B, Katz R. Malnutrition and dental caries: a review of the literature. Caries Res. 2005;39:441–4.
28. McArthur WP. Encyclopedia of immunology. Amsterdam: Elsevier; 1998. Oral Immunology. p. 1888–93.
29. Dodington DW, Young HE, Beaudette JR, Fritz PC, Ward WE. Improved healing after non-surgical periodontal therapy is associated with higher protein intake in patients who are non-smokers. Nutrients. 2021;13:3722.
30. Cheruvathoor DD, Thomas V, Kumar NR, Jose M. High prevalence of oral mucosal lesions in elderly: call for revolutionizing geriatric dental care strategies. J Fam Med Prim Care. 2020;9:4375–80.
31. Mulla S, Ansari A, Bhattacharjee M, Patil A, Methal S. Oral manifestations of nutritional deficiencies: a micro review of macro issues in the mouth. Oral Maxillofac Pathol J. 2023;14(2):217–9.

32. Karjalainen S, Sewón L, Söderling E, Larsson B, Johansson I, Simell O, Lapinleimu H, Seppänen R. Salivary cholesterol of healthy adults in relation to serum cholesterol concentration and oral health. J Dent Res. 1997;76(10):1637–43.
33. Joshi NV, Marawar PP. Hyperlipidemia-a link between periodontitis and coronary heart disease. J Indian Dent Assoc. 2011;5(2):183–6.
34. Gutierrez GA, Martinez-Mier EA. Chapter 6: vitamins and oral health. Monogr Oral Sci. 2020;28:59–67.
35. Antonenko O, Seijo M, Brito G, Gualtieri AF, Pellegrini G, Zeni SN. Low calcium intake and hypovitaminosis D negatively affect oral health in young men. Austin J Dent. 2017;4(7):1–8.
36. Bačun B, Galić D, Pul L, Tomas M, Kuiš D. Manifestations and treatment of hypovitaminosis in oral diseases: a systematic review. Dent J (Basel). 2024;12(6):152.
37. Elmadfa I, Meyer AL. The role of the status of selected micronutrients in shaping the immune function. Endocr Metab Immune Disord Drug Targets. 2019;19(8):1100–15.
38. Najeeb S, Zafar MS, Khurshid Z, Zohaib S, Almas K. The role of nutrition in periodontal health: an update. Nutrients. 2016;8(9):530.
39. Jilani T, Iqbal MP. Vitamin E deficiency in south Asian population and the therapeutic use of alpha-tocopherol (vitamin E) for correction of anemia. Pak J Med Sci. 2018;34(6):1571–5.
40. Halder M, Petsophonsakul P, Akbulut AC, Pavlic A, Bohan F, Anderson E, Maresz K, Kramann R, Schurgers L. Vitamin K: double bonds beyond coagulation insights into differences between vitamin K1 and K2 in health and disease. Int J Mol Sci. 2019;20(4):896.
41. Lam JR, Schneider JL, Zhao W, Corley DA. Proton pump inhibitor and histamine 2 receptor antagonist use and vitamin B12 deficiency. JAMA. 2013;310(22):2435–42.
42. Niafar M, Hai F, Porhomayon J, Nader ND. The role of metformin on vitamin B12 deficiency: a meta-analysis review. Intern Emerg Med. 2015;10(1):93–102.
43. Wiley KD, Gupta M. Vitamin B1 (Thiamine) deficiency. In: StatPearls. Treasure Island: StatPearls Publishing; 2025. Available from: https://www.ncbi.nlm.nih.gov/books/NBK537204/.
44. Bolat M, Trandafir L, Ciubara A, Diaconescu S. Oral manifestations of nutritional diseases in children. Rom J Oral Rehabil. 2016;8:56–60.
45. Sanvictores T, Chauhan S. Vitamin B5 (Pantothenic Acid). In: StatPearls. Treasure Island: StatPearls Publishing; 2025. Available from: https://www.ncbi.nlm.nih.gov/books/NBK563233/.
46. Brown MJ, Ameer MA, Daley SF, et al. Vitamin B6 deficiency. In: StatPearls. Treasure Island: StatPearls Publishing; 2025. Available from: https://www.ncbi.nlm.nih.gov/books/NBK470579/.
47. Saleem F, Soos MP. Biotin deficiency. In: StatPearls. Treasure Island: StatPearls Publishing; 2025. Available from: https://www.ncbi.nlm.nih.gov/books/NBK547751/.
48. Khan KM, Jialal I. Folic acid deficiency. In: StatPearls. Treasure Island: StatPearls Publishing; 2025. Available from: https://www.ncbi.nlm.nih.gov/books/NBK535377/.
49. Ankar A, Kumar A. Vitamin B12 deficiency. In: StatPearls. Treasure Island: StatPearls Publishing; 2025. Available from: https://www.ncbi.nlm.nih.gov/books/NBK441923/.
50. Kim J, Kim MJ, Kho HS. Oral manifestations in vitamin B12 deficiency patients with or without history of gastrectomy. BMC Oral Health. 2016;16(1):60.
51. Murererehe J, Uwitonze AM, Nikuze P, Patel J, Razzaque MS. Beneficial effects of vitamin C in maintaining optimal oral health. Front Nutr. 2022;8:805809.
52. Carr AC, Lykkesfeldt J. Vitamin C: from bench to bedside. Nutrients. 2021;13(4):1102.
53. Schlueter AK, Johnston CS. Vitamin C: overview and update. J Evid Based Complementary Altern Med. 2011;16(1):49–57.
54. Ghosh A, Pallavi SK, Nagpal B, Hegde U, Archana S, Nagpal J. Role of vitamins in oral health & disease: an overview. Indian J Appl Res. 2015;5:292–5.
55. Roop JK. Hypervitaminosis- an emerging pathological condition. Int J Health Sci Res. 2018;8(10):280–8.
56. Pacier C, Martirosyan DM. Vitamin C: optimal dosages, supplementation and use in disease prevention. Funct Food Health. 2015;5:89–107.

57. Li H, Zou Y, Ding G. Dietary factors associated with dental erosion: a meta-analysis. PLoS One. 2012;7:e42626.
58. Rathee M, Singla S, Tamrakar A. Calcium and oral health: a review. Int J Sci Res. 2013;2(9):335–6.
59. Hariharan R, Anitha N, Malathi L, Aravindha BN. Oral manifestations of hyperparathyroidism and its management-a review. Indian J Forensic Med Toxicol. 2020;14(4):1450–4.
60. Thomas DM, Mirowski GW. Nutrition and oral mucosal diseases. Clin Dermatol. 2010;28(4):426–31.
61. https://www.who.int/teams/environment-climate-change-and-health/chemical-safety-and-health/health-impacts/chemicals/inadequate-or-excess-fluoride
62. Lönnerdal B. Excess iron intake as a factor in growth, infections, and development of infants and young children. Am J Clin Nutr. 2017;106:1681S–7S.

Impact of Dietary Sugars on Dental Health

13

Anupama Ivaturi and Paula Moynihan

13.1 Introduction

Diet is a pivotal lifestyle factor impacting oral health [1]. Nutrition shapes jaw and tooth development, and malnutrition can exacerbate periodontal and infectious diseases including dental caries. The most profound impact occurs locally in the oral cavity, where dietary sugars are metabolised by acidogenic bacteria, causing a dysbiosis of the oral microbiome in favour of aciduric and acidogenic bacteria which favour disease. Moreover, if processed starches are retained in the mouth, salivary amylase hydrolyses them to maltose and glucose, which can be metabolised by bacteria. In this chapter, we turn our focus to the single most critical dietary element: sugars.

13.2 What Are Dietary Sugars?

The term 'sugars' refers to a range of biochemical components that include mono- and disaccharides, such as glucose, fructose, maltose, lactose, sucrose and galactose, which are found in various items of the human diet. The familiar white, brown or table sugar refers to sucrose, a disaccharide [2]. Sugars, or total sugars, are classified into two types. Figure 13.1 provides a detailed classification.

A. Ivaturi (✉)
Department of Human-Centred Computing, Faculty of IT, Monash University, Clayton, VIC, Australia
e-mail: Anu.Ivaturi@monash.edu

P. Moynihan
Adelaide Dental School, The University of Adelaide, Adelaide, SA, Australia
e-mail: paula.moynihan@adelaide.edu.au

S. R. Prabhu et al. (eds.), *Lifestyle in Oral Health and Disease*,
https://doi.org/10.1007/978-3-032-05888-1_13

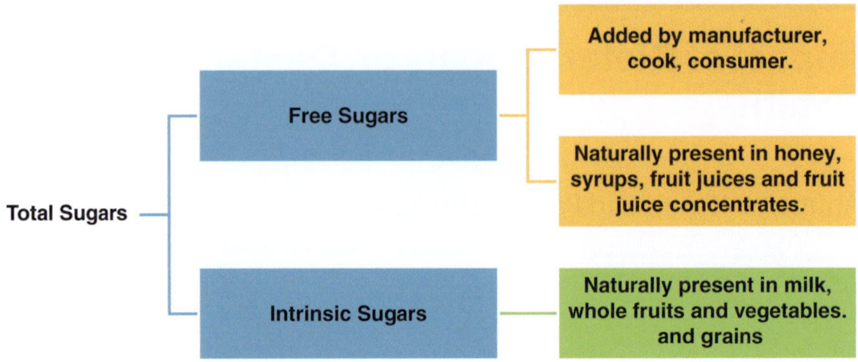

Fig. 13.1 Classification of dietary sugars

13.2.1 Definition of Total, Free and Added Sugars

Total sugars include free sugars and the sugars naturally present in whole fruits, vegetables, grains and milk, also referred to as intrinsic sugars [3]. Added sugars refer to sugars that are added during food processing or preparation. Free sugars include all added sugars, that is, monosaccharides and disaccharides added to foods and beverages by the manufacturer, cook or consumer, and sugars naturally present in honey, syrups, fruit juices and fruit juice concentrates [2].

13.3 What Are the Recommendations for the Intake of Sugars?

Free sugars make a sizeable contribution to total dietary sugars [3]. There is convincing evidence linking the amount of free sugars intake to dental caries [1]. Furthermore, intake of free sugars is a risk factor for overweight and obesity [4] and directly causes dental caries [1, 5]. In view of this governments, authoritative health bodies and agencies have made recommendations on the thresholds for consumption of free sugars.

In the 2015 Guideline on Sugars Intake for Adults and Children, the World Health Organization (WHO) [2] strongly recommends reducing the intake of free sugars throughout the life course, limiting this intake to less than 10% of total energy intake for both adults and children. The WHO also suggests that free sugars intake should be limited to less than 5% of total energy intake to help reduce dental caries over a lifetime. These recommendations were developed based on a systematic review of the evidence [6], which demonstrated that limiting free sugars intake is associated with a lower risk of dental caries, although even at the 10% threshold, dental caries is not eliminated. Recent evidence supports and strengthens these recommendations [7]. Furthermore, there is evidence indicating that dental caries could develop in both resistant and susceptible teeth of children whose free sugars intake is as low as 2–3% of energy intake, provided teeth are exposed to sugars for more than 3 years without changes in the environmental factors that confer protection, such as fluoride in water [8, 9].

An assessment by the European Food Safety Authority (EFSA) reviewed the evidence with the aim of defining a safe level of intake for sugars and considered the potential risks associated with sugar intake, including dental caries, weight gain and type 2 diabetes. The EFSA concluded that, based on available data, a tolerable upper intake level (UL) for dietary sugars could not be set and recommended that free sugar intake should be as low as possible within a nutritionally adequate diet [10]. The American Heart Association (AHA) recommends limiting added sugars to no more than 6% of calories (energy) per day. The national institutes of nutrition and health departments in other countries have either adopted the WHO recommendations or set a threshold that translates to household measures, as explained in Sect. 13.4.

13.4 What Do These Guidelines Mean, and How Do the Recommended Thresholds for Intake Translate?

Understanding the WHO guidelines for the recommended thresholds for the intake of free sugars is essential. Ideally, for dental health, the recommended threshold for free sugars intake should be less than 5% of total energy intake, meaning free sugars should account for less than 100 calories in a 2000-calorie diet (which is roughly appropriate for adolescents and adults, but children have a lower energy need). Each gram of sugar provides 4 calories, equivalent to less than 25 grams of free sugars per day, roughly equivalent to 6 level teaspoons. However, it is important to note that 'free sugars' are not just sucrose, that is, table sugar, but as described in Sect. 13.2, including all sugars added to food and drink by the manufacturer, cook or consumer, as well as those present in honey, syrups, fruit juices and fruit juice concentrates. This, however, does not mean a sugar-free diet. It means limited consumption of sugar-containing foods as part of a balanced diet [11].

13.4.1 Amount of Sugar Intake: The Contribution of Sugars to Daily Intake

Globally, the sugar intake of both adults and children exceeds the recommended thresholds, as indicated by reports on intake across various age groups in both high-income countries [12–14], including the USA (NHANES, 2020–25), the UK, Europe and Japan, as well as low-/lower-middle-income countries like Libya [15] and India [16], summarised in Table 13.1. Understanding how sugar intake is reported—whether in grams per day or as a percentage of daily energy intake—is valuable for dental professionals. Equally important is recognising the specific foods and beverages contributing to free sugar intake and, more relevant to dental

Table 13.1 Contribution of free sugars to energy intake by children and adolescents

Country	Age group (years)	Free sugars intake (% of energy)
United Kingdom (UK)	<10	12%
Lebanon	<10	12%
United States (USA)	2–5	14%
Japan	2–5	14%
France	3–6	16%
Germany	3–18	12%
Australia	4–8	14%
India	11–13	7.2%

health, identifying the timing and occasions when they are consumed. These aspects will be explored further in Sect. 13.5.

13.5 Beyond Table Sugar: Sources and Patterns of Free Sugars Intake and Relevance to Dental Health

13.5.1 Sources of Free Sugars

Nutrition epidemiological studies show that free sugars—beyond just table sugar—are present in a wide variety of foods and beverages (Table 13.2), with sources varying by region and age group [3, 11]. Oral hygiene standards, socio-economic status and fluoride exposure influence the relationship between sugars intake and caries [1]. Nevertheless, knowledge of the diverse sources of free sugars is essential to guide dietary behaviour change through chairside advice as well as public oral health education [17–19]. Epidemiological data show that intrinsic sugars have not been associated with dental caries, unlike free sugars [3]. Dental professionals can therefore encourage the intake of foods such as whole vegetables and fruits, whole grains and milk.

Sugar-sweetened beverages (SSBs), including cordials, fresh and canned fruit juices and carbonated as well as non-carbonated soft drinks, are significant contributors to free sugar intake, particularly among children and adolescents, leading to an increasing burden of dietary-related non-communicable diseases (NCDs) [20]. SSBs are acidic, contributing to the erosion of enamel and dentine. Both dental caries and erosion are costly to treat; therefore, prevention through changes in dietary behaviour is a practical approach to addressing the dental burden of disease.

Given the wide range of foods and beverages that contribute to free sugar intake, it is crucial for dental professionals to be aware and adopt creative, region-specific strategies for dietary assessment to address the intake of foods and beverages that are of relevance to dental health. Implementation of isolated public health strategies like fluoridation are not adequate to achieve prevention of caries if the intake of free sugars is not considered. This underscores the importance of addressing the root cause to reduce the risk of dental caries [20].

Table 13.2 Sources of free sugars across different populations

Region/population	Key sources of free sugars
United Kingdom (UK), United States of America (USA), Europe, Mexico	Sugar-sweetened beverages (SSBs: including sweetened juices), confectionery, biscuits, cakes, cereal bars and dried fruits
Portugal, Lebanon, China	Cakes, biscuits, cereal-based products and confectionery
Australia	SSBs, confectionery and cakes
USA	Ready-to-eat cereals, SSBs, sweet bakery products, confectionery, desserts (e.g. ice cream)
UK	SSBs, sugar and chocolate confectionery, biscuits and cakes
Brazil (Adolescents)	SSBs, cookies, confectionery, cakes, table sugar and honey
India	Table sugar, jaggery, sweetened milk products including fortified drink mixes, confectionery and sweet-baked products

13.5.2 Frequency and Patterns of Sugar Intake

Variations in the frequency and pattern of free sugars intake alter the plaque pH and salivary flow, thereby impacting the risk of dental caries [5]. Frequency refers to the number of times in a day free sugars are consumed, either as part of a main meal or as snacks between meals. The pattern encompasses intake during main meals (breakfast, lunch, dinner) and intake as snacks, that is, non-main meal occasions: in-between mealtimes, at bedtime, before breakfast and after dinner. Patterns of intake are also described as intake on weekdays compared with weekends [21], and intake during special occasions, for example, festivals and birthdays.

Intake of free sugars between main meals, when salivary flow is low, is a higher risk for dental caries. This is also true for bedtime intake of free sugars [1]. Foods and drinks containing free sugars are typically consumed as snacks [14]. Moreover, there is limited resource to educate patients especially children, adolescents, and their parents about lower salivary flow at bedtime and in-between meals, which is the primary reason that sugars intake at these times poses a greater risk for dental caries. Addressing the patterns of free sugars intake is crucial for efforts to prevent dental caries, which can be achieved within dental practices as described in Sect. 13.6.

Summary of evidence: Early animal studies demonstrated that both the frequency and amount of sugar intake are risk factors for dental caries. Systematic reviews reported a link between the number of daily or weekly servings of sugar-containing foods and caries in mixed and permanent dentition but found no association with the overall frequency of sugar intake from all sources. Human epidemiological studies found that both the amount and frequency of sugar intake contribute to caries risk [22].

Clinical Insight: amount versus frequency of sugars intake [22]. Intake of free sugars is linked to dental caries, obesity and increased of type 2 diabetes, cardiovascular disease, and some cancers. Reducing the frequency alone is insufficient to reduce the risk of caries and caries and other NCDs. The priority should be to reduce the total amount of sugars consumed from all sources. Goals set in terms of frequency may, however, be more tangible for patients to follow. Practical strategy would therefore be to advise reducing the number of times sugars are consumed in the day.

13.6 Leveraging Opportunities for Sugar Reduction Through Dental Settings

Dental practices are ideal settings for delivering dietary advice that aligns with general health recommendations. The negative health effects of dental caries are cumulative, tracking from childhood (permanent dentition) to adulthood. Despite robust evidence from epidemiological, microbiological and biochemical studies about the impact of free sugars on dental and overall health, many dental practitioners have not fully integrated dietary advice into routine care [18]. In recent efforts toward prevention, dental health organisations in high-income countries are collaborating with nutrition and dietetic professionals to create resources to support dental professionals in providing dietary advice [23]. The implementation, however, requires concerted efforts from all stakeholders, including government health agencies, consumer groups, parents, schoolteachers and the food industry. Beyond isolated chairside advice, dental professionals must encourage individuals to 'eat less' and take steps that lead to dietary behaviour change grounded in behaviour change theories (BCTs) based on behaviour feedback, social and environmental impact awareness, problem-solving and social comparison [18].

Dietary advice for caries prevention typically emphasises drinking water and avoiding SSB and foods containing free sugars, especially between meals, with little focus on long-term behaviour change [18]. Although dental professionals generally support integrating dietary advice into primary care, its implementation is hampered by a lack of clarity about the guidelines and recommended thresholds for sugars intake, as well as limited confidence, awareness, time and remuneration [24]. Therefore, better education of dentists on the thresholds for intake of free sugars and definitions of what constitutes 'low sugars' is needed, along with opportunities for adequate training and fostering multidisciplinary collaboration to ensure the effective and consistent delivery of dietary advice.

Dental professionals, especially public health and preventive dentistry specialists, must recognise the potential to transform dental practice into hubs for the prevention of diet-related non-communicable diseases, including dental caries. This transformation can be facilitated through co-created capacity-building efforts in consultation with dentists, nutritionists, dietitians and public policy experts. Furthermore, student dentists could be trained through the introduction of nutrition education in dental curricula to empower them in patient education that promotes a healthy balanced diet beyond just oral health.

Digital systems are now available for dental professionals to collect comprehensive data on dietary habits—including the types of food and beverages consumed, portion sizes, and timing of intake—to provide automated or tailored advice. With the limited need for professional training in nutrition and dietetics, these systems ensure that the advice provided by dentists is underpinned by robust dietary assessment, which factors in the amount and patterns of intake. An example of a validated digital system will be discussed in Sect. 13.7.

13.7 Approaches to Translating Guidelines on Sugars Intake into Actionable Advice

Integrating technology-driven approaches to support dietary behaviour change during regular dental visits offers numerous benefits. The most significant benefit is an increase in food literacy, enabling informed dietary choices that help prevent dental caries and other diet-related NCDs. Additionally, dentists can transition from paper-based dietary records to integrating dietary recall information with patient data. Furthermore, dentists and hygienists can easily review information, track progress in dietary behaviour change over the course of appointments and provide access to dietary data insights, helping patients understand and make a change.

Intake24 (https://intake24.com) is an open-source, low-cost, web-based dietary assessment tool designed for efficient and cost-effective dietary data collection and analysis [25]. Using a 24-h multiple-pass recall method, it helps create a digital record of food and drink intake. The system features prompts that enhance accuracy, check for missing items and uses food photographs and standard portion sizes for the estimation of the amount of intake. Optional tailored questions can be added to collect information on eating contexts relevant to dental health, for example, eating around bedtime and eating in between main meals. Intake24 automatically calculates nutrient and energy intake, streamlining data processing [26, 27].

Intake24: Clinical is an extension of the Intake24 system conceptualised after a series of co-creation workshops with nutritionists and dietitians. Intake24: Clinical uses one or multiple dietary recalls captured through Intake24 and conducts full nutritional analysis to provide condition specific dietary feedback. Dentists and other health professionals who are not trained dietitians or nutritionists can tailor this feedback minimising the need for detailed knowledge of nutrition and nutrition guidelines. Research indicates that dental professionals, including hygienists and oral health therapists, respond positively to training that enhances their confidence in promoting patient behaviour change [28]. This highlights the importance of equipping the dental workforce with the necessary skills to effectively use validated digital tools for providing dietary advice aimed at reducing free sugars intake to safeguard dental health.

13.8 Make Sugars Accountable

In conclusion, dental professionals must make the assessment and advice regarding free sugars an accountable part of patient care. This assessment should include the measurement of free sugars intake, consumption patterns that are relevant for developing patient-centred advice. Dental professionals should leverage existing digital tools to curate tailored dietary advice addressing the amount, sources and patterns of consumption to support dietary behaviour change.

Dental professionals are essential stakeholders in advocating for the reduction in free sugars, not only through chairside education but also by engaging in upstream approaches aimed at decreasing sugars consumption across broader systems. This includes advocating for the reformulation of sugar-containing foods and beverages. Additionally, dental professionals should support efforts to lower sugars consumption through active participation in the design of school menus and hospital food programmes to encourage healthier options. They play a crucial role in advocating for the taxation of SSBs and calling for restrictions on the sale of sugar-containing foods and SSBs school environments and urban settings, including businesses and workplaces, by collaborating with local governments on co-design of well-being programmes. Dental professionals could also work towards the development of trade regulations that limit the import and marketing of products containing free sugars.

References

1. Moynihan P, Petersen PE. Diet, nutrition and the prevention of dental diseases. Public Health Nutr. 2004;7(1A):201–26.
2. World Health Organization. Guideline: sugars intake for adults and children. Geneva: World Health Organization; 2015. Available from: https://www.who.int/publications/i/item/guideline-sugars-intake-for-adults-and-children.
3. Amoutzopoulos B, Steer T, Roberts C, Collins D, Page P, Nicholson S. Free and added sugar consumption and adherence to guidelines: the UK National Diet and Nutrition Survey (2014/15–2015/16). Nutrients. 2020;12(2):393.
4. World Health Organization. Diet, nutrition and the prevention of chronic diseases: report of a joint WHO/FAO expert consultation, Geneva, 28 January – 1 February 2002. Geneva: World Health Organization; 2003.
5. Sheiham A. Dietary effects on dental diseases. Public Health Nutr. 2001;4(2B):569–91.
6. Moynihan PJ, Kelly SA. Effect on caries of restricting sugars intake: systematic review to inform WHO guidelines. J Dent Res. 2014;93(1):8–18.
7. Moores CJ, Kelly SAM, Moynihan PJ. Systematic review of the effect on caries of sugars intake: ten-year update. J Dent Res. 2022;101(9):1034–45.
8. Sheiham A, James WP. A new understanding of the relationship between sugars, dental caries and fluoride use: implications for limits on sugars consumption. Public Health Nutr. 2014;17(10):2176–84.
9. Bernabé E, Vehkalahti MM, Sheiham A, Lundqvist A, Suominen AL. The shape of the dose-response relationship between sugars and caries in adults. J Dent Res. 2016;95(2):167–72.
10. Turck D, Bohn T, Castenmiller J, de Henauw S, Hirsch-Ernst KI, Kearney J, et al. Tolerable upper intake level for dietary sugars. EFSA J. 2022;20(1):e07074.
11. Moynihan P. Sugars and dental caries: evidence for setting a recommended threshold for intake. Adv Nutr. 2016;7(1):149–56.
12. Newens KJ, Walton J. A review of sugar consumption from nationally representative dietary surveys across the world. J Hum Nutr Diet. 2016;29(2):225–40.
13. Fujiwara A, Okada E, Okada C, Matsumoto M, Takimoto H. Association between free sugars intake and nutrient dilution among Japanese adults: the 2016 National Health and Nutrition Survey, Japan. Eur J Nutr. 2020;59(8):3827–39.

14. Perrar I, Alexy U, Nöthlings U. Intake of free sugar among children and adolescents in Germany declines—current results of the DONALD study. Eur J Nutr. 2024;63(7):2827–33.
15. Huew R, Maguire A, Waterhouse P, Moynihan P. Nutrient intake and dietary patterns of relevance to dental health of 12-year-old Libyan children. Public Health Nutr. 2014;17(5):1107–13.
16. Ivaturi A, Giles L, Do LG, Arora M, Rawal T, Moynihan PJ. Intake of free sugars by 11–13-year-old schoolchildren living in Delhi, India. Proc Nutr Soc. 2024;83(OCE1):E153.
17. Moynihan P, Miller C. Beyond the chair: public health and governmental measures to tackle sugar. J Dent Res. 2020;99(8):871–6.
18. Moynihan P. The content of dietary advice for young adolescents delivered in dental practice for caries prevention: a rapid scoping review. Curr Dev Nutr. 2024;8:nzad103248.
19. Moynihan PJ. Dietary advice in dental practice. Br Dent J. 2002;193(10):563–8.
20. World Health Organization. Sugars and dental caries. Geneva: World Health Organization; 2017. Available from: https://www.who.int/publications/i/item/sugars-and-dental-caries.
21. Svensson A, Larsson C, Eiben G, Lanfer A, Pala V, Hebestreit A, et al. European children's sugar intake on weekdays versus weekends: the IDEFICS study. Eur J Clin Nutr. 2014;68(7):822–8.
22. Moynihan P, Makino Y, Petersen PE, Ogawa H. Implications of WHO Guideline on sugars for dental health professionals. Community Dent Oral Epidemiol. 2018;46:1–7.
23. Australian Dental Association. Policy statement 2.2.2: diet and nutrition. 2023. Available from: https://ada.org.au/policy-statement-2-2-2-diet-nutrition.
24. O'Kane R, Watson S, Woodside J, McKenna GJ. Exploring the attitudes of general dental practitioners to providing dietary advice alongside oral rehabilitation for older adults. Gerodontology. 2024;41(1):101–10.
25. Foster E, Lee C, Imamura F, Hollis JL, Imamura M, Walton J, et al. Validity and reliability of an online self-report 24-h dietary recall method (Intake24): a doubly labelled water study and repeated-measures analysis. J Nutr Sci. 2019;8:e29.
26. Bradley J, Simpson E, Poliakov I, Matthews JN, Olivier P, Adamson AJ, et al. Comparison of INTAKE24 (an online 24-h dietary recall tool) with interviewer-led 24-h recall in 11–24-year-olds. Nutrients. 2016;8(6):358.
27. Simpson E, Bradley J, Poliakov I, Jackson D, Williams L, Olivier P, et al. Iterative development of an online dietary recall tool: INTAKE24. Nutrients. 2017;9(2):118.
28. Rogers KM, Arnett MC, Mays KA, Wang Q, Blue CM. Dental hygienists' use of motivational interviewing and perceptions of effectiveness in changing patient behaviours. J Dent Educ. 2022;86(8):909–17.

Impact of Sweetened and Acidic Soft Drinks on Dental Health

14

Rahena Akhter, Vickie Cai, and Rebecca Chen

14.1 Introduction

This chapter explores the impact of sugar-sweetened and acidic soft drinks (SSBs) on oral health. It discusses their definitions, global consumption trends and effects on oral health, particularly focusing on dental caries, erosion and periodontal disease. This chapter concludes with advice regarding managing the oral impact of SSBS from both public health and patient-level perspectives. SSBs, characterised by added caloric sweeteners or free sugars, pose significant health risks.

14.2 Definition of Sweetened and Acidic Soft Drinks

While there is currently no universal consensus on how sugar-sweetened beverages (SSBs) are defined, the World Health Organization (WHO) defined sugary drinks as 'all types of beverages containing free sugars, and these include carbonated or non-carbonated soft drinks, fruit/vegetable juices and drinks, liquid and powder concentrates, flavoured water, energy and sports drinks, ready-to-drink tea, ready-to-drink

R. Akhter (✉) · V. Cai · R. Chen
Sydney Dental School, Faculty of Medicine and Health, The University of Sydney, Camperdown, NSW, Australia
e-mail: rahena.akhter@sydney.edu.au; vickie.cai@sydney.edu.au; rebecca.chen@sydney.edu.au

S. R. Prabhu et al. (eds.), *Lifestyle in Oral Health and Disease*,
https://doi.org/10.1007/978-3-032-05888-1_14

coffee, and flavoured milk drinks' [1]. In terms of composition, some definitions include the addition of caloric sweeteners such as sucrose, high-fructose corn syrup (HFCS) or fruit juice concentrates added by beverage manufacturers or individuals themselves [2]. Some organisations have also established a sugar-to-liquid ratio; in the UK, this has been set as addition of >5 g per 100 mL, while in New York, it is defined as 6.25 g for 8 fl oz. (237 mL) [2].

14.3 Global Trends in SSB and Acidic Soft Drink Consumption

While sugar-sweetened beverage (SSB) consumption has decreased since the early 2000s, it remains high and is associated with increased incidence of chronic diseases like obesity and dental caries [3]. SSBs are concerning due to their links to obesity, cardiovascular disease (CVD), type 2 diabetes mellitus (T2DM), cancer and dental caries, as well as their contribution to health disparities. Despite limited national SSB intake estimates, a 2010 study attributed 184,000 global deaths to SSBs [4]. While high-income nations have shown some decrease, SSB intake remains high and may rise in non-Western countries. Research using Global Dietary Database data from 1990, 2005 and 2018 in 185 countries found the highest SSB intake among younger, urban, educated males [2] (Fig. 14.1). Sub-Saharan Africa experienced the most significant increase in intake, while Latin America/Caribbean saw a decrease, highlighting the need for targeted interventions (2).

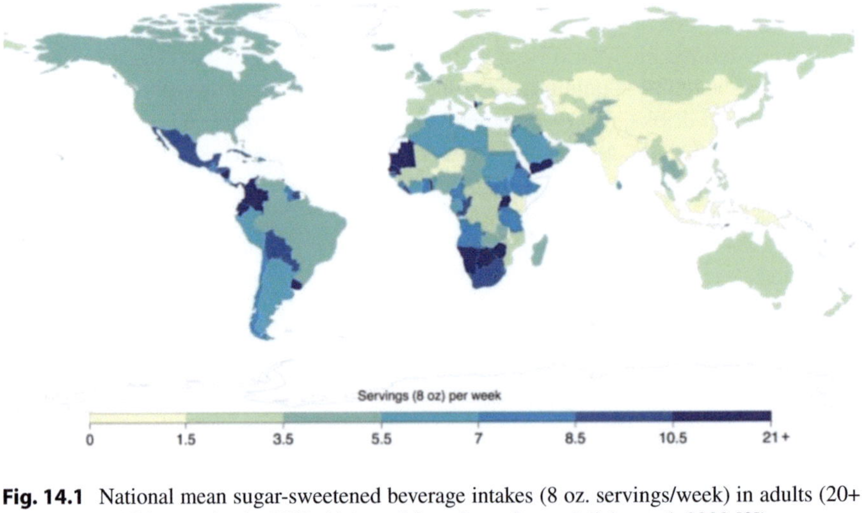

Fig. 14.1 National mean sugar-sweetened beverage intakes (8 oz. servings/week) in adults (20+ years) across 185 countries in 2018. (Adopted from Lara-Castor, Micha et al. 2023 [2])

14.4 Oral Health Impacts

14.4.1 Dental Caries

Dental caries is a biofilm-mediated, sugar-driven, multifactorial, dynamic disease that results in the phasic demineralisation and remineralisation of dental hard tissues [5]. Saliva's consistency and flow rate can affect its ability to flush away germs and substrates, thereby preserving dental hygiene. The intake of added sugar and fermentable carbohydrates is a well-known risk factor for dental caries. One significant source of added sugars is sugar-sweetened beverages (SSBs), which contribute about 47% of added sugar, primarily from soft drinks. The cariogenic potential of food is significantly influenced by its physical state. Liquid sugars, such as those in milkshakes and other sweetened beverages, move through the oral cavity very quickly and have little opportunity to cling to the surfaces of teeth. Dental caries develops because bacteria act on sugars for extended periods, producing acid as the sugar binds to the teeth. Since sugars from slowly dissolving sources are released gradually during the consumption of sweetened drinks or other products, their innate ability to flow, minimal or non-existent inclination to disperse, and comparatively high incompressibility account for developing dental caries.

Liquid carbohydrates are not retained in the mouth for very long; however, frequent consumption of carbohydrates throughout the day increases the risk of dental caries. Dental caries and erosion can result from bacterial acids remaining in the oral cavity for an extended period when teeth are continuously exposed to sugary liquids. A study by Virk et al., 2024, showed that the carbonated beverage they used was Red Bull, which contains carbonated water, sugar, caffeine, colouring agents and acidity regulator ingredients [6]. The sugar added is 11 g/100 g, which caused an instant decrease in salivary pH of up to 3.336 ± 0.46, below the critical pH level of 5.5, promoting demineralisation. Therefore, efforts to reduce frequency should also lead to a decrease in the quantity consumed [7].

Reasons that lead people to consume these drinks include parents' influence, peer pressure, diet fallacies, pleasure and taste [8]. One of the significant implications for dental health is the drinking habits of children and adults worldwide [9]. Extended and frequent consumption of an acidogenic drink causes recurrent bouts of low plaque pH, which eventually leads to demineralisation. The main factors that contribute to the damage caused by certain drinks to teeth are as follows: firstly, the low pH and titrable acidity of some drinks can cause enamel erosion; secondly, the fermentable carbohydrates in drinks are metabolised by plaque microorganisms to generate organic acids in the dental plaque, leading to demineralisation and progression to dental caries. The cariogenicity is related to the extent of acid production and the length of exposure to organic acids [10, 11].

14.4.2 Tooth Wear—Dental Erosion

Tooth wear is an umbrella term defined as the 'cumulative surface loss of mineralised tooth substance due to physical or chemo-physical processes (dental erosion, attrition, abrasion). It is not considered to be the result of dental caries, resorption, or trauma' [12].

Dental erosion is one aspect of tooth wear and occurs when acid not produced by oral bacteria dissolves the hard structure of the teeth [12, 13]. However, prolonged acid exposure will wear away the enamel and cause irreversible damage. The tooth surface's wearing away can result from intrinsic and extrinsic acids. Common intrinsic acids include those from acid reflux or other medical conditions that induce vomiting, such as bulimia. However, the extrinsic acids, primarily from SSBs, including carbonated soft drinks, acidic fruit juices and energy and sports drinks, contribute to the rise in erosion. Sugar-sweetened beverages have been the leading cause of extrinsic dental erosion over the past 20–30 years [14]. The critical pH at which dental erosion occurs is below 5.5 [15]. Most commercially available drinks have a pH below this critical level, with colas at a pH of 2.5 and sports drinks in Japan at a pH of 3.3 [16]. At the same time, a similar study in the United States found that 93% of common commercially available SSBs have a pH below 4.17. These drinks are widely accessible. The constant and frequent consumption of these SSBs has led to increased dental erosion globally, with 30–50% of baby teeth and 20–45% of adult teeth now affected by this condition [17].

The consequences of severe dental erosion can include tooth sensitivity, poor aesthetics due to a darkened tooth colour and the wearing away or chipping of the front edges of the tooth [18]. Continuous exposure to intrinsic or extrinsic acids eventually leads to tooth loss.

To diagnose and manage dental erosion, dentists and dental practitioners (oral health therapists [OHTs], dental therapists/hygienists) should conduct a thorough examination to identify signs of erosion (e.g. enamel texture loss, flattening on chewing surfaces), determine contributing factors and recommend strategies to minimise exposure to acidic foods and drinks.

14.4.3 Periodontal Disease

The periodontium is the collection of soft and hard tissues that surround, support and anchor the teeth, including the gingiva or gums, root cementum, periodontal ligament and alveolar bone. Periodontal diseases are immune-inflammatory conditions that affect the periodontal tissues, initiated by the accumulation of dental plaque (biofilm) in the space between the tooth and the gingiva.

In the early stages of inflammation (gingivitis), the gingiva becomes swollen and red and bleeds easily. With continued build-up, biofilm dysbiosis arises, causing an elevated hyperinflammatory state and the release of proteolytic enzymes (matrix metalloproteinases) along with bone-resorbing cells (osteoclasts) that degrade the periodontium tissues [19, 20]. In advanced stages (periodontitis), the progressive destruction of the connective tissue attachment and alveolar bone leads to tooth mobility and eventual loss.

Oral and periodontal health are critically important to overall health. Periodontal diseases are linked to a range of non-communicable diseases (NCDs), including cardiovascular disease, diabetes mellitus, neurodegenerative diseases and cancer [21–25]. While this may be attributed to common risk factors such as tobacco and alcohol consumption, literature has also pinpointed bidirectional relationships through inflammatory mechanisms, whereby periodontal and chronic systemic diseases may exacerbate each other's development and progression [23, 25]. Periodontal diseases have various risk and lifestyle factors, with recent studies highlighting the influence of dietary sugar intake. The consumption of sugary soft drinks triggers a hyper-inflammatory state, thus increasing the incidence of periodontal disease; however, evidence-based data are lacking in this regard.

A systematic review concluded that frequent intake of free sugars from foods or beverages was associated with periodontal diseases [26]. Another review analysed the impact of SSB consumption in particular, finding that it was linked to increased severity of gingival bleeding and periodontal disease [27]. Conversely, restricting free sugar consumption was associated with improved gingival health and lower dental plaque levels [28].

Dietary sugar intake may impact periodontal inflammation through several mechanistic pathways. Firstly, excess sugar increases pro-inflammatory cytokines and oxidative stress, inducing chronic systemic inflammation and exacerbating periodontal disease [29]. Furthermore, sugar-rich diets are linked to systemic risk factors for periodontal inflammation, including obesity, metabolic syndrome and diabetes [25, 29] mellitus. Additionally, dietary sugar may disrupt the diversity of the dental biofilm, leading to the proliferation of specific bacterial species that initiate and promote periodontitis [29].

14.5 Commercial Determinants of Health and the Impact of 'BIG Sugar'

To promote and maintain oral health, dental care systems must prioritise equity. Common risk factors such as sugar, alcohol and tobacco consumption contribute to various NCDs. Effective regulation and legislation are necessary to tackle these risk factors.

The sugar industry employs corporate and marketing strategies to increase consumption and profits, and it has, to some extent, influenced oral health research, policies and professional associations [30]. To combat this, transparent conflict of interest policies are essential to limit the industry's influence on research, policy and practice [31].

Public health policies must address common risk factors such as free sugar consumption, tobacco use and alcohol consumption that contribute to oral diseases and other non-communicable diseases (NCDs). The global sugar industry's strategies to boost sales often undermine public health initiatives to reduce sugar intake. In countries with stricter regulations on sugar taxation, like the UK and Mexico, the purchase and consumption of sugar-sweetened beverages (SSBs) have significantly decreased [32–34]. More countries must invest in upstream, policy-informed, population-wide strategies, including taxing sugary drinks and regulating advertising directed at children. Clinical preventive measures such as topical fluorides can help control caries; however, they should not overshadow the primary role of sugar in caries development, and transparent conflict of interest policies are urgently needed. The oral health community and the general public must address and shift the commercial determinants of oral health to reduce inequalities and improve overall public health.

14.6 Management for the Prevention of Oral Health Impacts Related to Sweetened and Acidic Soft Drinks

Evidence shows that both the frequency and amount of sugar consumed are associated with dental caries. Sugars that are potentially damaging to dental health are NMES (non-milk extrinsic sugar), which include all added sugars, sugars in fresh fruit juices, honey and syrups. The dietary reference value (DRV) for NMES is a maximum of 60 g/day, which equates to approximately 10% of daily energy intake [35].

Drinking sugary beverages with meals will reduce the chances of developing dental caries and erosion [36]. All patients should be advised to reduce acidic drink intake, keep acidic drinks to mealtimes and avoid them close to bedtime. If drinking acidic drinks, preventive measures should avoid behaviours that expose teeth to more acid (like swishing or sipping throughout the day) and instead drink them down in one go rather than sip over a long period. These acidic drinks should also be low in sugars wherever possible to minimise dental caries. The best drinks are, therefore, milk and water. Cow's milk is lower in sugar than formula milk and is higher in the protective factors, calcium and phosphorus.

Chewing gum to stimulate saliva may also be protective, and rinsing with sodium bicarbonate can support salivary health and promote remineralisation of teeth' enamel [37]. When toothbrushing, brush with soft-bristled and fluoride toothpaste, but avoid brushing immediately after acidic intake. SSB intake is a potentially modifiable lifestyle factor which contributes to the incidence of periodontal disease. Therefore, dietary modifications like restricting daily sugar intake to <10% of the total energy intake should be part of periodontal risk management [27, 29].

The soft drinks industry levy has the potential to reduce dental caries incidence. Oral health gains arising through raising the price of high-sugar and mid-sugar drinks and increasing the market share of low-sugar products will, at a population level, reduce the environmental determinants towards poor oral health [38].

14.7 Conclusion

The consumption of sweetened and acidic soft drinks remains a global health concern, contributing to dental caries, tooth erosion and periodontal diseases. Their high sugar and acid content lowers oral pH, leading to enamel demineralisation and increased oral inflammation. Preventive strategies include reducing the intake of SSBs or having them with meals; exposure to fluoride, saliva stimulation and dietary changes are essential. Policy interventions, including sugar taxes and advertising, are also necessary.

Restrictions can also reduce risk factors. Addressing individual behaviours and systemic factors is crucial for improving oral health and reducing related health disparities.

References

1. World Health Organization. Taxes on sugary drinks: why do it? [Internet]. World Health Organization; 2017. [cited 2025 14th Mar]. Available from: https://iris.who.int/bitstream/handle/10665/260253/WHO-NMH-PND-16.5Rev.1-eng.pdf
2. Lara-Castor L, Micha R, Cudhea F, Miller V, Shi P, Zhang J, et al. Sugar-sweetened beverage intakes among adults between 1990 and 2018 in 185 countries. Nat Commun. 2023;14(1):5957.
3. Malik VS, Popkin BM, Bray GA, Després JP, Hu FB. Sugar-sweetened beverages, obesity, type 2 diabetes mellitus, and cardiovascular disease risk. Circulation. 2010;121(11):1356–64.
4. Singh GM, Micha R, Khatibzadeh S, Lim S, Ezzati M, Mozaffarian D. Estimated global, regional, and national disease burdens related to sugar-sweetened beverage consumption in 2010. Circulation. 2015;132(8):639–66.
5. Pitts NB, Zero DT, Marsh PD, Ekstrand K, Weintraub JA, Ramos-Gomez F, et al. Dental caries. Nat Rev Dis Primers. 2017;3:17030.
6. Virk J, Malhan S, Sandhu GK, Sood H, Ishita PD. To assess the effect of selected locally available beverages on salivary pH, flow rate, and oral clearance rate among adults. J Conserv Dent Endod. 2024;27(8):833–7.
7. Moynihan PJ. Dietary advice in dental practice. Br Dent J. 2002;193(10):563–8.
8. Azrak B, Callaway A, Knözinger S, Willershausen B. Reduction of the pH-values of whole saliva after the intake of apple juice containing beverages in children and adults. Oral Health Prev Dent. 2003;1(3):229–36.
9. Verzeletti C, Maes L, Santinello M, Vereecken CA. Soft drink consumption in adolescence: associations with food-related lifestyles and family rules in Belgium Flanders and the Veneto Region of Italy. Eur J Pub Health. 2010;20(3):312–7.
10. Vartanian LR, Schwartz MB, Brownell KD. Effects of soft drink consumption on nutrition and health: a systematic review and meta-analysis. Am J Public Health. 2007;97(4):667–75.
11. Jerkovic K, Binnekade JM, van der Kruk JJ, van der Most JA, Talsma AC, van der Schans CP. Differences in oral health behaviour between children from high and children from low SES schools in The Netherlands. Community Dent Health. 2009;26(2):110–5.
12. Schlueter N, Amaechi Bennett T, Bartlett D, Buzalaf Marília Afonso R, Carvalho Thiago S, Ganss C, et al. Terminology of erosive tooth wear: consensus report of a workshop organized by the ORCA and the Cariology Research Group of the IADR. Caries Res. 2020;54(1):2–6.
13. Lussi A, Carvalho TS. Erosive tooth wear: a Multifactorial condition of growing concern and increasing knowledge. Monogr Oral Sci. 25:1–15.

14. Valenzuela MJ, Waterhouse B, Aggarwal VR, Bloor K, Doran T. Effect of sugar-sweetened beverages on oral health: a systematic review and meta-analysis. Eur J Pub Health. 2021;31(1):122–9.
15. Featherstone JD, Lussi A. Understanding the chemistry of dental erosion. Monogr Oral Sci. 2006;20:66–76.
16. Sato T, Fukuzawa Y, Kawakami S, Suzuki M, Tanaka Y, Terayama H, et al. The onset of dental erosion caused by food and drinks and the preventive effect of alkaline ionized water. Nutrients. 2021;13(10):3440.
17. Schlueter N, Luka B. Erosive tooth wear–a review on global prevalence and on its prevalence in risk groups. Br Dent J. 2018;224(5):364–70.
18. Mooney Y. How to manage tooth erosion. BDJ team. 2021;8(9):7–9.
19. Sapna G, Gokul S, Bagri-Manjrekar K. Matrix metalloproteinases and periodontal diseases. Oral Dis. 2014;20(6):538–50.
20. Hienz SA, Ivanovski S, Paliwal S, Mori G. Mechanisms of bone resorption in periodontitis. J Immunol Res. 2015;2015(2015):1–10.
21. Nadim R, Tang J, Dilmohamed A, Yuan S, Wu C, Bakre AT, et al. Influence of periodontal disease on risk of dementia: a systematic literature review and a meta-analysis. Eur J Epidemiol. 2020;35(9):821–33.
22. Nguyen ATM, Akhter R, Garde S, Scott C, Twigg SM, Colagiuri S, et al. The association of periodontal disease with the complications of diabetes mellitus. A systematic review. Diabetes Res Clin Pract. 2020;165:108244.
23. Hajishengallis G, Chavakis T. Local and systemic mechanisms linking periodontal disease and inflammatory comorbidities. Nat Rev Immunol. 2021;21(7):426–40.
24. Larvin H, Kang J, Aggarwal VR, Pavitt S, Wu J. Risk of incident cardiovascular disease in people with periodontal disease: a systematic review and meta-analysis. Clin Exp Dent Res. 2021;7(1):109–22.
25. Marruganti C, Suvan JE, D'Aiuto F. Periodontitis and metabolic diseases (diabetes and obesity): tackling multimorbidity. Periodontology. 2000:2023.
26. Kusama T, Nakazawa N, Takeuchi K, Kiuchi S, Osaka K. Free sugar intake and periodontal diseases: a systematic review. Nutrients. 2022;14(21):4444.
27. Gupta V, Dawar A, Bhadauria US, Purohit BM, Nilima N. Sugar-sweetened beverages and periodontal disease: a systematic review. Oral Dis. 2023;29(8):3078–90.
28. Woelber JP, Gebhardt D, Hujoel PP. Free sugars and gingival inflammation: a systematic review and meta-analysis. J Clin Periodontol. 2023;50(9):1188–201.
29. Shanmugasundaram S, Karmakar S. Excess dietary sugar and its impact on periodontal inflammation: a narrative review. BDJ open. 2024;10(1):78.
30. Kearns CE, Glantz SA, Schmidt LA. Sugar industry influence on the scientific agenda of the national institute of dental research's 1971 National caries program: a historical analysis of internal documents. PLoS Med. 2015;12(3):467–89.
31. Kearns CE, Schmidt LA, Glantz SA. Sugar industry and coronary heart disease research: a historical analysis of internal industry documents. JAMA Intern Med. 2016;176(11):1680–5.
32. Watt RG, Daly B, Allison P, Macpherson LMD, Venturelli R, Listl S, et al. Ending the neglect of global oral health: time for radical action. The Lancet (British edition). 2019;394(10194):261–72.
33. Arantxa Colchero M, Salgado JC, Unar-Munguía M, Molina M, Ng S, Rivera-Dommarco JA. Changes in prices after an excise tax to sweetened sugar beverages was implemented in Mexico: evidence from Urban Areas. PLoS One. 2015;10(12):e0144408-e.
34. Scarborough P, Adhikari V, Harrington RA, Elhussein A, Briggs A, Rayner M, et al. Impact of the announcement and implementation of the UK soft drinks industry levy on sugar content, price, product size and number of available soft drinks in the UK, 2015–19: a controlled interrupted time series analysis. PLoS Med. 2020;17(2):e1003025-e.

35. Department of Health. Dietary reference values for food energy and nutrients for the United Kingdom: report of the panel on dietary reference values of the committee on medical aspects of food policy. London: HMSO; 1991.
36. Nielsen SJ, Popkin BM. Changes in beverage intake between 1977 and 2001. Am J Prev Med. 2004;27(3):205–10.
37. Li H, Zou Y, Ding G. Dietary factors associated with dental erosion: a meta-analysis. PLoS One. 2012;7(8):e42626.
38. Briggs ADMD, Mytton OTMPH, Kehlbacher AP, Tiffin RP, Elhussein ABA, Rayner MP, et al. Health impact assessment of the UK soft drinks industry levy: a comparative risk assessment modelling study. Lancet Public Health. 2017;2(1):e15–22.

Fluoride and Oral Health

15

Christopher Sexton and Nicole Stormon

15.1 Introduction

Fluoride has played a crucial role in oral health for over a century, significantly contributing to the prevention of oral diseases worldwide. It is arguably the most impactful intervention for preventing dental caries available.

Fluoride for the prevention of oral disease first came into use in the mid-twentieth century when Grand Rapids, Michigan, United States of America, became the first city to introduce community water fluoridation in 1945 [1, 2]. The Grand Rapids water fluoridation study was a breakthrough in public health and a landmark study design for its time [3]. The study was the first controlled long-term community trial to assess the effects of fluoride on dental health [1, 2]. Researchers compared Grand Rapids, where fluoride was added to the public water supply, to the nearby city of Muskegon, which initially served as a non-fluoridated control group [1, 2]. This design allowed scientists to measure the direct impact of fluoride on dental caries while accounting for external variables. The study enrolled children over several years, systematically recording dental health outcomes and demonstrating a significant reduction in cavities among those exposed to fluoridated water [1, 2]. At a time when most medical studies were conducted in controlled laboratory settings or clinical trials, the Grand Rapids community-based study provided robust epidemiological evidence of fluoride's preventive benefits. The overwhelming success of the study led to the widespread adoption of water fluoridation policies across the United States and internationally [3].

C. Sexton (✉)
The University of Queensland, Poche Centre for Indigenous Health and The University of Queensland, School of Dentistry, Brisbane, QLD, Australia
e-mail: c.sexton@uq.edu.au

N. Stormon
The University of Queensland, School of Dentistry and Queensland Health, Metro North Health, Community and Oral Health, Brisbane, QLD, Australia

S. R. Prabhu et al. (eds.), *Lifestyle in Oral Health and Disease*,
https://doi.org/10.1007/978-3-032-05888-1_15

In a contemporary context, fluoride is commonly found in drinking water, toothpaste, topical gels, mouth rinses and professional dental treatments, making it one of the most widely used preventive measures in modern dentistry. Despite its evidence-based benefits, fluoride has been the subject of controversy [4, 5]. While excessive fluoride exposure can increase an individual's risk for dental fluorosis, some opponents argue that exposure to fluoride leads directly to systemic health risks, while others raise concerns about mass medication and individual consent. Extensive scientific evidence supports its safety and effectiveness in preventing dental decay, with leading health organisations advocating for its continued use [6–8].

> *'Adequate exposure to fluoride is an essential factor in the prevention of dental caries'.*
> *World Health Organisation, Oral Health (March 17, 2025)*

Fluoride's importance in oral health prevents lifestyle-related oral diseases like dental caries. Lifestyle-related oral diseases are those conditions influenced by diet, oral hygiene and environmental factors [9]. Dental caries is among the most prevalent non-communicable diseases worldwide and can be prevented by managing lifestyle-related risk factors. Fluoride plays a crucial role in communities with high sugar consumption and limited access to professional dental care, serving as a cost-effective preventive measure for individuals and entire populations. This chapter will outline how fluoride prevents dental caries and discuss its application for individuals, dental practitioners, public health and policy.

15.2 Fluoride: Mechanisms of Action Within the Oral Cavity

Fluoride is crucial in maintaining enamel integrity by regulating demineralisation and remineralisation processes. Fluoride facilitates remineralisation directly onto the tooth surface through sources such as fluoridated toothpaste, mouth rinses and professional applications. This is also known as topical fluoride.

There is a continuing shift and balance occurring in the oral cavity due to various factors, including microorganisms, saliva and lifestyle elements such as oral hygiene, diet and smoking behaviours [10]. The demineralisation and remineralisation balance in teeth refers to the dynamic equilibrium between mineral loss and gain at the enamel surface [10, 11]. Tooth structure demineralisation occurs when acids dissolve calcium and phosphate from hydroxyapatite crystals [10, 11]. Remineralisation restores these minerals to maintain enamel integrity and prevent caries formation and is often enhanced using fluoride (Fig. 15.1) [10, 11].

When exposed to an acidic environment, enamel undergoes demineralisation, where calcium and phosphate ions are lost from the hydroxyapatite crystalline structure [10, 11]. The critical pH at which enamel begins to dissolve is approximately 5.5 [12–14]. Dentin, however, has a lower mineral content and a higher critical pH of 6.2–6.5, making it more susceptible to demineralisation [12–14].

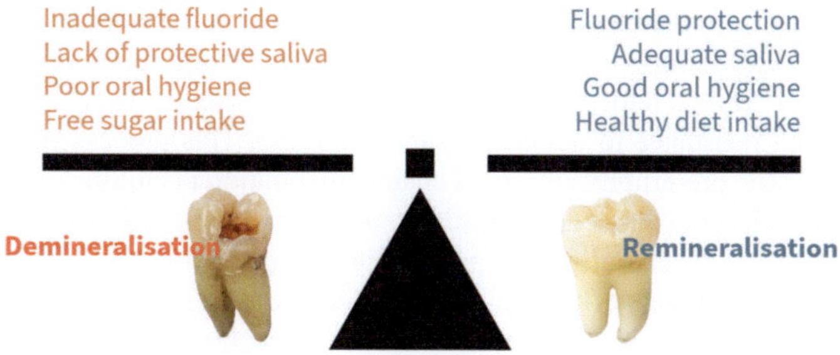

Fig. 15.1 The balance of demineralisation and remineralisation in the dental caries process. (Adapted from Pitts et al. [10])

Fluoride mitigates this process by facilitating remineralisation, enhancing the redeposition of lost minerals and incorporating into the enamel as fluorapatite ($Ca_5(PO_4)_3F$) [15, 16]. Fluorapatite has a lower critical pH of approximately 4.5 and significantly increases enamel resistance to acid dissolution, providing a robust defence against cariogenic challenges [15, 16]. Fluoride inhibits demineralisation by forming a protective surface layer on enamel, reducing mineral solubility and buffering against acid exposure [17, 18].

Fluoride notably influences the oral microbiome by modulating bacterial metabolism and biofilm composition [19]. Research has demonstrated that fluoride interferes with glycolytic pathways in cariogenic bacteria (such as Streptococcus mutans) by inhibiting enolase, an essential enzyme in bacterial carbohydrate metabolism [20, 21]. This disruption reduces lactic acid production, which lowers the overall acidity of the biofilm environment and decreases the risk of enamel demineralisation [22]. Fluoride has been shown to impair bacterial adhesion and biofilm formation, thereby limiting the proliferation of acidogenic and aciduric species [23]. While fluoride does not function as a broad-spectrum antimicrobial agent, its selective impact on metabolic pathways helps maintain a less cariogenic oral environment. Emerging research continues to explore fluoride's broader ecological effects on oral microbial diversity and its role in promoting a microbiome conducive to oral health [24].

As opposed to topical fluoride, systemic fluoride is primarily ingested through fluoridated water, food and dietary supplements [25, 26]. Through this pathway, it is absorbed in the gastrointestinal tract and incorporated into developing dental structures [25, 26]. Once consumed, fluoride is rapidly absorbed in the stomach and small intestine, with bioavailability influenced by factors such as gastric pH, dietary composition and the presence of divalent cations, which can reduce fluoride absorption by forming insoluble complexes [27]. Following absorption, fluoride is distributed via the bloodstream, reaching peak plasma levels within 30–60 min post-ingestion [25, 26].

A portion of circulating fluoride is incorporated into developing teeth during enamel and dentine formation which occurs before the age of 6 years [28, 29]. Hydroxyapatite crystal lattice forms fluorapatite, thereby reducing enamel solubility and enhancing resistance to demineralisation [28, 29]. This process is particularly critical during the pre-eruptive phase of enamel maturation in children under 6 years of age, where fluoride exposure optimises enamel hardness and stability [28, 29]. Excessive fluoride intake during this period can disrupt ameloblast activity. This can result in dental fluorosis which is a condition characterised by hypomineralisation and enamel opacity [30, 31]. The extant literature indicates appropriate uses of fluoride reduce the risk of dental fluorosis and adverse effects on the teeth [30, 31].

Beyond its role in enamel formation, systemic fluoride contributes to a dynamic fluoride reservoir in saliva and dental plaque, where it continuously interacts with tooth surfaces to promote remineralisation and inhibit demineralisation [8, 20]. While systemic fluoride was historically considered the primary mechanism for caries prevention, contemporary research underscores the predominant role of topical fluoride, obtained from sources such as fluoridated toothpaste, mouth rinses and professional applications. These topical agents exert a more immediate protective effect by facilitating remineralisation directly at the tooth surface. Systemic fluoride remains integral to public health strategies during tooth development in children, preventing dental caries.

15.3 Sources of Fluoride

Fluoride occurs naturally in various environmental sources and has been extensively integrated into public health initiatives and consumer products to improve oral health. Its availability through multiple pathways guarantees both systemic and topical benefits in the prevention of caries.

15.3.1 Natural Sources of Fluoride

Fluoride naturally occurs in groundwater, surface water and certain foods. The concentration of fluoride in water sources varies geographically and is influenced by geological composition. Natural fluoride levels in drinking water can range from trace amounts to over 10 mg/L, and excessive prolonged exposure to high levels may lead to dental or skeletal fluorosis. Foods such as tea, seafood and some vegetables can also contribute to dietary fluoride intake.

15.3.2 Water Fluoridation

Water fluoridation is a well-established public health measure aimed at reducing dental caries at the population level. The process involves adjusting the fluoride concentration in public water supplies to an optimal level that balances caries prevention with minimal risk of dental fluorosis. Implementation requires a combination of infrastructure, regulatory oversight and ongoing monitoring to ensure safe and effective fluoride delivery.

The fluoridation process begins with a water quality assessment, determining the natural fluoride content and identifying whether supplementation is necessary. Fluoride is typically added in the form of sodium fluoride (NaF), fluorosilicic acid (H_2SiF_6) or sodium fluorosilicate (Na_2SiF_6), each selected based on solubility, cost and compatibility with existing water treatment systems. The fluoridation system must integrate with water treatment facilities, ensuring precise fluoride dosing, continuous monitoring and compliance with safety regulations.

Water treatment plants often utilise automated dosing systems equipped with real-time fluoride sensors to maintain fluoride at optimal levels. These systems allow for continuous adjustments, ensuring that fluoride concentrations remain within the recommended range. Regular water testing and quality assurance protocols are essential for safeguarding public health.

Public health authorities provide guidelines on optimal fluoride levels. These guidelines vary from country to country but share similarities based on evidence of optimal preventive outcomes balanced with mitigating effects such as dental fluorosis [8]. The recommended fluoride concentration in drinking water typically ranges from 0.6 to 1.1 mg/L, with 0.7 mg/L widely accepted as the standard in temperate climates. In regions with higher water consumption due to hotter climates, fluoride concentrations may be adjusted downward to minimise the risk of excessive intake.

Fluoridation programmes require governmental policy support, public consultation and collaboration between health and water management agencies. Despite strong scientific backing, implementation remains contentious in some regions, with debates surrounding individual choice, ethical considerations and the potential for adverse health effects. However, comprehensive reviews by global health organisations consistently reaffirm the safety and effectiveness of community water fluoridation in reducing dental caries and improving oral health equity.

15.3.3 Fluoride-Containing Products

Topical fluoride products are a primary means of delivering fluoride directly to the tooth surface, enhancing remineralisation and reducing demineralisation [6]. These include the following:

- Toothpaste: The most common fluoride delivery system, with concentrations typically ranging from 1000 to 1500 ppm fluoride in over-the-counter formulations and up to 5000 ppm in prescription-based products [32].
- Mouthwashes: Used adjunctively for fluoride exposure, often containing 225 to 900 ppm fluoride for daily or weekly use [33].

- Gels and foams: Applied in clinical settings for intensive fluoride delivery, often in concentrations of 12,300 ppm fluoride (e.g. acidulated phosphate fluoride gels) [34].
- Fluoride varnishes: High-concentration formulations (typically 22,600 ppm fluoride) applied professionally for targeted, sustained fluoride release [35].

15.3.4 Professional Fluoride Treatments in Clinical Settings

Dental practitioners can provide high-dose fluoride applications to patients at increased risk for caries. Professional fluoride treatments consist of varnishes, gels and foams, which offer prolonged fluoride contact with enamel and dentin, enhancing remineralisation and inhibiting demineralisation. These treatments are especially beneficial for individuals with xerostomia, orthodontic appliances or extensive restorations, as well as for children in high-risk caries populations.

Due to the high fluoride concentration in these products, their use is often regulated by local health authorities. They restrict application to dental professionals to ensure appropriate dosing and minimise the risk of fluorosis or toxicity. This regulation ensures that professional fluoride applications are tailored to individual patient needs, particularly those with active caries or a history of frequent caries progression.

The International Caries Classification and Management System (ICCMS™) recognises fluoride as a fundamental component of caries prevention and management [36, 37]. The ICCMS emphasises that fluoride should be used as part of a comprehensive, risk-based caries management approach, integrating professional fluoride applications with behavioural modifications, dietary counselling and at-home fluoride use [36, 37]. According to the ICCMS guidelines, professional fluoride treatments, such as fluoride varnish applications at least twice per year, are essential for individuals at moderate to high risk of developing caries [36, 37].

15.4 Types of Fluoride

Fluoride is available in various formulations, each with distinct properties and applications for oral health. These fluoride compounds are utilised in consumer dental products and professional treatments to prevent and manage dental caries. Each type of fluoride serves specific clinical and preventive purposes, contributing to comprehensive caries management strategies tailored to the individual needs of patients.

Sodium fluoride (NaF) is one of the most widely used fluoride compounds in oral health products. It is found in toothpaste, mouth rinses and professional fluoride applications. NaF offers high bioavailability and is utilised in both over-the-counter and prescription formulations. Its high solubility in water enables effective fluoride ion release, and it is commonly applied in fluoride varnishes and topical treatments [38].

Stannous fluoride (SnF_2) has both anticaries and antimicrobial properties, offering additional benefits beyond enamel remineralisation. It inhibits bacterial metabolism and biofilm formation, reducing the risk of gingivitis and dental caries. Unlike NaF, SnF_2 has a lower pH, enhancing fluoride uptake but increasing the risk of enamel erosion. SnF_2 can cause tooth staining due to its interaction with dietary chromogens and requires stabilising agents in toothpaste formulations to maintain efficacy [38].

Sodium monofluorophosphate (Na_2PO_3F) is often included in fluoride toothpaste, where it undergoes enzymatic hydrolysis in the mouth to release fluoride ions. Sodium monofluorophosphate is less reactive with calcium-containing compounds in saliva, enhancing its stability in formulations. However, unlike NaF, MFP requires enzymatic activation by salivary phosphatases to release fluoride, which may slightly delay its bioavailability compared to directly ionized fluoride sources.

Acidulated phosphate fluoride (APF) is a clinically applied fluoride formulation, often used in professional gels and foams. It combines fluoride with phosphoric acid to enhance enamel uptake, leading to greater fluoride incorporation into hydroxyapatite. APF solutions typically contain 1.23% fluoride (12,300 ppm) and have a pH of approximately 3.5, which increases fluoride absorption but may etch ceramic and composite restorations, limiting its use in some patients [39].

Silver fluoride (AgF) and silver diamine fluoride ($Ag(NH_3)_2F$) are specialised fluoride formulations used primarily to arrest caries in high-risk populations [40]. Silver diamine fluoride (SDF) contains 38% silver diamine fluoride (44,800 ppm fluoride) and combines the antimicrobial properties of silver with the remineralising effects of fluoride, effectively halting caries progression by disrupting bacterial metabolism and promoting dentin remineralisation [40]. SDF is commonly used in minimally invasive dentistry, particularly for non-restorative caries management in children, elderly patients and individuals with limited access to dental care [40, 41]. SDF causes permanent black staining of arrested caries lesions, which may limit its aesthetic acceptance. To mitigate staining, potassium iodide (KI) can be applied after SDF treatment, although its efficacy remains debated.

15.5 Fluoride and Lifestyle Behaviours

Dietary and lifestyle choices play a critical role in oral health, influencing the risk of dental caries and erosion. Sugar consumption is the primary dietary factor contributing to dental decay, as oral bacteria metabolise free sugars and produce acids that demineralise enamel. The frequency and quantity of sugar intake directly impact caries risk, prompting global recommendations to reduce sugar intake for both dental and overall health benefits.

Beyond sugar, acidic foods and beverages also pose significant risks to enamel integrity. Citrus fruits, soft drinks and alcoholic beverages lower the pH in the oral cavity, leading to enamel erosion that weakens teeth and increases their susceptibility to dental caries. When acidic foods are combined with high sugar content, the risk is exacerbated, accelerating both erosion and bacterial acid production.

Lifestyle factors such as smoking and alcohol consumption further compromise oral health. Smoking reduces salivary flow, limiting fluoride distribution and increasing caries risk, while alcohol's acidity erodes enamel and exacerbates fluoride inefficacy. Understanding the interaction between these dietary and behavioural factors is essential for developing effective prevention strategies to maintain optimal oral health.

15.6 Sugar Consumption and Dental Caries

Dietary free sugars are the main nutritional risk factors for dental caries (see Callout 1). When free sugars are consumed, oral bacteria metabolise them and produce acids as by-products, which demineralise the outer protective layer of tooth enamel, leading to the onset or progression of dental caries. The frequency and amount of sugar intake are directly linked to caries risk. Regular consumption of foods and beverages high in sugar increases the duration of acid exposure, thus raising the risk of enamel demineralisation (see Sect. 15.2).

Foods with low levels of sugar have a cumulative effect on dental health. The World Health Organisation strongly recommends reducing the intake of free sugars (see Callouts 1 and 2) to a maximum of 10% of total energy intake throughout a person's life and conditionally recommends a further reduction to below 5% (approximately 25 grams or 6 tablespoons per day) of total energy consumption. The WHO recommendations are based on the overall health benefits, such as lower body weight and reduced diabetes risk, and they note the advantages for dental health.

Callout 1: What are free sugars, and what foods are they found in?

Free sugars are mono- or disaccharides added to foods and beverages by manufacturers, cooks or consumers. They include sugars naturally present in honey, syrups, fruit juices and fruit juice concentrates. These sugars are frequently added to foods to increase the sweet taste, but they provide limited nutritional benefits beyond additional energy intake.

Contrastingly, *intrinsic sugars* are found in whole fruits, vegetables and dairy products, where they are bound within cellular structures. They are digested more slowly and have a lower cariogenic potential. Whole foods provide dietary fibre and other nutrients that mitigate their impact on oral health.

Callout 2: Major sources of free sugars include the following:

Sugar-sweetened beverages: Soft drinks, energy drinks, fruit juices, sports drinks, flavoured milks and flavoured waters.

Processed and packaged foods: Cakes, biscuits, pastries, cereals and confectionery.

Condiments and sauces: Sauces and salad.

Dairy-based desserts and sweetened yogurts: Many yogurts and flavoured dairy.

Alcoholic beverages: Alcoholic drinks, particularly cocktails and mixed beverages but prevalent in all alcohol beverages.

Snack, muesli or granola bars: Have added sugar content while frequently marketed as a healthier option.

15.7 Acidic Foods and Beverages

Acidic foods and beverages, such as citrus fruits, soft drinks and wine, erode tooth enamel. The acids in these items lower the pH in the oral cavity, leading to the dissolution of hydroxyapatite crystals in enamel. Enamel erosion weakens the teeth and makes them more susceptible to dental caries. This process differs from caries, as dental erosion is a chemical process rather than a result of bacterial growth in the oral cavity. Foods and beverages with lower pH and higher acidic erosion risk, balanced with elevated levels of free sugars for taste, are particularly harmful to dental health. The lower pH causes dental enamel erosion, and the sugar creates a favourable environment for bacteria to multiply, releasing more acid as a by-product (see Chapter).

15.8 Smoking and Tobacco Products

Smoking and tobacco products are strongly associated with oral health deterioration due to their negative effect on salivary function, which prevents the distribution of fluoride throughout the oral cavity. Tobacco use, particularly cigarette smoking, has been linked to reduced salivary flow (xerostomia). Saliva is the transporter of fluoride within the oral cavity, and a reduction in saliva decreases the availability and distribution of fluoride across the oral cavity. Consequently, there is an increased risk of demineralisation and reduced remineralisation from available fluoride. The harmful effect of smoking on oral health is further exacerbated as smoking alters the composition of the oral microbiome and increases the prevalence of pathogenic bacteria, resulting in a higher caries risk. These impacts due to smoking are independent of the other harms strongly associated with smoking and tobacco use (see Chapter).

15.9 Efficacy and Safety of Fluoride

The benefits of fluoride access to oral health are well-documented and continue to be a focus of research in dental literature. Multiple reviews have found consistent evidence for the efficacy of fluoride in preventing dental caries [8, 32, 42]. However, fluoride is not without controversy. Health concerns surround fluoride, along with proposed associations with adverse health outcomes due to misinformation and fears related to potential toxicity [43].

15.9.1 Effectiveness of Fluoride in Reducing Dental Caries

There is consolidated evidence from multiple systematic reviews that consistently demonstrates the efficacy of fluoride in caries prevention. Water fluoridation has been identified and is considered one of the most effective public health interventions for reducing the incidence of dental caries [44]. Contemporary evidence for the efficacy of water fluoridation indicates that the effect size of water fluoridation has decreased; however, it is still considered effective in reducing the prevalence of caries in children [8]. Similarly, fluoride toothpaste has been shown to substantially reduce caries incidence, with studies indicating a reduction of 15–30% in children and 20–40% in adults.

15.9.2 Known Adverse Events Associated with Fluoride

There is an increased risk of dental fluorosis with the growing availability of fluoride from sources like toothpaste and water. Exposure to fluorides during tooth development is linked to dental fluorosis, so only children under the age of eight are at risk of developing this condition due to fluoride exposure. Dental fluorosis is characterised by hypocalcification of tooth enamel and can appear as opaque or white enamel at mild levels or as brown and pitted stains at more severe levels. Recent studies have identified that mild levels of dental fluorosis in children may disappear over time, and that dental fluorosis does not negatively affect perceptions of oral health [45, 46]. Early studies of community water fluoridation investigated the optimal concentration of fluorides to balance the benefits of dental caries prevention with the risk of developing dental fluorosis.

There is evidence of adverse health outcomes from ongoing exposure to high concentrations of fluorides beyond recommended levels. For example, evidence suggests that skeletal fluorosis is associated with water fluoridation in India, China and other countries; however, fluoride concentration in the water often far exceeds the recommended maximum of 1.5 mg/L of fluoride [47, 48].

15.10 The Origins of Controversies and Misinformation Regarding Fluoride

Despite a substantial body of scientific evidence endorsing fluoride's benefits for dental health, its use remains contentious. Misinformation about fluoride's risks has been widely and sometimes systematically disseminated. A large part of the opposition to fluoride arises from concerns regarding potential health risks purported to be linked to fluoride's presence in drinking water. These concerns originate from misinterpretation and the spread of unsubstantiated claims.

One common argument posits that fluoride exposure may lead to severe health issues, such as cancer or neurological impairments. However, comprehensive studies and reviews, including those from the World Health Organization (WHO), the Centers for Disease Control and Prevention (CDC) and Australia's National Health and Medical Research Council (NHMRC), have consistently found no credible evidence linking fluoride to these adverse health outcomes when used at the levels recommended in public health guidelines. When administered in appropriate quantities, fluoride is safe and beneficial.

Misinformation often arises from extrapolating associations from studies where fluoride concentrations in community water sources are much higher than recommended guidelines. Research from regions with naturally elevated fluoride levels in drinking water has shown evidence of adverse health effects. It is crucial to note that these fluoride levels vastly exceed those used in controlled water fluoridation programmes. They do not reflect the levels found in standard dental products or those recommended by national or international organisations [44].

Callout 3: World Health Organisation recommendations for fluoride intake [49]

Water fluoridation: The recommended optimal fluoride concentration in drinking water generally ranges from 0.7 to 1.5 mg/L. The optimal target concentration is normally between 0.5 and 1.0 mg/L to optimize caries prevention while minimizing the risk of fluorosis and is dependent on local conditions.

Fluoride toothpaste: Fluoride toothpaste with concentrations of 1000–1500 ppm is commonly recommended for both children and adults, with specific guidelines for children under the age of six. Recommendations also emphasize the need for parental supervision to ensure that children do not ingest excessive amounts of toothpaste.

Professional fluoride treatments: For individuals at higher risk of developing dental caries, professional fluoride treatments, including fluoride varnishes, are often recommended.

Natural fluoride exposure: In regions with naturally high fluoride concentrations in drinking water, interventions to mitigate the risks of excess fluoride exposure include the provision of low-fluoride bottled water, and public health campaigns to raise awareness about proper fluoride use. Mothers are encouraged to breastfeed as breast milk is optimal for infant health and usually low in fluoride, even if the mother has high fluoride intake. Discourage the use of fluoride-rich coal for cooking purposes to avoid additional exposure.

15.11 Patient Education

Dental practitioners play a crucial role in educating patients about fluoride and advocating for its use in preventing dental caries. As trusted sources of evidence-based information, they are responsible for addressing patient concerns, dispelling myths and reinforcing the importance of fluoride in maintaining optimal oral health. Effective patient education fosters informed decision-making, empowering individuals to incorporate fluoride into their daily oral hygiene practices.

Research consistently demonstrates that patient education significantly improves adherence to preventive measures, including fluoride use. Studies show that individuals who receive clear, personalised fluoride guidance from dental professionals exhibit better oral hygiene habits, reduced caries incidence and increased acceptance of professional fluoride treatments [50, 51]. Educational interventions targeting parents and caregivers are instrumental in preventing early childhood caries by promoting appropriate fluoride use in young children.

15.12 Integrating Patient Education into Clinical Practice

Incorporating fluoride discussions into routine dental visits ensures that patients understand its benefits and receive tailored recommendations based on their risk level. Regular reinforcement of fluoride messaging enhances long-term adherence to preventive measures. Establishing a structured approach to fluoride education within clinical workflows promotes consistent patient engagement and emphasises the importance of fluoride as a key preventive strategy.

Ensuring all dental team members provide uniform fluoride-related guidance is essential for effective patient education. Conducting team training sessions on communication strategies guarantees that fluoride recommendations are conveyed consistently. A well-trained team enhances patient trust and engagement, improving adherence to fluoride use.

Documenting patient interactions regarding fluoride use, concerns and recommendations in their records is essential for continuity of care. Proper documentation enables practitioners to monitor patient adherence and address ongoing questions or misconceptions during subsequent visits. This practice ensures that fluoride education remains a crucial aspect of preventive care and allows personalised follow-ups tailored to each patient's needs.

Effective patient education depends on clear communication, cultural awareness and active listening to ensure fluoride recommendations are well understood and adopted (Table 15.1).

Table 15.1 Strategies to effectively integrate fluoride education into clinical practice

Principle	Description	Discussion points
Clarity and simplicity	Explaining fluoride's benefits and safety in a manner that is easily understandable for patients of all literacy levels. Avoiding technical jargon while maintaining scientific accuracy to foster patient comprehension.	How fluoride works The safety of fluoride Most suitable options available for individual needs
Cultural sensitivity	Recognising and respecting diverse cultural beliefs about fluoride use. Adapting communication styles to align with patients' cultural perspectives, addressing concerns with empathy and respect.	How can evidence-based fluoride uses be integrated with your belief and practices?
Active listening	Identifying patient misconceptions, fears and barriers to fluoride use. Engaging patients with open-ended questions to assess their understanding and address concerns effectively.	Acknowledge and respect differing views and beliefs Offer alternatives Explain the risks of choosing not to use fluorides

15.13 Addressing Misconceptions in Patients

Despite strong scientific evidence supporting fluoride's role in caries prevention, misconceptions and resistance persist among some patients. Addressing these concerns requires a patient-centred approach combining scientific rigour and empathetic communication. One common concern is fluoride safety and toxicity. Patients may be apprehensive about fluoride exposure due to misinformation circulated in media and online platforms. Dental practitioners should emphasise fluoride's extensive safety record when used appropriately and clarify that regulatory agencies support its use within recommended guidelines.

Dental fluorosis is often a misunderstood issue. Although excessive fluoride intake during enamel formation can result in mild fluorosis, its effects are mostly cosmetic and do not affect tooth function. Clinicians should reassure patients by explaining the balance between optimal fluoride exposure for caries prevention and minimising the risk of fluorosis, especially for children.

Dispelling misinformation requires providing patients with credible, peer-reviewed sources that counter pseudoscientific claims. Many fluoride-related myths arise from misinterpretations of research or isolated studies lacking scientific consensus. Healthcare professionals should guide patients to evidence-based resources and remain open to addressing their questions.

Fostering trust and confidence in fluoride recommendations involves engaging patients in open discussions rather than outright dismissing their concerns. Visual aids, pamphlets and trusted online resources can reinforce key messages. Encouraging a dialogue where patients feel heard and understood enhances compliance and promotes informed decision-making regarding fluoride use.

15.14 Fluoride Policies and Public Health

The implementation and acceptance of population-level fluoride delivery methods vary widely across global regions and populations. Providing fluoride to the population depends on the infrastructure, local conditions, political will, regulations and the socioeconomic status of the country and its residents.

15.14.1 Water Fluoridation

Water fluoridation has been adopted as a cornerstone of dental public health in countries like the United States, Australia and Ireland. In the United States, approximately 73% of the population with access to public water systems receives fluoridated water [52]. Australia has achieved similar coverage, with nearly 90% of the population benefiting from water fluoridation, depending on the state or territory [53]. Ireland, a long-time proponent of fluoridation, has mandated it since 1960s and continues to maintain high levels of coverage [54].

In contrast, countries in Europe, as well as low- and middle-income nations, do not fluoridate their water supplies. The reasons for this include a lack of infrastructure for centralised water systems, especially in rural or remote areas with dispersed populations, public resistance based on perceptions of safety or individual autonomy and conflicting health priorities. Western European nations, such as Germany and the Netherlands, have either halted or never initiated a water fluoridation programme due to philosophical and political concerns.

In some regions, including China, India and Sub-Saharan Africa, naturally occurring concentrations of fluoride in groundwater exceed recommended limits. The high concentration of fluoride in water sources poses a health risk rather than a benefit. In other regions, the natural fluoridation levels are too low to provide protection, and artificial fluoridation is logistically or politically unfeasible.

15.14.2 Salt and Milk Fluoridation

Where water fluoridation is not feasible, salt fluoridation has emerged as a viable alternative. Salt fluoridation involves adding fluoride to table salt at concentrations that mirror the protective effect of fluoridated water [55, 56]. This strategy has been implemented successfully in countries such as Switzerland and across Latin America, including Mexico, Colombia and Costa Rica.

Salt fluoridation is particularly effective in regions with decentralised water systems or where bottled water is widely consumed [57, 58]. It can be easier to regulate and distribute through existing food supply chains, allowing for targeted population-level interventions [57, 58]. However, challenges include ensuring consistent salt consumption across demographics, public education on fluoride sources and managing potential interactions with salt-reduction campaigns aimed at addressing cardiovascular disease [56, 58].

Milk fluoridation programmes have been trialled or implemented in countries like the United Kingdom, Thailand and Chile. These programmes are often school-based and aim to reach children who may not have access to fluoridated water or toothpaste. While milk fluoridation can effectively reduce dental caries in younger populations, it poses other logistical challenges. Distribution must be consistent, and the fluoride must be bioavailable in the milk matrix. The reach of such programmes is limited by school attendance, lactose intolerance and dietary practices, raising questions about equity and sustainability.

15.14.3 Fluoride in Toothpaste

Toothpaste is the most common and accessible fluoride delivery method globally. However, actual concentrations and availability vary widely across countries due to regulatory frameworks, local production practices and cost. Some countries permit low-fluoride or even fluoride-free toothpaste to be sold, often due to affordability concerns. Mislabelled or counterfeit products also pose risks in some markets. Additionally, low-fluoride toothpaste marketed for children can contribute to suboptimal protection if used exclusively and beyond the recommended age ranges.

Access to fluoride toothpaste is significantly influenced by socioeconomic status, with lower-income families often unable to afford the regular use of high-quality products. In some regions, toothpaste is viewed as a luxury rather than a necessity, highlighting the need for public health policies that subsidise or provide fluoride products to vulnerable populations.

15.15 Socioeconomic Disparities in Access to Fluoride

Fluoride access and use are strongly influenced by socioeconomic factors. Individuals and communities with lower income levels are less likely to have access to fluoridated water, fluoride toothpaste or professional dental care. In such settings, the burden of dental disease is disproportionately high, exacerbating existing health inequities.

Even in countries with established fluoridation programmes, coverage gaps persist in rural, remote or Indigenous communities due to infrastructure limitations or historical underinvestment [59, 60]. Targeted efforts are necessary to ensure that fluoride reaches those most at risk of dental disease, as these groups are likely to experience higher levels of dental disease as well.

15.16 Cultural and Political Resistance

Fluoridation has long faced opposition from groups concerned about personal liberty, government overreach and potential health risks [59–62]. While the scientific consensus supports the safety and efficacy of fluoride at recommended levels, misinformation continues to shape public perception and influence policy decisions. Public policies are not always based on scientific evidence; thus, coordinated efforts are needed to maintain or initiate population-level fluoridation programmes. In some regions, fluoridation debates are framed as environmental or ethical issues rather than health interventions. Building public trust, engaging communities and transparently addressing concerns are essential for gaining acceptance of fluoridation programmes.

15.17 Geographic and Environmental Challenges

Geography plays a key role in determining the feasibility of fluoride strategies. In areas with naturally high fluoride levels, fluorosis presents a serious health challenge. Conversely, in areas with naturally low fluoride levels and dispersed populations, implementing fluoridation through centralised systems is technically difficult and costly. Innovative solutions such as household de-fluoridation units, fluoride varnish programmes or school-based oral health initiatives can be employed in these contexts. However, sustainability remains a concern.

15.18 Cost-Effectiveness of Fluoride Programmes

Water fluoridation is widely recognised as one of the most cost-effective public health measures for preventing dental caries. Estimates from the United States and Australia show that every dollar invested in water fluoridation yields between $20 and $40 in dental treatment savings in these countries. The benefits are particularly pronounced in children and low-income populations, where fluoridation reduces the need for costly restorative procedures.

Salt and milk fluoridation provides good cost–benefit ratios, although they may be less efficient due to extra programme logistics. Fluoride toothpaste, while inexpensive individually, can become less accessible in lower-income settings without policy support or subsidies.

Strong policy frameworks, government commitment and public trust in health authorities have contributed to the successful implementation of a public fluoridation programme. Fluoridation is a preventive health intervention regarded as a cost-effective and equitable strategy for reducing dental caries. The evidence strongly supports increased access to fluorides, particularly for populations with limited access to dental care.

References

1. Arnold FA Jr. Grand rapids fluoridation study—results pertaining to the eleventh year of fluoridation. Am J Public Health Nations Health. 1957;47(5):539–45.
2. Arnold FA Jr, Dean HT, Knutson JW. Effect of fluoridated public water supplies on dental caries prevalence: seventh year of Grand Rapids-Muskegon study. Public Health Rep. 1953;68(2):141.

3. Horowitz HS. The effectiveness of community water fluoridation in the United States. J Public Health Dent. 1996;56(5):253–8.
4. Aoun A, Darwiche F, Al Hayek S, Doumit J. The fluoride debate: the pros and cons of fluoridation. Prev Nutr Food Sci. 2018;23(3):171.
5. Johnson J. "A man's mouth is his castle": the midcentury fluoridation controversy and the visceral public. Q J Speech. 2016;102(1):1–20.
6. Marinho V. Cochrane reviews of randomized trials of fluoride therapies for preventing dental caries. Eur Arch Paediatr Dent. 2009;10:183–91.
7. Wong M, Clarkson J, Glenny A-M, Lo E, Marinho V, Tsang B, et al. Cochrane reviews on the benefits/risks of fluoride toothpastes. J Dent Res. 2011;90(5):573–9.
8. Iheozor-Ejiofor Z, Walsh T, Lewis SR, Riley P, Boyers D, Clarkson JE, et al. Water fluoridation for the prevention of dental caries. Cochrane Database Syst Rev. 2024;10:CD010856.
9. Wen P, Chen M, Zhong Y, Dong Q, Wong H. Global burden and inequality of dental caries, 1990 to 2019. J Dent Res. 2022;101(4):392–9.
10. Pitts NB, Zero DT, Marsh PD, Ekstrand K, Weintraub JA, Ramos-Gomez F, et al. Dental caries. Nat Rev Dis Primers. 2017;3(1):1–16.
11. Featherstone J. The continuum of dental caries—evidence for a dynamic disease process. J Dent Res. 2004;83(1_suppl):39–42.
12. Bowen WH. The Stephan curve revisited. Odontology. 2013;101:2–8.
13. Shellis RP, Barbour ME, Jesani A, Lussi A. Effects of buffering properties and undissociated acid concentration on dissolution of dental enamel in relation to pH and acid type. Caries Res. 2013;47(6):601–11.
14. West NX, Joiner A. Enamel mineral loss. J Dent. 2014;42:S2–S11.
15. Amaechi BT, AbdulAzees PA, Okoye LO, Meyer F, Enax J. Comparison of hydroxyapatite and fluoride oral care gels for remineralization of initial caries: a pH-cycling study. BDJ Open. 2020;6(1):9.
16. Queiroz CS, Hara AT, Paes Leme AF, Cury JA. pH-cycling models to evaluate the effect of low fluoride dentifrice on enamel de-and remineralization. Braz Dent J. 2008;19:21–7.
17. Kensche A, Buschbeck E, König B, Koch M, Kirsch J, Hannig C, et al. Effect of fluoride mouthrinses and stannous ions on the erosion protective properties of the in situ pellicle. Sci Rep. 2019;9(1):5336.
18. García-Godoy F, Hicks MJ. Maintaining the integrity of the enamel surface: the role of dental biofilm, saliva and preventive agents in enamel demineralization and remineralization. J Am Dent Assoc. 2008;139:25S–34S.
19. Grigalauskienė R, Slabšinskienė E, Vasiliauskienė I. Biological approach of dental caries management. Stomatologija. 2015;17(4):107–12.
20. Buzalaf MAR, Pessan JP, Honório HM, Ten Cate JM. Mechanisms of action of fluoride for caries control. Monogr Oral Sci. 2011;22:97–114.
21. Pandit S, Kim J-E, Jung K-H, Chang K-W, Jeon J-G. Effect of sodium fluoride on the virulence factors and composition of Streptococcus mutans biofilms. Arch Oral Biol. 2011;56(7):643–9.
22. Zwemer JD. Lactic acid formation by lactobacilli exposed to fluoridized enamel. J Dent Res. 1957;36(2):182–91.
23. Loskill P, Zeitz C, Grandthyll S, Thewes N, Müller F, Bischoff M, et al. Reduced adhesion of oral bacteria on hydroxyapatite by fluoride treatment. Langmuir. 2013;29(18):5528–33.
24. ten Cate J. Contemporary perspective on the use of fluoride products in caries prevention. Br Dent J. 2013;214(4):161–7.
25. Hellwig E, Lennon A. Systemic versus topical fluoride. Caries Res. 2004;38(3):258–62.
26. Cho HJ, Jin BH, Park DY, Jung SH, Lee HS, Paik DI, et al. Systemic effect of water fluoridation on dental caries prevalence. Community Dent Oral Epidemiol. 2014;42(4):341–8.
27. Henschler D, Büttner W, Patz J. Absorption, distribution in body fluids, and bioavailability of fluoride. Calcium metabolism, bone and metabolic. bone diseases: Springer; 1975. p. 111–21.
28. Hargreaves J. The level and timing of systemic exposure to fluoride with respect to caries resistance. J Dent Res. 1992;71(5):1244–8.

29. Robinson C, Connell S, Kirkham J, Brookes SJ, Shore RC, Smith AM. The effect of fluoride on the developing tooth. Caries Res. 2004;38(3):268–76.
30. Akuno M, Nocella G, Milia E, Gutierrez L. Factors influencing the relationship between fluoride in drinking water and dental fluorosis: a ten-year systematic review and meta-analysis. J Water Health. 2019;17(6):845–62.
31. Ismail AI, Hasson H. Fluoride supplements, dental caries and fluorosis: a systematic review. J Am Dent Assoc. 2008;139(11):1457–68.
32. Walsh T, Worthington HV, Glenny AM, Marinho VCC, Jeroncic A. Fluoride toothpastes of different concentrations for preventing dental caries. Cochrane Database Syst Rev. 2019;3:CD007868.
33. Marinho VCC, Chong LY, Worthington HV, Walsh T. Fluoride mouthrinses for preventing dental caries in children and adolescents. Cochrane Database Syst Rev. 2016;7:CD002284.
34. Marinho VCC, Worthington HV, Walsh T, Chong LY. Fluoride gels for preventing dental caries in children and adolescents. Cochrane Database Syst Rev. 2015;6:CD002280.
35. Marinho VCC, Worthington HV, Walsh T, Clarkson JE. Fluoride varnishes for preventing dental caries in children and adolescents. Cochrane Database Syst Rev. 2013;7:CD002279.
36. Pitts NB, Ekstrand KR, ICDAS Foundation. International Caries Detection and Assessment System (ICDAS) and its International Caries Classification and Management System (ICCMS)–methods for staging of the caries process and enabling dentists to manage caries. Community Dent Oral Epidemiol. 2013;41(1):e41–52.
37. Pitts NB, Ismail AI, Martignon S, Ekstrand K, Douglas GV, Longbottom C, et al. ICCMS™ guide for practitioners and educators. 2014. Available from: https://www.iccms-web.com/uploads/asset/59284654c0a6f822230100.pdf.
38. Paepegaey A, Day T, Boulding A, Harris R, Barker M, Bellamy P. In vitro comparison of stannous fluoride, sodium fluoride, and sodium monofluorophosphate dentifrices in the prevention of enamel erosion. J Clin Dent. 2013;24(3):73–8.
39. Danelon M, Takeshita EM, Peixoto LC, Sassaki KT, Delbem ACB. Effect of fluoride gels supplemented with sodium trimetaphosphate in reducing demineralization. Clin Oral Investig. 2014;18:1119–27.
40. Oliveira BH, Rajendra A, Veitz-Keenan A, Niederman R. The effect of silver diamine fluoride in preventing caries in the primary dentition: a systematic review and meta-analysis. Caries Res. 2019;53(1):24–32.
41. Hendre AD, Taylor GW, Chávez EM, Hyde S. A systematic review of silver diamine fluoride: effectiveness and application in older adults. Gerodontology. 2017;34(4):411–9.
42. Marinho VC, Higgins JP, Sheiham A, Logan S. Combinations of topical fluoride (toothpastes, mouthrinses, gels, varnishes) versus single topical fluoride for preventing dental caries in ch2 Water fluoridation statiildren and adolescents. Cochrane Database Syst Rev. 2004;1:CD002781.
43. Armfield JM. When public action undermines public health: a critical examination of antifluoridationist literature. Aust New Zealand Health Policy. 2007;4:25.
44. National Health and Medical Research Council (NHMRC). Information paper—water fluoridation: dental and other human health outcomes. Canberra; 2017.
45. Chankanka O, Levy SM, Warren JJ, Chalmers JM. A literature review of aesthetic perceptions of dental fluorosis and relationships with psychosocial aspects/oral health-related quality of life. Community Dent Oral Epidemiol. 2010;38(2):97–109.
46. Do LG, Ha DH, Spencer AJ. Natural history and long-term impact of dental fluorosis: a prospective cohort study. Med J Aust. 2016;204(1):25.
47. Del Bello L. Fluorosis: an ongoing challenge for India. Lancet Planet Health. 2020;4(3):e94–e5.
48. Srivastava S, Flora SJS. Fluoride in drinking water and skeletal fluorosis: a review of the global impact. Curr Environ Health Rep. 2020;7(2):140–6.
49. World Health Organization. Everybody's business: strengthening health systems to improve health outcomes: WHO's framework for action; 2007.
50. Ko A, Chi DL. Fluoride hesitancy: a mixed methods study on decision-making about forms of fluoride. Community Dent Oral Epidemiol. 2023;51(5):997–1008.

51. Koh M, Kerr D, Hill CM, Chi DL. A mixed-methods study on topical fluoride beliefs and refusal behaviors for caregivers of children with special health care needs. Matern Child Health J. 2024;28(1):104–15.
52. Centres for Disease Control. 2022 Water fluoridation statistics; 2022. Available from: https://www.cdc.gov/fluoridation/php/statistics/2022-water-fluoridation-statistics.html.
53. Senevirathna L, Ratnayake HE, Jayasinghe N, Gao J, Zhou X, Nanayakkara S. Water fluoridation in Australia: a systematic review. Environ Res. 2023;237:116915.
54. James P, Harding M, Beecher T, Parnell C, Browne D, Tuohy M, et al. Fluoride and caring for children's teeth (FACCT): clinical fieldwork protocol. HRB Open Res. 2018;1:4.
55. Yeung CA. Efficacy of salt fluoridation. Evid Based Dent. 2011;12(1):17–8.
56. Marthaler TM. Increasing the public health effectiveness of fluoridated salt. Schweiz Monatsschr Zahnmed. 2005;115(9):785–92.
57. Gillespie GM, Baez R. Development of salt fluoridation in the Americas. Schweiz Monatsschr Zahnmed. 2005;115(8):663–9.
58. Bergmann KE, Bergmann RL. Salt fluoridation and general health. Adv Dent Res. 1995;9(2):138–43.
59. Knox MC, Garner A, Dyason A, Pearson T, Pit SW. Qualitative investigation of the reasons behind opposition to water fluoridation in regional NSW, Australia. Public Health Res Pract. 2017;27:2711705.
60. Griffin M, Shickle D, Moran N. European citizens' opinions on water fluoridation. Community Dent Oral Epidemiol. 2008;36(2):95–102.
61. Armfield JM, Akers HF. Risk perception and water fluoridation support and opposition in Australia. J Public Health Dent. 2010;70(1):58–66.
62. Armfield JM, Akers HF. Community water fluoridation support and opposition in Australia. Community Dent Health. 2011;28(1):40–6.

Obesity and Oral Health

16

S. Rajasekharan and Luc Martens

16.1 Introduction

Obesity has emerged as a significant health epidemic of the twenty-first century, with its prevalence rising at an alarming rate. The World Health Organization (WHO) reports that approximately one-third of the global population is affected by obesity, with a notable increase among adolescents (13–17 years) and young adults (18–30 years) [1]. This condition arises from a complex interplay of genetic predisposition, environmental influences and lifestyle choices. Factors such as the widespread consumption of calorie-dense foods, sedentary behaviour and heightened stress levels have significantly contributed to the growing obesity crisis.

Obesity is commonly classified using the body mass index (BMI), which assesses weight relative to height. BMI was introduced by a Belgian astronomer, mathematician and statistician named Adolphe Quetelet in 1835, and it was previously referred to as the Quetelet's index. A BMI of 30 or higher is generally categorised as obese. Additionally, waist circumference and body fat percentage are often used to evaluate obesity further. These classifications go beyond mere statistics; they serve as indicators of health risks, with higher BMI levels linked to increased morbidity and mortality rates.

Over the past 50 years, obesity has risen globally, emerging as a significant social concern with negative impacts on both general health and oral health [2]. Recent research has uncovered a compelling link between obesity and oral health, demonstrating how excess weight can exacerbate or predispose individuals to various oral health issues.

S. Rajasekharan (✉) · L. Martens
Paediatric Dentistry, ELOHA (Equal Lifelong Oral Health for All) Research Group, Oral Health Sciences, Ghent, Belgium
e-mail: Sivaprakash.Rajasekharan@ugent.be; luc.martens@ugent.be

S. R. Prabhu et al. (eds.), *Lifestyle in Oral Health and Disease*,
https://doi.org/10.1007/978-3-032-05888-1_16

16.2 The Interplay Between Lifestyle Factors, Obesity and Oral Health

Obesity is linked to specific lifestyle factors, including poor dietary habits, smoking, alcohol consumption, insufficient physical activity and psychological stress, all of which can indirectly affect oral health. These influences may lead to reduced dental visits or stress-related conditions like bruxism. Unhealthy eating patterns, particularly the frequent intake of sugary beverages and snacks, are key contributors to both obesity and deteriorating oral health [3]. Such diets not only promote weight gain but also heighten the risk of dental caries, gingival issues and periodontal disease. Additionally, processed foods, typically rich in refined sugars and unhealthy fats, further exacerbate obesity and compromise oral health [4].

Smoking is frequently associated with obesity and can worsen periodontal disease. Furthermore, the combined influence of smoking and poor dietary habits can have a synergistic effect, resulting in more severe oral health issues [5]. In addition, a lack of physical activity contributes to obesity and neglect of proper oral hygiene. People with obesity are often less inclined to follow consistent dental care routines, which further deteriorate their oral health. Physical inactivity also impairs the body's ability to manage systemic inflammation, which can indirectly affect oral health. Psychological stress, commonly linked to obesity, worsens oral health by intensifying conditions like bruxism and periodontitis. Stress-related hormonal changes can alter immune responses, making individuals more susceptible to oral infections and inflammation [6].

16.3 The Interplay Between Systemic Health Conditions

Obesity is associated with certain systemic health conditions, such as diabetes, sleep apnoea, cardiovascular health and inflammation, which can have a direct and/or indirect influence on oral health. These diseases often share common risk factors, such as inflammation, dietary patterns and lifestyle behaviours, which can exacerbate their impact on obesity and oral health.

Diabetes, strongly associated with obesity, is a significant risk factor for oral health problems. Elevated blood sugar levels impair wound healing and increase susceptibility to infections, leading to complications such as periodontal disease and edentulism [7]. The bidirectional relationship between diabetes and periodontal disease indicates that managing one condition can have a positive impact on the other.

Obstructive sleep apnoea, commonly associated with obesity, can impact oral health by causing dry mouth. Dry oral conditions can lead to dental caries, erosive tooth wear and gingival inflammation. Additionally, obstructive sleep apnoea can disrupt normal sleep patterns, contributing to stress-related oral conditions such as oral ulceration, bruxism and temporomandibular joint disorders [8].

Obesity contributes to cardiovascular diseases, which are also linked to oral health conditions such as periodontitis. Inflammation is a common pathway connecting these disparate systemic disorders [9]. Systemic inflammation associated with obesity disrupts the immune response in the oral cavity, making it harder to combat infections and heal tissues. This exacerbates the risk of periodontal disease and other oral health disorders. The interplay between obesity and oral health reflects broader systemic interactions, emphasising the need for integrated healthcare approaches.

16.4 The Interplay Between Obesity and Oral Health

Oral health problems, including periodontitis and dental caries, remain widespread yet often neglected as part of broader health concerns. In addition to poor periodontal health and associated caries risk, individuals with obesity had poor compliance towards oral hygiene. Obese individuals frequently consumed a diet high in fat and low in vegetables, exhibited elevated intake of added sugars, increased oral microbial counts, reduced salivary flow rates, lower salivary pH levels, and higher concentrations of immune globulins [10].

16.4.1 Obesity and Periodontitis

Periodontitis is a chronic inflammatory condition affecting the supporting structures of the teeth. It arises from the interaction between pathogenic bacteria and the host's immune response, potentially leading to the partial or complete loss of teeth [11]. In the United States, data from the National Health and Nutrition Examination Survey (2009–2014) reveal that periodontitis is especially prevalent among adults aged 30 and older. Over 47% of all adults had periodontitis, distributed as 8.7, 30.0 and 8.5% with mild, moderate and severe periodontitis respectively [12]. The increasing social and health burden of periodontitis highlights the urgent need for global public health interventions [13].

Obesity, which is associated with chronic low-grade inflammation, can worsen other inflammatory conditions, including periodontitis [9]. Obesity induces a hyper-inflammatory state, with T-lymphocyte and monocyte/macrophage changes that could affect response to the microbial challenge [14]. Numerous studies conducted globally have consistently shown a positive correlation between obesity and the prevalence of periodontitis (Table 16.1).

Excessive consumption of added sugars, high-sugar diets, elevated levels of periodontal pathogens and inflammatory cytokines are significant factors linking obesity and periodontitis. Added sugars, rich in glucose, contribute to postprandial hyperglycaemia and prolonged inflammatory responses lasting up to 16 h [15]. These repeated spikes in blood sugar levels induce oxidative stress, perpetuating a hyper-inflammatory state that is linked to both obesity and periodontal disease [10].

Table 16.1 Summary of systematic reviews and meta-analyses evaluating the relationship between obesity and periodontitis

Sl. no.	Author	Year	Study design	Number of included studies	Conclusion
1	Kandaswamy et al. [16]	2024	SR with MA	17	Obesity definition (body mass index cut-off value >25 or >30) was significant for serum resistin ($p<0.05$) and gingival crevicular fluid resistin ($p<0.05$) between obese patients with periodontitis and normal weight patients with periodontitis.
2	Foratori-Junior et al. [17]	2022	SR with MA	11	A positive association between overweight/obesity and periodontitis in pregnant women was found, with overall random-effects relative risk and 95% CI of 2.21 (1.53–3.17).
3	Cruz-Ávila et al. [18]	2022	SR	10	Interleukin-6 and CRP levels increased in obese individuals with periodontitis.
4	Abu-Shawish et al. [19]	2022	SR	15	Fourteen studies reported a positive association between increased body mass index and clinical attachment loss, probing pocket depth or both. Eight studies report higher odds of obese adults having periodontitis and a dose–response relationship between obesity and periodontitis was seen in three studies
5	Khan et al. [10]	2018	SR	25	Seventeen studies showed an association between obesity and periodontitis (OR: 1.1–4.5). The obesity indicators of body mass index, waist circumference, waist-hip ratio and body fat percentage were significantly associated with measures of periodontitis of bleeding on probing, plaque index, probing depths, clinical attachment loss, calculus, oral hygiene index and community periodontal index
6	Keller et al. [11]	2015	SR	13	Overweight, obesity, weight gain and increased waist circumference may be risk factors for the development of periodontitis or worsening of periodontal measures such as periodontal disease, alveolar bone loss, attachment loss and plaque index
7	Li et al. [20]	2015	SR with MA	16	Obesity (measured by body mass index) was significantly associated with visible plaque index (OR: 4.75; 95% CI: 2.42, 9.34), bleeding on probing (OR: 5.41; 95% CI: 2.75, 10.63), subgingival calculus (OR: 3.07; 95% CI: 1.10, 8.62), probing depth (OR: 14.15; 95% CI: 5.10, 39.25) and flow rate of salivary secretion (SMD: –0.89; 95% CI: –1.18, –0.61)

(continued)

Table 16.1 (continued)

Sl. no.	Author	Year	Study design	Number of included studies	Conclusion
8	Nascimento et al. [21]	2015	SR with MA	5	Overweight and obese patients presented higher risk to develop new cases of periodontitis (RR: 1.13; 95% CI: 1.06–1.20 and RR: 1.33 95% CI: 1.21–1.47 respectively) compared with normal weight patients
9	Papageorgiou et al. [22]	2015	SR with MA	15	Systemically healthy overweight/obese patients were associated with higher decrease in tumour necrosis factor- alpha levels (1 study) and higher decrease in HbA1c levels (1 study) compared to systemically healthy normal-weight patients
10	Suvan et al. [23]	2011	SR	33	Statistically significant associations between periodontitis and body mass index category obese OR 1.81(1.42, 2.30), overweight OR 1.27(1.06, 1.51) and obese and overweight combined OR 2.13(1.40, 3.26)

SR Systematic review, *MA* meta-analysis, *OR* odds ratio, *RR* risk ratio, *SMD* standardised mean difference, *CI* confidence interval, *HbA1c* haemoglobin A1c, *CRP* C-reactive protein

16.4.2 Obesity and Gingival Inflammation

'Periodontal disease' and 'periodontitis' are often used interchangeably in the literature. However, they are not identical, as 'periodontal disease' encompasses both periodontitis and gingivitis [24]. Periodontal disease, characterised by gum inflammation and tissue destruction, is significantly more prevalent in individuals with obesity. A proposed bidirectional link between obesity and oral disease highlights the central role of altered inflammation, a key factor in both obesity and periodontal disease [25]. Specifically, while individuals who are obese or overweight are more susceptible to periodontal disease, the presence of periodontal disease may also worsen dyslipidaemia [26].

Chronic inflammation driven by excess adipose tissue weakens the body's ability to combat bacterial infections in the gums, leading to disease progression [27]. Most studies demonstrate that obese individuals are at a significantly greater risk of developing periodontal disease compared to those with a healthy weight (Table 16.2). This elevated risk is attributed to the increased production of inflammatory mediators, such as interleukin-6 (IL-6) and tumour necrosis factor-alpha (TNF-α), which accelerate the destruction of periodontal tissue [23].

In addition to higher rates of periodontal disease, obese individuals often demonstrate poor oral hygiene practices that further exacerbate periodontal health challenges [28]. Key factors such as ethnicity, gender, age, socio-economic status, parental education level, medications, oral hygiene practices, dietary habits,

Table 16.2 Summary of systematic reviews and meta-analyses evaluating the relationship between obesity and periodontal disease

Sl. no.	Author	Year	Study design	Number of included studies	Conclusion
1	Arbildo-Vega et al. [31]	2024	Umbrella review	14	All studies reported that periodontal disease was associated with obesity, with an OR and RR ranging from 1.1 to 1.46 and 1.64 to 2.21, respectively.
2	Mirzaei et al. [32]	2022	SR with MA	34	Periodontal disease increased the odds of dyslipidaemia by 15% (OR: 1.15, 95% CI: 1.04, 1.26). No statistically significant association of periodontal disease with low HDL, high LDL, hypertriglyceridemia and hypercholesteremia.
3	Kim et al. [13]	2022	SR with MA	37	Obesity conferred increased odds of periodontal disease with an OR (1.35, 95% CI: 1.05–1.75). The OR was the highest in the 18–34 years group (2.21, 95% CI: 1.26–3.89. and in European countries (2.46, 95% CI: 1.11–5.46).
4	Da Silva et al. [33]	2021	SR with MA	90	Significantly higher levels of gingival inflammation are observed in those with obesity when compared to those who were not obese (SMD: 0.26; 95% CI: 0.07–0.44).
5	Martens et al. [14]	2017	SR with MA	12	Significantly positive association between periodontal disease and obesity in children.
6	Martinez-Herrera et al. [9]	2017	SR	28	Twenty-six studies described an association between obesity and periodontal disease, while two studies reported no such association.
7	Chaffee & Weston [34]	2010	SR with MA	70	A greater mean clinical attachment loss among obese individuals, a higher mean body mass index among periodontal patients and a trend of increasing odds of prevalent periodontal disease with increasing body mass index were found.

SR systematic review, *MA* meta-analysis, *OR* odds ratio, *RR* risk ratio, *SMD* standardised mean difference, *CI* confidence interval smoking and blood pressure are essential variables to be considered when examining the relationship between obesity and periodontal disease [29, 30].

16.4.3 Obesity and Non-surgical Periodontal Therapy

Non-surgical periodontal therapy (NSPT) is widely regarded as the gold standard for treating chronic periodontitis. It aims to address or eliminate the microbial causes and contributing factors of gum and periodontal diseases. Key components of NSPT typically include plaque management, caries prevention and scaling and root planning [35]. Studies have shown improved clinical outcomes in non-obese patients following NSPT compared to their obese counterparts (Table 16.3).

However, the combination of non-surgical periodontal therapy with azithromycin, chlorhexidine and cetylpyridinium chloride resulted in lowered blood pressure and reduced serum levels of HbA1c, hsCRP, IL-1β and TNF-α. Additionally, salivary resistin levels decreased in patients with obesity and periodontitis following therapy and the use of chlorhexidine mouth rinse. Pre- and post-treatment data indicate improvements in metabolic biomarkers (total cholesterol, LDL, triglycerides, insulin resistance, C3 and GCF levels of TNF-α, chemerin, vaspin, omentin-1 and visfatin, 8-OHd) along with reductions in periodontal pathogen counts [36].

Table 16.3 Summary of systematic reviews and meta-analyses evaluating the impact of non-surgical periodontal therapy in obese patients

Sl. no.	Author	Year	Study design	Number of included studies	Conclusion
1	Menezes et al. [36]	2024	SR	18	Non-surgical periodontal therapy can reduce inflammation and improve metabolic markers.
2	Zhang et al. [26]	2023	SR with MA	17	Non-surgical periodontal therapy reduces pro-inflammatory cytokines in obese patients.
3	Akram et al. [37]	2016	SR with MA	5	In three studies, non-surgical periodontal therapy resulted in a significantly better clinical periodontal outcome among non-obese subjects than obese subjects.
4	Gerber et al. [38]	2016	SR	8	Three of eight studies failed to show an influence of obesity on pocket depth reduction after non-surgical therapy. The remaining five studies documented a negative effect on the outcome of non-surgical periodontal therapy.
5	Nascimento et al. [39]	2016	SR with MA	5	No differences on periodontal healing between obese and non-obese subjects were observed after periodontal treatment.

SR systematic review, *MA* meta-analysis

16.4.4 Obesity and Dental Caries

Similar to obesity, dental caries is a complex, global, multifactorial condition. Dental caries result from cariogenic bacteria in dental plaque producing organic acids that metabolise fermentable carbohydrates and demineralise tooth enamel. In addition to direct factors like pathogenic bacteria, fermentable carbohydrates, saliva and time, other elements such as oral hygiene habits and socioeconomic conditions also influence the development of caries [2].

Diets high in sugar and acidic foods, commonly associated with obesity, significantly contribute to dental caries [40]. These dietary patterns promote the proliferation of pathogenic bacteria, increasing the risk of cavities. Additionally, the connection between obesity and dental caries may be influenced by factors such as low socioeconomic status, limited access to healthcare services and poor health literacy [41]. Furthermore, conditions like xerostomia and reduced salivary flow, which are often linked to obesity, exacerbate susceptibility to caries by compromising the protective function of saliva [42]. Several studies have evaluated the association between overweight/obesity and dental caries, considering the various common risk factors present in both obesity and caries [43] (Table 16.4).

Although most studies show a significant association between obesity and dental caries, contradictory results have also been published. The results from various studies appear to be influenced by the non-uniformity of assessments, poor reporting, variations in the definitions of obesity and overweight and the assessment of dental caries, as well as unstandardised protocols, settings, procedures of measurements and the age and ethnicity of participants [52]. This is true not only for studies evaluating dental caries risk in obese patients but also for all studies reporting an association between obesity and various aspects of oral health. Hence, these results should be interpreted with utmost caution.

Table 16.4 Summary of systematic reviews and meta-analyses examining the relationship between obesity and dental caries

Sl. no.	Reference	Year	Study design	Number of included studies	Conclusion
1	Bakhoda MR et al. [41]	2024	SR with MA	22	Children at the highest body mass index category were 44% more likely to have early childhood caries than those at the bottom (OR: 1.44; 95% CI: 1.16–1.78)—a significant direct association between BMI and the risk of dental caries in children.
2	Garrocho-Rangel A et al. [44]	2024	Umbrella review	9	The relationship between obesity and dental caries in children is inconclusive and likely to be complex.
3	Pizzi JF et al. [45]	2024	SR with MA	41	No association between overweight and/or obesity and dental caries in Brazilian children/ adolescents for most anthropometric reference curves using body mass index.
4	Silveira MG et al. [46]	2022	SR	7	Association between obesity and dental caries remains undefined; better-designed studies with standardised methods needed.
5	Alshehri YFA et al. [47]	2020	SR	14	For children, two studies resulted in a positive association between high body mass index and caries, six studies resulted in a negative association and two studies had a non-significant association. For adults, two studies resulted in a positive association between high body mass index and dental caries, and two studies had a non-significant association.
6	Manohar N et al. [43]	2020	SR with MA	9	Children with overweight and obesity had a significantly higher dental caries experience compared with children with normal weight.
7	Angelopoulou MV et al. [48]	2019	SR with MA	12	Overweight/obese children are at greater risk of early childhood caries; evidence inconsistency noted.
8	Paisi M et al. [49]	2019	SR	84	Twenty-six studies showed a positive relationship between body mass index and caries, 19 showed a negative association and 43 found no association.
9	Carson SJ [50]	2018	SR with MA	14	Five studies showed no association between body mass index and dental caries, five studies found a positive association and three an inverse association. Meta-analysis showed no differences in dental caries between underweight and normal weight children.

(continued)

Table 16.4 (continued)

Sl. no.	Reference	Year	Study design	Number of included studies	Conclusion
10	Chen D et al. [51]	2018	SR with MA	14	Obese group had more caries than the normal-weight group in their primary teeth. More caries was found among the overweight and obese children in both primary and permanent teeth in high-income countries, but not in low- and middle-income countries.
11	Li LW et al. [52]	2015	SR	17	Two studies found an inverse association between anthropometric measurements and dental caries while 15 studies showed inconsistent association.
12	Hayden C et al. [53]	2013	SR with MA	14	A significant relationship between childhood obesity and dental caries (effect size = 0.104, $p = 0.049$) was found.
13	Silva AE et al. [54]	2013	SR	28	The positive association between obesity and dental caries in permanent teeth was identified in six studies, a negative association was found in one, and eight showed no association. For studies evaluating mixed dentition, four of them found a positive association, one found positive correlation and seven showed no association. There was no correlation between obesity and caries in one study in which permanent dentition was analysed.
14	Hooley M et al. [55]	2012	SR	49	Twenty-three studies found no association between BMI and dental caries, 17 found a positive relationship between BMI and dental caries and nine found an inverse relationship.
15	Kantovitz KR et al. [56]	2006	SR	3	Only one study showed direct association between obesity and dental caries.

SR systematic review, *MA* meta-analysis, *OR* odds ratio, *CI* confidence interval, *BMI* body mass index)

16.5 Obesity and Salivary Profile

Saliva plays a crucial role in maintaining oral health by neutralising acids, maintaining oral pH, physically removing food debris and moisturises oral mucosa [57]. Saliva sampling is a pragmatic method for diagnosing and monitoring diseases, as it can be collected easily and non-invasively [58]. Studies have shown that the saliva of obese and normal-weight people differs in terms of salivary pH, flow rate, bacterial profile and inflammatory biomarkers (Table 16.5) [2]. The salivary concentration of adipokines and cytokines such as adiponectin, leptin, resistin, waspin,

Table 16.5 Summary of meta-analyses assessing the association between obesity and salivary profile

Sl. no.	Author	Year	Study design	Number of included studies	Conclusion
1	Habobe HA et al. [60]	2025	SR	16	Key salivary biomarkers were consistently elevated in individuals with medically unhealthy obesity, including 8-OHdG, IL-6, IL-8, resistin, TNFR1, PTX-3, AEA, OEA, TNF-α and sICAM-1.
2	Deng Q et al. [61]	2024	SR with MA	50	Children and adolescents with obesity had significantly higher gingival crevicular fluid TNF-α, leptin, adiponectin and IL-1β levels than those with normal weight.
3	Deng et al. [2]	2023	SR with MA	15	Children and adolescents with obesity had significantly higher gingival crevicular fluid levels of tumour necrosis factor-alpha (SMD: 0.56; 95% CI: 0.07, 1.04), adiponectin (SMD: 0.33; 95% CI: 0.06, 0.60), leptin (SMD: 0.52; 95% CI: 0.15, 0.90) and interleukin-1 beta (SMD: 0.71; 95% CI: 0.44, 0.99) than those with normal weight.
4	Hatipoglu O et al. [42]	2022	SR with MA	24	Salivary flow rate decreases significantly with obesity notably when saliva is stimulated; the decrease in salivary flow rate is much more prominent in adolescence and adulthood than in childhood; no significant differences in pH or buffer capacity.
5	Duffles L et al. [62]	2019	SR with MA	34	Individuals with obesity presented higher levels of TNF-α in saliva than individuals without obesity.

SR systematic review, *MA* meta-analysis, *IL* interleukin, *OHdG* 8-hydroxy-2'-deoxyguanosine, *TNFR* tumour necrosis factor receptor, *PTX* pentraxin, *AEA* anandamide, *OEA* oleoylethanolamide, *TNF* tumour necrosis factor, *sICAM* soluble intercellular adhesion molecule

interleukin 1β (IL-1β), IL-6, IL-8, IL-10, TNF-α, monocyte chemotactic factor, CD40/CD40L and other inflammatory markers like matrix metalloproteinase 2 (MMP-2), plasminogen activator inhibitor (PAI-1), soluble intercellular adhesion molecule 1 (sICAM-1) and pentraxin 3 (PTX3) are potential biomarkers for early diagnosis of obesity [59].

16.6 Obesity and Oral Microbiota

A healthy oral microbiome is characterised by the intricate balance between species diversity and their relative proportions. Oral microbes contribute significantly to both oral and systemic health by supporting colonisation resistance, aiding nutrient digestion and regulating immune responses [63]. Chronic inflammation alters the oral microbiome, increasing the prevalence of pathogenic bacteria [64]. Studies

Table 16.6 Summary of systematic reviews assessing the association between obesity and oral microbiota

Sl. no.	Author	Year	Study design	Number of included studies	Conclusion
1	De Lemos et al. [66]	2024	SR	11	Nine of the selected articles showed an association between oral microbiota and overweight and obesity in children and adolescents.
2	Alarcón-Sánchez et al. [65]	2024	SR	8	Evident alterations in the composition of the subgingival microbiota in subjects with obesity and periodontitis.

SR systematic review

profiling subgingival bacterial communities in overweight/obese and non-obese individuals have identified several oral bacteria significantly linked to obesity (Table 16.6). An increased bacterial count and a higher proportion of *Campylobacter gracilis, Eubacterium nodatum, Fusobacterium nucleatum spp. vincentii, Streptococcus intermedius, Actinomyces gerencseriae, Aggregatibacter actinomycetemcomitans and Treponema socransky* species in patients with both obesity and periodontitis compared to those who are obese but periodontally healthy have been observed [65]. Although apparent alterations in microbial diversity are noted, identifying a distinct microbiota pattern remains elusive.

16.7 Obesity and Other Oral Health Conditions

A positive correlation between obesity and dental eruption was also identified, with earlier eruptions of first and second permanent molars [67]. Obesity is significantly associated with poorer mastication [68], and compared to normal-weight individuals, being overweight or obese decreases the risk of temporomandibular joint disorders (OR: 0.66, 95% CI: 0.46–0.95). Obesity alone significantly reduced this risk (OR: 0.58) [69]. Furthermore, a bidirectional association between obesity and tooth loss/edentulism has been confirmed [70].

16.8 The Interplay Between Bariatric Surgery and Oral Health

The primary approaches to weight loss include dietary therapy, physical activity, medication and bariatric surgery. In patients with morbid obesity (body mass index of ≥ 40 or ≥ 35 kg/m^2) who have associated co-morbidities, bariatric surgery is currently regarded as the only effective treatment. Procedures such as gastric bypass, sleeve gastrectomy, adjustable gastric banding and biliopancreatic diversion aim to reduce the stomach's capacity or limit nutrient absorption. While these surgeries effectively promote weight loss and improve obesity-related health conditions, they can also have implications for oral health [71].

After bariatric surgery, patients are at risk of nutritional deficiencies, including vitamins and minerals essential for oral health, such as calcium, vitamin D and vitamin B12 [72]. These deficiencies have been shown to increase susceptibility to dental caries and periodontal disease (Table 16.7). Additionally, some bariatric

Table 16.7 Summary of systematic reviews and meta-analyses evaluating the connection between bariatric surgery and oral health

Sl. no.	Reference	Year	Study design	Number of included studies	Conclusion
1	Ferraz et al. [77]	2023	SR with MA	30	Bariatric surgery caused no difference in the index of decayed, missing or filled teeth. Salivary flow and probing depth presented a slight increase after bariatric surgery. Post-surgery patients showed an increase (%) in tooth wear at the dentin level (MD=–6.23; CI 95%=–8.45–4.01).
2	Čolak et al. [78]	2021	SR with MA	4	All studies showed significant worsening of bleeding on probing (4.21% (95% CI: 0.32, 8.11)), clinical attachment loss (0.16 mm (95% CI: 0.05, 0.27)), periodontal pocket depth (0.14 mm (95% CI: 0.06, 0.23)) and percentage of percentage of periodontal pocket depth 4–5 mm: 1.72% (95% CI: 0.11, 3.34) 6 months after bariatric surgery, but no change after 12 months.
3	Franco et al. [79]	2020	SR	5	Bariatric surgery does not reduce the incidence of periodontal disease.
4	Quintella et al. [73]	2020	SR	5	Patients undergoing bariatric surgery had a significantly higher incidence of dental erosion.
5	Dos Santos et al. [80]	2019	SR with MA	6	Bariatric surgery does not influence bleeding on probing or probing pocket depth, but leads to a worsening of clinical attachment loss.
6	Fontanille et al. [81]	2018	SR with MA	10	Six-month follow-up after bariatric surgery showed significantly increased periodontal inflammation and periodontal destruction. However, 12 months after bariatric surgery, the difference between bariatric patients and control was no longer significant indicating a transient nature.
7	Maria de Souza et al. [82]	2018	SR with MA	9	Plaque index was lower after than before bariatric surgery (MD: –1.29; CI 95% –2.34 to –0.24). There was no significant difference in clinical attachment level, gingival index, percentage of bleeding sites and pocket probing depth before and after bariatric surgery.
8	Salgado-Peralvo AO et al. [83]	2017	SR	9	Bariatric surgery is associated with increased dental caries risk.

SR systematic review, *MA* meta-analysis, *MD* mean difference, *CI* confidence interval surgery patients experience acid reflux as a side effect, which can contribute to erosive tooth wear and hypersensitivity [73].

Furthermore, bariatric surgery often necessitates changes in eating habits, including more frequent, smaller meals [74]. This eating pattern can increase the number of eating moments, raising the risk of caries. To mitigate these effects, patients should be encouraged to maintain diligent oral hygiene practices. Patients undergoing bariatric surgery have shown altered salivary buffering capacity and reduced unstimulated salivary flow due to xerostomia [75]. This may partly be attributed to medications prescribed post-surgery, including appetite suppressants and painkillers. Reduced saliva production compromises the natural defence mechanisms of the oral cavity, increasing the risk of dental caries and periodontal disease. Dentists may recommend artificial salivary agents [57] or saliva-stimulating agents [76] to alleviate decreased salivary flow and xerostomia.

Comprehensive dental care is essential for bariatric surgery patients. Regular dental checkups help monitor and address oral health challenges related to the surgery. Collaboration between dentists and bariatric surgeons ensures a holistic approach to patient care, addressing both systemic and oral health needs.

Figure 16.1 shows a flowchart illustrating the bidirectional and unidirectional relationships between lifestyle factors, systemic health conditions, obesity and oral health.

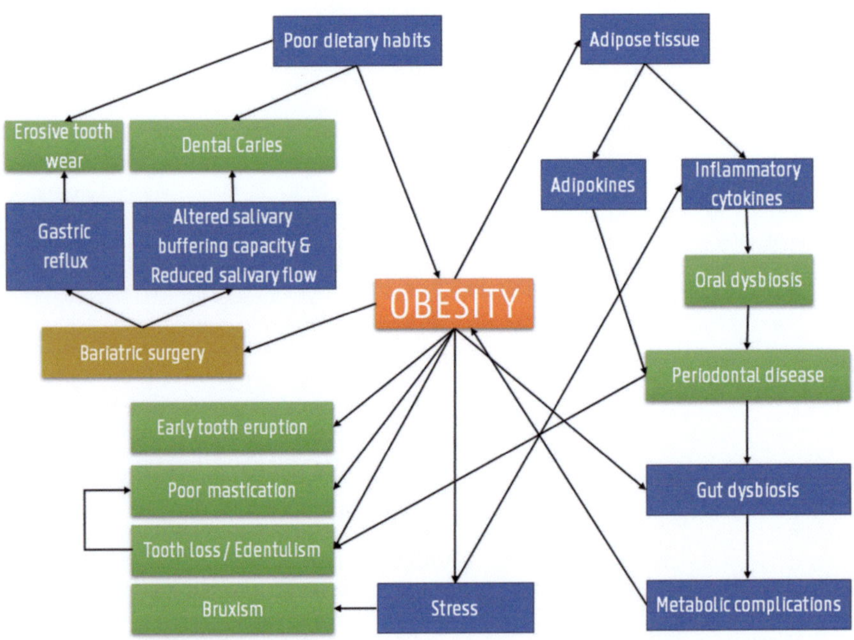

Fig. 16.1 Flowchart depicting the interplay between lifestyle factors, systematic health conditions, obesity and oral health

16.9 Implications for Clinical Practice

Oral health professionals play a vital role in raising awareness and educating patients about the link between overweight and obesity and the heightened risk of periodontal disease. Encouraging good oral hygiene practices, such as regular brushing, flossing and using mouthwash, is essential to prevent plaque accumulation and reduce the risk of gum disease. In personalised medicine, integrating body mass index measurements into routine risk assessments is recommended to help patients understand the multifaceted, systemic nature of obesity.

Preventive strategies should address modifiable risk factors, including diet, physical activity and weight management, to lower the chances of obesity and periodontal disease. Establishing a monitoring plan with regular dental visits and targeted evaluations can aid in the early detection and treatment of periodontal issues in obese patients. Furthermore, collaboration with endocrinologists, dietitians and other healthcare specialists is critical for a holistic approach to managing obesity. This coordinated care ensures that patients receive comprehensive medical and dental support [31].

16.10 Conclusion

The association between obesity and oral health seems significant. Obesity contributes to various oral health issues, particularly periodontal disease and dental caries. Addressing this relationship requires a comprehensive approach that includes advocating for nutritious diets, promoting consistent oral hygiene practices and managing systemic health conditions. By tackling the interplay between obesity and oral health, healthcare professionals can significantly enhance patients' overall health and quality of life.

Future research should prioritise exploring the molecular pathways that link obesity to oral health and developing innovative strategies that address both conditions simultaneously. Public health initiatives aimed at reducing obesity rates and enhancing oral health awareness can potentially deliver long-term benefits at both individual and community levels.

References

1. Collaboration NCDRF. Worldwide trends in underweight and obesity from 1990 to 2022: a pooled analysis of 3663 population-representative studies with 222 million children, adolescents, and adults. Lancet. 2024;403(10431):1027–50.
2. Deng Q, Wong HM, Peng S. Salivary and gingival crevicular fluid biomarkers of periodontal health and/or obesity among children and adolescents: a systematic review and meta-analysis. Heliyon. 2024;10(1):e23782.
3. Mahmoud SA, El Moshy S, Rady D, Radwan IA, Abbass MMS, Al Jawaldeh A. The effect of unhealthy dietary habits on the incidence of dental caries and overweight/obesity among Egyptian school children (A cross-sectional study). Front Public Health. 2022;10:953545.

4. Monda A, de Stefano MI, Villano I, Allocca S, Casillo M, Messina A, et al. Ultra-processed food intake and increased risk of obesity: a narrative review. Foods. 2024;13(16):2627.
5. Beklen A, Sali N, Yavuz MB. The impact of smoking on periodontal status and dental caries. Tob Induc Dis. 2022;20:72.
6. Macri M, D'Albis G, D'Albis V, Antonacci A, Abbinante A, Stefanelli R, et al. Periodontal health and its relationship with psychological stress: a cross-sectional study. J Clin Med. 2024;13(10):2942.
7. Ghanem AS, Nagy AC. Oral health's role in diabetes risk: a cross-sectional study with sociodemographic and lifestyle insights. Front Endocrinol (Lausanne). 2024;15:1342783.
8. Maniaci A, Lavalle S, Anzalone R, Lo Giudice A, Cocuzza S, Parisi FM, et al. Oral health implications of obstructive sleep apnea: a literature review. Biomedicines. 2024;12(7):1382.
9. Martinez-Herrera M, Silvestre-Rangil J, Silvestre FJ. Association between obesity and periodontal disease. A systematic review of epidemiological studies and controlled clinical trials. Med Oral Patol Oral Cir Bucal. 2017;22(6):e708–e15.
10. Khan S, Barrington G, Bettiol S, Barnett T, Crocombe L. Is overweight/obesity a risk factor for periodontitis in young adults and adolescents?: a systematic review. Obes Rev. 2018;19(6):852–83.
11. Keller A, Rohde JF, Raymond K, Heitmann BL. Association between periodontal disease and overweight and obesity: a systematic review. J Periodontol. 2015;86(6):766–76.
12. Eke PI, Dye BA, Wei L, Thornton-Evans GO, Genco RJ. Cdc periodontal disease surveillance workgroup: James Beck GDRP. Prevalence of periodontitis in adults in the United States: 2009 and 2010. J Dent Res. 2012;91(10):914–20.
13. Kim CM, Lee S, Hwang W, Son E, Kim TW, Kim K, et al. Obesity and periodontitis: a systematic review and updated meta-analysis. Front Endocrinol (Lausanne). 2022;13:999455.
14. Martens L, De Smet S, Yusof MY, Rajasekharan S. Association between overweight/obesity and periodontal disease in children and adolescents: a systematic review and meta-analysis. Eur Arch Paediatr Dent. 2017;18(2):69–82.
15. Lula EC, Ribeiro CC, Hugo FN, Alves CM, Silva AA. Added sugars and periodontal disease in young adults: an analysis of NHANES III data. Am J Clin Nutr. 2014;100(4):1182–7.
16. Kandaswamy E, Lee CT, Gururaj SB, Shivanaikar S, Joshi VM. Association of adipokine levels with obesity in periodontal health and disease: a systematic review with meta-analysis and meta-regression. J Periodontal Res. 2024;59(4):623–35.
17. Foratori-Junior GA, Pereira PR, Gasparoto IA, de Carvalho Sales-Peres SH, Storniolo de Souza JM, Khan S. Is overweight associated with periodontitis in pregnant women? Systematic review and meta-analysis. Jpn Dent Sci Rev. 2022;58:41–51.
18. Cruz-Avila J, Hernandez-Perez E, Gonzalez-Gonzalez R, Bologna-Molina R, Molina-Frechero N. Periodontal disease in obese patients; Interleukin-6 and C-reactive protein study: a systematic review. Dent J (Basel). 2022;10(12):225.
19. Abu-Shawish G, Betsy J, Anil S. Is obesity a risk factor for periodontal disease in adults? a systematic review. Int J Environ Res Public Health. 2022;19(19):12684.
20. Li LW, Wong HM, Sun L, Wen YF, McGrath CP. Anthropometric measurements and periodontal diseases in children and adolescents: a systematic review and meta-analysis. Adv Nutr. 2015;6(6):828–41.
21. Nascimento GG, Leite FR, Do LG, Peres KG, Correa MB, Demarco FF, et al. Is weight gain associated with the incidence of periodontitis? A systematic review and meta-analysis. J Clin Periodontol. 2015;42(6):495–505.
22. Papageorgiou SN, Reichert C, Jager A, Deschner J. Effect of overweight/obesity on response to periodontal treatment: systematic review and a meta-analysis. J Clin Periodontol. 2015;42(3):247–61.
23. Suvan J, D'Aiuto F, Moles DR, Petrie A, Donos N. Association between overweight/obesity and periodontitis in adults. A systematic review. Obes Rev. 2011;12(5):e381–404.

24. Watanabe K, Cho YD. Periodontal disease and metabolic syndrome: a qualitative critical review of their association. Arch Oral Biol. 2014;59(8):855–70.
25. Mervish NA, Hu J, Hagan LA, Arora M, Frau C, Choi J, et al. Associations of the oral microbiota with obesity and menarche in inner city girls. J Child Obes. 2019;4(1):2.
26. Zhang Y, Jia R, Zhang Y, Sun X, Mei Y, Zou R, et al. Effect of non-surgical periodontal treatment on cytokines/adipocytokines levels among periodontitis patients with or without obesity: a systematic review and meta-analysis. BMC Oral Health. 2023;23(1):717.
27. Hajishengallis G, Chavakis T. Local and systemic mechanisms linking periodontal disease and inflammatory comorbidities. Nat Rev Immunol. 2021;21(7):426–40.
28. Marro F, De Smedt S, Rajasekharan S, Martens L, Bottenberg P, Jacquet W. Associations between obesity, dental caries, erosive tooth wear and periodontal disease in adolescents: a case-control study. Eur Arch Paediatr Dent. 2021;22(1):99–108.
29. Reeves AF, Rees JM, Schiff M, Hujoel P. Total body weight and waist circumference associated with chronic periodontitis among adolescents in the United States. Arch Pediatr Adolesc Med. 2006;160(9):894–9.
30. Nascimento GG, Seerig LM, Vargas-Ferreira F, Correa FO, Leite FR, Demarco FF. Are obesity and overweight associated with gingivitis occurrence in Brazilian schoolchildren? J Clin Periodontol. 2013;40(12):1072–8.
31. Arbildo-Vega HI, Cruzado-Oliva FH, Coronel-Zubiate FT, Aguirre-Ipenza R, Meza-Malaga JM, Lujan-Valencia SA, et al. Association between periodontal disease and obesity. Umbrella Review. Medicina (Kaunas). 2024;60(4):621.
32. Mirzaei A, Shahrestanaki E, Malmir H, Ejtahed HS, Tajbakhsh D, Seif E, et al. Association of periodontitis with lipid profile: an updated systematic review and meta-analysis. J Diabetes Metab Disord. 2022;21(2):1377–93.
33. da Silva FG, Pola NM, Casarin M, Silva CFE, Muniz F. Association between clinical measures of gingival inflammation and obesity in adults: systematic review and meta-analyses. Clin Oral Investig. 2021;25(7):4281–98.
34. Chaffee BW, Weston SJ. Association between chronic periodontal disease and obesity: a systematic review and meta-analysis. J Periodontol. 2010;81(12):1708–24.
35. Tajik Z, Mehrafarid H, Bayani M, Almasi-Hashiani A. Comparison of visfatin levels before and after non-surgical periodontal therapy: a systematic review and meta-analysis. PLoS One. 2025;20(2):e0315035.
36. Menezes CC, Barbirato DDS, Fogacci MF, Maranon-Vasquez GA, Carneiro JRI, Maia LC, et al. Systemic benefits of periodontal therapy in patients with obesity and periodontitis: a systematic review. Braz Oral Res. 2024;38:e031.
37. Akram Z, Safii SH, Vaithilingam RD, Baharuddin NA, Javed F, Vohra F. Efficacy of non-surgical periodontal therapy in the management of chronic periodontitis among obese and non-obese patients: a systematic review and meta-analysis. Clin Oral Investig. 2016;20(5):903–14.
38. Gerber FA, Sahrmann P, Schmidlin OA, Heumann C, Beer JH, Schmidlin PR. Influence of obesity on the outcome of non-surgical periodontal therapy – a systematic review. BMC Oral Health. 2016;16(1):90.
39. Nascimento GG, Leite FR, Correa MB, Peres MA, Demarco FF. Does periodontal treatment have an effect on clinical and immunological parameters of periodontal disease in obese subjects? A systematic review and meta-analysis. Clin Oral Investig. 2016;20(4):639–47.
40. Cheever VJ, Mohajeri A, Patel K, Burris RC, Hung M. Impact of free sugar consumption on dental caries: a cross-sectional analysis of children in the United States. Dent J (Basel). 2025;13(2):48.
41. Bakhoda MR, Haghighat Lari MM, Khosravi G, Khademi Z, Abbasi F, Milajerdi A. Childhood obesity in relation to risk of dental caries: a cumulative and dose-response systematic review and meta-analysis. BMC Oral Health. 2024;24(1):966.

42. Hatipoglu O, Maras E, Hatipoglu FP, Saygin AG. Salivary flow rate, pH, and buffer capacity in the individuals with obesity and overweight; A meta-analysis. Niger J Clin Pract. 2022;25(7):1126–42.
43. Manohar N, Hayen A, Fahey P, Arora A. Obesity and dental caries in early childhood: A systematic review and meta-analyses. Obes Rev. 2020;21(3):e12960.
44. Garrocho-Rangel A, Martinez-Lopez I, Butron-Tellez Giron C, Pozos-Guillen A, Zavala-Alonso V. Obesity/overweight and dental caries experience in children and adolescents: an umbrella review. Eur Arch Paediatr Dent. 2024;25(6):779–89.
45. Pizzi JF, Carrada CF, Zeferino MVS, Doriguetto PVT, Abreu LG, Scalioni FAR, et al. Overweight/obesity and dental caries in Brazilian children and adolescents: a systematic review and meta-analysis. Braz Oral Res. 2024;38:e015.
46. Silveira MG, Schneider BC, Tillmann TF, Silva AE. Excess weight and dental caries throughout childhood and adolescence: systematic review of longitudinal studies. Int J Clin Pediatr Dent. 2022;15(6):691–8.
47. Alshehri YFA, Park JS, Kruger E, Tennant M. Association between body mass index and dental caries in the Kingdom of Saudi Arabia: systematic review. Saudi Dent J. 2020;32(4):171–80.
48. Angelopoulou MV, Beinlich M, Crain A. Early childhood caries and weight status: a systematic review and meta-analysis. Pediatr Dent. 2019;41(4):261–72.
49. Paisi M, Kay E, Bennett C, Kaimi I, Witton R, Nelder R, et al. Body mass index and dental caries in young people: a systematic review. BMC Pediatr. 2019;19(1):122.
50. Carson SJ. No consistent association found between dental caries and body mass index in children. Evid Based Dent. 2018;19(2):38–9.
51. Chen D, Zhi Q, Zhou Y, Tao Y, Wu L, Lin H. Association between dental caries and BMI in children: a systematic review and meta-analysis. Caries Res. 2018;52(3):230–45.
52. Li LW, Wong HM, Peng SM, McGrath CP. Anthropometric measurements and dental caries in children: a systematic review of longitudinal studies. Adv Nutr. 2015;6(1):52–63.
53. Hayden C, Bowler JO, Chambers S, Freeman R, Humphris G, Richards D, et al. Obesity and dental caries in children: a systematic review and meta-analysis. Community Dent Oral Epidemiol. 2013;41(4):289–308.
54. Silva AE, Menezes AM, Demarco FF, Vargas-Ferreira F, Peres MA. Obesity and dental caries: systematic review. Rev Saude Publica. 2013;47(4):799–812.
55. Hooley M, Skouteris H, Boganin C, Satur J, Kilpatrick N. Body mass index and dental caries in children and adolescents: a systematic review of literature published 2004 to 2011. Syst Rev. 2012;1:57.
56. Kantovitz KR, Pascon FM, Rontani RM, Gaviao MB. Obesity and dental caries–a systematic review. Oral Health Prev Dent. 2006;4(2):137–44.
57. Alhejoury HA, Mogharbel LF, Al-Qadhi MA, Shamlan SS, Alturki AF, Babatin WM, et al. Artificial Saliva for therapeutic management of Xerostomia: a narrative review. J Pharm Bioallied Sci. 2021;13(Suppl 2):S903–S7.
58. Chielle EO, Casarin JN. Evaluation of salivary oxidative parameters in overweight and obese young adults. Arch Endocrinol Metab. 2017;61(2):152–9.
59. Zysk B, Ostrowska L, Smarkusz-Zarzecka J. Salivary adipokine and cytokine levels as potential markers for the development of obesity and metabolic disorders. Int J Mol Sci. 2021;22(21):11703.
60. Habobe HA, Pieters RHH, Bikker FJ. Investigating the salivary biomarker profile in obesity: a systematic review. Curr Obes Rep. 2025;14(1):25.
61. Deng Q, Wong HM, Peng S. Alterations in salivary profile in individuals with dental caries and/or obesity: a systematic review and meta-analysis. J Dent. 2024;151:105451.

62. Duffles LF, Hermont AP, Abreu LG, Pordeus IA, Silva TA. Association between obesity and adipokines levels in saliva and gingival crevicular fluid: a systematic review and meta-analysis. J Evid Based Med. 2019;12(4):313–24.
63. Yang Y, Cai Q, Zheng W, Steinwandel M, Blot WJ, Shu XO, et al. Oral microbiome and obesity in a large study of low-income and African-American populations. J Oral Microbiol. 2019;11(1):1650597.
64. Leng Y, Hu Q, Ling Q, Yao X, Liu M, Chen J, et al. Periodontal disease is associated with the risk of cardiovascular disease independent of sex: a meta-analysis. Front Cardiovasc Med. 2023;10:1114927.
65. Alarcon-Sanchez MA. Influence of obesity on subgingival microbiota composition in subjects with different periodontal status: a systematic review. Rev Cient Odontol (Lima). 2024;12(1):e187.
66. de Lemos GM, Resende CMM, Campello CP, Ribeiro IS, Mendes AK, de Lima ELS, et al. Is oral microbiota associated with overweight and obesity in children and adolescents? A systematic review. Crit Rev Food Sci Nutr. 2024;64(13):4275–85.
67. Mohamedhussein N, Busuttil-Naudi A, Mohammed H, UlHaq A. Association of obesity with the eruption of first and second permanent molars in children: a systematic review. Eur Arch Paediatr Dent. 2020;21(1):13–23.
68. Tada A, Miura H. Association of mastication and factors affecting masticatory function with obesity in adults: a systematic review. BMC Oral Health. 2018;18(1):76.
69. Wang X, Yang Y, Lin L, Yao Q, Zhang J. Obesity and temporomandibular joint disorders: a systematic review and meta-analysis. BMC Oral Health. 2023;23(1):607.
70. Nascimento GG, Leite FR, Conceicao DA, Ferrua CP, Singh A, Demarco FF. Is there a relationship between obesity and tooth loss and edentulism? A systematic review and meta-analysis. Obes Rev. 2016;17(7):587–98.
71. de Moura-Grec PG, Yamashita JM, Marsicano JA, Ceneviva R, de Souza Leite CV, de Brito GB, et al. Impact of bariatric surgery on oral health conditions: 6-months cohort study. Int Dent J. 2014;64(3):144–9.
72. Lupoli R, Lembo E, Saldalamacchia G, Avola CK, Angrisani L, Capaldo B. Bariatric surgery and long-term nutritional issues. World J Diabetes. 2017;8(11):464–74.
73. Quintella MCM, Farias T, SoutoMaior JR, Casado B, Leao RS, Moraes SLD. Relationship between bariatric surgery and dental erosion: a systematic review. Surg Obes Relat Dis. 2020;16(9):1283–90.
74. Nikiforova I, Barnea R, Azulai S, Susmallian S. Analysis of the association between eating behaviors and weight loss after laparoscopic sleeve gastrectomy. Obes Facts. 2019;12(6):618–31.
75. Kogawa EM, Melo FF, Pires RG, Caetano PCC, de Lima RJ, Benito LAO, et al. The changes on salivary flow rates, buffering capacity and chromogranin A levels in adults after bariatric surgery. Clin Oral Investig. 2024;28(3):159.
76. Dodds MWJ, Haddou MB, Day JEL. The effect of gum chewing on xerostomia and salivary flow rate in elderly and medically compromised subjects: a systematic review and meta-analysis. BMC Oral Health. 2023;23(1):406.
77. Ferraz AX, Goncalves FM, Ferreira-Neto PD, Santos RS, Guariza-Filho O, Zeigelboim BS, et al. Impact of bariatric surgery on oral health: a systematic review and meta-analysis. Clin Oral Investig. 2023;27(5):1869–84.
78. Colak D, Gaspersic R, Kucic AC, Pintar T, Gaspirc B. The effect of bariatric surgery on periodontal health: systematic review and meta-analyses. Arch Med Sci. 2021;17(4):1118–27.

79. Franco R, Barlattani A Jr, Perrone MA, Basili M, Miranda M, Costacurta M, et al. Obesity, bariatric surgery and periodontal disease: a literature update. Eur Rev Med Pharmacol Sci. 2020;24(9):5036–45.
80. Dos Santos MCM, Pellizzer EP, SoutoMaior JR, Casado B, Luna Gomes JM, Vasconcelos B, et al. Clinical periodontal conditions in individuals after bariatric surgery: a systematic review and meta-analysis. Surg Obes Relat Dis. 2019;15(10):1850–9.
81. Fontanille I, Boillot A, Range H, Carra MC, Sales-Peres SHC, Czernichow S, et al. Bariatric surgery and periodontal status: A systematic review with meta-analysis. Surg Obes Relat Dis. 2018;14(10):1618–31.
82. Maria de Souza G, Douglas W, dc Oliveira D, Santos Lages F, Andrade Fernandes I, Falci GM, S. Relationship between bariatric surgery and periodontal status: a systematic review and meta-analysis. Surg Obes Relat Dis. 2018;14(8):1205–16.
83. Salgado-Peralvo AO, Mateos-Moreno MV, Arriba-Fuente L, Garcia-Sanchez A, Salgado-Garcia A, Peralvo-Garcia V, et al. Bariatric surgery as a risk factor in the development of dental caries: a systematic review. Public Health. 2018;155:26–34.

Eating Disorders and Oral Health

17

Rene Panico, Gerado Marcelo Gilligan,
Eduardo David Piemonte, and Jeronimo Pablo Lazos

17.1 Introduction

Eating disorders are characterised by abnormal eating habits that affect the overall health of an individual. They are complex and life-impacting conditions affecting physical, mental and social aspects of health. Millions of people worldwide suffer from eating disorders. Eating disorders can occur at any age, gender or race. A person with an eating disorder will have health risks affecting nearly every organ in the body, including the oral cavity. Genetics, brain chemistry, environment and social influences have a significant role to play in the causation of eating disorders. Eating disorders often run in families. Various trends, such as dieting, the media or fashion, can trigger an underlying predisposition for an eating disorder. Eating disorders are conscious lifestyle choices made by people.

17.2 Types of Eating Disorders

Anorexia nervosa (AN): In this disorder, individuals restrict the number of calories and the types of food they consume. Sometimes, they use extreme measures such as excessive exercise or vomiting after eating because they perceive themselves as overweight even when they are underweight. Bulimia nervosa (BN): This disorder is characterised by episodes of binge eating, where individuals consume large amounts of food, followed by efforts to eliminate the extra calories through unhealthy methods like vomiting or using laxatives. Binge eating disorder: In this

R. Panico (✉) · G. M. Gilligan · E. D. Piemonte · J. P. Lazos
Department of Oral Medicine, Facultad de Odontologia, Universidad Nacional de Cordoba, Córdoba, Argentina
e-mail: rene.panico@unc.edu.ar; ggilligan@unc.edu.ar; eduardo.piemonte@unc.edu.ar; jerolazos@unc.edu.ar

S. R. Prabhu et al. (eds.), *Lifestyle in Oral Health and Disease*,
https://doi.org/10.1007/978-3-032-05888-1_17

disorder, individuals lose control over their eating and frequently overeat, even when they feel uncomfortably full or are not hungry.

Anorexia nervosa (AN) and bulimia nervosa (BN) are complex psychiatric conditions that affect both physical and psychological health. These disorders are characterised by abnormal behaviours related to food intake, leading to chronic malnutrition or cyclical episodes of binge eating followed by purging. While systemic manifestations are widely recognised, oral manifestations in both hard and soft tissues are also common and may be among the first signs dentists can detect during a routine dental/oral examination [1, 2]. For several years, eating disorders and oral health conditions have been extensively studied, and it is now clear that there is a strong correlation between specific oral manifestations and these disorders. Although these oral signs and symptoms could assist in the early diagnosis of the underlying disorder, their identification and the eventual establishment of a correlation are currently heavily limited to the clinician's experience [3]. This chapter focuses on the clinical oral manifestations of these disorders, providing an essential tool for general dentists to identify early signs, collaborate in the early diagnosis of these conditions and facilitate timely intervention.

17.3 Systemic Manifestations of Anorexia Nervosa and Bulimia Nervosa

Eating disorders encompass various conditions, such as anorexia nervosa (AN), bulimia nervosa (BN), avoidant/restrictive food intake disorder, binge eating disorder, pica, rumination disorder, other specified feeding or eating disorder and unspecified feeding or eating disorders. These conditions lead to clinically significant compromises in physical health, psychological well-being and social functioning, typically manifesting as alterations in the quantity, quality or frequency of ingested food, often accompanied by concerns regarding body weight, shape or size [3, 4]. Individuals with eating disorders face high morbidity and mortality risks due to factors like malnutrition (causing cardiac and bone health issues, reduced immune system function, leading to increased susceptibility to infections, muscular weakness and reduced ability to perform daily tasks, impaired wound healing), overnutrition (leading to obesity and metabolic syndrome), compensatory behaviours (triggering electrolyte imbalances and cardiovascular or neurological problems) and mood disturbances (negative effects on brain function, including apathy, depression and deterioration in social interactions raising suicide risk) [3]. Eating disorders affect multiple body systems, with consequences that include electrolyte imbalances typically associated with dehydration, extreme weight loss, cardiac arrhythmias, osteoporosis and hormonal disturbances. Among these, hormonal alterations in women are often accompanied by amenorrhea [5, 6]. Repeated episodes of self-induced vomiting in BN can also lead to dehydration, metabolic alkalosis and erosions of teeth.

The multifactorial aetiology of eating disorders, which likely involves a combination of sociocultural, neurobiological, genetic, psychological and interpersonal factors, underscores the complexity of causality. Sociocultural influences, such as societal pressures for thinness and media portrayals of idealised body standards, can shape body image concerns and leads to eating behaviours. Neurobiological factors, including dysregulation of neurotransmitters like serotonin and dopamine, may affect mood, appetite and reward processing. Genetic predispositions also play a role, as familial studies suggest a heritable component to vulnerability [7]. Psychological factors, such as perfectionism, low self-esteem and coexisting mental health conditions like anxiety or depression, further contribute to the risk. Interpersonal dynamics, including family conflicts, loss of loved ones, history of trauma or peer influences, can exacerbate these vulnerabilities. The interplay of these diverse factors creates a highly individualised and intricate path to the development of eating disorders, complicating efforts to establish a clear causal framework [1, 3, 8].

17.4 Dental and Oral Manifestations of Anorexia Nervosa and Bulimia Nervosa

Dental manifestations are common in patients with eating disorders due to the repeated exposure of the oral cavity to gastric juices and associated oral habits. Although dental manifestations in patients with BN and AN are the most described and recognised in the literature, some studies suggest that these are late expressions of the disease. In this context, it has been reported that soft tissue lesions may precede complex dental (hard) tissue lesions [1]. The dentist's role is pivotal in recognising the possible implications of some of these findings, approaching the patient sensitively and communicating empathetically to engage them in a treatment plan, reducing the risk of further tooth erosion and improving oral health and hygiene [9]. Some of the main manifestations include the following:

- *Dental Erosion*: Frequent vomiting in bulimia and chronic regurgitation of gastric juices result in the progressive demineralisation of enamel (Fig. 17.1). The lingual surfaces of the maxillary anterior teeth are usually the most affected. As the condition progresses, erosion may extend to all tooth surfaces, leaving dentin exposed, which increases dental sensitivity and the risk of fractures. Interestingly, digestive enzymes (e.g. pepsin, trypsin) that can reach the oral cavity and saliva during reflux or vomiting can partially degrade the dentine matrix. This degradation could influence the stability of the dentine matrix against mechanical forces and the susceptibility of eroded dentine to combined chemo-mechanical impacts [10].

- *Rampant Caries*: Enamel loss due to erosion, combined with xerostomia (dry mouth) associated with dehydration, increases susceptibility to dental caries. Additionally, binge-eating episodes characterised by consuming sugar-rich foods exacerbate this process.

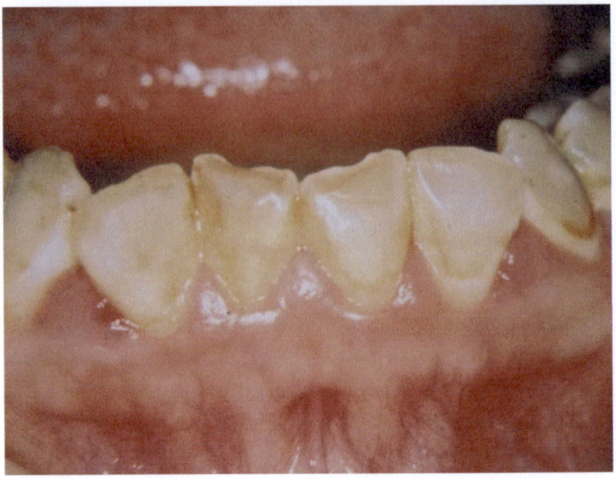

Fig. 17.1 Loss of mineralised tissue (enamel and dentin) leads to dental hypersensitivity in a patient with bulimia. This loss of mineralised tissue is due to the demineralising effect of the acids in vomit

- *Enamel Hypoplasia*: In severe cases of anorexia nervosa, chronic malnutrition during adolescence and dental development periods can interfere with proper enamel mineralisation, leading to hypoplasia in permanent teeth.
- *Xerostomia*: Daily dehydration and diuretics or laxatives in patients with AN and BN reduce salivary flow, contributing to dry mouth. Saliva protects teeth by neutralising acids and remineralising enamel; its reduction creates an environment more conducive to dental caries and erosion [11].
- *Salivary Gland Hypertrophy and Parotidomegaly*: Repeated vomiting and frequent stimulation of the salivary glands to neutralise gastric acid can cause visible and palpable enlargement of the parotid glands, known as Sialedenosis (or sialosis). This hypertrophy is a common feature in bulimic patients and can result in a characteristic facial appearance with cheek swelling [12].

Oral soft tissue alterations are another key area of manifestation in eating disorders, often overlooked or underdiagnosed by clinicians.

- *Petechiae and Haematomas in the Vomiting Induction Zone*: Frequent manoeuvres to induce vomiting cause mechanical trauma to the mucosa of the hard palate, soft palate and uvula. This results in petechiae (small red spots caused by capillary rupture) (Fig. 17.2a) and ecchymotic lesions (Figs. 17.2b, c), signs of recurrent tissue damage. These lesions are typically painless, and their severity correlates with the intensity and frequency of self-inflicted trauma during vomiting induction. Recognition of these lesions requires diascopy. Due to capillary rupture and blood extravasation, these lesions do not disappear during the diascopy manoeuvre [1, 13] (Fig. 17.2b). In bulimia nervosa, severe episodes of self-induced vomiting can result in extensive ecchymotic lesions on the uvula (Fig. 17.3).

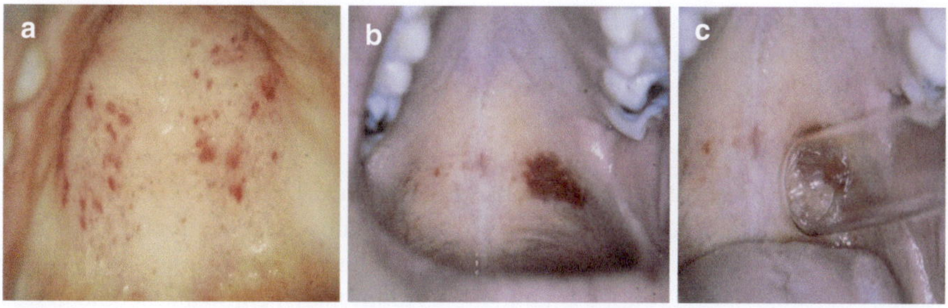

Fig. 17.2 (**a–c**) Petechiae and ecchymotic lesions: Palatal petechiae and purpuric lesions on the hard palate, with a lenticular shape and a reddish or purplish appearance (**a**), which do not fade with diascopy. These lesions are found in the areas associated with the induction of vomiting. Reddish and purplish lesions are caused by blood extravasation into the submucosal tissue due to the rupture of blood vessels, resulting in an ecchymosis (**b**). On the right (**c**), through the procedure of diascopy, it is observed that when pressure is applied with a transparent device, the red lesion does not fade

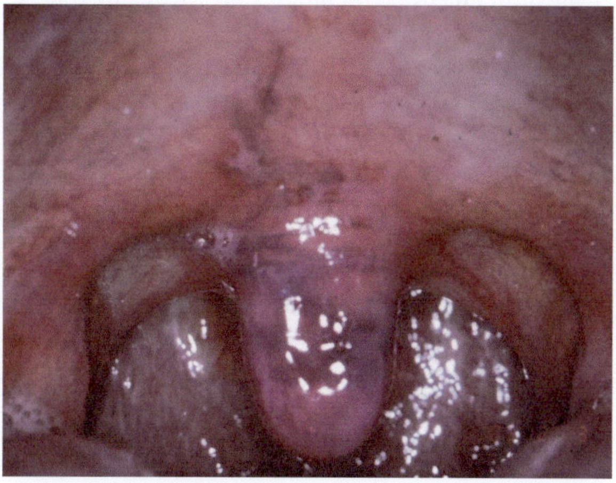

Fig. 17.3 Lesion due to blood extravasation in a patient with severe bulimia nervosa, characterised by numerous episodes of self-induced vomiting. An extensive ecchymosis is observed affecting the soft palate and uvula

- *Atrophic Glossitis*: Mucosal atrophy is commonly observed and is primarily attributed to a reduced intake of essential nutrients, particularly B-group vitamins (B1, B6 and B12), which are crucial for cell turnover, and iron, whose deficiency can lead to anaemia. This condition is often linked to a burning sensation, most notably on the tongue (glossodynia) [14]. The burning sensation may also be influenced by underlying psychological factors, such as anxiety, depression and stress, as well as neurological disorders [1]. In patients with anorexia nervosa, chronic nutritional deficiencies can lead to a smooth, shiny and painful tongue (atrophic glossitis) with a depapillated surface. A full blood count should be undertaken to confirm anaemic status and referral to the general practitioner or medical facility. In such cases, clinicians should also rule out *Candida* spp. infection and consider the possibility of atrophic candidiasis of the tongue. Fungal proliferation can be caused partly by the acidic environment and high carbohydrate intake in bulimic patients and, in part, by nutritional deficiencies. Chronic candidiasis has also been associated with the onset of angular cheilitis, although the latter can also be caused by superinfection by *Staphylococcus* [14].

Moreover, in several cases, anaemia is highly associated with iron, folate and vitamin B12 deficiencies due to chronic malnutrition. This condition can lead to generalised pallor of the entire oral mucosa. Clinically, anaemia manifests as oral mucosal pallor, fatigue and delayed healing of oral lesions. This clinical sign can be visually detected during routine examination. Additionally, clinicians should assess the conjunctival mucosa for further evaluation [6, 15]. A complete blood count and serological tests for iron, vitamin B12 and folate should be performed to confirm these haematological deficiencies.

- *Necrotising sialometaplasia*: Although rare, this condition can be triggered by recurrent vomiting and dehydration episodes, leading to ischemic necrosis in minor salivary glands. It presents as a painful ulcer, typically located on the palate or in mucosa with minor salivary glands (Fig. 17.4), with an acute onset and a necrotic appearance. Its clinical correlation with local factors, such as BN, is critical for diagnosis [16]. Due to its clinical similarity to malignant or infectious entities, a biopsy is recommended for definitive diagnosis.

- *Exfoliative or Desquamative Cheilitis and Angular Cheilitis Associated with Self-Induced Vomiting:*

Desquamative and angular cheilitis cases have been reported, often associated with nutritional deficiencies and/or generalised dehydration. In desquamative cheilitis, scales can be observed on the vermilion border, usually affecting the lower lip (Fig. 17.5) While not typically painful, these lesions can cause discomfort, leading

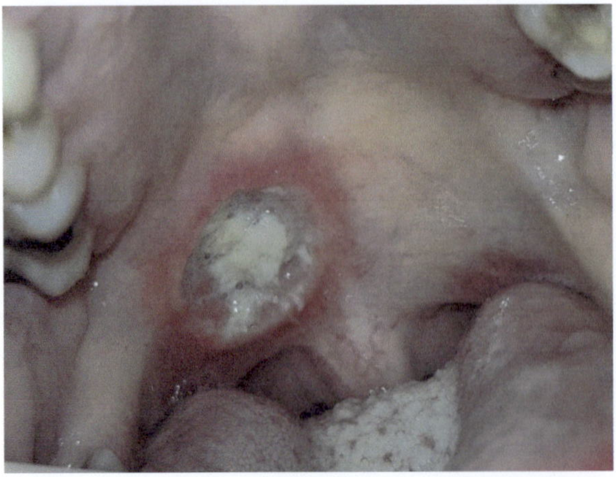

Fig. 17.4 Ulcer on the palate with a necrotic base and erythema. While the clinical appearance often resembles a malignant ulcer, acute evolution is key in differentiating diagnoses from malignant entities (such as squamous cell carcinoma) or infections (such as deep mycoses)

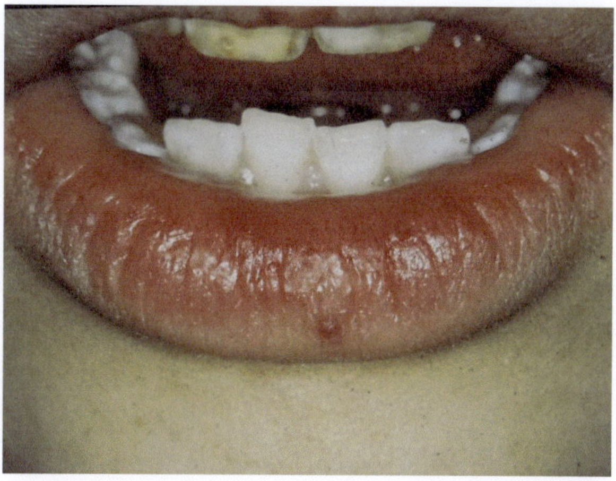

Fig. 17.5 Exfoliative cheilitis due to dehydration in an anorexia nervosa patient

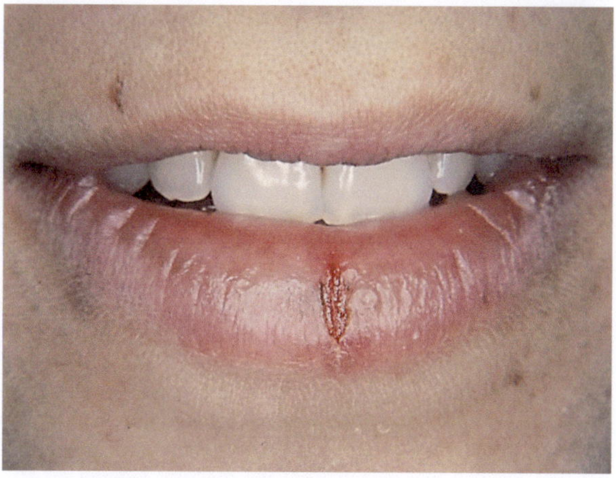

Fig. 17.6 A linear fissure in the medial region of the lip in a patient with anorexia nervosa with lip biting due to self-injury

to erosions and bleeding. Factitious habits often accompany this type of cheilitis, where individuals inflict self-harm, including lip biting (Fig. 17.6) or the removal of lip scales, onychophagia and trichophagia. Conversely, angular cheilitis usually present with bilateral fissures [17], x which can cause pain, particularly during mouth-opening movements associated with vomiting or self-induced vomiting [1]. Self-induced vomiting may also cause epithelial atrophy of the palatal mucosa (Fig. 17.7).

- *Mucositis*: Repeated episodes of vomiting and the use of medications or diuretics can result in chronic inflammation of the oral mucosa, with the appearance of painful ulcers and mucositis. Mucositis may present as generalised erythema of the oral mucosa in response to gastric acids and abrupt changes in salivary pH. These lesions, combined with poor healing due to malnutrition, can be recurrent and challenging to manage.

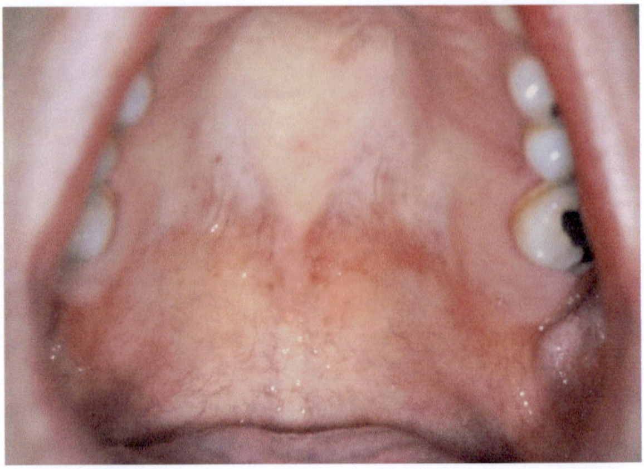

Fig. 17.7 Palatal epithelial atrophy due to trauma caused by self-induced vomiting

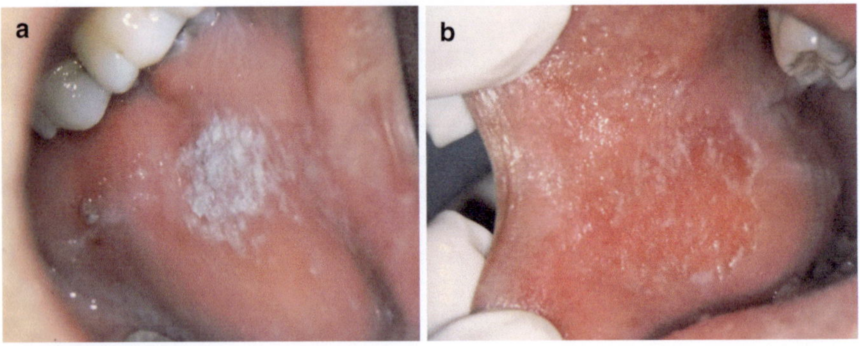

Fig. 17.8 (**a**, **b**). A patient with anorexia nervosa developed lesions due to self-inflicted trauma from biting the buccal mucosa, presenting this condition known as morsicatio buccarum. Clinically, bilateral white lesions resembling hyperkeratosis are observed, along with the presence of epithelial tags (scales) that detach from the mucosa, leaving an atrophic bed, sometimes erosive or ulcerated

- *Oral Hyperkeratosis*: Chronic friction between the teeth and soft tissues due to repeated regurgitation or vomiting-inducing manoeuvres can lead to mucosal thickening, hyperkeratosis, particularly on the soft palate and dorsal surface of the tongue clinically appearing as white plaques.
- *Bite Marks on the Mucosa—Morsicatio buccarum*: A common manifestation in patients with bulimia and anorexia nervosa is the presence of bite marks on the oral mucosa, particularly on the buccal mucosa (Fig. 17.8a, b), lips or tongue. These lesions occur due to self-inflicted trauma from repeated biting or chewing, often linked to stress, anxiety or attempts to control the urge to eat. The appearance of cheek biting may vary, ranging from superficial indentations to deeper ulcerations. These lesions may cause discomfort and, if left untreated, can lead to further complications, such as infections or chronic inflammation [1, 18].

- *Yellow Palate:* Yellowish discolouration of the oral mucosa in patients with eating disorders is an underreported condition. However, one study indicated that one in three patients may present this type of lesion [1]. A yellowish or orange discolouration may be observed on the soft palate and floor of the mouth (as well as in other areas such as the palms of the hands), resulting from hypercarotenaemia. Carotene is a lipochrome that naturally contributes to skin and mucosae pigmentation. When blood carotene levels are elevated, the extent of yellowish discolouration increases. Pigmentation typically first appears on the tip of the nose, palms and soles, gradually spreading throughout the body, with the most pronounced involvement in the palms, soles and nasolabial folds. The sclera remains unaffected, which helps differentiate carotenaemia from jaundice. However, in some cases, carotenaemia may manifest as palatal mucosal discoloration (Fig. 17.9a, b). It is important to note that the conjunctiva and oral mucosa lack a stratum corneum, which may influence the presentation of hypercarotenaemia in these areas [19, 20]. Hypercarotenaemia in anorexia nervosa may result from either increased carotene and vitamin A intake or an acquired defect in vitamin A metabolism or utilisation. Reducing carotene intake eventually leads to the resolution of skin pigmentation. Patients should be advised that various green vegetables, such as green beans and spinach, are rich in carotene and should therefore be avoided. Consultation with a nutritionist and the development of a structured meal plan can be beneficial [19].

- *Pica*: The current version of the Diagnostic and Statistical Manual of Mental Disorders (DSM-5) defines *pica* as persistent eating of non-nutritive substances for at least 1 month that is inappropriate to the developmental level of the individual and is not part of a culturally supported or socially normative practice.

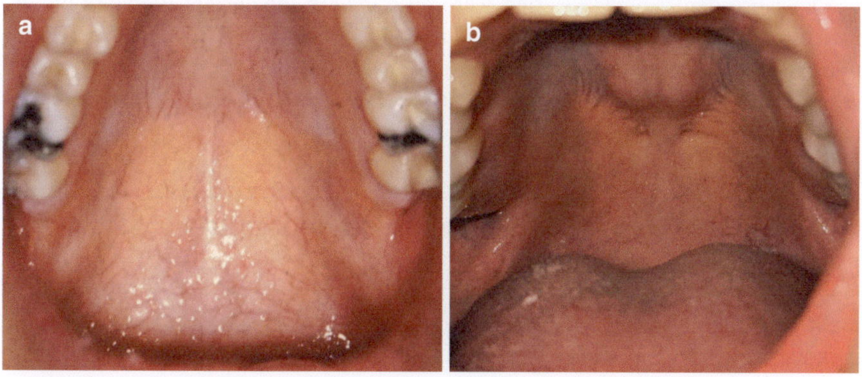

Fig. 17.9 (**a**, **b**). Yellowish pigmentation of the mucous membranes, especially in the soft palate and floor of the mouth, accompanied by marked hyperplasia of the palatine salivary glands (**a**) and the yellowish lesion, is represented by a hypercarotenaemia patch on the palatal mucosa in a young female patient with severe anorexia nervosa, malnutrition and high consumption of carotenoid-rich vegetables (**b**)

The term pica originates from the Latin name for the magpie—a bird rumoured to have a penchant for eating almost anything. There are many different subtypes of pica, such as trichophagia (eating of hair), geophagia (eating of dirt and soil) or even coprophagia (eating of faeces). In the case of trichophagia, ingested hair can form an indigestible mass (a trichobezoar) which is a potential cause of gastric outlet obstruction. Complications include obstruction, perforation and poisoning [21, 22]. Pica could be also associated with other mental disturbances such as autism and schizophrenia.

Although there is no evidence that pica presents with oral lesions fully associated with this condition, there are some cases in the literature where the ingestion of non-nutritive substances triggers pathogenic phenomena. Among these, a case of gingival enlargement, macrocheilia and Miescher's granulomatous cheilitis was associated with allergens resulting from ingesting a foreign substance in a patient with a pica-related eating disturbance [23].

17.5 Other Associated Oral Manifestations

In addition to the most common manifestations, there are other oral signs that dentists should consider:

- *Halitosis*: Patients with bulimia may suffer from chronic reflux due to recurrent vomiting episodes, contributing to damage to the oral, pharyngeal and oesophageal mucosa. Bad breath may result from several factors associated with eating disorders, including xerostomia, food debris remaining in the oral cavity after binge episodes and gastroesophageal reflux.

Other oro-dental outcomes that were described in the current literature among patients suffering from eating disorders included hypersensitivity, temporomandibular disorders, parafunctional habits and malocclusion. These individuals also reported a higher frequency of muscle disorders, facial pain, earache, headache and burning sensations in the mouth [3].

17.6 Importance of Early Recognition for Dentists

Dentists are uniquely positioned to detect the early signs of eating disorders, as many oral manifestations occur before the patient seeks medical help for systemic complications. Dental erosion, rampant caries, salivary gland hypertrophy (sialosis) and soft tissue lesions should alert oral health professionals to the potential presence of an underlying eating disorder. School-based programmes play a crucial role in early detection, where the involvement of school dental therapists and paediatric dentists is particularly important, as adolescents are a high-risk group for developing eating disorders. These professionals can serve as an early point of contact for identifying oral health signs and facilitating timely referrals to multidisciplinary care teams.

Early detection allows for timely intervention, prevention of irreversible oral damage and referral of the patient to a multidisciplinary team that includes psychologists, nutritionists and physicians. Early intervention improves the patient's oral health and can be a key factor in enhancing their overall health and well-being.

Training of dentists plays a critical role in the early identification and management of eating disorders. Incorporating a dedicated teaching topic on eating disorders within the dental curriculum is essential to equip future professionals with the knowledge and skills to recognise oral manifestations and provide appropriate care. Given these conditions' increasing prevalence, integrating this training into undergraduate and continuing education programmes is important. Additionally, web-based training for dentists can be an effective tool to ensure that dental professionals remain up-to-date with the latest knowledge and diagnostic strategies. Online platforms can offer flexible learning opportunities, enabling dentists to enhance their understanding of eating disorders, recognise the signs early and collaborate with multidisciplinary teams to benefit patients. By prioritising this training, dental professionals can play a significant role in improving outcomes for individuals with eating disorders [24].

17.7 Conclusion

The oral manifestations of eating disorders are numerous and varied, affecting both hard and soft tissues of the oral cavity. As part of the healthcare team, dentists play a critical role in the early recognition of these signs, facilitating prompt intervention. Accurate history-taking is essential in these cases, as patients may be reluctant to disclose their disordered eating behaviours due to feelings of shame. Dentists must approach these conversations with sensitivity and care, creating an environment where patients feel comfortable sharing vital information. A thorough history and awareness of the common oral symptoms associated with eating disorders enable dental professionals to identify potential issues early and make appropriate referrals for further evaluation and treatment. Collaborating with other healthcare professionals, comprehensive treatment of these patients can significantly improve long-term outcomes and quality of life.

References

1. Panico R, Piemonte E, Lazos J, Gilligan G, Zampini A, Lanfranchi H. Oral mucosal lesions in Anorexia Nervosa, Bulimia Nervosa and EDNOS. J Psychiatr Res. 2017;96:178–82.
2. Monda M, Costacurta M, Maffei L, Docimo R. Oral manifestations of eating disorders in adolescent patients. A review. Eur J Paediatr Dent junio de. 2021;22(2):155–8.
3. Valeriani L, Frigerio F, Piciocchi C, Piana G, Montevecchi M, Donini LM, et al. Oro-dental manifestations of eating disorders: a systematic review. J Eat Disord. 2024;12(1):87.

4. DSM Library [Internet]. [citado 13 de enero de 2025]. Diagnostic and statistical manual of mental disorders | psychiatry online. Disponible en.: https://psychiatryonline.org/doi/book/10.1176/appi.books.9780890425787
5. Rallis E, Lotsaris K, Grech VS, Tertipi N, Sfyri E, Kefala V. The nutrient–skin connection: diagnosing eating disorders through dermatologic signs. Nutrients. 2024;16(24):4354.
6. Forney KJ, Buchman-Schmitt JM, Keel PK, Frank GKW. The medical complications associated with purging. Int J Eat Disord. 2016;49(3):249–59.
7. Berrettini W. The genetics of eating disorders. Psychiatry (Edgmont). 2004;1(3):18–25.
8. Udo T, Grilo CM. Psychiatric and medical correlates of DSM-5 eating disorders in a nationally representative sample of adults in the United States. Int J Eat Disord. 2019;52(1):42–50.
9. Anderson K, Ismaila N, Flynn PJ, Halabi S, Jagannath S, Ogaily MS, et al. Role of bone-modifying agents in multiple myeloma: American Society of Clinical Oncology clinical practice guideline update. J Clin Oncol. 10 de marzo de. 2018;36(8):812–8.
10. Schlueter N, Glatzki J, Klimek J, Ganss C. Erosive-abrasive tissue loss in dentine under simulated bulimic conditions. Arch Oral Biol. 2012;57(9):1176–82.
11. Vieira Esteves C, Gushiken de Campos W, Gallo RT, Ebling Artes G, Shimabukuro N, Witzel AL, et al. Oral profile of eating disorders patients: case series. Spec Care Dentist. 2019;39(6):572–7.
12. Santoro V, Grulliero P, Tartaro GP, Colella G. A case of parotidomegaly associated with eating disorders (anorexia/bulimia). Minerva Stomatol. 1998;47(10):565–71.
13. Mitchell JE, Crow S. Medical complications of anorexia nervosa and bulimia nervosa. Curr Opin Psychiatry. 2006;19(4):438–43.
14. Giannini G, Gehrke SA, Tari SR, Lorusso F, Scarano A. Oral mucosae manifestation in patients with eating disorders: an overview. Annal Stomatol [Internet]. 2024. [citado 13 de enero de 2025];4(2) Disponible en: https://www.labpublishers.com/ann-stomatol/article/oral-mucosae-manifestation-in-patients-with-eating-disorders-an-overview/
15. Walsh K, Blalock DV, Mehler PS. Hematologic findings in a large sample of patients with anorexia nervosa and bulimia nervosa. Am J Hematol abril de. 2020;95(4):E98–101.
16. Salvado F, de Nobre MA, Gomes J, Maia P. Necrotizing Sialometaplasia and bulimia: a case report. Medicina (Kaunas). 2020;56(4):188.
17. Warnakulasuriya KA, Samaranayake LP, Peiris JS. Angular cheilitis in a group of Sri Lankan adults: a clinical and microbiologic study. J Oral Pathol Med. 1991;20(4):172–5.
18. Limeres J, Feijoo JF, Baluja F, Seoane JM, Diniz M, Diz P. Oral self-injury: an update. Dent Traumatol. 2013;29(1):8–14.
19. Robboy MS, Sato AS, Schwabe AD. The hypercarotenemia in anorexia nervosa: a comparison of vitamin A and carotene levels in various forms of menstrual dysfunction and cachexia. Am J Clin Nutr. 1974;27(4):362–7.
20. Priyadarshani AMB. Insights of hypercarotenaemia: a brief review. Clin Nutr ESPEN. 2018;23:19–24.
21. Khosravi M. Pica behaviors in schizophrenia: a call for further research. J Eat Disord. 2021;9(1):117.
22. Xiang H, Han J, Ridley WE, Ridley LJ. Pica: eating disorder. J Med Imaging Radiat Oncol. 2018;62(Suppl 1):97–8.
23. Dayanarayana U, Shastry SP, Kempegowda RT, Sridhar N, Kumar NN, Srinivasreddy MB. Management of Cheilitis Granulomatosa with pica disorder: a rare case report. Int J Clin Pediatr Dent. 2024;17(4):483–9.
24. DeBate RD, Severson H, Zwald ML, Shaw T, Christiansen S, Koerber A, et al. Development and evaluation of a web-based training program for oral health care providers on secondary prevention of eating disorders. J Dent Educ. 2009;73(6):718–29.

Obstructive Sleep Apnoea and Oral Health

18

Ananda P. Dasanayake, Dulip Ratnasoma, Meena Singh, Pankaj Singh, and Richard McGowan

18.1 Introduction

Obstructive sleep apnoea (OSA) is a serious sleep disorder characterised by repeated airway obstructions leading to systemic health risks and significant oral health implications. This cessation of breathing during sleep for various durations is a considerable problem, mainly in adults and, to some extent, in children. Continuous positive airway pressure (CPAP) machines are essential devices used to treat obstructive sleep apnoea (OSA). The US market for these devices has experienced notable growth over the past decade, driven by increasing awareness and diagnosis of sleep disorders. Forecasts indicate continued growth, with the US market expected to reach around $2.24 billion by 2030, reflecting a compound annual growth rate of 6.2%. In this chapter, we will discuss the epidemiology of sleep apnoea in relation to oral health, which are bidirectionally related, meaning certain oral structures can lead to OSA, and OSA and CPAP use, in return, can affect oral health.

A. P. Dasanayake (✉) · M. Singh
Department of Epidemiology & Health Promotion, New York University, New York, USA
e-mail: ad75@nyu.edu; ms13643@nyu.edu

D. Ratnasoma
First Physicians Group, Sarasota, FL, USA
e-mail: dRatnasoma@gmail.com; Dulip-ratnasoma@smh.com

P. Singh
APP-NEA, New York,, NY, USA

Advanced Dentistry of Long Island, Woodbury, NY, USA
e-mail: drpankajsingh@app-nea.com

R. McGowan
New York University Health Sciences Library, New York, NY, USA
e-mail: Richard.McGowan@nyulangone.org

S. R. Prabhu et al. (eds.), *Lifestyle in Oral Health and Disease*,
https://doi.org/10.1007/978-3-032-05888-1_18

18.2 Sleep Apnoea

The word apnoea comes from the Greek word ápnoia, which is composed of prefix—a, meaning without or lack of, and pnoē, meaning breath or breathing, so apnoea means without breath or cessation of breathing [1]. Obstructive sleep apnoea (OSA), a common and chronic medical condition, is one of over 70 sleep disorders characterised by repeated airway obstructions during sleep, involving hypopnoeas progressing into apnoea resulting in hypoxemia, excessive hypoventilation and respiratory effort-related arousals as a response to upper airway collapse [2]. Sleep apnoea is characterised by an obstructed airflow for 10 s or longer during sleep, accompanied by arterial oxygen desaturation of more than 4% above baseline [3]. These episodes of airway occlusion occur during sleep, when muscles surrounding the pharynx relax as a result of decreased neural tone. This muscle relaxation, in combination with a negative intrathoracic pressure, causes a collapse in the pharynx, blocking the airway. Most airway collapses last between 10 and 30 s, with some apnoeas lasting for more than a minute before the brain senses the lack of oxygen in the body and causes a brief arousal from sleep. This pattern can happen hundreds of times in one night and can lead to sudden reductions in blood oxygen levels, with blood oxygen concentration decreasing to 40% in severe cases [3].

During sleep, when the muscles at the back of the throat relax, the tongue falls back into the oropharynx when the patient is lying back. A crowded oropharynx secondary to enlarged tonsils or low draping soft palate blocking the airway, breathing stops and starts during sleep repeatedly. These breathing interruptions caused by repetitive upper airway collapses result from a combination of anatomical, physiological and lifestyle factors.

The most common type of apnoea is OSA, first described over 30 years ago [4], and has gained broad interest as several health-related conditions are implicated with it. If left untreated, it can lead to dementia, diminished neurocognitive function, decreased immune response to acute infections and chronic diseases, increased risk of motor vehicle accidents, reduced quality of life, hypertension, insulin resistance and cardiovascular diseases [5–7].

There are varying estimates of the commonality of OSA. In a systematic review, the overall global population prevalence of OSA ranged from 9 to 38%, according to 24 studies done in North America, Latin America, Europe, Australia, New Zealand and Asia [8]. OSA was higher in men and increased with increasing age, and in some elderly groups, it was as high as 90% in men and 78% in women. The reported occurrence of OSA in the overall adult population has increased over time as well, which has been correlated with rising rates of obesity [9].

18.3 Diagnostic Tools for OSA

The diagnosis of OSA relies on objective sleep studies. Polysomnography (PSG), the gold standard for diagnosis, is an overnight sleep study that records various physiological parameters to assess sleep architecture and breathing abnormalities

[2]. Key measurements in PSG include the apnoea–hypopnoea index (AHI), which quantifies the number of apnoea (complete airflow cessation for ≥10 s) and hypopnoea (partial airflow reduction of ≥30% with oxygen desaturation ≥3–4%) events per hour of sleep [10]. The oxygen desaturation index (ODI) tracks the frequency of oxygen drops ≥3% per hour, correlating with the severity of intermittent hypoxia [11]. PSG also records electroencephalography (EEG) to monitor brain activity and sleep stages, electromyography (EMG) to detect muscle activity and limb movements and electrooculography (EOG) to track eye movements, which is crucial for identifying rapid eye movement (REM) sleep. Additionally, thoracoabdominal respiratory effort is assessed using respiratory inductance plethysmography, while airflow is measured via nasal pressure transducers and thermistors. Combining these techniques helps differentiate between obstructive and central sleep apnoea, determine sleep efficiency and guide appropriate treatment recommendations. Despite PSG's comprehensive diagnostic capability, home sleep apnoea testing (HSAT) has emerged as a practical alternative for patients with a high likelihood of moderate to severe OSA. Unlike PSG, HSAT is conducted in a home setting and primarily focuses on measuring airflow, respiratory effort and oxygen saturation levels to confirm an OSA diagnosis [12]. While HSAT offers increased accessibility and cost-effectiveness, it may be less reliable in detecting mild OSA or distinguishing among different types of sleep-disordered breathing.

The apnoea–hypopnoea index, or AHI, is a key measure used to diagnose and assess the severity of OSA. It represents the average number of apnoea (complete stoppage of airflow) and hypopnoea (partial airway collapse) events per hour of sleep. For instance, if a person has 100 apnoea/hypopnoea events over 5 h of sleep, their AHI would be 100/5 or 20. Data from Switzerland [13] show that the median AHI was 6. 6.9 events per hour in women and 14. 9 per hour in men. The prevalence of moderate-to-severe sleep-disordered breathing (≥15 events per hour) was 23.4, 4% (95% confidence interval [CI]: 20. 9–26.0. 0) in women and 49.7. 7% (46.6–52. 8) in men.

Central sleep apnoea (CSA) is related to impaired brain signalling, leading to irregular breathing patterns. This occurs due to brainstem dysfunction [14]. When the brain fails to send the correct signals to the respiratory muscles, it can lead to CSA [15]. In addition, heart failure, stroke and other conditions affecting brain and heart function can increase the CSA risk. Certain medications such as opioids can also suppress the brain's breathing control, potentially causing CSA, as a direct relation is shown between the AHI and the daily dosage of methadone [16].

Among the symptoms of OSA are loud and persistent snoring, excessive daytime sleepiness, headaches in the morning, dry mouth or sore throat upon waking, bruxism or teeth grinding, difficulty concentrating and mood changes. Some of the oral health effects are discussed in detail below.

18.4 Causes of Sleep Apnoea

As previously mentioned, OSA is caused by partial or complete airway blockage during sleep, leading to repeated breathing pauses [17]. The known causes of OSA are a combination of anatomical, physiological, lifestyle, genetic and medical conditions. The main causes include the excessive relaxation of throat muscles during sleep, causing the airway to collapse and narrow airways due to enlarged tonsils, adenoids, enlarged tongue, enlarged uvula and low draping soft palate. Obesity contributes to fat deposits below the tongue and around the neck and throat, narrowing the airway [18, 19]. Some people naturally have a smaller airway, increasing their risk of collapse. Weak muscles in the throat, often due to aging or neurological conditions, can also contribute to airway obstruction.

18.5 Unmodifiable and Modifiable Risk Factors for Sleep Apnoea

Risk factors for OSA can be put into several categories, as below.

- Anatomical (e.g. enlarged tonsils, adenoids, a low-hanging soft palate or a retruded jaw can contribute to airway obstruction).
- Physiological (e.g. muscle tone, aging effects). Aging reduces upper airway muscle tone, increasing the likelihood of collapse.
- Lifestyle (e.g. obesity, alcohol use, smoking). Obesity increases fat deposits around the airway, alcohol relaxes throat muscles and smoking promotes inflammation, all of which raise OSA risk.

Age increases the risk of OSA due to reduced upper airway muscle tone and changes in fat distribution [20]. Men are two to three times more likely to have OSA, although the risk in women also rises after menopause. The occurrence of OSA shows a significant positive correlation with both age and obesity, affecting 90% of elderly men and 78% of elderly women [7]. OSA becomes increasingly common with age and varies between men and women.

Lifestyle and medical conditions such as alcohol and sedative use relax throat muscles, increase airway collapse [16] and can suppress the central arousal response leading to OSA [21]. Smoking causes inflammation in the respiratory tract and fluid retention in the airway, decreasing inspiratory effort and volume [22].

Sex and hormonal differences can also lead to OSA, as males are at higher risk than premenopausal females, possibly due to differences in fat distribution and hormonal protection in females. Family history, genetic predisposition to craniofacial abnormalities such as narrow mandible and maxilla and obesity are also important factors [23]. Genetic predisposition and family history increase the risk due to inherited traits like airway structure and fat distribution [15]. Nasal conditions such as deviated nasal septum, enlarged nasal turbinate, chronic nasal congestion and obstruction can increase airway resistance and predisposition to OSA [24].

Among the modifiable physical and biological risk factors are obesity, large neck circumference, enlarged tonsils or adenoids, nasal congestion, small/narrow jaws and recessed chin or retrognathia [25]. The most significant risk factor for OSA is obesity, which increases fat accumulation around the pharyngeal structures, leading to airway collapse [5, 26]. A large neck circumference greater than 17 inches (43 cm) in men and 16 inches (40 cm) in women also increases the risk [27]. Enlarged tonsils or adenoids are common in children with OSA [25]. Nasal congestion or chronic nasal obstruction from allergies or structural issues such as a deviated septum can worsen OSA. Small/narrow jaws, recessed chins or retrognathia affect airway size and stability, especially in children, where the effects can present as ADHD, excessive sleepiness in class and restlessness.

18.6 Dental/ Oral Causes

High lingual frenum contributes to impaired mandible growth, poor tongue function of swallowing and speech and dental crowding, all contributing to the risk of apnoeic events. Malocclusion and jaw structure are related to sleep apnoea as the jaw size position, and airway size is key factors in sleep apnoea. People with narrow jaws or setback mandibles are at higher risk. The palate is at the nasal base, and a narrow palate is typically seen in children with unilateral or bilateral dental crossbite. There is a high incidence of snoring and sleep apnoea in children. A narrow mandible typically leads to dental crowding and a narrow oral cavity where the tongue will rest above the occlusal plane and exhibit ridges (imprints of the lingual surfaces of the posterior mandibular teeth) on the lateral borders of the tongue, increasing the likelihood of tongue falling back into the oropharynx when supine and compounded with lack of neural tone during sleep, increases the risk for an apnoeic event.

While oral structures can influence OSA as described above, there are considerable oral health implications related to OSA as well. These include dry mouth or xerostomia caused by mouth breathing, a protective response to the physiologic need for maintaining aerobic cellular metabolism by sustainable blood oxygen saturation in the absence of nasal inspiration. Mouth breathing due to blocked airways increases the risk of cavities, gum disease and bad breath.

Bruxism or teeth grinding also often leads to the development of mandibular lingual tori and worn-down teeth, prone to tooth fracture, jaw and orofacial pain and temporomandibular joint (TMJ) disorders. Gastroesophageal reflux disease (GERD) is a common condition resulting from hypoventilation efforts putting pressure on the stomach, causing gastric acids to spill into the oesophagus and oral cavity right after an arousal event. It is linked to Barrett's oesophagus, erosion and enamel weakening. People with sleep apnoea are more prone to gum inflammation and periodontal disease due to an impaired immune response to chronic inflammation and dry mouth so that they may experience gum disease. Finally, oral appliance-related effects can also be seen in the mouth. Wearing oral appliances for sleep apnoea can be protective and decrease bruxism and TMJ-related symptoms. Still, if oral appliance therapy is not calibrated/titrated or not monitored properly, it can cause bite changes, tooth movement or TMJ issues, which are discussed later.

18.7 Sleep Apnoea and Other Diseases

OSA is strongly linked to various systemic health conditions. Understanding these connections is crucial for the holistic and overall management of OSA. Sleep apnoea increases the risk of severe cardiovascular conditions. Diabetes and hypertension are strongly associated with OSA as shown in a study from Switzerland [13] in which, after multivariable adjustment, the upper quartile for the AHI (>20.6 events per hour) was associated independently with the presence of hypertension (odds ratio: 1.60, 95% CI: 1.14–2.26; $p = 0.0292$ for trend across severity quartiles), diabetes (odds ratio: 2.00, 95% CI: 1.05–3.99; $p = 0.0467$), metabolic syndrome (odds ratio: 2.80, 95% CI: 1.86–4.29; $p < 0.0001$) and depression (odds ratio: 1·92, 95% CI: 1.01–3-64; $p = 0.0292$). Heart disease and stroke can both contribute to and result from OSA.

The repeated drops in oxygen during sleep lead to oxidative stress, inflammation and sympathetic nervous system activation, all of which can damage the cardiovascular system. Fifty per cent of sleep apnoea patients have high blood pressure. Atrial fibrillation (AFib) is strongly associated with untreated sleep apnoea [28]. Obstructive sleep apnoea doubles the risk of stroke and coronary artery disease and is the leading cause of stroke, heart attack and death during sleep [29]. Type 2 diabetes and metabolic syndrome are related to sleep apnoea [30] as it is an independent risk factor for insulin resistance and glucose intolerance. Poor sleep quality disrupts the production and release of certain hormones and metabolic processes, increasing the likelihood of obesity (nearly 70% of sleep apnoea patients are overweight or obese), dyslipidaemia or elevated cholesterol and triglyceride levels, and fatty liver disease, which is common in sleep apnoea due to chronic low oxygen levels. Cognitive decline and brain health are related to chronic oxygen deprivation, beta-amyloid plaque formation and fragmented sleep, which negatively affect brain health and function. Memory loss is linked to hippocampal atrophy, the brain area responsible for memory. Increased risk of Alzheimer's disease can be seen in sleep apnoea patients [31] as it may accelerate the buildup of beta-amyloid plaques. There is also a strong connection with mood disorders such as depression, anxiety and irritability.

Apnoea can also lead to oral and systemic inflammation as apnoea results in decreased immune function, which promotes a chronic inflammatory state that can worsen periodontal disease and vice versa. Cancer risk may also be higher among apnoea patients as the chronic intermittent hypoxia caused by sleep apnoea may promote tumour growth and metastasis, particularly in lung, breast and colon cancers. Immune system dysregulation is also affected by apnoea as poor sleep quality and can compromise immune function, making sleep apnoea patients more susceptible to infections and chronic inflammatory conditions. Sleep apnoea during pregnancy can increase the risk of gestational diabetes, pre-eclampsia and preterm birth and low birth weight, conditions that are also associated with poor oral health [32–35].

18.8 Sleep Apnoea and Oral Health

Dentists are often the first to identify sleep apnoea symptoms, and they can collaborate with sleep physicians for diagnosis and treatment. Dentists can also screen for apnoea and identify the individual risk factors such as enlarged tongue or tonsils, narrow or high-arched palate, dental crowding and lingually tipped mandibular posterior teeth, low draping soft palate, enlarged or elongated uvula, worn teeth from bruxism, mandibular lingual tori, TMJ disorders and jaw positioning issues. They can then recommend a home sleep study or an in-lab polysomnography to confirm the severity of sleep apnoea and when medically appropriate and based on practice parameters and guidelines set by the American Academy of Sleep Medicine and Dental Sleep Medicine [2], use oral appliance therapy such as mandibular advancement devices (MADs).

These custom-made devices are based on the fundamental premise that cardiopulmonary resuscitation (CPR) is highly effective in establishing and maintaining a patent upper airway by repositioning the jaw and, consequently, the tongue forward to prevent airway collapse. This approach is effective and comparable to CPAP therapy for mild-to-moderate sleep apnoea. It serves as a viable alternative for those who cannot tolerate CPAP machines, and before surgical interventions are considered. Limited evidence suggests long-term use of mandibular advancement devices (MAD) might improve comorbidities and healthcare outcomes. Adjunctive treatments, such as dentofacial orthopaedics and orthodontics, can expand the mandible and palate, enhancing nasal breathing and airway space. Myofunctional therapy, which includes tongue and facial muscle exercises, can strengthen the airway muscles. Additionally, as described below, surgical options such as orthognathic surgery or soft palate reduction may be necessary in severe cases.

18.9 Interventions

Mild, moderate and severe OSA based on OHI scores are shown in Table 18.1 with treatment options.

18.10 Continuous Positive Air Pressure or CPAP Machines and OSA

CPAP machines (Fig. 18.1) are highly effective for severe sleep apnoea when recommended. Still, they can cause oral health issues such as dry mouth, lip and gum irritation or swelling, risk of cavities due to changes in salivary flow and lip and mouth sores from the CPAP mask. Dentists often help manage these side effects by

Table 18.1 Mold, moderate, and severe OSA based on OHI scores

AHI Score	OSA severity	Symptoms
0–4.9	Normal	No significant airway obstruction
5–14.9	Mild[a]	Snoring & Occasional daytime sleepiness
15–29.9	Moderate[b]	Loud snoring, frequent awakening, daytime fatigue
>=30	Severe[b]	Oxygen desaturation, high risk of heart disease & daytime sleepiness

[a]Mild: May not always need CPAP. Life cycle changes can help
[b]Moderate to Severe: AHI>15, usually requires CPAP or another treatment

Fig. 18.1 Oral appliances: continuous positive air pressure machine

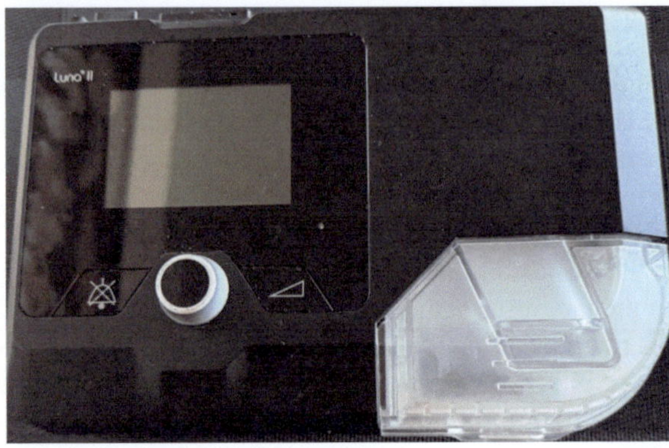

prescribing saliva substitutes, fluoride treatments and other oral health interventions. When it comes to treating sleep apnoea, oral appliances and surgery are key alternatives or adjuncts to CPAP, especially for those who cannot tolerate CPAP. Oral appliances are considered the best nonsurgical and reversible treatment option for mild-to-moderate sleep apnoea, especially for patients who cannot tolerate CPAP. Surgery is ideal for severe sleep apnoea or when anatomical abnormalities are the primary cause. In some cases, combining multiple treatments—such as oral appliances, CPAP, surgery and lifestyle changes—yields the best outcomes.

CPAP users should check their mask fit regularly as a poorly fitted mask can cause air leaks, increasing mouth breathing and dryness. This can be prevented by working with the sleep therapist or provider to adjust the fit and reduce side effects. Mask choices are numerous as well. For those who primarily breathe through the mouth, a full-face mask (covering both nose and mouth) may help prevent dry mouth. In any event, seeing the dentist regularly (every 6 months or more often if needed) to discuss CPAP use can help them monitor for signs of dry mouth, cavities or gum disease. Those who experience mouth sores, gum irritation or signs of infection, their sleep doctor and the dentist can intervene quickly.

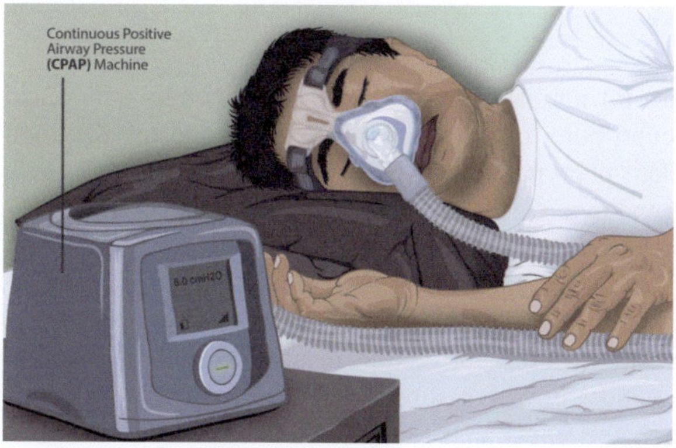

18.11 Oral Appliances: Continuous Positive Air Pressure Machine

Oral appliances for sleep apnoea are patient-specific, custom-made and worn during sleep to help keep the airway open by repositioning the jaw, tongue or soft tissues. These include mandibular advancement devices (MADs), the most common type for sleep apnoea [36]. These appliances move the mandible slightly forward to prevent airway collapse, resembling a sports mouthguard or orthodontic retainer. Among the pros of these devices are that they are comfortable and easy to use compared to CPAP, effective for mild-to-moderate obstructive sleep apnoea, and non-motorised, portable and silent. However, they are not without cons, such as jaw pain, tooth movement or bite changes over time, and these devices are not as effective for severe sleep apnoea. These side effects are easily mitigated by properly fitted and titrated oral appliance, a morning repositioner/aligner and periodic follow-ups. Tongue retaining devices (TRDs) hold the tongue forward to prevent it from blocking the airway and are often recommended for patients who are edentulous or with fewer than three teeth per quadrant, with large tongues or those who cannot tolerate MADs. Among the pros of TRDs is that they have a simple design, and no jaw repositioning is required. Among the cons are that they are less comfortable than MADs for some users and might cause drooling or tongue soreness. The oral appliances are made after a thorough initial evaluation where the dentist examines the airway, jaw structure and teeth and takes custom impressions using either digital scans or physical moulds of teeth and a construction bite that defines the protrusive and vertical position of the jaws for the lab to fabricate the oral appliance. Then, as in dentures, the appliance is fitted and adjusted for maximum comfort and effectiveness, followed by regular check-ups to monitor for bite changes, appliance wear or TMJ issues.

Combination therapy is better for some patients when oral appliances are used along with CPAP at lower pressures or adjunctive therapies like myofunctional therapy.

18.12 Surgical Options

Surgery is considered when oral appliances and CPAP fail or when anatomical abnormalities significantly contribute to airway obstruction. Among the common surgical options is uvulo-palato-pharyngoplasty (UPPP), in which excess tissue is removed from the soft palate and uvula to widen the airway. This method effectively reduces snoring and mild sleep apnoea but may cause swallowing difficulties or changes in voice. Genioglossus advancement (GA) is the tongue repositioning by pulling the tongue muscle attachment forward, preventing airway collapse and is often combined with other procedures for better results. Maxillomandibular advancement (MMA) is the most effective surgical treatment for moderate-to-severe sleep apnoea in which the upper and lower jaws are moved forward to increase airway space. It has shown a high success rate (up to 90%), but recovery can take longer. Hypoglossal nerve stimulation (inspire therapy) is an implantable device that stimulates the hypoglossal nerve, keeping the tongue from blocking the airway. It is activated during sleep with a remote control. This technique is minimally invasive with a growing success rate. Septoplasty and turbinate reduction can correct a deviated nasal septum or reduce enlarged turbinates to improve nasal breathing. They are often combined with other treatments for sleep apnoea. Finally, tonsillectomy and adenoidectomy are common in children with sleep apnoea caused by enlarged tonsils or adenoids, and these significantly improve airway and breathing.

18.13 The Dentist's Role in Systemic Health

Considering the significant overlap between oral health conditions and systemic health issues, dentists are essential in identifying at-risk patients and referring them to specialists for diagnosis and, when medically appropriate, for the overall management of sleep apnoea patients.

The dentist's role is essential as CPAP therapy can also lead to oral health issues like dry mouth, gum irritation and an increased risk of cavities. Dry mouth or xerostomia is usually due to reduced salivary flow that can lead to cavities, gum disease and bad breath. A dry mouth makes growing bacteria easier, leading to tooth decay. The air pressure or friction from the CPAP mask usually causes gum inflammation or irritation. Mouth sores or ulcers occur due to poorly fitting masks or straps. CPAP therapy can also result in retrusion of the anterior maxillary teeth and impaired maxillary growth and development, especially in the paediatric patient. Among the ways of reducing these risks are regular dental checkups to identify the oral symptoms related to sleep apnoea early, maintaining good oral hygiene by brushing teeth twice a day and flossing daily, using fluoride toothpaste and mouthwash to prevent cavities, and staying hydrated to combat dry mouth. Custom night guards can help with bruxism and protect teeth from damage. Collaborating among specialists such as sleep doctors, ENT specialists, dentists and orthodontists for comprehensive care is often advisable.

18.14 Oral Healthcare in Sleep Apnoea Patients

Oral healthcare tips for CPAP users include staying hydrated by drinking plenty of water throughout the day and avoiding alcohol and caffeine, which can worsen dry mouth. A humidifier may be necessary unless the CPAP machine has a built-in humidifier. Increased humidity can reduce dry mouth and nasal irritation. A heated humidifier may provide even more moisture. Maintaining excellent oral hygiene, even with the above measures, is essential. Patients should brush twice a day with fluoride toothpaste, floss daily to remove plaque between teeth or use microinterdental brushes, use a fluoride mouthwash or prescription fluoride gel to strengthen teeth and prevent cavities and use an alcohol-free mouthwash to avoid further drying. To overcome xerostomia, one can try over-the-counter saliva substitutes. Evidence shows that xylitol-based products may also promote saliva flow and prevent cavities.

18.15 Conclusion

In conclusion, OSA is a growing problem in the ageing population that can lead to many unwanted comorbidities. Several modifiable risk factors can be corrected. Treatment options are many, and teams of specialists can help OSA patients lead comfortable lives. There are also clear guidelines to follow regarding OSA and the chosen treatment modalities.

References

1. Demko BG. The history behind the mechanics of Oral appliance therapy for treating obstructive sleep apnea. J Dent Sleep Med. 2019;6(1)
2. AASM. Obstructive sleep apnea. In: Obstructive Sleep Apnea; 2008. 2025(February 20).
3. Eckert DJ, Malhotra A. Pathophysiology of adult obstructive sleep apnea. Proc Am Thorac Soc. 2008;5(2):144–53.
4. Young T, Palta M, Dempsey J, Skatrud J, Weber S, Badr S. The occurrence of sleep-disordered breathing among middle-aged adults. N Engl J Med. 1993;328(17):1230–5.
5. Young T, Skatrud J, Peppard PE. Risk factors for obstructive sleep apnea in adults. JAMA. 2004;291(16):2013–6.
6. George CF. Sleep apnea, alertness, and motor vehicle crashes. Am J Respir Crit Care Med. 2007;176(10):954–6.
7. Heinzer R, Petitpierre NJ, Marti-Soler H, Haba-Rubio J. Prevalence and characteristics of positional sleep apnea in the HypnoLaus population-based cohort. Sleep Med. 2018;48:157–62.
8. Senaratna CV, Perret JL, Lodge CJ, Lowe AJ, Campbell BE, Matheson MC, et al. Prevalence of obstructive sleep apnea in the general population: a systematic review. Sleep Med Rev. 2017;34:70–81.
9. Peppard PE, Young T, Barnet JH, Palta M, Hagen EW, Hla KM. Increased prevalence of sleep-disordered breathing in adults. Am J Epidemiol. 2013;177(9):1006–14.
10. Ruehland WR, Rochford PD, O'Donoghue FJ, Pierce RJ, Singh P, Thornton AT. The new AASM criteria for scoring hypopneas: impact on the apnea hypopnea index. Sleep. 2009;32(2):150–7.

11. Varghese L, Rebekah G, Priya N, Oliver A, Kurien R. Oxygen desaturation index as alternative parameter in screening patients with severe obstructive sleep apnea. Sleep Sci. 2022;15(Spec 1):224–8.
12. Kapur VK, Auckley DH, Chowdhuri S, Kuhlmann DC, Mehra R, Ramar K, et al. Clinical practice guideline for diagnostic testing for adult obstructive sleep apnea: an American Academy of sleep medicine clinical practice guideline. J Clin Sleep Med. 2017;13(3):479–504.
13. Heinzer R, Vat S, Marques-Vidal P, Marti-Soler H, Andries D, Tobback N, et al. Prevalence of sleep-disordered breathing in the general population: the HypnoLaus study. Lancet Respir Med. 2015;3(4):310–8.
14. Rajeswari J, Jagannath M. Brain connectivity analysis based classification of obstructive sleep apnea using electroencephalogram signals. Sci Rep. 2024;14(1):5561.
15. Redline S, Young T. Epidemiology and natural history of obstructive sleep apnea. Ear Nose Throat J. 1993;72(1):20–1. 4–6
16. Webster LR, Choi Y, Desai H, Webster L, Grant BJ. Sleep-disordered breathing and chronic opioid therapy. Pain Med. 2008;9(4):425–32.
17. Dempsey JA, Xie A, Patz DS, Wang D. Physiology in medicine: obstructive sleep apnea pathogenesis and treatment—considerations beyond airway anatomy. J Appl Physiol. 2014;116(1):3–12.
18. Peppard PE, Young T, Palta M, Skatrud J. Prospective study of the association between sleep-disordered breathing and hypertension. N Engl J Med. 2000;342(19):1378–84.
19. Choudhury N, Deshmukh P. Obstructive sleep apnea in adults and ear, nose, and throat (ENT) health: a narrative review. Cureus. 2023;15(10):e47637.
20. Vgontzas AN, Li Y, He F, Fernandez-Mendoza J, Gaines J, Liao D, et al. Mild-to-moderate sleep apnea is associated with incident hypertension: age effect. Sleep. 2019;42(4):zsy265.
21. Issa FG, Sullivan CE. Alcohol, snoring and sleep apnea. J Neurol Neurosurg Psychiatry. 1982;45(4):353–9.
22. Ioannidou D, Kalamaras G, Kotoulas SC, Pataka A. Smoking and obstructive sleep apnea: is there an association between these Cardiometabolic risk factors?–gender analysis. Medicina. 2021;57(1137):1–13.
23. Redline S, Tishler PV, Tosteson TD, Williamson J, Kump K, Browner I, et al. The familial aggregation of obstructive sleep apnea. Am J Respir Crit Care Med. 1995;151(3 Pt 1):682–7.
24. Kim HY, Jeong JI, Dhong HJ, Sohn JH, Hong SD, Kim JH, et al. Nasal obstruction and palate-tongue position on sleep-disordered breathing. Clin Exp Otorhinolaryngol. 2013;6(4):226–30.
25. Mangat D, Orr WC, Smith RO. Sleep apnea, hypersomnolence, and upper airway obstruction secondary to adenotonsillar enlargement. Arch Otolaryngol. 1977;103(7):383–6.
26. Young T, Peppard PE, Gottlieb DJ. Epidemiology of obstructive sleep apnea: a population health perspective. Am J Respir Crit Care Med. 2002;165(9):1217–39.
27. Davies RJ, Stradling JR. The relationship between neck circumference, radiographic pharyngeal anatomy, and the obstructive sleep apnoea syndrome. Eur Respir J. 1990;3(5):509–14.
28. Gami AS, Pressman G, Caples SM, Kanagala R, Gard JJ, Davison DE, et al. Association of atrial fibrillation and obstructive sleep apnea. Circulation. 2004;110(4):364–7.
29. Redline S, Yenokyan G, Gottlieb DJ, Shahar E, O'Connor GT, Resnick HE, et al. Obstructive sleep apnea-hypopnea and incident stroke: the sleep heart health study. Am J Respir Crit Care Med. 2010;182(2):269–77.
30. Liu J, Xu J, Guan S, Wang W. Effects of different treatments on metabolic syndrome in patients with obstructive sleep apnea: a meta-analysis. Front Med (Lausanne). 2024;11:1354489.
31. Andrade AG, Bubu OM, Varga AW, Osorio RS. The relationship between obstructive sleep apnea and Alzheimer's disease. J Alzheimer's Dis. 2018;64(s1):S255–S70.
32. Facco FL, Parker CB, Reddy UM, Silver RM, Koch MA, Louis JM, et al. Association between sleep-disordered breathing and hypertensive disorders of pregnancy and gestational diabetes mellitus. Obstet Gynecol. 2017;129(1):31–41.
33. Chokwiriyachit A, Dasanayake AP, Suwannarong W, Hormdee D, Sumanonta G, Prasertchareonsuk W, et al. Periodontitis and gestational diabetes mellitus in non-smoking females. J Periodontol. 2013;84(7):857–62.

34. Dasanayake AP, Chhun N, Tanner AC, Craig RG, Lee MJ, Moore AF, et al. Periodontal pathogens and gestational diabetes mellitus. J Dent Res. 2008;87(4):328–33.
35. Dasanayake AP. Poor periodontal health of the pregnant woman as a risk factor for low birth weight. Ann Periodontol. 1998;3(1):206–12.
36. Yu M, Ma Y, Han F, Gao X. Long-term efficacy of mandibular advancement devices in the treatment of adult obstructive sleep apnea: a systematic review and meta-analysis. PLoS One. 2023;18(11):e0292832.

Risky Sexual Behaviour and Oral Health 19

Siddharth Sarkar, Rajkumar Sanahan, and S. R. Prabhu

19.1 Risky Sexual Behaviours

Risky sexual behaviours have traditionally been defined as those associated with higher chances of pregnancy or higher chances of transmission of sexually transmitted infections (STIs) [1]. While precisely defining risky sexual behaviour may be challenging, risky sexual behaviours include actions such as having multiple sexual partners, interacting with sex workers and engaging in sexual activities with individuals who inject drugs, as these increase the risk of STIs. Additionally, scenarios like unprotected sex and sex influenced by substances also fall under the category of risky sexual behaviours [2–7].

Risky sexual behaviour is not always dangerous; it simply increases risk. This increase in risk implies that some risk may already exist. Additionally, uncertainty remains regarding whether the sexual act may result in adverse consequences, such as sexually transmitted infections. Defining absolutes is challenging in this context. The 'risk appetite' also plays a role, since life (and sexual intercourse) probably often presents risks worth taking. Nonetheless, risky sexual behaviours are an important construct from a public health perspective, as they can sometimes lead to health damage and necessitate care. In times of accelerated human immunodeficiency virus (HIV) spread, determining and reducing risk hold pragmatic value. When a significant portion of the community engages in high-risk sexual behaviour,

S. Sarkar (✉) · R. Sanahan
National Drug Dependence Treatment Centre, All India Institute of Medical Sciences, New Delhi, India

S. R. Prabhu
School of Dentistry, University of Queensland, Brisbane, QLD, Australia
e-mail: r.prabhu@uq.edu.au

S. R. Prabhu et al. (eds.), *Lifestyle in Oral Health and Disease*,
https://doi.org/10.1007/978-3-032-05888-1_19

the overall risk of contracting STIs becomes a public health issue that must be addressed [8].

Apart from the public health aspect, other lenses can be used to examine risky sexual behaviours. One of these is the moral and religious perspective, where many such behaviours are proscribed [9]. Another lens is popular or 'pop' culture, wherein certain sexual behaviours that were previously abhorred are subsequently normalised. Yet another lens is a subaltern expression of hedonism, where risky sexual experiences are desired or celebrated [10, 11]. Substances of abuse often reduce inhibitions and cloud judgement, leading to risky sexual behaviours [6].

This chapter discusses the oral health manifestations of risky sexual behaviours, the direct effects of oral sexual behaviours (both infectious and non-infectious) and the indirect effects of risky sex on oral health.

19.2 Risky Oral Sexual Behaviours and Oral Health Vulnerabilities

Sexual acts that involve stimulating the genitalia with the mouth, teeth, tongue or throat are referred to as oral sex [12]. Partners of all sexual orientations, both homosexual and heterosexual, frequently engage in oral sex, which can occur as part of foreplay, and during or after sexual activity.

Three kinds of oral sex [12–14] exist, namely:

- Cunnilingus (refers to oral vaginal contact): Stimulation of the vagina or the vulva of a woman, especially her clitoris, using lips and tongue by the partner.
- Fellatio (refers to oral penile contact): Stimulation of penis of a man through licking or sucking by the partner's mouth.
- Analingus (refers to oral anal contact): Stimulation of anus of a sexual partner using tongue or lips.

People of any sexual orientation can engage in oral sex. According to reports, over 85% of sexually active adults between the ages of 18 and 44 have had at least one oral sexual encounter with a partner of the opposite sex, compared to 41% of teenagers aged 15–19 years [15]. A sizable fraction of teenagers participates in oral sex and other noncoital sexual practices. Research shows that between 14% and 50% of teenagers engaged in oral sex before their first sexual encounter, that oral sex is more common than vaginal sex and that few teenagers use barrier protection during oral sex [16–21].

Sexually transmitted infections (STIs) can result from oral sex, but pregnancy does not. Adults and teenagers who engage in oral sex must be aware that it is linked to HIV and other STIs, including gonorrhoea [22, 23], herpes [24], syphilis [25] and HIV [26]. Oral sex can also potentially spread human papillomavirus virus (HPV) [23] and chlamydia [23] infections.

The oral cavity and oral mucosa harbour several distinct types of microbiota. Many of these are commensals and non-pathogenic. However, they may become pathogenic if present in excessive numbers. Generally, intact mucous membranes protect the body from infections caused by harmful microbes, such as those leading to STIs. A virus can enter systemic circulation through various channels in the oral cavity, acting as entry points for infections from the mouth to the bloodstream, including abrasions, wounds, open sores and bleeding gum disease (gingivitis, periodontitis) [27]. Pre-cum, semen, vaginal fluids, menstrual blood and even saliva can be introduced into the mouth during oral sex [28]. The risk of infection increases with the quantity of these bodily fluids to which one is exposed. Factors associated with heightened rates of transmission of infections through the oral route include having multiple sexual partners and sustaining injuries or abrasions during the sexual act [27, 29]. Furthermore, it is well recognized that oral ulcers, such as those caused by an STI, heighten the risk of acquiring and transmitting HIV [30]. Patients with an STI may initially present with lesions in the oral cavity, which can be noticeable and can impede speech or swallowing, among other basic tasks. It is crucial to remember that STIs manifesting in the oral cavity are often asymptomatic, creating opportunities for future transmission of infections. Consequently, oral health can be affected by risky oral sexual behaviours [12, 28, 31–35]. Generally, the rates of transmission of various blood-borne viruses are significantly lower through oral sexual contact, but the risk still exists.

19.3 Oral Bacterial Infections Due to Risky Oral Sexual Behaviours

19.3.1 Syphilis

Treponema pallidum is the causative agent of syphilis, primarily spread through sexual contact. Chancres develop where the bacterium has penetrated the mucosa and typically occur in the anogenital area. Occasionally, they may also appear in the oral mucosa, presumably as a consequence of unprotected sexual intercourse. The chancres are painless, indurated ulcers that are infective and last for about 4 weeks. Lymphadenopathy may also accompany chancres. Although chancres are more common in the anogenital region, 12–14% of cases have been documented in extragenital areas [36]. Of these, between 40% and 75% are thought to arise in the mouth [37], with extragenital primary syphilis most commonly occurring in the oral mucosa. With a reported transmission rate of 18–80% during sexual contact, oral lesions in this context are extremely contagious [38].

Analingus, cunnilingus and fellatio are frequent oral sex modes of transmission [12]. Secondary syphilis may also have oral manifestations, which are polymorphous, like condyloma lata, that develop in the vicinity of the primary chancre. The oral manifestations of secondary syphilis may not necessarily result from oral sex. Tertiary syphilis is rare and presents with gumma, which are granulomatous lesions with a necrotic core that may range from a few millimetres to a centimetre in diameter. Oral intercourse is not directly linked to the development of secondary or tertiary syphilis symptoms [38].

19.3.2 Chlamydia Trachomatis

Chlamydia trachomatis serovars L1–L3 are the causative agents of lymphogranuloma venereum, a systemic illness transmitted through sexual contact. Proctitis is often associated with lymphogranuloma venereum; however, documented cases of infections in other sites, including the urethra and pharynx, have been reported [39, 40]. Consequently, a pharyngeal venereal lymphogranuloma may act as an infection reservoir [37, 40]. These chlamydia serovars can lead to pharyngeal infections, which may present with nonspecific symptoms such as sore throats, cervical adenopathies, odynophagia or tongue ulcers [40]. Conversely, lesions in the pharynx are rare, and pharyngeal *C. trachomatis* infections typically remain asymptomatic [41]. Chlamydial infections do not exhibit specific oral symptoms.

Fellatio, cunnilingus and analingus are common forms of oral sex transmission [12]. Infertility is known to result from genital tract chlamydia infection, and recent research suggests that oral sex may also be associated with this undesirable outcome. Chlamydia transmitted through oral sex colonise the gastrointestinal tract, where they remain undetected by the human host and are tolerated by the immune system for extended periods. This could lead to pelvic inflammatory disease and other serious side effects [42].

In these situations, molecular biology methods can be used to identify *C. trachomatis* in the oropharynx. Since pharyngeal chlamydia is far less prevalent than pharyngeal gonorrhoea [43], several nations advise screening for pharyngeal *C. trachomatis* in specific circumstances; however, it is not a widely accepted practice globally [43, 44]. A study revealed that 53% of men who have sex with men (MSM) and 32% of female patients with pharyngeal *C. trachomatis* did not also have an anogenital *C. trachomatis* infection, underscoring the potential for missing cases if screening is restricted to the anogenital area [44]. Prospective research is needed to assess the necessity and financial viability of routine screening for non-rectal lymphogranuloma venereum among MSM.

19.3.3 Neisseria Gonorrhoeae

The organism causing gonorrhoea, a sexually transmitted infection, is *Neisseria gonorrhoeae*. It is associated with ectopic pregnancy and tubal infertility in women, urethritis and proctitis in men, and increased HIV susceptibility and transmissibility in both sexes [45]. The columnar epithelium of the cervix and urethra, along with the transitional epithelium of the oropharynx and rectum, are common entry points for gonorrhoea infection, although the stratified squamous epithelium that constitutes the skin and the mucosal lining of the oral cavity appears to be more resistant to *N. gonorrhoeae* [37].Since the first description of oropharyngeal colonisation by *N. gonorrhoeae* in 1944, numerous investigations have been conducted on this topic.

Oropharyngeal infection with *N. gonorrhoeae* is less frequent than genital colonisation, but it can still present as pharyngitis, tonsillitis, gingivitis, stomatitis or glossitis [46, 47]. It is crucial to remember that only 15% of people with pharyngeal gonococcal infections exhibit symptoms, including sore throats and cervical adenopathies; the majority of cases are asymptomatic. Molecular biology methods are the most effective means of detecting *N. gonorrhoeae* in the oropharynx of asymptomatic patients [47]. When symptoms are present, acute ulcerative inflammation, which is quite painful, is typically the outcome of a gonococcal infection of the oral cavity; these numerous ulcers are accompanied by non-adherent pseudo-particles, a bright red oral mucosa that bleeds readily and pseudo-membranes that can be yellow, grey or white. These lesions are nonspecific and present a broad differential diagnosis, including immune-bullous diseases, erythema multiforme and herpes simplex virus (HSV) infection [27, 38]. According to recent investigations, extragenital *N. gonorrhoeae* infections are significantly more common among MSM. The risk of complications and potential disease reservoirs increases when gonococcal infections at anorectal or oropharyngeal areas go undetected, as they are generally asymptomatic and often occur without a concurrent urogenital infection [30]. In addition to behavioural risk factors for both STIs (such as having multiple sexual partners and insufficient condom use), gonococcal infections at extragenital sites are thought to facilitate HIV transmission and/or acquisition due to a higher biological susceptibility to inflammation and immunosuppression [30].

The most common mode of oral sex transmission for gonorrhoea is fellatio [12]. The International Union against Sexually Transmitted Infections (IUSTI) [48] and the Centers for Disease Control and Prevention (CDC) [49] typically recommend screening for oropharyngeal and/or anorectal gonorrhoea in MSM based on reported histories of anal and/or oral sexual encounters. Other organizations, however, suggest annual screening for MSM at all sites (or every 3–6 months for high-risk MSM).

19.4 Oral Viral Infections Due to Risky Oral Sexual Behaviours

19.4.1 Human Papillomavirus Virus (HPV)

HPV is transmitted from the genitalia to the oral cavity through orogenital contact. HIV can cause squamous cell carcinoma, condylomata acuminata, oral warts and squamous papillomas in the mouth. Low-risk HPV subtypes 6 and 11 are responsible for condylomata acuminata because they are less likely to lead to squamous cell carcinoma. These are benign lesions that primarily affect the anogenital area, although they may also be found in the oral mucosa due to sexual contact. HPV subtypes such as 16, 18, 31 and 33 are associated with an increased risk of cervical cancers, as well as other penile, oropharyngeal and anal cancers. Oropharyngeal squamous cell carcinomas (OPSCCs) are linked to HPV-16. Having multiple sex partners and engaging in oral sex are examples of high-risk sexual behaviours associated with HPV-related oropharyngeal squamous cell carcinomas. There is a slight risk of contracting hepatitis C and HPV infection during receptive orogenital intercourse [12].

Previous research has established a strong and now recognized link between oropharyngeal HPV infection and oral sex [50]. The majority of patients with HPV-associated oropharyngeal squamous cell carcinomas are white men under 60 who have minimal tobacco exposure, good performance status and high-risk sexual practices such as having multiple partners and engaging in more oral sex [27, 29, 51]. Oral intercourse with multiple partners, a history of prior sexually transmitted infections or HPV-related genital cancer, marijuana use starting at a younger age, ongoing immunosuppression (such as being HIV-positive) and possibly a French kiss are also considered risk factors [52]. It is believed that HPV-positive OPSCC is a sexually acquired condition contracted through direct orogenital contact. The number of oral sex partners a patient has had throughout their life is the greatest risk factor for HPV-positive OPSCC patients. HPV infects the basal epithelial cells through mucosal sores or abrasions [53]. Fellatio, cunnilingus and analingus are common modes of oral sex transmission [12].

19.4.2 Herpes Simplex Virus (HSV)

Herpes labialis is primarily caused by the type 1 herpes simplex virus (HSV). Typically, childhood mucocutaneous contact with an infected individual leads to primary infections. The virus remains dormant in the sensory ganglia after the initial infection. Reactivation can occur spontaneously or in response to stress. Fever, sore throat and painful vesicles in the gingival and buccal mucosa are common clinical manifestations. Dysphagia and lymphadenopathy may occasionally accompany gingivostomatitis. HSV-2 primarily causes genital herpes, but it can also sometimes produce oral herpes, which is similar to HSV-1 in its presentation. Sexual contact is the main route of HSV-2 transmission, mostly occurring among young adults and can result in genital or, less frequently, oral lesions [38]. A significant risk factor for HSV-1 acquisition is insertional orogenital contact. Fellatio, cunnilingus and analingus are common modes of oral sex transmission [12].

19.4.3 Molluscum Contagiosum

Molluscum contagiosum (MC) is caused by a poxvirus transmitted through autoinoculation, sexual contact or via fomites. In adults, the lesions of molluscum contagiosum are located at the site of inoculation and typically arise from oral and anal sexual intercourse. Commonly found on the lips and in the perioral areas, the lesions may also occasionally appear on the palate and buccal mucosa. In individuals with HIV, the lesions can be widespread and typically present in clusters [12].

19.4.4 HIV (Human Immunodeficiency Virus)

HIV is a well-known sexually transmitted infection, but concerning sexual transmission, it is recognised that oral sex has a very low risk of HIV infection than other sexual practices. Patients should be informed, however, that there is a possibility of orogenital transmission [37, 54]. Cunnilingus, fellatio and analingus are common modes of oral sex transmission of HIV [12].

Numerous factors are likely linked to the biological risk of HIV transmission or acquisition through oral sexual contact. These include the integrity and mechanical characteristics of the sexual mucosa, mucosal immunity, local inhibitory factors, the presence or absence of cofactors that may facilitate transmission, the presence or absence of the virus at sexual sites (oral, vaginal, anal and penile) and the viral load (if present). The significance of oral sex in HIV transmission depends on several factors, including the prevalence of HIV in the community where oral sex occurs, the infectivity of oral secretions and how oral pathology influences them, resistance to infection from inhibitory compounds in saliva, the role of high-activity antiretroviral therapy, the extent to which personal prophylaxis is practised and the relative frequency of oral sex compared to other activities [55].

The most frequently reported sexual activity among patients with a first HIV infection was unprotected oral–genital contact. In every situation, receptive anal intercourse was found to be more dangerous than insertive anal intercourse, which was, in turn, deemed more dangerous than oral sex, while oral sex with ejaculation was considered riskier than oral sex without ejaculation [56]. According to the available data, orogenital intercourse between the penis and the mouth, as well as between the vagina and the mouth, may spread HIV. Although it seems less likely, case reports reveal an apparent risk of transmission from the mouth to the penis. Compared to vaginal and anal intercourse, the risk of HIV transmission via orogenital contact is significantly lower [12].

19.5 Other Infections/Conditions Associated with Risky Oral Sexual Behaviours

19.5.1 Nonspecific Urethritis (NSU)

NSU may cause penile discharge or a burning sensation during urination. The modes of transmission for oral sex include fellatio and cunnilingus. A sore throat can indicate a throat infection. HIV may spread more easily if NSU increases the viral load in semen [12].

19.5.2 Hepatitis A and E

Analingus, or oral sex, is a means of spreading both of these diseases. Both hepatitis A and hepatitis E are infectious viral liver illnesses. Fever, loss of appetite, diarrhoea, vomiting, black urine, jaundice and abdominal pain are typical signs of hepatitis. There is a vaccine for prevention [23].

19.5.3 Hepatitis B

Most frequently, infected blood is used to spread the virus; virus particles are present in blood, semen, stool and saliva. There is undeniable evidence that the virus can be transmitted through vaginal and anal intercourse, but it remains unproven if it can be transmitted through oral sex (fellatio, cunnilingus and analingus). Common presenting complaints include weakness, jaundice (yellowing of skin and eyes), dark urine and an enlarged liver. Vaccination is available for prevention [23].

19.5.4 Bowel Organisms and Worms

Shigella, *Campylobacter* and *Salmonella* can spread through analingus or oral sex. Diarrhoea and abdominal pain are initial symptoms. Following a microbiological stool analysis, treatment is administered [12].

19.5.5 Intestinal Parasites

These include *Cryptosporidium*, *Giardia* and *Amoeba*. Analingus, or oral sex, may be the means of transmission. Unknown diarrhoea, stomach cramps, bloating, increased gas and nausea are some of the symptoms. Following a microbiological stool analysis, treatment is administered [12].

19.6 Oral Non-infective Conditions Due to Risky Oral Sexual Behaviours

Due to their often asymptomatic nature, the danger of oral traumatic lesions linked to oral intercourse seems to have received less attention. The patient may not recognise the aetiology of the lesions until they become symptomatic. The doctor might not obtain an oral sex history even if the patient is aware of the cause of the oral sores. A few reports of oral sex-related traumatic lesions exist in the dentistry [57–59] and medical [60–63] literature. Although fellatio-related palatal lesions have been observed in individuals aged 18–59, they have primarily affected young women in their early 20s [57, 59]. Additionally, young children, typically around the age of three, have been reported to have mouth lesions caused by sexual abuse [58, 64].

Palatal ecchymoses, palatal erythema, palatal haemorrhage, palatal petechiae and palatal purpura are all examples of fellatio-linked traumatic blood vessel injuries of the palate [60, 62, 63, 65]. Due to blunt trauma from oral sex, the palate blood vessels may dilate, which could lead to haemorrhage. Multiple factors contribute to the aetiology of fellatio-associated palatal haemorrhagic lesions. A severe reflex palatopharyngeal spasm occurring during fellatio may cause mucosal damage with submucosal vascular rupture and bleeding, or it may result from direct and intense contact between the distal penis and palate. One of the main contributing factors to the mechanism of harm is the contemporaneous negative pressure produced by irrumation, which is the entry of a mouth with a penis.

Submucosal haemorrhages can be detected during tooth brushing, flossing or oral cavity examinations despite typically being asymptomatic. During sexual intercourse, the lingual frenulum is susceptible to ulcers due to frequent contact (cunnilingus tongue). The lingual frenulum often scrapes against the incisal edges of the mandibular central incisors as the tongue is thrust forward during the sexual act, causing horizontal ulceration [66]. This lesion usually corresponds to the contact of the ventral tongue with the incisal edge of the mandibular incisor teeth when the tongue is in its most forward position and the lingual frenulum is stretched [66].

Submucosal haemorrhages can be detected during tooth brushing, flossing or oral cavity examinations, despite typically being asymptomatic. During sexual intercourse, the lingual frenulum is susceptible to ulcers due to frequent contact (cunnilingus tongue). As the tongue is thrust forward during the sexual act, the lingual frenulum repeatedly scrapes against the incisal margins of the mandibular central incisors, resulting in horizontal ulceration [66]. When the tongue is in its most forward position and the lingual frenulum is stretched, this lesion typically correlates with the ventral tongue's contact with the incisal edge of the mandibular incisor teeth [66]. The ulceration is coated in a fibrinous exudate and appears nonspecific. Although ulcers typically resolve within 7–10 days, they can recur after several episodes. Visible oral injuries are uncommon, even though children frequently experience sexual abuse in the oral cavity [67]. Petechiae, erythema and/or erosions, especially in the region where the hard and soft palates meet, are some oral indicators of sexual abuse that are caused by forced oral intercourse.

To make an accurate diagnosis, a thorough history and oral examination are necessary. Treatment is typically not required for fellatio-induced palatal lesions [68–70]. Without frequent fellatio, lesions often heal within a week. New bouts of receptive oral sex may cause the lesions to reappear. A topical anaesthetic cream may be used to treat ulcers of the frenulum associated with cunnilingus to alleviate discomfort. Surgical removal of fibrous lesions may be necessary [66, 71].

19.7 Oral Manifestations of Non-oral Risky Sexual Behaviours

Most oral manifestations in individuals affected by sexually transmitted diseases, except for HIV, mainly occur when transmitted via oral sex, autoinoculation or intimate physical contact that involves direct or indirect contact of the oral mucosa with the affected lesion. The oral lesions typically appear at the site of inoculation [37]. Autoinoculation can also occur, for example, from primary vaginal lesions, although orogenital contact is by far the most common method through which HPV is transmitted to the oral mucosa [27, 38]. The primary method of HSV transmission is through sexual intercourse—vaginal, anal or oral sex—primarily during young adulthood, which may result in oral or, less frequently, vaginal lesions when there is mucocutaneous contact [38]. Buccal lesions caused by Molluscum contagiosum (MC) may appear when the disease is spread by fomites, close physical contact or autoinoculation. Sexual contact, particularly vaginal and anal sex, is the main means of infection in adults, and lesions are typically found at the site of inoculation [72]. HIV can spread through unprotected vaginal or anal sex or through contact with HIV-infected blood on mucous membranes or non-intact skin [37]. HIV patients with weakened immune systems may present with oral conditions such as necrotizing ulcerative gingivitis, oropharyngeal infection with HSV, HPV or *Candida species*, oral hairy leukoplakia and Kaposi sarcoma [73]. Syphilis spreads through direct contact with a syphilis sore (chancre) during sexual activity—vaginal, anal or oral. These sores, whether primary, secondary or tertiary, can appear on the genitals, anus, mouth or lips [38]. Transmission of chlamydial and gonorrhoeal infections occurs through sexual contact of all kinds, but oral manifestations (nonspecific symptoms) may appear via oral sex [46, 47].

19.8 Measures That Can Be Taken to Address Oral Manifestation of Risky Sexual Behaviours

It is advisable to take appropriate precautions before engaging in or receiving oral, penetrative vaginal or anal sex with a partner due to the illness risks stated above. Risky oral sexual behaviours have the potential to spread HIV and other venereal illnesses and infections. Below are various ways to reduce the likelihood of acquiring diseases caused by dangerous oral sexual behaviours [12, 14].

19.8.1 Physical Precautionary Measures/Barriers

For fellatio and vaginal or anal penetrative sex, latex or polyurethane condoms (flavoured condoms also available) could be utilised.

For cunnilingus, cut-open condoms, dental dams and latex squares are recommended.

During analingus, the use of plastic wraps (if authorised) is advisable.

19.8.2 Other Health Hygiene Measures

If one of the partners has any open sores or wounds on their mouth or genitalia, bleeding gums or STIs, avoid oral intercourse.

Another precaution is to limit the number of sexual partners a person engages with.

Other measures include steering clear of 'casual' sex with a stranger, and routine screenings and health examinations, including dental examinations.

It is crucial to consult a specialist for more information and to get medical advice as soon as possible if there is any doubt.

Due to the risk of disease, many medical practitioners recommend using condoms or dental dams when engaging in oral intercourse with a partner whose STI status is unknown. Although a condom can serve as a temporary dental dam, it is preferable to use an actual one. Any potential bleeding should not be exposed in the oral cavity. Plastic wrap can be utilised as a barrier during oral sex, although many people find that its thickness diminishes sensation [14]. Additionally, it is advisable to use barrier techniques during anal or vaginal intercourse to prevent HIV transmission and reduce the risk of oral immunocompromise symptoms.

19.9 Conclusion

Regardless of their prior experience with penetrative intercourse, young people are very likely to engage in oral sex. Giving or receiving oral stimulation—such as sucking or licking—of the penis, vagina and/or anus is known as oral sex. Oral intercourse with an infected partner can transmit sexually transmitted diseases, including genital warts (HPV), gonorrhoea, syphilis, genital herpes, HIV, intestinal parasites and hepatitis.

The hazards of oral sex can be decreased in several ways. Generally speaking, the risk of HIV and other STIs spreading during oral intercourse can be reduced by using a physical barrier. The likelihood of infection transmission between partners engaging in oral sex is significantly decreased when there is a healthy mouth free of wounds, damaged skin, lip sores, bleeding gums and oral epithelium. Individuals who engage in oral intercourse frequently must have regular oral health examinations; therefore, maintaining good oral hygiene is essential for preserving oral integrity, as the quality of life is significantly impacted by oral integrity.

References

1. Wellings K, Collumbien M, Slaymaker E, Singh S, Hodges Z, Patel D, et al. Sexual behaviour in context: a global perspective. Lancet. 2006;368(9548):1706–28.
2. Kebede A, Molla B, Gerensea H. Assessment of risky sexual behavior and practice among Aksum University students, Shire Campus, Shire Town, Tigray, Ethiopia, 2017. BMC Res Notes. 2018;11(1):88.
3. Chanakira E, O'Cathain A, Goyder EC, Freeman JV. Factors perceived to influence risky sexual behaviours among university students in the United Kingdom: a qualitative telephone interview study. BMC Public Health. 2014;14(1):1055.
4. Spice W. Management of sex workers and other high-risk groups. Occup Med. 2007;57(5):322–8.
5. Stoner BP. Avoiding risky sex partners: perception of partners' risks v partners' self reported risks. Sex Transm Infect. 2003;79(3):197–201.

6. Chawla N, Sarkar S. Defining "high-risk sexual behavior" in the context of substance use. J Psychosexual Health. 2019;1(1):26–31.
7. Ritchwood TD, Ford H, DeCoster J, Sutton M, Lochman JE. Risky sexual behavior and substance use among adolescents: a meta-analysis. Child Youth Serv Rev. 2015;52:74–88.
8. Kann L, McManus T, Harris WA, Shanklin SL, Flint KH, Queen B, et al. Youth risk behavior surveillance—United States, 2017. MMWR Surveill Summ. 2018;67(8):1–114.
9. Asekun-Olarinmoye OS, Asekun-Olarinmoye EO, Adebimpe WO, Omisore AG. Effect of mass media and internet on sexual behavior of undergraduates in Osogbo metropolis, Southwestern Nigeria. Adolesc Health Med Ther. 2014;5:15–23.
10. Dotson-Blake KP, Knox D, Zusman ME. Exploring social sexual scripts related to oral sex: a profile of college student perceptions. Prof Couns. 2012;2(1):1–11.
11. Pakpahan C, Darmadi D, Agustinus A, Rezano A. Framing and understanding the whole aspect of oral sex from social and health perspectives: a narrative review. F1000Res. 2022;11:177.
12. Saini R, Saini S, Sharma S. Oral sex, oral health and orogenital infections. J Global Infect Dis. 2010;2(1):57–62.
13. Ramanathan V. Risky sexual Behaviours. In: Prabhu SR, Wagoner N, Hill J, Sawleshwarkar S, editors. Sexually transmissible Oral diseases [Internet]. 1st ed. Wiley; 2023. p. 91–5. Available from: https://onlinelibrary.wiley.com/doi/10.1002/9781119826781.ch8.
14. Kumar T, Puri G, Aravinda K, Arora N, Patil D, Gupta R. Oral sex and oral health: an enigma in itself. Indian J Sex Transm Dis AIDS. 2015;36(2):129–32.
15. Dalby J, Stoner BP. Sexually transmitted infections: updates from the 2021 CDC guidelines. Am Fam Physician. 2022;105(5):514–20.
16. Schwartz IM. Sexual activity prior to coital initiation: a comparison between males and females. Arch Sex Behav. 1999;28(1):63–9.
17. Boekeloo BO, Howard DE. Oral sexual experience among young adolescents receiving general health examinations. Am J Health Behav. 2002;26(4):306–14.
18. Gates GJ, Sonenstein FL. Heterosexual genital sexual activity among adolescent males: 1988 and 1995. Fam Plan Perspect. 2000;32(6):295–7, 304.
19. Schuster MA, Bell RM, Kanouse DE. The sexual practices of adolescent virgins: genital sexual activities of high school students who have never had vaginal intercourse. Am J Public Health. 1996;86(11):1570–6.
20. Prinstein MJ, Meade CS, Cohen GL. Adolescent oral sex, peer popularity, and perceptions of best friends' sexual behavior. J Pediatr Psychol. 2003;28(4):243–9.
21. Halpern-Felsher BL, Cornell JL, Kropp RY, Tschann JM. Oral versus vaginal sex among adolescents: perceptions, attitudes, and behavior. Pediatrics. 2005;115(4):845–51.
22. Huengsberg M. Sexually transmitted diseases: 3rd ed. Ed King K Holmes, P Frederick Sparling, Per-Anders Mardh, Stanley M Lemon, Walter E Stamm, Peter Piot, Judith N Wasserheit. $170.50. New York: McGraw Hill, 1999. ISBN 0-07-029688-X. Sex Transm Infect. 2000;76(6):498.
23. Edwards S, Carne C. Oral sex and the transmission of viral STIs. Sex Transm Infect. 1998;74(1):6–10.
24. Jin F, Prestage GP, Mao L, Kippax SC, Pell CM, Donovan B, et al. Transmission of herpes simplex virus types 1 and 2 in a prospective cohort of HIV-negative gay men: the health in men study. J Infect Dis. 2006;194(5):561–70.
25. Centers for Disease Control and Prevention (CDC). Transmission of primary and secondary syphilis by oral sex—Chicago, Illinois, 1998–2002. MMWR Morb Mortal Wkly Rep. 2004;53(41):966–8.
26. Hawkins DA. Oral sex and HIV transmission. Sex Transm Infect. 2001;77(5):307–8.
27. Bruce AJ, Rogers RS. Oral manifestations of sexually transmitted diseases. Clin Dermatol. 2004;22(6):520–7.
28. Pai V, Prabhu SR. Oral and genital microbiota. In: Prabhu SR, Wagoner N, Hill J, Sawleshwarkar S, editors. Sexually transmissible Oral diseases [internet]. 1st ed. Wiley; 2023. p. 83–9. Available from: https://onlinelibrary.wiley.com/doi/10.1002/9781119826781.ch7.

29. Tanaka TI, Alawi F. Human papillomavirus and oropharyngeal cancer. Dent Clin N Am. 2018;62(1):111–20.
30. Valejo Coelho MM, Matos-Pires E, Serrão V, Rodrigues A, Fernandes C. Extragenital Gonorrhoea in men who have sex with men: a retrospective study in a STI clinic in Lisbon, Portugal. Acta Med Port. 2018;31(5):247–53.
31. Limeres Posse J, Diz Dios P, Scully C. Viral diseases transmissible by kissing. In: Saliva protection and transmissible diseases [Internet]. Elsevier; 2017. p. 53–92. Available from: https://linkinghub.elsevier.com/retrieve/pii/B9780128136812000044.
32. Glynn TR, Operario D, Montgomery M, Almonte A, Chan PA. The duality of oral sex for men who have sex with men: an examination into the increase of sexually transmitted infections amid the age of HIV prevention. AIDS Patient Care STDs. 2017;31(6):261–7.
33. Turek EM, Fairley CK, Tabesh M, Phillips TR, Bradshaw CS, Rodriguez E, et al. HIV, sexually transmitted infections and sexual practices among male sex workers attending a sexual health Clinic in Melbourne, Australia: 2010 to 2018. Sex Transm Dis. 2021;48(2):103–8.
34. Drake VE, Fakhry C, Windon MJ, Stewart CM, Akst L, Hillel A, et al. Timing, number, and type of sexual partners associated with risk of oropharyngeal cancer. Cancer. 2021;127(7):1029–38.
35. Prabhu SR, Wagoner N, Hill J, Sawleshwarkar S, editors. Sexually transmitted disease risk and oral sex. In: Sexually transmissible oral diseases [Internet]. 1st ed. Wiley; 2023. p. 97–104. Available from: https://onlinelibrary.wiley.com/doi/10.1002/9781119826781.ch9.
36. Yu X, Zheng H. Syphilitic chancre of the lips transmitted by kissing: a case report and review of the literature. Medicine (Baltimore). 2016;95(14):e3303.
37. Queirós C, da Costa JB. Oral transmission of sexually transmissible infections: a narrative review. Acta Medica Port. 2019;32(12):776–81.
38. Fernández-López C, Morales-Angulo C. Lesiones otorrinolaringológicas secundarias al sexo oral. Acta Otorrinolaringol Esp. 2017;68(3):169–80.
39. de Vries HJC. The enigma of lymphogranuloma venereum spread in men who have sex with men: does ano-oral transmission plays a role? Sex Transm Dis. 2016;43(7):420–2.
40. Dosekun O, Edmonds S, Stockwell S, French P, White JA. Lymphogranuloma venereum detected from the pharynx in four London men who have sex with men. Int J STD AIDS. 2013;24(6):495–6.
41. Hamasuna R, Hoshina S, Imai H, Jensen JS, Osada Y. Usefulness of oral wash specimens for detecting Chlamydia trachomatis from high-risk groups in Japan. Int J Urol. 2007;14(5):473–5.
42. Bavoil PM, Marques PX, Brotman R, Ravel J. Does active Oral sex contribute to female infertility? J Infect Dis. 2017;216(8):932–5.
43. Nash JL, Hocking JS, Read TRH, Chen MY, Bradshaw CS, Forcey DS, et al. Contribution of sexual practices (other than anal sex) to bacterial sexually transmitted infection transmission in men who have sex with men: a cross-sectional analysis using electronic health records. Sex Transm Infect. 2014;90(1):55–7.
44. van Rooijen MS, van der Loeff MFS, Morré SA, van Dam AP, Speksnijder AGCL, de Vries HJC. Spontaneous pharyngeal chlamydia trachomatis RNA clearance. A cross-sectional study followed by a cohort study of untreated STI clinic patients in Amsterdam, The Netherlands. Sex Transm Infect. 2015;91(3):157–64.
45. Chow EPF, Tabrizi SN, Phillips S, Lee D, Bradshaw CS, Chen MY, et al. Neisseria gonorrhoeae bacterial DNA load in the pharynges and saliva of men who have sex with men. J Clin Microbiol. 2016;54(10):2485–90.
46. Osborne NG, Grubin L. Colonization of the pharynx with Neisseria gonorrhoeae: experience in a clinic for sexually transmitted diseases. Sex Transm Dis. 1979;6(4):253–6.
47. Wiesner PJ, Tronca E, Bonin P, Pedersen AH, Holmes KK. Clinical spectrum of pharyngeal gonococcal infection. N Engl J Med. 1973;288(4):181–5.
48. Bignell C, Unemo M, European STI. Guidelines editorial board. 2012 European guideline on the diagnosis and treatment of gonorrhoea in adults. Int J STD AIDS. 2013;24(2):85–92.
49. Workowski KA, Bolan GA, Centers for Disease Control and Prevention. Sexually transmitted diseases treatment guidelines, 2015. MMWR Recomm Rep. 2015;64(RR-03):1–137.

50. D'Souza G, Kreimer AR, Viscidi R, Pawlita M, Fakhry C, Koch WM, et al. Case-control study of human papillomavirus and oropharyngeal cancer. N Engl J Med. 2007;356(19):1944–56.
51. Ang KK, Harris J, Wheeler R, Weber R, Rosenthal DI, Nguyen-Tân PF, et al. Human papillomavirus and survival of patients with oropharyngeal cancer. N Engl J Med. 2010;363(1):24–35.
52. Gargano JW, Unger ER, Liu G, Steinau M, Meites E, Dunne E, et al. Prevalence of genital human papillomavirus in males, United States, 2013–2014. J Infect Dis. 2017;215(7):1070–9.
53. Budu VA, Decuseară T, Balica NC, Mogoantă CA, Rădulescu LM, Chirilă M, et al. The role of HPV infection in oropharyngeal cancer. Romanian J Morphol Embryol. 2019;60(3):769–73.
54. Robinson EK, Evans BG. Oral sex and HIV transmission. AIDS. 1999;13(6):737–8.
55. Rothenberg RB, Scarlett M, del Rio C, Reznik D, O'Daniels C. Oral transmission of HIV. AIDS. 1998;12(16):2095–105.
56. Suarez TP, Kelly JA, Pinkerton SD, Stevenson YL, Hayat M, Smith MD, et al. Influence of a partner's HIV serostatus, use of highly active antiretroviral therapy, and viral load on perceptions of sexual risk behavior in a community sample of men who have sex with men. J Acquir Immune Defic Syndr. 2001;28(5):471–7.
57. Damm DD, White DK, Brinker CM. Variations of palatal erythema secondary to fellatio. Oral Surg Oral Med Oral Pathol. 1981;52(4):417–21.
58. Shanel-Hogan KA. What is this red mark? J Calif Dent Assoc. 2004;32(4):304–5.
59. Hupp WS. Palatal erythema. J Am Dent Assoc. 2009;140(5):555–7.
60. Worsaae N, Wanscher B. Oral injury caused by fellatio. Acta Derm Venereol. 1978;58(2):187–8.
61. Aloi FG. Suffused ecchymosis of the palate caused by fellatio. G Ital Dermatol Venereol. 1984;119(5):351–2.
62. van Wyk CW. The oral lesion caused by fellatio. Am J Forensic Med Pathol. 1981;2(3):217–9.
63. Muthu K, Kannan S, Muthusamy S, Sidhu P. Palatal ecchymosis associated with irrumation. Indian J Dermatol Venereol Leprol. 2015;81(5):505–7.
64. Heitzler GD, Cranin AN, Gallo L. Sexual abuse of the oral cavity in children. N Y State Dent J. 1994;60(2):31–3.
65. Bellizzi R, Krakow AM, Plack W. Soft palate trauma associated with fellatio: case report. Mil Med. 1980;145(11):787–8.
66. Neville BW, Damm DD, Allen CM, Chi AC. Color atlas of oral and maxillofacial diseases [Internet]. Amsterdam: Elsevier; 2019. Available from: https://linkinghub.elsevier.com/retrieve/pii/C2016001896X.
67. Parte-Serna ACDL, Oliván-Gonzalvo G, Fratila CR, Hermoso-Vallespí M, Peiró-Aubalat A, Ortega-Soria R. The dark side of Paediatric dentistry: child abuse. Iberoam J Med. 2020;3:194–200. Available from: https://zenodo.org/record/3739084.
68. Cohen PR, Miller VM. Fellatio-associated petechiae of the palate: report of purpuric palatal lesions developing after oral sex. Dermatol Online J. 2013;19(7):18963.
69. De Barros Pinto Grifoni L, Navarro CM. Oral lesion secondary to oral sex. Oral Surg Oral Med Oral Pathol Oral Radiol. 2020;129(1):e67.
70. Giansanti JS, Cramer JR, Weathers DR. Palatal erythema: another etiologic factor. Oral Surg Oral Med Oral Pathol. 1975;40(3):379–81.
71. Prabhu SR. Oral traumatic lesions associated with Oral sex. In: Prabhu SR, Wagoner N, Hill J, Sawleshwarkar S, editors. Sexually transmissible oral diseases [Internet]. 1st ed. Wiley; 2023. p. 105–13. Available from: https://onlinelibrary.wiley.com/doi/10.1002/9781119826781.ch10.
72. Fornatora ML, Reich RF, Gray RG, Freedman PD. Intraoral molluscum contagiosum: a report of a case and a review of the literature. Oral Surg Oral Med Oral Pathol Oral Radiol Endod. 2001;92(3):318–20.
73. Glick M, Muzyka BC, Lurie D, Salkin LM. Oral manifestations associated with HIV-related disease as markers for immune suppression and AIDS. Oral Surg Oral Med Oral Pathol. 1994;77(4):344–9.

Impact of Chronic Stress and Mental Illness on Oral Health

20

Cameron L. Randall and Tamanna Tiwari

20.1 Introduction

The associations between chronic stress, mental illness and poor oral health outcomes are not only well documented but also critically important to understand. These intricate relationships reflect a bidirectional interplay among biological, behavioural, psychological and social factors. Moreover, shared social determinants significantly contribute to both mental health challenges and oral health issues. This chapter offers essential concepts and insights into chronic stress and mental disorders, empowering oral healthcare providers to excel in multidisciplinary, comprehensive and person-centred care environments. Specifically, this chapter reviews key definitions and background information about stress and mental illness. It also reviews contemporary literature on the complex associations between stress, mental health and oral health. By understanding these connections, providers can better address the holistic needs of their patients and improve overall health outcomes.

C. L. Randall (✉)
Department of Oral Health Sciences, University of Washington School of Dentistry, Seattle, WA, USA
e-mail: CLR333@uw.edu

T. Tiwari
Department of Primary Dental Care, School of Dentistry, University of Minnesota, Minneapolis, MN, USA
e-mail: ttiwari@umn.edu

S. R. Prabhu et al. (eds.), *Lifestyle in Oral Health and Disease*,
https://doi.org/10.1007/978-3-032-05888-1_20

20.2 Impact of Chronic Stress and Mental Illness on Oral Health

Dental providers comprehensively consider patients' cases and histories in an increasingly person-centred oral healthcare era. Stress and mental health are essential features of a patient's health history. These phenomena may play a key role in oral health and other health outcomes, so they should be thoroughly and thoughtfully considered, along with dental-related implications.

20.2.1 Stress: Definitions, Foundational Concepts and Key Background

Generally, *stress* or the *stress response* represents any disruption in homeostasis as a function of physical or psychological stimuli, which are referred to as *stressors* [1]. The stress response involves nervous, endocrine and immune mechanisms, and it is understood to play an adaptive role, preparing the body to handle challenges (i.e. stressors) [1]. The contemporary science of stress and its modern conceptualisations have roots in a 1936 article by physician and chemist Hans Selye [2, 3]. In that article, Selye described a three-phase physiologic response to injury [4]. The framework, known as 'general adaptation syndrome' or 'Selye's syndrome', posited that the stress response involves an initial alarm phase, a resistance or adaptation phase and an exhaustion or death phase [2, 4]. The framework was applied extensively to research in the decades that followed, giving rise to much more complex models of stress [2].

Considering the human experience of stress, the World Health Organization defines stress as 'a state of worry or mental tension caused by a difficult situation… a natural human response that prompts us to address challenges and threats in our lives' [5]. Researchers and clinicians distinguish between acute stress and chronic stress, as well as a range of other categories of stress. *Acute stress* is short-term stress experienced secondary to immediate stressors or challenges; it often involves a strong physiological component, including activation of the sympathetic system [1]. Conversely, *chronic stress* is experienced over an extended period of time secondary to a stressor that is present over that same period; it also involves a physiological component and can involve a prominent cognitive component, too (e.g. worry and rumination) [1]. While acute stress can be considered in the dental context, chronic stress may be most relevant to oral health outcomes. Chronic stress has cumulative effects that increase the risk of physical and psychological health problems [1, 6].

Chronic stress can be caused by any number of challenges or other stimuli present over an extended period (including positive stimuli). Common examples include physiological stressors such as food insecurity and associated poor nutrition, ongoing sleep deprivation or chronic illness or pain; environmental stressors such as noise, pollution or unsafe conditions; and psychological stressors such as worries, perceptions or negative cognitions related to school/work, social or other demands

[1]. Daily, family and caregiving stressors also contribute to chronic stress [7]. All people will experience some of these stressors, and all people will experience some chronic stress. However, there are individual differences in how people cope with these stressors to mitigate chronic stress [8]. Further, individual differences exist in the number and magnitude of these stressors experienced by anyone. Thus, some people are at much higher risk than others for experiencing chronic stress and its consequences.

Importantly, disparities have been observed in the prevalence of chronic stress and associated health outcomes [7]. Disparities in chronic stress may be partially accounted for by differential experience of environmental, neighbourhood, family, socioeconomic and other stressors, with some groups more vulnerable to exposure than others [7]. Moreover, chronic stress has been suggested as a mechanism by which social determinants of health influence health outcomes and account for health disparities [9]. Chronic stress increases *allostatic load*—'the cumulative [biological] burden of stress on the body' [10]—which is a risk factor for systemic and psychiatric diseases such as heart disease, diabetes, depression and cognitive impairment [7, 11, 12]. Recently, in a rapidly growing body of literature, classism, racism and other forms of discrimination have been identified as chronic stressors that account at least partially for health disparities across a range of diseases, disorders and other health outcomes [13–18].

20.2.2 Mental Health: Definitions, Foundational Concepts and Key Background

The World Health Organisation defines *mental health* as 'a state of mental well-being that enables people to cope with the stresses of life, realise their abilities, learn well, and work well' [19]. The U.S. Substance Abuse and Mental Health Services Administration describes mental health as comprising emotional, psychological and social well-being—'it affects how we think, feel and act, and helps determine how we handle stress, relate to others and make choices' [20]. Importantly, people experience mental health along a continuum from good to poor. Moreover, mental health can change over time, varying as a function of stress, behavioural and biological factors, among other influences. Towards the poor end of the mental health continuum, people may experience a *mental disorder*, which the World Health Organisation defines as 'a clinically significant disturbance in an individual's cognition, emotional regulation, or behaviour…usually associated with distress or impairment in important areas of functioning' [21]. The terms mental disorder, *mental health condition* and *mental illness* are often used interchangeably, though 'mental illness' is a broader term that captures the wide range of mental disorders and other health conditions that affect cognition, emotion and behaviour. Mental disorders can range from mild to severe, and one person's experience of a particular disorder may be quite different from another person's experience of the same disorder in terms of symptoms and impact [22].

A comprehensive review of the dozens of mental disorders that exist is beyond the scope of this chapter. However, it is important that oral healthcare providers have a basic appreciation of the most prevalent or serious disorders. *Anxiety disorders* represent the most common class of mental disorders. These disorders are characterised by excessive, distressing and impairing fear or anxiety, which may include physiological reactivity (i.e. sympathetic response), worry and avoidance or other behavioural disturbance [21, 23]. *Generalised anxiety disorder* involves frequent and uncontrollable worry (about many things, not necessarily specific) that interferes with academic/occupational, social and other activities [24]. Sometimes, generalised anxiety disorder includes physical symptoms like poor concentration, restlessness or muscle tension [24]. *Specific phobia* involves excessive and persistent fear of a specific stimulus, and the fear is often understood by the person with the phobia to be irrational (i.e. the feared object or situation is not threatening) [24]. Phobias are impairing because they often involve extreme avoidance of feared stimuli (e.g. missing important life events because of an excessive fear of flying). *Social anxiety disorder* involves excessive and persistent fear of negative evaluation by others (e.g. embarrassment and humiliation) and associated distress and avoidance of academic/occupational or social situations where one might encounter such evaluation [24]. *Panic disorder* involves recurrent panic attacks, which may include rapid heart rate, shortness of breath, sweating, trembling, feeling faint, nausea or feeling detached [24]. The panic attacks may happen reliably in the context of a feared stimulus or unexpectedly and seemingly randomly. *Agoraphobia* involves excessive and persistent fear of being in a situation where it would be difficult to escape if a panic attack were to occur, resulting in avoidance of such situations or, in some cases, avoidance of most places outside the home [24].

Another common class of mental disorders is mood disorders. *Major depressive disorder* is the most common of these and involves experiencing several symptoms most of the day, most every day, for two or more weeks. Those symptoms include feeling sad, down or hopeless; experiencing a loss of enjoyment in previously interesting or pleasurable activities; changes in appetite and/or sleep; decreased energy; irritability; difficulty concentrating; feelings of worthlessness or inappropriate guilt; or suicidal ideation or behaviour [24]. Less common but potentially very serious is *bipolar disorder*, which involves experiencing fluctuating episodes of intense emotional states [24]. Episodes can be depressive (which involve symptoms similar to major depressive disorder) or manic (excessively happy, energetic mood, often with decreased need for sleep and increased activity and/or risk-taking). Other serious mental illnesses include *schizophrenia*, which includes periods when people experience psychosis, delusions, hallucinations, disorganised thinking/speech or marked changes in motor behaviour [24]. Schizophrenia is relatively rare, affecting less than 1% of the population [25].

Other less prevalent disorders include *post-traumatic stress disorder*, which occurs in individuals who have experienced a traumatic event and involves re-experiencing the event (e.g. flashbacks or nightmares), changes in mood and concentration, physiological reactivity (e.g. easily startled and feeling on edge) and avoidance of reminders of the event [24]. *Obsessive-compulsive disorder* involves recurring, uncontrollable thoughts (i.e. obsessions) and excessive behaviours that are repeated (i.e. compulsions); the obsessions and compulsions are emotionally distressing and impair functioning in academic/occupational, social and/or other domains [24]. *Eating disorders* involve abnormal eating behaviours that impact physical and mental health, and the most common of these are *anorexia nervosa* (characterised by restricted eating) and *bulimia nervosa* (characterised by a cycle of binge eating followed by purging) [24]. *Substance use disorders* involve compulsive misuse or abuse of substances despite harmful consequences [24]. All of these disorders cause significant distress and impairment, and they can be very serious, even life-threatening. There are many other mental disorders, including those with onset in or experienced primarily during childhood (e.g. attention deficit hyperactivity disorder, separation anxiety disorder and behaviour disorders).

Globally, approximately one in eight people are living with a mental disorder, with anxiety disorders and major depressive disorder accounting for the greatest proportion of those experienced [21]. Among children and adolescents aged 5–24 years, specifically, the prevalence of any mental disorder was 11.6% in 2019 [26]. The global burden of mental disorders is high. In 2019, the disability-adjusted life years (DALY) rate for mental disorders was 1426.5 and 1703.3 per 100,000 for males and females respectively, with the highest rates observed in Australasia, Tropical Latin America and high-income North America [27]. The incidence and DALY rate for mental disorders have decreased over the last two decades, but the number of new cases of and deaths associated with mental disorders has increased [28]. That trajectory and an increasing global prevalence are expected to continue [28, 29].

Comorbidity within mental disorders is common. For instance, results from a recent large study of adults from 27 countries indicated that each prior lifetime mental disorder assessed was associated with risk of subsequent onset of the other disorders [30]. Comorbidity has also been demonstrated between mental disorders and substance abuse, especially among patients with serious mental disorders [31, 32]. Additionally, comorbidity has been demonstrated between mental disorders and general medical disorders and pain, and especially among patients with serious mental disorders [33–35]. In fact, mental disorders are associated with increased risk of a subsequent medical problem in a longitudinal manner [36].

As noted above, mental disorders can have a wide range of consequences, some of which can be very serious. For instance, all mental disorders involve some level of emotional distress and impairment in functioning in academic/occupational, social, family and other domains and/or activities of daily living. Depending on their severity, some mental disorders also have consequences related to physical health, finances and mortality. Thankfully, there are numerous effective interventions for treating mental disorders. A full review of such interventions is beyond the scope of this chapter, but oral healthcare providers should be aware of some of the most common practical intervention approaches.

Nonpharmacological approaches include various forms of psychotherapy or 'talk therapy.' The reality is that psychotherapy often involves much more than just talking. For instance, *behavioural therapy* includes applying evidence-based strategies like reinforcement, shaping and modelling to promote behaviour change; behavioural activation to increase activity and improve mood; and habituation through systematic desensitisation to reduce fear, anxiety and avoidance [37]. *Cognitive therapy* includes evidence-based strategies for changing maladaptive thinking patterns that contribute to mental disorders [37]. And *cognitive behaviour therapy* integrates relevant cognitive and behavioural strategies; it has been shown to be effective for the treatment of mood disorders, anxiety disorders, post-traumatic stress disorder, obsessive-compulsive disorder, eating disorders and substance use disorders [37–39]. These approaches can be delivered by various mental health clinicians, including psychiatrists, clinical psychologists, clinical social workers, counsellors, community health workers and others.

There are also numerous pharmacological approaches, with medications indicated for mood disorders, anxiety disorders, bipolar disorder, schizophrenia and psychosis, post-traumatic stress disorder, obsessive-compulsive disorder, attention-deficit hyperactivity disorder and more. These medications are typically prescribed by a psychiatrist or other physician, physician assistant, nurse practitioner or similar clinicians (see textbook by Sadek [2021] or a similar offering tailored to psychotropic medications commonly prescribed in your region) [40]. In the case of nonpharmacological and pharmacological approaches for treating mental disorders, care is most often provided one-on-one in general medical (i.e. primary care) or psychiatric/psychological practices. However, integrated behavioural healthcare is becoming more common. Such a healthcare model involves the provision of primary healthcare and the provision of behavioural healthcare (i.e. mental healthcare) in an integrated system, with referrals and communication facilitated easily between providers and, in most cases, the colocation of primary care and behavioural health clinic spaces [41, 42]. This model makes it easier for patients to receive behavioural health services and allows for comprehensive healthcare; in both paediatric and adult populations, it is associated with improved clinical outcomes and a range of other benefits [42–45].

20.2.3 Stress, Mental Health and Oral Health

Research on the associations between stress, mental health and oral health is still in its relative infancy. However, the available literature clearly shows bidirectional and complex relationships between psychological well-being and oral health.

The earliest work in this area addressed chronic stress and oral health. One of the first studies on the topic found that work-related mental demand was positively associated with periodontal health but not dental caries [46]. Subsequent studies demonstrated associations between perceived stress and poorer oral health across adolescence and adulthood, with one finding that the association is modified by dental insurance and socioeconomic position [47, 48]. In other studies, higher chronic stress levels were associated with poorer oral hygiene behaviour, less healthy dietary habits and poorer oral health outcomes (e.g. plaque and gingivitis), suggesting that the relationship between stress and oral health may be through oral health behaviours [49–52]. In more recent studies, associations between academic/occupational stress and oral health and quality of life have been confirmed [52–56]. Chronic stress has been posited as a key driver that helps explain social inequities in oral health outcomes [57, 58].

Some studies have addressed the associations between mental health and oral health. Most of those studies have focused on patients with serious mental illness or severe mental disorders. One review concluded that 61% of adults with serious mental illness had suboptimal oral health (i.e. xerostomia, caries, decayed teeth and/or periodontal disease), with poor oral hygiene, diets high in carbohydrates, poor perception of oral health needs, psychotropic medication use and poor access to dental care identified as potential drivers [59]. Findings from other studies are in general agreement—oral health is suboptimal among those with serious mental illness, and routine assessment and treatment may be lacking [60, 61].

Among people with anxiety and depressive disorders, a systematic review found that all disorders within these two classes were associated with increased dental decay and tooth loss, but not periodontal disease [62]. Data from a recent study involving a nationally representative cohort in the U.S. demonstrate that all six different oral health conditions related to periodontal disease were greater in prevalence among participants with internalising problems, and that most were greater in prevalence among participants with externalising problems or substance abuse [63]. In another recent U.S. nationally representative study involving a path analysis, socioeconomic position was associated with dental treatment seeking, oral health behaviours and mental health, and all of those factors were associated with self-rated oral health [64]. Finally, in one other recent study, poor mental health was associated with lower likelihood to visit the dentist within the last year, unmet oral health need and self-reported oral health status [65]. Taken together, these and other studies make it clear that mental health and oral health are related across a range of mental health problems and severity of those problems [66–68].

There has been some work addressing the oral healthcare of patients with mental illness. For instance, the British Society for Disability and Oral Health published guidelines and recommendations that include approaches for patients living in institutional care, residential community care or general community settings [69]. Those guidelines also provide consideration of access to care, oral health screening, oral health promotion and additional training [69]. Unfortunately, they have not been updated since 2000. A Cochrane review found no evidence that oral health education and advice help patients with serious mental illness achieve clinically meaningful oral health outcomes; the conclusion was to follow the British Society for Disability and Oral Health's guidelines and recommendations until better evidence is generated [70]. A recent scoping review found that, for patients with a range of mental disorders, four types of interventions demonstrated positive effects on oral health knowledge, behaviours and outcomes: educational interventions, physical interventions, behavioural and educational interventions and educational and physical interventions [71]. Another recent paper suggested that a 'psychiatric dental consultation liaison service' may benefit the management of dental patients with mental health problems, and such a framework may fit well into existing special care dentistry practice models [72].

Additional work certainly is needed to identify the most effective approaches for providing dental care to people with mental disorders. That work should build upon recent narrative review and qualitative studies that identified barriers and enablers for oral healthcare for people with mental disorders [73–75]. Moreover, that work should consider recent suggestions that good oral health is a prerequisite for good mental health—'no mental health without oral health' (i.e. that, due to the bidirectional relationship that exists, the focus should be on more than just the oral health consequences of mental health problems) [76].

Indeed, the associations between mental health and oral health are complex, and a better understanding of that complexity may yield increasingly effective approaches for prevention and intervention. A recent review highlights an interplay of factors related to microbiome dysregulation, translocated bacteria and systemic inflammation that may partially explain associations between stress, mental health and oral health [77]. Another recent review suggests that bidirectional mechanisms involving biological, behavioural, psychological and social processes are at play in the relationship between mental health and oral health [78]. For example, low motivation and poor concentration—hallmarks of depression—may result in poorer than usual oral hygiene behaviours and a drift towards a more cariogenic diet. In turn, worsening oral health and oral health-related quality of life may exacerbate depressive symptomatology in a vicious cycle. New or increased tobacco or alcohol use that is comorbid with depressive or other mental disorder symptomatology may also contribute to worsening oral health. In addition to these behavioural and psychological processes, shared social determinants likely play an important role. For instance, lower socioeconomic position, housing insecurity, food insecurity, lack of access to primary healthcare and dental care and discrimination-related stress can influence a range of health behaviours (e.g. diet, oral hygiene, use of preventive care and timely dental treatment seeking when there are restorative needs) and other factors that drive both mental health and oral health outcomes [78, 79].

Finally, there is an important and complex role of psychotropic medications in the mental health and oral health connection. Common side effects of psychotropic medications frequently prescribed for the treatment of mental disorders have oral manifestations that may increase one's risk for oral health problems. A review of therapeutic guidelines and a medicines handbook identified 57 drugs used to treat mental disorders, including antidepressants, antipsychotics and anxiolytics/sedatives. Of those, xerostomia was the most commonly indicated side effect (91%) across all classes of drugs [80]. Xerostomia increases one's risk for caries and more rapid caries development [81]. So, patients with mental disorders who are taking psychotropic medications may be more likely to develop oral health problems, which in turn may exacerbate stress and mental health problems. Other common side effects of psychotropic medications include dysgeusia (antidepressants), tardive dyskinesia and increased salivation (antipsychotic medications) [80]. Dysgeusia may affect dietary behaviour (and caries risk if the new diet is more cariogenic), nutrition and quality of life [82]. Increased salivation may result in social difficulties and withdrawal, skin irritation and reduced quality of life [83]. Oral healthcare providers must be aware of any psychotropic medications being taken by their patients as well as any oral side effects experienced; treatment plans should be considered accordingly.

20.2.4 Training in Integrated Oral and Behavioural Healthcare

Given the associations between stress, mental health and oral health, oral healthcare providers must have at least a foundational awareness of key definitions and concepts related to stress and mental health. It is also imperative for oral healthcare providers to consider how they might integrate behavioural healthcare with the oral healthcare they provide. Such an approach mirrors what is already happening in medicine (specifically, primary care) [41, 42]. Moreover, and perhaps most critically though, it facilitates the provision of person-centred care. Once referred to as patient-centred care, the expanded and refined concept of person-centred care is based on the premise that 'patients are persons and should not be reduced to their disease alone, but rather that their subjectivity and integration within a given environment, their strengths, their future plans and their rights should also be taken into account' [84]. Person-centred care involves appreciation and consideration of 'all' of the patient, including their medical history, psychological profile, issues related to stress and mental illness and environment, including relevant social determinants of health. In dentistry, this means: (1) exploring disease and its context; (2) the patient as a whole person (importantly, 'seek[ing]' to understand illness within the person's bio*psycho*social circumstances); (3) the doctor–patient relationship ethos and (4) the doctor-patient relationship—common ground and sharing responsibility (see Kristensen et al. 2023 for full review and detailed description) [85].

To be clear, oral healthcare providers are not expected to be mental health experts, nor are they expected to provide behavioural healthcare. However, while keeping within their scope of practice, oral healthcare providers could benefit their patients by finding ways to consider stress and mental illness as part of regular diagnosis and treatment planning. Further, they could help their patients by working towards integrating oral and behavioural healthcare, as relevant. Because discoveries related to the oral health and mental health connection are relatively recent, it is likely that many practising oral healthcare providers did not have explicit training in mental health and behavioural healthcare. Thus, current trainees and practising providers may benefit from training in integrating oral and behavioural healthcare.

The dental student, resident and continuing education curricula should cover research on the connection between mental health and oral health. Such instruction may include content related to the epidemiology of mental health and oral health problems and the associations between mental health and oral health outcomes; the mechanisms that explain the complex interplay between mental health and oral health; disparities in oral health outcomes experienced by people living with mental illness; and approaches for tailored treatment planning for patients with a mental disorder, as well as relevant skills for behaviour change counselling and oral health promotion. Curricula should also provide opportunities for meaningful, person-centred application of appropriate skills, which may be facilitated by skills/simulation training exercises and other experiential learning, interprofessional education and clinical experiences with embedded mental healthcare providers, social workers and similar professionals. A recently published framework for integrating behavioural health and oral health in predoctoral dental education provides specific guidance for training in this area [79].

The framework includes three domains: education, organisation and community [79]. In the education domain, trainees should be taught how mental and oral health are related. Instruction in dentally relevant behavioural health topics should also be provided. For example, training should cover mental illness (e.g. anxiety disorders, mood disorders, severe mental disorders and substance use disorders), neurodevelopment, domestic violence, dental care-related fear and anxiety, acute and chronic pain, psychotropic pharmacology, oral health-related quality of life, comprehensive health history gathering (including psychosocial and behavioural history) and social determinants of health [79]. Importantly, background information and opportunities for clinical skill development should be provided. Also within the education domain, trainees should be taught about patient behaviour, oral health promotion and the dentist–patient interaction, including basic communication skills and more advanced health counselling skills [79]. A supportive organisational environment that includes champions and facilitators of integrated behavioural health and oral health should be fostered, with involvement of a behavioural health or health behaviour expert when possible [79]. Finally, the priorities of the community (i.e. patients experiencing mental illness) should be centred, and there should be inclusive engagement with community members [79]. Refer to Tiwari and Randall [79] for complete details.

20.3 Conclusions

Readers should consider the following:

1. There are well-documented associations between stress, oral health and mental health. These associations involve bidirectional and complex relationships that are influenced by biological, behavioural, psychological and social factors, all of which should be considered in the treatment of patients with mental health problems.
2. A basic understanding of chronic stress and its associations with oral health may benefit oral healthcare providers in formulating case conceptualisations and treatment plans as part of comprehensive dental care.
3. A basic understanding of common mental disorders will help prepare oral healthcare providers to work with patients with these disorders. Communication approaches and treatment planning should be adapted to meet patients' needs, and the integration of mental healthcare and oral healthcare should be facilitated to the extent possible.

References

1. Chu B, Marwaha K, Sanvictores T, Awosika AO, Ayers D. Physiology, stress reaction [Updated 2024 May 7]. In: StatPearls [Internet]. Treasure Island: StatPearls Publishing; 2025. Available from: https://www.ncbi.nlm.nih.gov/books/NBK541120/.
2. Jackson M. Evaluating the role of Hans Selye in the modern history of stress. In: Cantor D, Ramsden E, editors. Chapter 1: Stress, shock, and adaptation in the twentieth century. Rochester: University of Rochester Press; 2014.
3. Tan SY, Yip A. Hans Selye (1907–1982): founder of the stress theory. Singapore Med J. 2018;59(4):170–1.
4. Selye H. A syndrome produced by diverse nocuous agents. Nature. 1936;138:32.
5. World Health Organization. Stress [Updated 2023 February 21]. 2023. Available from: https://who.int/news-room/questions-and-answers/item/stress.
6. Mariotti A. The effects of chronic stress on health: new insights into the molecular mechanisms of brain-body communication. Future Sci OA. 2015;1(3):FS023.
7. American Psychological Association. Fact sheet: health disparities and stress [Updated 2012]. 2012. Available from: https://www.apa.org/topics/racism-bias-discrimination/health-disparities-stress.
8. Parkes KR, Hughes EL. Individual differences in coping with stress. In: Carducci BJ, Nave CS, Mio JS, Riggio RE, editors. The Wiley encyclopedia of personality and individual differences. Hoboken: Wiley; 2020. p. 377–81.
9. Bailey ZD, Williams DR. Stress, health, and disparities. In: Zigmond MJ, Rowland LP, Coyle JT, editors. Neurobiology of brain disorders. London: Elsevier Academic; 2015. p. 765–79.
10. Rodriquez EJ, Kim EN, Sumner AE, Nápoles AM, Pérez-Stable EJ. Allostatic load: importance, markers, and score determination in minority and disparity populations. J Urban Health. 2019;96(Suppl 1):3–11.
11. Djuric Z, Bird CE, Furumoto-Dawson A, Rauscher GH, Ruffin MT, Stowe RP, et al. Biomarkers of psychological stress in health disparities research. Open Biomark J. 2018;1:7–19.
12. Guidi J, Lucente M, Sonino N, Fava GA. Allostatic load and its impact on health: a systematic review. Psychother Psychosom. 2021;90(1):11–27.
13. Williams DR, Gonzalez HM, Williams S, Mohammed SA, Moomal H, Stein DJ. Perceived discrimination, race and health in South Africa. Soc Sci Med. 2008;67(3):441–52.
14. Pengpid S, Peltzer K. Perceived discrimination and health outcomes among middle-aged and older adults in India: results of a national survey in 2017–2018. BMC Geriatr. 2021;21:559.
15. Cavalhieri KE, Wilcox MM. The compounded effects of classism and racism on mental health outcomes for African Americans. J Couns Psychol. 2022;69(1):111–20.
16. Murkey JA, Watkins BX, Vieira D, Boden-Albala B. Disparities in allostatic load, telomete length and chronic stress burden among African American adults: a systematic review. Psychoneuroendocrinology. 2022;140:105730.
17. Cavalhieri KE, Willyard A, Phillippi JC. The effects of different types of classism on psychological outcomes: preliminary findings. Int J Adv Couns. 2023 May;3:1–19.
18. Hines AL, Albert MA, Blair JP, Crews DC, Cooper LA, Long L, et al. Neighborhood factors, individual stressors, and cardiovascular health among black and white adults in the US. JAMA Netw Open. 2023;6(9):e2336207.
19. World Health Organization. Mental health [Updated 2022 June 17]. 2022. Available from: https://www.who.int/news-room/fact-sheets/detail/mental-health-strengthening-our-response.
20. Substance Abuse and Mental Health Services Administration. Mental health [Updated 2024 November 8]. 2024. Available from: https://www.samhsa.gov/mental-health.
21. World Health Organization. Mental disorders [Updated 2022 June 8]. 2022. Available from: https://www.who.int/news-room/fact-sheets/detail/mental-disorders.
22. National Institute of Mental Health. Mental illness [Updated 2024 September]. 2024. Available from: https://www.nimh.nih.gov/health/statistics/mental-illness.

23. American Psychiatric Association. What are anxiety disorders? [Updated 2023 June]. 2023. Available from: https://www.psychiatry.org/patients-families/anxiety-disorders/what-are-anxiety-disorders.
24. American Psychiatric Association. Diagnostic and statistical manual of mental disorders. 5th ed., text revision. Washington, DC: American Psychiatric Association; 2022.
25. World Health Organization. Schizophrenia [Updated 2022 January 10]. 2022. Available from: https://www.who.int/news-room/fact-sheets/detail/schizophrenia.
26. Kieling C, Buchweitz C, Caye A, Silvani J, Ameis SH, Brunoni AR, et al. Worldwide prevalence and disability from mental disorders across childhood and adolescence: evidence from the global burden of disease study. JAMA Psychiatry. 2024;81(4):347–56.
27. GBD 2019 Mental Disorders Collaborators. Global, regional, and national burden of 12 mental disorders in 204 countries and territories, 1990–2019: a systematic analysis for the global burden of disease study 2019. Lancet Psychiatry. 2022;9(2):137–50.
28. Wu Y, Lu W, Tao M, Cao H, Yuan H, Minguan Y, et al. Changing trends in the global burden of mental disorders from 1990 to 2019 and predicted levels in 25 years. Epidemiol Psychiatr Sci. 2023;32:e63.
29. Richter D, Wall A, Bruen A, Whittington R. Is the global prevalence rate of adult mental illness increasing? Systematic review and meta-analysis. Acta Psychiatr Scand. 2019;140(5):393–407.
30. McGrath JJ, Lim CCW, Plana-Ripoll O, Holtz Y, Agerbo E, Momen NC, et al. Comorbidity within mental disorders: a comprehensive analysis based on 145990 survey respondents from 27 countries. Epidemiol Psychiatr Sci. 2020;29:e153.
31. Siegfried N. A review of comorbidity: major mental illness and problematic substance use. Aust N Z J Psychiatry. 1998;32(5):707–17.
32. Weaver T, Madden P, Charles G, Renton A, Tyrer P, Barnes T, et al. Comorbidity of substance misuse and mental illness in community mental health and substance misuse services. Br J Psychiatry. 2003;183(4):304–13.
33. Walker ER, Druss BG. A public health perspective on mental and medical comorbidity. JAMA. 2016;316(10):1104–5.
34. Bahorik AL, Satre DD, Kline-Simon AH, Weisner CM, Campbell CI. Serious mental illness and medical comorbidities: findings from an integrated health care system. J Psychosom Res. 2017;100:35–45.
35. Bondesson E, Pardo FL, Stigmar K, Ringqvist Å, Petersson IF, Jöud A, et al. Comorbidity between pain and mental illness—evidence of a bidirectional relationship. Eur J Pain. 2018;22(7):1304–11.
36. Momen NC, Plana-Ripoll O, Agerbo E, Benros ME, Børglum AD, Christensen MK, et al. Association between mental disorders and subsequent medical conditions. N Engl J Med. 2020;382:1721–31.
37. Opland C, Torrico TJ. Behavioral therapy [Updated 2024 November 13]. In: StatPearls [Internet]. Treasure Island: StatPearls Publishing; 2025. Available from: https://www.ncbi.nlm.nih.gov/books/NBK609098.
38. Chand SP, Kuckel DP, Huecker MR. Cognitive behavior therapy [Updated 2023 May 23]. In: StatPearls [Internet]. Treasure Island: StatPearls Publishing; 2025. Available from: https://www.ncbi.nlm.nih.gov/books/NBK470241.
39. Hofmann SG, Asnaani A, Vonk IJJ, Sawyer AT, Fang A. The efficacy of cognitive behavioral therapy: a review and meta-analysis. Cogn Ther Res. 2012;36(5):427–40.
40. Sadek J. Clinician's guide to psychopharmacology. Cham: Springer Nature; 2021.
41. American Psychiatric Association. Integrated behavioral healthcare [Updated 2024 January]. 2024. Available from: https://www.psychiatry.org/patients-families/integrated-behavioral-healthcare.
42. Schrager S. Integrating behavioral health into primary care. Fam Pract Manag. 2021;28(3):3–4.
43. Asarnow JR, Rozenman M, Wiblin J, Zeltzer L. Integrated medical-behavioral care compared with usual primary care for child and adolescent behavioral health: a meta-analysis. JAMA Pediatr. 2015;169(10):929–37.

44. Padwa H, Teruya C, Tran E, Lovinger K, Antonini VP, Overholt C, et al. The implementation of integrated behavioral health protocols in primary care settings in project care. J Subst Abus Treat. 2016;62:74–83.
45. Thapa BB, Laws MB, Galárraga O. Evaluating the impact of integrated behavioral health intervention: evidence from Rhode Island. Medicine. 2021;100(34):e27066.
46. Marcenes WS, Sheiham A. The relationship between work stress and oral health status. Soc Sci Med. 1992;35(12):1511–2.
47. Arman K, Petruninaitė A, Grigalauskienė R, Slabšinskienė E. Stress experience and effect on self-perceived oral health status among high school students. Stomatologija. 2016;18(3):75–9.
48. Vasiliou A, Shankardass K, Nisenbaum R, Quiñonez C. Current stress and poor oral health. BMC Oral Health. 2016;16:88.
49. Deinzer R, Hilpert D, Bach K, Schawacht M, Herforth A. Effects of academic stress on oral hygiene—a potential link between stress and plaque-associated disease. J Clin Periodontol. 2001;28(5):459–64.
50. Deinzer R, Granrath N, Spahl M, Linz S, Waschul B, Herforth A. Stress, oral health behaviour and clinical outcome. Br J Health Psychol. 2005;10(2):269–83.
51. Lee MY, Choi EM, Son JH, Chang SJ. The effects of perceived stress on dietary habits and oral health behaviors of Korean adolescents. J Dent Hyg Sci. 2013;13(4):440–8.
52. Choi JS. The relationship between stress perception and oral health status. J Korean Soc Dent Hyg. 2014;14(4):555–61.
53. da Cunha Scalo GP, Abegg C, Celeste RK, Hökerberg YHM, Faerstein E. Occupational stress and self-perceived oral health in Brazilian adults: a pro-Saude study. Ciénc Saúde Colet. 2013;18(7):2069–74.
54. Acharya S, Pentapati KC. Work stress and oral health-related quality of life among Indian information technology workers: an exploratory study. Int Dent J. 2012;62(3):132–6.
55. Hong MH. The effects of occupational stress on oral health impact profile (OHIP) in local government workers. J Korean Soc Dent Hyg. 2012;12(3):471–83.
56. Kim JE, Lee ST, Kim YE, Bae SH, Shin HJ, Jo JE, et al. Influence of stress on the oral health and quality of life of university students. J Korean Soc Dent Hyg. 2018;18(5):797–806.
57. Sisson KL. Theoretical explanations for social inequalities in oral health. Community Dent Oral Epidemiol. 2007;35(2):81–8.
58. Gomaa N, Tenenbaum H, Glogaur M, Quiñonez C. The biology of social adversity applied to oral health. J Dent Res. 2019;98(13):1442–9.
59. Matevosyan NR. Oral health of adults with serious mental illnesses: a review. Community Ment Health J. 2010;46:553–62.
60. Edward KL, Felstead B, Mahoney AM. Hospitalized mental health patients and oral health. J Psychiatr Ment Health Nurs. 2012;19(5):419–25.
61. Turner E, Berry K, Aggarwal VR, Quinlivan L, Villanueva T, Palmier-Claus J. Oral health self-care behaviours in serious mental illness: a systematic review and meta-analysis. Acta Psychiatr Scand. 2022;145(1):29–41.
62. Kisely S, Sawyer E, Siskind D, Lalloo R. The oral health of people with anxiety and depressive disorders—a systematic review and meta-analysis. J Affect Disord. 2016;200:119–32.
63. Kalaigian A, Chaffee BW. Mental health and oral health in a nationally representative cohort. J Dent Res. 2023;102(9):1007–14.
64. Heaton LJ, Santoro M, Tiwari T, Preston R, Schroeder K, Randall CL, et al. Mental health, socioeconomic position, and oral health: a path analysis. Prev Chronic Dis. 2024;21:E76.
65. Tiwari T, Kelly A, Randall CL, Tranby E, Franstve-Hawley J. Association between mental health and oral health status and care utilization. Front Oral Health. 2022;2:732882.
66. O'Neil A, Berk M, Venugopal K, Kim SW, Williams LJ, Jacka FN. The association between poor dental health and depression: findings from a large-scale, population-based study (the NHANES study). Gen Hosp Psychiatry. 2014;36(3):266–70.
67. Nguyen VH, Lin SC, Cappelli DP, Nair S. The association between dental, general, and mental health status among underserved and vulnerable populations served at health centers in the US. J Public Health Dent. 2018;78(1):41–8.

68. Choi J, Price J, Ryder S, Siskind D, Solmi M, Kisely S. Prevalence of dental disorders among people with mental illness: an umbrella review. Aust N Z J Psychiatry. 2022;56(8):949–63.
69. British Society for Disability and Oral Health. Oral health care for people with mental health problems: guidelines and recommendations. London: British Society for Disability and Oral Health; 2000.
70. Khokhar MA, Khokhar WA, Clifton AV, Tosh GE. Oral health education (advice and training) for people with serious mental illness. Cochrane Database Syst Rev. 2016;2016(9):CD008802.
71. Kuipers S, Boonstra N, Kronenberg L, Keuning-Plantinga A, Castelein S. Oral health interventions in patients with a mental health disorder: a scoping review with critical appraisal of the literature. Int J Environ Res Public Health. 2021;18(5):8113.
72. Poornachitra P, Narayan V. Management of dental patients with mental health problems in special care dentistry: a practical algorithm. Cureus. 2023;15(2):e34809.
73. McKibbin CL, Kitchen-Andren KA, Lee AA, Wykes TL, Bourassa KA. Oral health in adults with serious mental illness: needs for and perspectives on care. Community Ment Health J. 2015;51:222–8.
74. Slack-Smith L, Hearn L, Scrine C, Durey A. Barriers and enablers for oral health care for people affected by mental health disorders. Aust Dent J. 2017;62(1):6–13.
75. Scrine C, Durey A, Slack-Smith L. Enhancing oral health for better mental health: exploring the view of mental health professionals. Int J Ment Health Nurs. 2018;27(1):178–86.
76. Kisely S. No mental health without oral health. Can J Psychiatr. 2016;61(5):277–82.
77. Skallevold HE, Rokaya N, Wongsirichat N, Rokaya D. Importance of oral health in mental health disorders: an updated review. J Oral Biol Craniofac Res. 2023;13(5):544–52.
78. Joury E, Kisely S, Watt RG, Ahmed N, Morris AJ, Fortune F, et al. Mental disorders and oral disease: future research directions. J Dent Res. 2023;102(1):5–12.
79. Tiwari T, Randall CL. A framework for the integration of behavioral health and oral health in predoctoral dental education. J Calif Dent Assoc. 2024;52(1):2353747.
80. Cockburn N, Pradhan A, Taing MW, Kisely S, Ford PJ. Oral health impacts of medications used to treat mental illness. J Affect Disord. 2017;223:184–93.
81. Su N, Marek CL, Ching V, Grushka M. Caries prevention for patients with dry mouth. J Can Dent Assoc. 2011;77:b85.
82. Jafari A, Alaee A, Ghods K. The etiologies and considerations of dysgeusia: a review of the literature. J Oral Biosci. 2021;63(4):319–26.
83. Bavikatte G, Sit PL, Hassoon A. Management of drooling of saliva. Br J Med Pract. 2012;5(1):a507.
84. Ekman I, Swedberg K, Taft C, Lindseth A, Norberg A, Brink E, et al. Person-centered care—ready for prime time. Eur J Cardiovasc Nurs. 2011;10:248–51.
85. Kristensen CB, Asimakopoulou K, Scambler S. Enhancing patient-centered care in dentistry: a narrative review. Br Med Bull. 2023;148:79–88.

Effects of Chronic Sun Exposure on the Labial Mucosa

21

Eduardo David Piemonte, Rene Panico,
Gerado Marcelo Gilligan, and Jeronimo Pablo Lazos

21.1 Introduction

21.1.1 Solar Radiation as a Fundamental Component of the Environment and as a Source of Life and Energy

The sun is a fundamental energy source that is crucial for maintaining the human environment. From a biological perspective, it plays a primary role in photosynthesis, an essential process for recycling oxygen, converting CO2 into biomass and supporting the food chain, which includes human nutrition [1]. Additionally, solar radiation contributes to climate, temperature patterns and seasonal cycles, influencing ecosystems, agriculture and water resources [2]. Moreover, solar energy is a renewable source that can be harnessed cleanly and sustainably, reducing dependency on fossil fuels and decreasing pollution [3].

21.1.2 Environmental, Occupational or Recreational Conditions that Increase Exposure to Solar UV Radiation—Other Sources of UV Radiation

Most solar radiation that reaches the Earth's surface has a wavelength within 300–2500 nm, encompassing ultraviolet radiation (UVR) (<400 nm), visible light (400–780 nm, also known as sunlight) and near-infrared (NIR) light (>780 nm). UVR is a form of non-ionising radiation with a wavelength ranging from 100 to

E. D. Piemonte (✉) · R. Panico · G. M. Gilligan · J. P. Lazos
Department of Oral Medicine, Facultad de Odontología, Universidad Nacional de Córdoba, Córdoba, Argentina
e-mail: epiemonte@yahoo.com; renepanico@hotmail.com; ggilligan@unc.edu.ar; jerolazos@gmail.com

S. R. Prabhu et al. (eds.), *Lifestyle in Oral Health and Disease*,
https://doi.org/10.1007/978-3-032-05888-1_21

400 nm and is classified into three main types: UVA (320–400 nm), UVB (280–320 nm) and UVC (100–280 nm) [4].

Solar UVR can vary according to specific conditions. Primarily, the amount of solar radiation that reaches the Earth's surface is influenced by atmospheric, geographical and climatic factors (Fig. 21.1). Exposure increases during summer, especially around midday, and living near the equator results in higher UVR exposure due to the sun's direct position. At higher altitudes, UVR levels rise, with mountainous regions providing more significant exposure. In areas experiencing ozone layer depletion or lacking clouds, the absorption of solar UVR decreases, leading to increased exposure [5, 6]. Similarly, the reflection of solar UVR is higher on surfaces such as sand, water, snow and cement, which amplifies exposure. UVR intensity is categorised using specific guidelines, such as the UV index, which ranges from 1 to 11 or higher. This prediction is based on a combination of latitude, the day of the year, total ozone overhead, elevation above sea level and cloud cover [7].

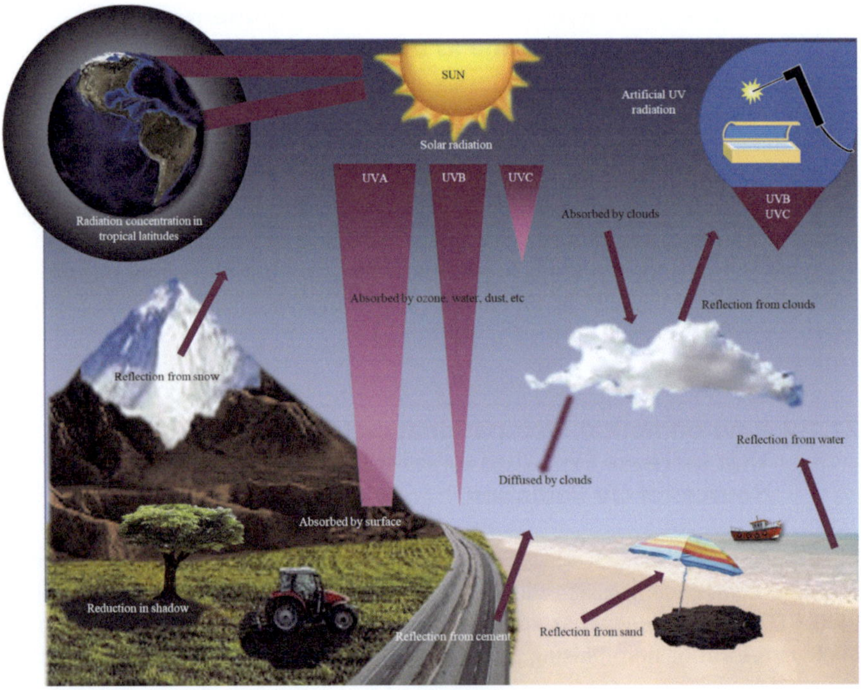

Fig. 21.1 UV radiation: Atmospheric, geographical and climatic factors influencing ultraviolet radiation (UVR). The primary source of UVR is the sun, but there are also artificial sources (arc welders, sunbeds etc.). In areas where UVR strikes the Earth's surface more perpendicularly, the amount of radiation is greater, which is influenced by latitude, season and time of day. UVR is absorbed or reflected in the atmosphere by ozone, clouds and suspended dust. UVR-C is fully immersed in the atmosphere; a small proportion of UVR-C reaches the surface, while UVR-A predominantly reaches the Earth's surface. UVR is reflected by certain surfaces such as water, sand and snow, increasing exposure levels that affect humans

Meteorological services report the UV index and is available in various applications, although not in all regions, limiting its application. Human activities also affect the intensity of exposure to solar UVR. Outdoor jobs (e.g. agriculture, construction, fishing and oil extraction) expose workers to long hours in the sun. Likewise, outdoor recreational activities like swimming, skiing, hiking and surfing imply significant sun exposure. Exposure increases further when clothing is inadequate, such as not wearing a hat [8–10]. Aside from the sun, other sources of UVR can be harmful. Tanning beds and lamps utilise UVR to tan the skin but can considerably raise the risk of skin cancer [11]. Germicidal lamps, growth lamps for indoor plants, welding machines, foundry furnaces and other artificial sources can emit intense UVR, necessitating proper protection to prevent ocular and skin burns [8, 12–17].

21.1.3 Biological Conditions of the Human Being that Facilitate the UVR Effects

Several biological conditions can render specific individuals—particularly those with less melanin in the lip vermilion—more vulnerable to the harmful effects of UV radiation. Racial phototypes with lower levels of melanin have less protection against UV radiation and are more susceptible to its effects [18, 19]. The Fitzpatrick scale is used to classify racial phototypes. It is based on the response to 45–60 minutes of midday solar exposure in northern latitudes (20–45 degrees) during early summer.

This response is evaluated based on two parameters: erythema or inflammatory signs after 24 hours and tanning after one week. The erythema is more pronounced in individuals with lighter phototypes, and the acquired tan (or skin colour) is less significant (Table 21.1). The Fitzpatrick classification does not relate to skin colour

Table 21.1 Fitzpatrick's skin phototypes

Skin phototypes	Unexposed skin colour	Sunburn susceptibility	Time to MED[a]	Tanning capacity	Tanned skin
I	Pale white	Very high (always burns)	21	Never	No tan
II	White	High (almost always burns)	26	Sometimes and minimally	Light tan
III	Light brown	Moderate (sometimes burns)	32	Usually and uniformly	Medium tan
IV	Medium brown, olive	Low (rarely burns)	48	Always tans easily	Dark tan
V	Dark brown	Very low (very rarely burns)	64	Always tans very easily	Very dark tan
VI	Dark brown, black	Extremely low (almost never burns)	64	Always tans intensely	Extremely dark tan

Data from: Aguilera J, et al. Actas Dermosifiliogr (Engl Ed). 2020 Nov;111(9):799–801. https://doi.org/10.1016/j.adengl.2020.06.004

[a]Time to MED: Minutes to reach minimal erythemal dose in summer with an UV index of 9–10

but rather to the skin's protection against solar radiation. A high or dark phototype does not imply total protection against solar radiation; rather, it indicates that the patient has better protection when exposed to solar UVR, as outlined in the Fitzpatrick study. Therefore, when a person with phototype V or VI is exposed for an extended period at a different latitude, in the mountains or on highly reflective terrain, they will inevitably experience the harmful effects of solar UVR, albeit with less intensity than individuals with lighter racial phototypes [20]. Thus, assessing UVR risk solely based on phototype categories may provide both patients and physicians with a false sense of security, as individuals of colour can also develop skin cancer [21].

Unfortunately, this and other classifications of racial phototypes refer to the skin and not to the lip vermilion. Since it has a thinner epithelium with less keratinisation and fewer melanocytes than the skin [22], the racial phototype of the lip will always be less than the skin. The lower thickness of the vermilion epithelial allows a deeper penetration of UVR, therefore increasing damage. This occurs primarily in children and elderlies, as well as more in the lip vermilion compared to the skin in the same person [19, 23]. Certain medications—such as tetracyclines, retinoids and others—can increase the skin's sensitivity to UVR [24–26]. Some people have a genetic predisposition that could increase susceptibility to UVR's harmful effects, for example, xeroderma pigmentosum and lupus erythematosus, among others [27, 28].

21.1.4 Direct Beneficial Effects of Solar Radiation on Humans

Solar radiation has numerous beneficial effects on human health. Sun exposure is essential for synthesising vitamin D in the skin, which is vital for bone health because it facilitates calcium absorption. It also influences immune function, cardiovascular health and mood regulation [29, 30]. Sun exposure can alleviate symptoms of seasonal affective disorder and enhance overall mood by impacting serotonin regulation [31, 32]. Sunlight helps regulate the body's circadian rhythms, the 24-hour biological cycles that influence sleep and wakefulness. Sun exposure can improve sleep quality and reset the biological clock [33]. Although excessive exposure may be harmful, moderate amounts can also assist in treating conditions like psoriasis and vitiligo [34–36].

21.1.5 Solar Radiation Harmful to Humans: UVR

Despite the benefits of the sun, excessive exposure can also harm human health, primarily due to UV radiation (Table 21.2). Approximately 90–99% of UVA reaches the Earth's surface because the atmosphere does not filter it. Due to its longer wavelength, UVA can penetrate deeper into the skin, but its low energy makes it hazardous only with prolonged exposure. It causes skin ageing and dyschromias and induces both immediate and persistent tanning. Approximately 1–10% of UVB reaches the Earth's surface as the ozone layer filters it. Because of its shorter wavelength, UVB penetrates only the upper layer of the epidermis, but its high energy can cause

Table 21.2 UVR main harmful effects on human health

	Acute effects	Chronic effects
Skin	Sunburn	Premature aging
	Photoallergy	Actinic keratosis
	Phototoxicity	Basal cell carcinoma
		Squamous cell carcinoma
		Skin melanoma
		Dyschromias
Lip	Acute actinic cheilitis	Chronic actinic cheilitis/actinic keratosis
	Photoallergy	Lip squamous cell carcinoma
	Phototoxicity	Lip melanoma(?)
		Dyschromias
Eyes	Photoconjunctivitis	Cataracts
	Photokeratitis	Pterygium
		Macular degeneration
		Blindness
Immune system	Viral reactivation human papilloma virus (HPV); herpes simplex virus 1 (HSV1); others)	Immunosuppression
Other disorders worsen by UVR	Xeroderma pigmentosum	
	Vitiligo	
	Lupus erythematosus	
	Porphyrias	
	Melasma	

sunburn, tanning, wrinkles, photoaging and skin cancer. Solar UVC is entirely filtered by the atmosphere, with major artificial sources including arc welders and germicidal lamps. Its shorter wavelength has shallow penetration, but its high energy makes it the most dangerous, being responsible for burns and skin cancer [37].

In general, all UVRs penetrate the superficial layer of the skin and may cause damage, depending on whether the exposure is acute or chronic. Short-term exposure beyond an individual' s tolerance can result in sunburn of varying severity; however, drug- mediated photosensitivity can occur even with minimal exposure [38, 39]. Photosensitivity phenomena can be classified as phototoxicity and photoallergy. Phototoxicity is more common and typically acute. It results from direct tissue injury, clinically presenting as sunburn, erythema, oedema, bullae and vesicles. Common systemic medications associated with this include chlordiazepoxide, griseofulvin, voriconazole, ketoconazole, ciprofloxacin, tetracyclines, furosemide, amiodarone, quinidine, thiazides, benzydamine, sulfonamide, ketoprofen, naproxen and ibuprofen, especially when administered in high doses. Conversely, photoallergic responses are due to delayed hypersensitivity reactions, presenting as papular or eczematous eruptions. Drugs linked to photoallergy include benzophenone- 3, padimate O, homosalate, para- aminobenzoic acid, avobenzone, 6-methylcoumarin, dapsone, benzydamine, hydroxychloroquine, piroxicam and musk ambrette, even at low doses [40, 41]. Additionally, dyes used in the textile industry, photosensitising agents in agriculture and some inks in the printing industry may contain photosensitisers [17]. Chronic exposure to UVR can lead to more severe and often irreversible effects related to oxidative stress, DNA mutations and epigenetic changes [42–45]. Cumulative exposure to UVR increases the risk of skin cancer, including melanoma, which is why solar and UVR, in general, are classified as carcinogens for humans by the International Agency for Research on Cancer (IARC; [46, 47]). UVR can accelerate the skin' s aging process, resulting in wrinkles, sunspots and loss of elasticity [48, 49]. UVR-related skin damage, including cancer, is significantly less prevalent in individuals with darker phototypes compared to those with fair skin. However, skin malignancies in people with dark skin are often detected at a more advanced stage, which consequently leads to a worse prognosis. Photodamage caused by UVR is more readily identified in light skin phototypes; in those with darker phototypes, it is more likely to manifest as pigmentary changes, including uneven skin tone, post-inflammatory hyperpigmentation or melasma [50]. Unprotected exposure to intense sunlight can harm the eyes, leading to cataracts, pterygium and macular degeneration. Chronic UVR exposure can suppress the skin' s immune response, diminishing the body' s ability to defend against certain infections and even skin cancer [48, 51, 52].

21.2 Lip Diseases Associated with Exposure to Solar and/or UV Radiation

The entire spectrum of UVR can damage the exposed surfaces of the human body, including the lip vermilion, although UVB rays are the most significant [43]. The skin reflects 70% of UVR, primarily due to melanin, compared to only 5–10% for the lip. This difference is due to the thinner epithelium and keratin layer, a lower amount of melanin and minimal-to-non-existent secretion from sebaceous and sweat glands. The lower lip vermilion is more susceptible to UV damage than the skin [53]. Initial exposure may result in acute cheilitis, and with chronic exposure, actinic cheilitis or actinic keratosis of the lip vermilion (AC/AKL) can develop, potentially leading to lip squamous cell carcinoma (LSCC). These three diseases can be regarded as part of a spectrum of the same process. Furthermore, the activation of melanocytes can lead to pigmented lesions.

21.2.1 Acute Actinic Cheilitis

Cheilitis refers to a group of inflammatory diseases that affect the lips, characterised by a broad spectrum of causes and clinical manifestations. Acute actinic cheilitis is the most common type, primarily affecting the lower lip in children, adolescents and young adults. It can be exacerbated by nutritional deficiencies, factitious causes or medication [54, 55]. The most frequent clinical feature is multiple and recurring dryness and scaling of the lips, which patients often peel off, leading to erosions and crusts that can be painful (Fig. 21.2). In some instances, fissures, red spots due to atrophy and lip oedema may also be observed. In the absence of predisposing factors, cheilitis may resolve quickly with treatment; however, repeated sun exposure

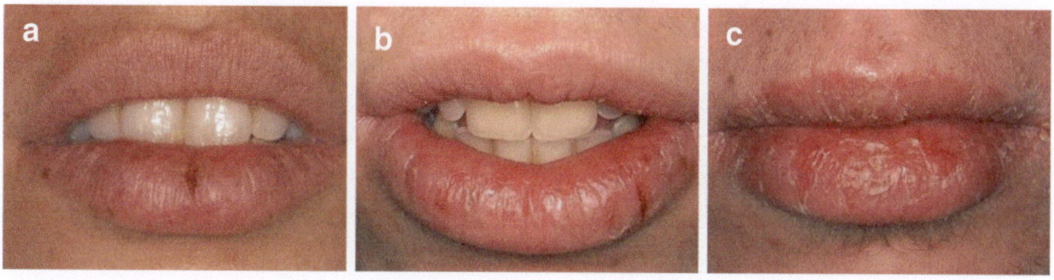

Fig. 21.2 Acute actinic cheilitis in young patients: (**a**) Initial lesions located exclusively on the lower lip, with a central linear fissure. (**b**) More extended alterations with part of the lower mucosa exposed. (**c**) Multiple desquamations and oedema on the lips, noting that lesions are more extended even to the upper lip

can lead to recurrence. Among the acute cheilitis associated with UV radiation, those caused by phototoxicity and photoallergic reactions can affect only the lips or be part of a broader skin condition [56]. Cheilitis, due to phototoxicity, typically has an acute onset and presents with erythema, blisters, erosions and crusts. Over time, this may result in the development of melanotic macules as a sequel. In contrast, cheilitis, due to photoallergy, often appears with scales, is sometimes accompanied by eczema on the lips and usually does not leave scars [57]. Photoallergy due to medications can occur when a drug is applied directly to or briefly contacts the lips, triggered by various mouthwashes, lipstick ingredients, sunscreen agents, toothpaste components, nail polish and cosmetics [58–61].

21.2.2 Actinic Cheilitis or Actinic Keratosis of the Lip Vermilion

21.2.2.1 Epidemiology and Aetiology of Actinic Cheilitis and Actinic Keratosis

Actinic cheilitis (AC) and actinic keratosis of the lip (AKL) are chronic inflammatory conditions of the lip that result from excessive exposure to solar ultraviolet radiation, primarily affecting the lower lip [62]. Some authors consider AC/AKL to be misnomers and prefer terms such as solar cheilitis, solar cheilosis, solar keratosis or actinic cheilitis of the lip [63]. In patients with prolonged UVR exposure over the years, genetic, tissue and clinical changes can develop in the lip vermilion. These changes are directly related to both the individual's skin phototype and cumulative UVR exposure, affecting individuals of any phototype. However, they are more frequent among fair-skinned, middle-aged to elderly individuals who are exposed to intense sources of UVR, whether natural or artificial, for occupational or recreational purposes. Furthermore, there is a higher incidence among people living near the equator, at high altitudes or in areas with reflective surfaces such as water, sand, snow or cement. Typically, those affected do not use lip sunscreen or hats. Thus, high-risk groups include fishermen (sailor's lip), construction workers, agricultural workers, gardeners, soldiers and athletes. The male- to- female ratio is 10: 1, related to the higher frequency of the aforementioned activities and lower sunscreen use

[64, 65]. A meta-analysis demonstrated that the factors from highest to lowest risk for AC are having a light skin phototype, being over 50 years old, experiencing daily high cumulative sun exposure throughout life, and being male. Additionally, being a drinker or smoker is also considered a risk factor for AC/AKL [66]. The aetiology and physiopathogenic mechanisms for AC are similar to those of actinic keratosis of the skin. Moreover, AC/AKL may also be associated with arsenic exposure and certain genetic disorders (e.g. xeroderma pigmentosum, porphyria cutanea or albinism) [64, 67–70]. The global prevalence of AC/AKL has been estimated at 2. 08% [71], while in high-risk groups, it can reach values close to 45% [72].

21.2.2.2 Clinical Manifestations of AC/AKL

AC/AKL is a slowly developing, typically asymptomatic lesion that exhibits a wide range of clinical features (Fig. 21.3). Patients are often unaware of the potential risk of damage, believing that these changes may arise from their occupation or ageing. A clinical examination of the lips may reveal dryness, atrophy, scaly lesions, swelling, erythema, vertical fissures, ulceration and blurred demarcation between the vermilion border and the skin. White or yellowish spots or plaques (with sharp or diffuse delimitation), a mottled appearance that indicates the simultaneous presence of erythema and white patches, loss of elasticity and a crenated surface can also be observed [64, 73–76]. Initial findings include atrophy, evidenced by blotchy and pale areas, dryness and occasionally fissures. Blurring of the margin between the vermilion and the adjacent skin is common. AC/AKL is often accompanied by melanotic macules, likely a reaction to the inflammatory process [77, 78]. As it progresses, scales and rough areas develop, affecting parts or even most of the lip vermilion. Occasionally, it may present as a single plaque with some scales. Patients frequently remove the plaque or scales repeatedly, causing further damage, only for them to reappear. Changes in surface texture, generalised or localised thickening of the epithelium (plaques), chronic ulceration, atrophy, nodules, bleeding and failure of conservative treatment all indicate early malignant transformation, thus necessitating a biopsy [62, 64, 73, 79, 80].

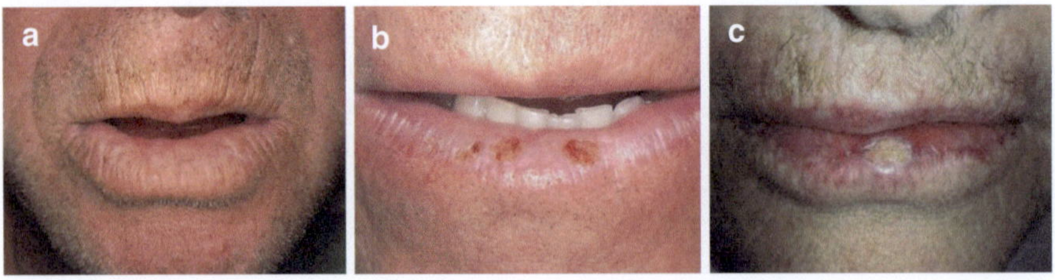

Fig. 21.3 Clinical features of AC/AKL. (**a**) Generalised loss of definition of the lower lip vermilion border; notice that the colour is also similar to the skin, which is atrophy and dryness. (**b**) A fair-skinned male developing small, round, chronic ulcerations and generalised lower lip atrophy. (**c**) A more advanced case with a larger rough keratotic area, also having atrophy and dryness; again, the vermillion appearance is beginning to look similar to the skin

Due to the heterogeneous nature of AC/AKL and the lack of correspondence between clinical and histological modifications, it is recommended to address treatment *only* when a histopathological analysis is available, preferably from multiple areas [63]. This is true even in cases without apparent alterations to avoid underdiagnosing dysplasia or LSCC.

Integrating non-invasive diagnostic techniques with visual inspection and palpation of the lips can be helpful and well tolerated during the diagnosis, treatment and follow-up of patients with AC/AKL [81]. Nevertheless, these complementary methods seem to be poorly studied. Three well-conducted systematic reviews on the accuracy of non-invasive diagnostic tests for detecting malignant transformation did not find any articles applying this technique in AC/AKL [82–84]. In this regard, although vital staining with toluidine blue and Lugol's iodine is one of the most commonly used non-invasive procedures in oral potential malignant disorder (OPMD) (including narrow-band imaging), we have not encountered studies with specific data for AC/AKL. Due to the ease of visual access, optical or digital image amplification can be achieved with a dermatoscope or videodermatoscope. The dermatoscope allows for direct viewing of images, whereas a videodermatoscope requires the image to be viewed on a computer screen [85]. Image amplification facilitates the detection of smaller lesions and details not visible with routine visual inspection, thereby enabling the identification of more suspicious lesions for biopsy [76, 86, 87]. Certain features visible under magnification, such as red and white mottled lesions, diffusely distributed polymorphic vessels, ulceration and blood spots, are frequently observed in AC/AKL. It is worth noting that the overlap of such variations with other forms of cheilitis complicates identifying lesions that are pathognomonic for AC/AKL [88]. Nonetheless, a scaly lesion exhibiting exophytic growth, ulceration or showing red and white mottled lesions with linear and hairpin vessels on dermoscopy may have a high probability of being an LSCC [87]. Autofluorescence induced by LED lamps emitting at wavelengths of 400 to 460 nm reveals a heterogeneous pattern, characterised by both loss and increase of fluorescence in the lip vermilion in AC/AKL, facilitating the detection of areas with moderate to severe epithelial dysplasia [89, 90]. Reflectance confocal microscopy (RCM) permits examination of the epidermis and superficial dermis at resolutions comparable to those achieved with light optical microscopy. It provides detailed images of tissue architecture and cellular morphology in vivo and in real time. With RCM, the stratum granulosum and spinosum of normal epithelium exhibit a consistent honeycomb pattern [76, 91–93]. In cases of AC/AKL with dysplasia, this honeycomb pattern becomes irregular, which is also consistent with histopathological evaluation [82]. However, evident inflammation poses a diagnostic challenge, making it necessary to perform a biopsy in uncertain cases [92]. RCM can be employed to monitor AC/AKL cases, locate biopsy sites and identify the early progression of AC/AKL to SCC with good sensitivity and specificity, though it is expensive [94].

21.2.2.3 Histopathological Findings in AC/AKL

In histopathological studies, the epithelium in AC/AKL almost always presents acanthosis and hyperparakeratosis, although hyperorthokeratosis is also often present. However, it is common to find epithelial atrophy and/or granulosis. In the connective tissue, a basophilic degeneration of collagen fibres, called *solar elastosis,* is usually detected. A chronic inflammatory infiltrate varying from mild-to-severe can be seen, composed mainly of lymphocytes, some plasma cells and eosinophils. Blood vessels can be seen dilated because of the increase in endothelial cells. Histological changes of AC/AKL can be presented unevenly, disregarding the clinical presentation [65, 74, 79, 80]. The epithelium can display different degrees of dysplasia, and the potential for malignant transformation increases with more severity. When there is ulceration and severe inflammation, cellular atypia can be found, making the distinction between proper LSCC and AC/AKL challenging [95, 96] (Fig. 21.4).

21.2.2.4 Malignant Transformation of AC/AKL

A lesion must meet certain criteria to be classified as an OPMD, and AC/AKL fulfils these criteria. In longitudinal studies, areas of tissue with specific clinical alterations that were initially identified as 'precancerous' have undergone malignant transformation during follow-up. The potential for malignant change of AC/AKL into

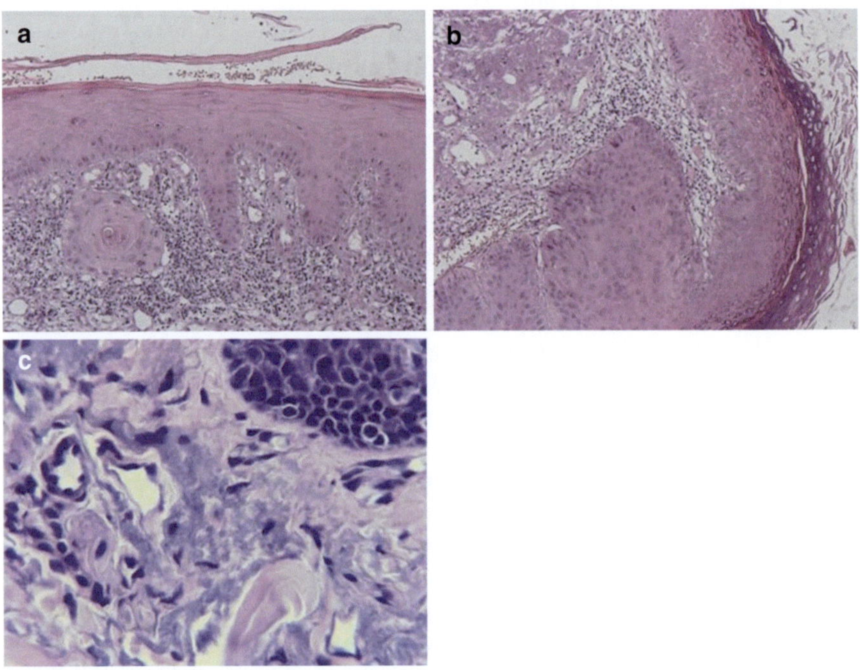

Fig. 21.4 Histopathological features of AC/AKL. (**a**) Epithelial atrophy, with a dense chronic inflammatory cell infiltrate and dilated blood vessels. (**b**) Hyperorthokeratosis with some hyperchromatism and nuclear pleomorphism on the basal and parabasal epithelium, basophilic degeneration of collagen and mononuclear infiltrate within the connective tissue. (**c**) Often the underlying connective tissue reveals a band of amorphous, acellular, basophilic change known as solar elastosis, as shown in the image. (Images **a** and **b** courtesy of Prof. Benjamin Martinez-Rondanelli)

Box 21.1 AC/AKL as an Oral Potentially Malignant Disorder

- Longitudinal studies show that between 3.07 and 16.9% of AC/AKL undergo malignant transformation to squamous cell carcinoma.
- With an AC/AKL global prevalence of approximately 2%, more than 70% of lip vermilion squamous cell carcinomas occur on lips with AC/AKL.
- Moderate or severe dysplasia can be observed in more than 40% of AC/AKL.
- Several biomarkers associated with carcinogenesis have shown elevated expression in AC/AKL.

LSCC is unquestionable; however, evidence of its transformation rate is scarce. While two studies with rigorous follow-up reported transformation rates of 12.05% and 16.9% [65, 97] (Box 21.1), a recent systematic review estimated the rate at 3. 3.07% [72]. AC/AKL can coexist at the margins of evident oral squamous cell carcinomas, with LSCC developing in lips affected by actinic cheilitis in over 70% of cases [98]. Some AC/AKL may exhibit morphological and cytological changes analogous to those seen in epithelial malignancies but without overt invasion. AC/AKL may display mild, moderate or severe dysplasia, or even no dysplasia at all. The frequency of dysplasia grades varies across studies, but the combined instances of moderate and severe dysplasia (or high- grade dysplasia, according to the binary system) may exceed 40% of cases [74, 99–101] (Box 21.1). Most studies report no correlation between the degree of dysplasia and clinical variables. One study utilising both the binary and World Health Organization (WHO) systems identified that the presence of erosions, ulcers and crusts is linked to high-grade, moderate and severe dysplasia, while the blurring of the border between the labial vermilion and the skin correlates with low-grade, mild or no dysplasia [102, 103]. Certain chromosomal, genomic and molecular alterations detected in clearly invasive oral cancers are also observed in these potential 'premalignant' phases. Changes in the activity of various carcinogenic biomarkers are associated with AC/AKL. Some of the reported biomarkers include p 53, p 63, cyclin D 1, bcl- 2, Ki- 67, murine double minute 2 (MDM-2), programmed cell death protein 1 (PD-1), transforming growth fator beta 1 (TGF-β1), β-catenin, cyclooxygenase, signal transducer and activator of transcription protein, fibroblast growth factor, cytokeratin, syndecan, laminin, integrins, mast cells and natural and cytotoxic killer cells [64, 80, 104–113]. Although these may contribute to the molecular evolution of AC/AKL to LSCC, their reliability as clinical predictive markers or for staging purposes remains uncertain [64]. The malignant transformation of AC/AKL, whether treated surgically or non- surgically, is absent or exceedingly rare [114, 115].

21.2.2.5 Treatment of AC/AKL

Most of the alterations produced by AC/AKL are considered irreversible [116]. Removal of the dysplastic epithelium is recommended with prior histopathological confirmation always, either by surgical or non-surgical interventions, even in the case of homogeneous lesions [63]. Vermilionectomy, a lip shaving considered an excisional biopsy (complete surgical removal), is the preferred choice because it allows adequate histological evaluation of the resected tissue and accurate diagnosis [117], at the same time eliminating epithelial dysplasia [118]. All the other treatment options do not allow a complete anatomopathological evaluation and detection of possible areas of LSCC [79, 119]. The surgical approach (laser ablation or vaporisation, partial surgery, vermilionectomy) offered complete clinical resolution in more than 90% of the cases, while non-surgical treatment was lower than 70%. In addition, the recurrence rate was lower for surgical (8.4%) than for non-surgical treatment (12.6–19.2%) [114, 117, 120, 121]. Adverse effects were also lower for surgical treatment, with laser surgery having the least. Those include pain, swelling, bruising, paraesthesia, infection, necrosis, bleeding, haematomas and difficulty eating immediately after surgery [76]. Among non-surgical treatments, options include photodynamic therapy, 3% diclofenac in 2.5% hyaluronic acid, photodynamic treatment with 5% imiquimod, aminolaevulinic acid, 5% imiquimod, fluorouracil, 0.015% ingenol mebutate and 50% trichloroacetic acid. Some common adverse effects for those are pain, burning, erythema, oedema, bleeding and swelling [76]. Despite its moderate clinical efficacy, non-surgical procedures elicited outstanding cosmetic outcomes [114, 120, 121], with very low rates of malignant transformation after treatment in all studies. Therapy selection should be made on an individual basis. This ought to be guided by the pathological findings and the potential for malignant transformation, considering the side effects, the patient's cosmetic wishes and the available scientific evidence. In cases with severe or extended moderate dysplasia, a surgical approach is recommended. Non-surgical treatments are endorsed in lesions with mild-to-moderate dysplasia. Regardless of the chosen therapy, preventive measures and regular follow-up after treatment are *mandatory* [114].

21.2.3 Lip Cancer

21.2.3.1 Histological Types of Lip Cancer

The term lip cancer (LC) refers specifically to carcinomas originating in the *lip vermilion*, not skin or mucosa [122]. Its features—particularly prognostic ones—are often intermediate between oral squamous cell carcinoma (OSCC) and cutaneous squamous cell carcinoma (CSCC). Still, it is usually grouped with OSCC in epidemiological records, making it difficult to find specific data on LSCC [123]. The predominant histological type among LC is LSCC, which is 80–90% [124–126]. LSCC generally affects the lower lip in 70–95% of cases, probably because its anatomical position exposes it more directly to UVR [87, 101, 124, 127, 128]. According to different studies, most LSCCs are well or moderately differentiated, accounting for 90% or more of cases [101, 127]. This attribute is strongly linked to a better prognosis [129, 130]. Verrucous carcinomas are very rare, are generally associated with tobacco use and arise where the cigarette rests on the lower lip. Lip basal cell carcinoma is also very unusual, affecting mainly the upper lip in women, at an older age than LSCC and without association with UVR [124, 128, 131].

21.2.3.2 Epidemiology and Aetiology of LSCC

LSCC and OSCC represented 2.9% of all cancers among males and 1% among females [132], though the incidence rate and proportion of LSCC regarding mouth cancers are variable. The estimated global incidence of LC in 2012 was 0.3 per 100,000 (0.4 in men and 0.2 in women) [133]. Countries or regions with a significant amount of fair-skinned population, those exposed to UVR for long periods and/or living in tropical or subtropical regions tend to have higher incidence. In 2012, the countries with the highest incidence of LC were Australia, Serbia, Ukraine and the south of Spain, with rates higher than 2.3/100,000. Other countries with relatively high incidence rates included the Nordic, Baltic and Eastern European countries. The incidence of LSCC is also relatively high in Iceland, Canada, the United States, Mexico, Brazil, Cuba, South Africa, New Zealand, Tunisia, Turkey, Iraq, and Georgia, with values ranging from 0.4 to 2.3/100,000 [133]. It is estimated that LC constitutes nearly 11% of all oral cancers in both men and women [133], but then in countries with high incidence -like Australia-, LC can represent up to 49% [134]. Most countries have shown a decrease in LC incidence, especially those with a Caucasian population, likely associated with a lower proportion of people working outdoors, better measures for UV protection and reduced smoking [132].

Similar to other oral malignancies, carcinogenesis does not seem to be limited to a single agent, but rather to a complex multistep process of interactions between putative risk factors [122]. For decades, it has been recognised that LC has a multifactorial aetiology. For LSCC, UVR and racial phototype are the main risk factors. Tobacco and/or alcohol use are relatively less important compared to OSCC [101, 122, 135, 136]. Family predisposition, educational level and poor oral health are also considered to a lesser extent [122]. Exceptionally, predisposing systemic diseases such as albinism, xeroderma pigmentosum and lupus erythematosus can have a role [137, 138]. As in AC/AKL, the risk is strongly related to early and cumulative sunlight exposure, based primarily on two facts [46, 136]. Firstly, risk factors are essentially the same as those for AC/AKL, meaning any condition allowing greater time or intense UVR exposure (outdoor work in areas with high UVR or for long periods lacking solar protection) [46, 134, 135]. Secondly, while OSCC originates in precursor lesions in 30–50% of cases [139], LSCC develops on actinic cheilitis in more than 70% of cases, disregarding those that may evolve from leukoplakias [98]. Furthermore, AC/AKL and LSCC share a similar expression of mutations and biomarkers associated with carcinogenesis [140, 141]. LSCC can affect individuals with *any phototype*, even though it is more common in individuals with lighter skin. LSCC affects predominantly men, not due to sex-related features, but rather because of sociocultural factors which increase men's exposure to UVR [98, 124]. Regarding age, LSCC ordinarily appears after 50 years, the average age is higher than AC/AKL, reinforcing the concept that cumulative UVR over time increases the risk of LSCC [124, 142]. LSCC is uncommon in younger patients, with case series reported on patients undergoing immunosuppressive therapy for renal transplant [143].

21.2.3.3 Clinical Manifestations of LSCC

LSCC is a readily detectable cancer due to the easy visual and tactile access, both for professionals and patients. LSCC can occur anywhere on the lip, primarily the lower lip when related to AC/AKL. If it is associated with tobacco use, it usually occurs at the site where the cigarette is placed. The clinical appearance of LSCC can vary considerably depending on size, ranging from a small lesion of no more than 5 mm to involving the entire vermillion, skin and mucosa of the lip and buccal mucosa (Figs. 21.5 and 21.6). LSCC T2, T3 and T4 can show as tumours with an irregular surface, verrucous or vegetative appearance, well-defined margins or even as deep ulcers with raised and indurated edges, partly covered with crusts. Bleeding and pain might occur, but usually only in advanced cases. They too can appear as flat lesions, with a slightly irregular sandpaper-like surface, and tend to occupy the entire lip vermilion. Palpation of the mucosal and skin surfaces helps define the clinical depth of invasion. The biggest challenge for clinical diagnosis is T1, which can be confused with a manifestation of AC/AKL or leukoplakia, seeming a benign lesion, initially being asymptomatic. The appearance of red spots, fissures, scales, white or yellowish plaques, erosions, ulcers, nodules (even smaller than 1 cm) and being persistent in the *same* site for more than a month can be an indicator of LSCC. The lesions grow gradually into large tumours or ulcers. Palpation is an important clinical assessment because induration and perceptible thickening are also indicators of a potential malignant transformation. When finding any of those clinical manifestations, a biopsy is essential to ensure histopathological diagnosis. In cases of heterogeneous and extensive lesions, taking multiple samples is recommended [79, 87, 143–145]. Examination of neck lymph node metastasis should initially be done by palpation, but it has a high false positive and false negative result, rendering decreased accuracy and low sensitivity [146]. Clinical assessment alone, based on visual examination and palpation, often fails to detect occult metastases, leading to overtreatment or undertreatment [147]. To improve the accuracy of lymph node metastasis detection in LSCC, imaging methods such as computed tomography, magnetic resonance, positron emission tomography/computed tomography and ultrasonography with or without fine needle aspiration could be used.

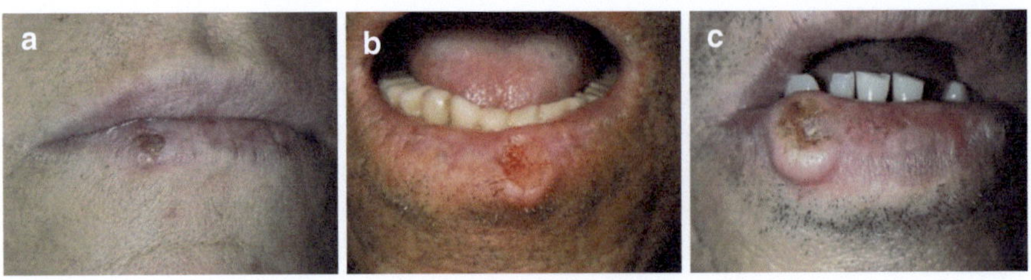

Fig. 21.5 Initial lip squamous cell carcinoma (SCC). (**a**) Woman of ≤50 years, with a loss of exposure throughout her life as an athlete. The lesion began as a small rough patch that slowly grew and became thicker, and the biopsy proved it to be SCC. (**b**) Early invasive SCC emerging on a patient with AC of the lower lip. An asymptomatic, round chronic ulceration gradually increasing its size over the years, in a lip with blurring borders and atrophy. (**c**) Patient with a long-standing actinic cheilitis with a chronic ulcer. Biopsy revealed early invasive squamous cell carcinoma

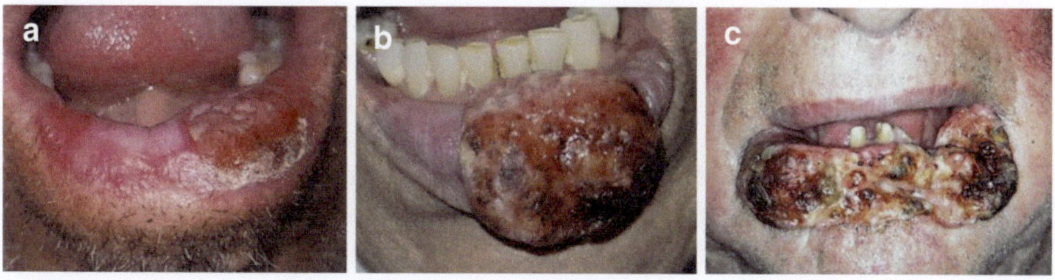

Fig. 21.6 Advanced lip SCC. (**a**) Lower lip macrocheilia, erythema, white plaques in the middle and a large ulcer on the left, with irregular patches, the latter being indurated to palpation. (**b**) An exophytic, round, of about 6 cm, and well-circumscribed tumour on the lower lip, presenting several crusts and atrophic areas, also indurated. (**c**) An advanced case involving the skin and vermilion of the lip, including the oral mucosa, showing a lesion that had developed several years earlier was observed, growing to the point of an irregular, exophytic tumor, very firm to palpation, accompanied by crusts and erosions. The patient had trouble talking, swallowing and eating, having lost a great deal of weight

Each of these procedures has advantages and disadvantages, but the integration of these imaging modalities provides a more comprehensive evaluation, allowing better staging and treatment planning [147].

21.2.3.4 Prognosis and Treatment of LSCC

The relatively low incidence of metastasis and slow growth should not induce an underestimation of LSCC evolution [144]. In patients with LSCC, lymph node metastasis occurs in 3–20% of the cases, which is lower than in the oral cavity, although higher than skin [98, 135, 143]. LSCC related to AC/AKL has a lower frequency of lymph node metastasis compared to LSCC without AC/AKL (10% vs. 50%), which suggests that AC/AKL is an indicator of better prognosis [98]. A tumour thickness larger than 5 mm also increases the risk of lymph node metastasis [148]. Rates of lymph node metastasis range from 3.4% to 7% for T1 tumours, 11% to 35% for T2 tumours and 17% to 100% for T3 and T4 tumours [135, 144]. LSCC seldom produces distant metastases, with an overall incidence of 0.5–3%. Distant metastasis could occur in up to 10% of patients with poorly differentiated LSCC of advanced size and lymph node metastasis, or locoregional recurrence [149]. Overall, LSCC survival is around 80% [135]. Diagnosed and treated in early stages, the survival rate rises to 90%, but with lymph node metastasis, survival decreases to 30–70% [143, 144].

In stages I and II, surgical excision for LSCC is the first line of treatment unless contraindicated by the patient's comorbidities. Surgical excision with 1 cm margins or Mohs surgery is indicated, demonstrating clearance rates of 92 and 100% [135, 150]. Mohs surgery is a micrographic procedure that has become the gold standard for certain types of skin cancer, including lip cancer. It involves removing the affected tissue in layers while performing immediate microscopic analysis. The process is repeated until no more malignant cells are found. The main advantage of Mohs surgery is that it allows the preservation of as much healthy tissue as possible. This is especially important in visible or functionally sensitive areas such as the face, as well as having a high survival rate and very low recurrence rates [130, 151, 152]. Radiation therapy (RT) is considered adjuvant therapy for cases when clear margins cannot be obtained or for high-risk tumours (poorly differentiated, thickness larger than 5 mm) [79, 153]. Decision to use RT should be taken with special care, considering adverse effects such as soft tissue induration, functional impairment, increased difficulty of future surgery and aesthetic impairment [79, 154]. Stage III and IV require surgery combined with RT, chemotherapy combined with RT or surgery following the Mohs method. In stages III and IV, excision of regional lymph nodes is performed as routine, and in stages I and II it is performed only when the clinical or imaging procedures generate suspicion. Despite recent advances in LSCC treatments, the patient would likely have affected diverse functions (phonation, chewing, swallowing), and could have severe aesthetical consequences, deteriorating the self-image, and subsequently affecting patients' quality of life profoundly [155, 156].

21.2.4 Lip Melanoma

Skin melanoma constitutes 1% of skin cancers, but accounts for 75% of skin cancer deaths [157], and like LSCC, it is also associated with cumulative exposure to UVR [158, 159]. The number of melanocytes is lower in the vermilion than in the skin, so it would be expected lip melanoma (LM) to have a higher frequency than the oral mucosa. However, including mucosa and vermilion, LM is very rare [160]. LM is more frequent in the upper lip, unlike LSCC. Initially, LM can be shown as a small ulcerated dark brown nodule [160, 161], or as a dark spot on the lip vermilion. Melanocytic nevus and oral melanotic macule may be indistinguishable from early LM lesions. More advanced lesions can have irregular and poorly defined borders, sometimes ulcerated. It can easily extend to the mucosa and skin of the lip, even presenting satellite lesions [160, 162]. At this stage, it must be differentiated from other dark lesions common on the lip, such as melanocytic nevi, reactive melanosis and vascular malformations. LM can then grow and generate exophytic or ulcerated tumours, sometimes larger than 4 cm, with a very poor prognosis [160]. Less frequently, LMs can present as the desmoplastic (amelanotic melanoma) type, observable as ulcers or lip swellings of various sizes *without* melanin formation, making its clinical and histopathological diagnosis even more challenging [163, 164].

21.2.5 Lip Dyschromias

While low phototypes have a higher risk of AC/AKL and LSCC, patients with intermediate and high phototypes have higher risk of presenting dyschromias. Both hyper or hypochromias are plausibly caused or aggravated by UVA and visible light solar radiation [50, 165]. Among those caused by sunlight, the lentigo solar or senile, post-inflammatory pigmentations or melanotic macules [38], melanoacanthoma and labial lentigo in the lip vermilion can be mentioned [22, 78, 166, 167].

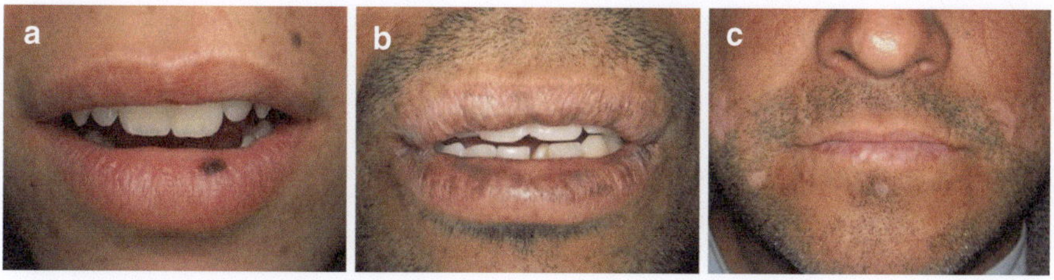

Fig. 21.7 Lip dyschromias. (**a**) Reactive hyperchromia in the lower lip, here showing uniform brown coloration and a sharply demarcated limit. (**b**) Reactive hyperchromia is seen as multiple, flat and poorly demarcated lesions on the lower lip, extended to both vermillion and mucosa. (**c**) Hypomelanotic spots can be seen on the lip and face of the patient with vitiligo

Vitiligo is among those aggravated by sunlight, often in the context of autoimmunity, and can be expressed on the vermilion lips [168]. Independently of the aesthetic factor, such lesions do not carry risk of LM, but they can be an indicator of chronic exposure to solar radiation (Fig. 21.7). It is important to consider differential diagnoses, especially for hyperchromic lesions, among which various syndromes, hormonal alterations and drug-induced hyperpigmentation stand out [22].

21.3 Prevention of UVR-Induced Lip Damage

Cutaneous response to UVR exposure is spectrally and dose dependent. Prevention measures can be implemented depending on UVR intensity, which increases according to atmospheric, geographic and climatic conditions. UVR intensity is higher at latitudes closer to the Earth's equator, on clear days, at times closer to noon, at higher altitudes above sea level and when the ground is highly reflective. The reason and duration of UVR exposure and skin phototype must also be considered to assess UVR damage [18].

Due to the relatively few studies addressing preventive measures for UVR-related LSCC and AC, some concepts in this section are based on research regarding UVR-related skin cancer. Unlike OSCC, LSCC and AC are primarily attributed to a single risk factor: UVR. Similar to skin cancer and precancer, this makes identifying individuals or groups at risk easier. This theoretically establishes the primary preventive measure: reducing UVR exposure on the lip. However, UVR-related cancer is not merely a biological phenomenon. Instead, it should be viewed as a complex set of sociobiological variables influencing UVR exposure and the implementation of preventive measures [169]. Sociocultural factors may include:

- Population ageing.
- Human ecological factors: residing in areas with high UVR levels and/or a depleted ozone layer and/or arsenic in the water.
- Large-scale European migration to more equatorial latitudes.
- Social structures maximised segregation for centuries.

- Gender-based differences in occupational choice, sunbathing, tanning, sunscreen use and clothing choice.
- Occupational ultraviolet exposure.
- The complex interplay of socioeconomic status, race and urbanisation on skin cancer incidence and mortality.
- The effects of war on skin cancer.
- Cultural shifts in clothing, travel, outdoor sports, recreation and UVR exposure protection.
- Religion's effects on clothing and sun exposure.

Those variables should be considered when a patient is received or a prevention measure is designed at the population level.

Photoprotective agents can be categorised into natural agents (such as ozone, clouds, fog, pollutants and the skin itself), physical agents (like clothes, hats, and sunglasses), sunscreens and antioxidants (primarily from diet, which reduce the oxidative effects caused by UV radiation). The various methods of photoprotection can work together to provide maximum protection against UV radiation (see Table 21.3).

21.3.1 Control of UVR/Sun Exposure

Understanding the optimal timing and duration of sunlight exposure is crucial for enhancing its beneficial effects while minimising harmful consequences by adopting appropriate sun protection measures. Exposure to morning and evening sunlight, when the UV index is below 3, is recommended for harnessing its positive effects. When the UV index is 3 or higher, harmful effects can occur [171]. Avoiding high or intense UV exposure is the most important approach to UV protection. Approximately 50–75% of daily UV flux occurs two hours before and after solar noon. Therefore, people should seek shade during those hours of the day when the UV index ranges from 3 to 7. If the UV index is 8 or higher, individuals should stay indoors [172]. Similarly, it is advisable to avoid the use of tanning beds or exposure to other sources of UV radiation unless necessary.

21.3.2 UVR Protection with Clothing

Physical protection by clothing, with a hat and sunglasses, is the second line in UV protection, being even more effective measure than sunscreens on areas that can be covered. It is the most important protection measure for those individuals who cannot or do not want to avoid sun exposure for work or recreational reasons. In a few cultures, the lip is permanently covered with clothing. To protect the face, specifically the lip *vermilion*, the use of wide-brimmed hats is suggested. Narrow-brimmed hats or caps can leave areas of the lip uncovered, especially when the UVR falls laterally or obliquely. More importantly, the hat protects against direct UVR, but not against that reflected by the ground [173], so in areas with high reflectance, this method should be complemented with photoprotective barriers applied directly to the lip.

Table 21.3 Preventive measures for UV radiation-induced damage to the lips

	UV-index				
Risk group	0-2 low	3-5 moderate	6-7 high	8-10 Very high	11+ extreme
Very high-risk people**	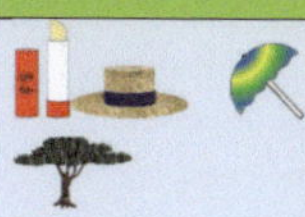	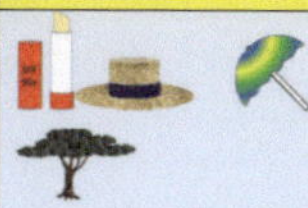	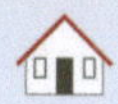	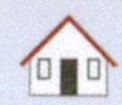	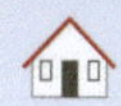
High-risk people*	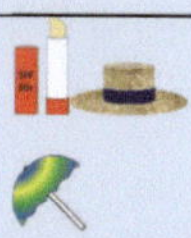	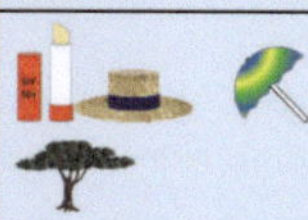	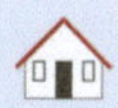	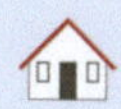	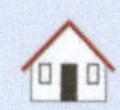
SPh-I	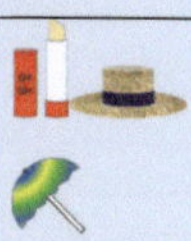	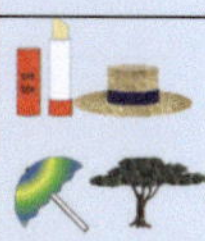	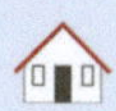	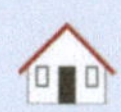	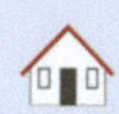
SPh-II	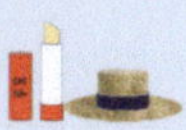	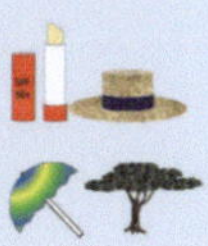		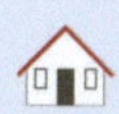	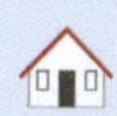
SPh-III	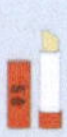	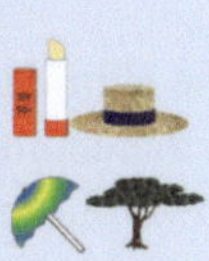		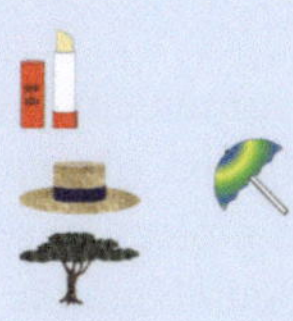	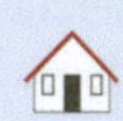
SPh-IV	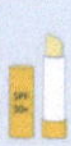	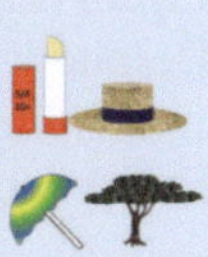		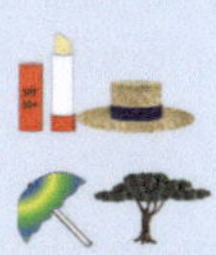	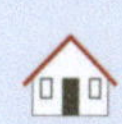

(Continued)

Tab. 21.3 (continued)

SPh-V	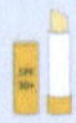	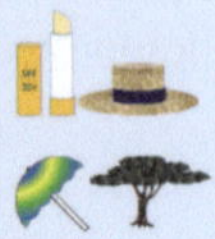	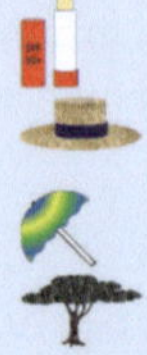	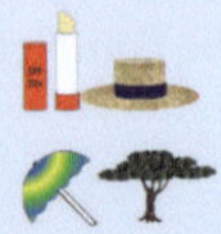	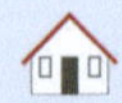
SPh-VI	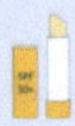	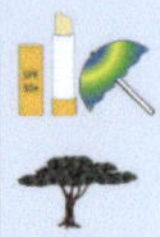		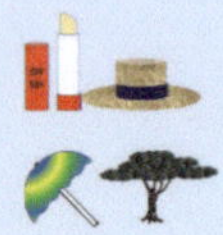	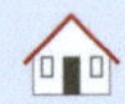
 Avoid sun between 10 am-2 pm	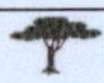 Seek shade near noon	 Reduce exposure time	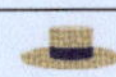 Hat use	 Lip balm SPF 50 Filter UVB UVA	 Lip balm SPF 30 Filter UVB UVA

SPh: Skin phototypes according to Fitzpatrick

* Children over 6 months, adolescents, elderly

** Children under 6 months, conditions that can exacerbate with UVR exposure (xeroderma pigmentosum, vitiligo, lupus erythematosus, etc…)

SPF: Solar Protection Factor

On reflective surfaces (snow, sand, water, etc.) increase UV index by 50%

These protective measures do not apply to skin or eyes

21.3.3 UVR Protection with Sunscreens

Commercial sunscreens protect against the skin-damaging effects of UVR, and its use reduces the risk of squamous cell and melanoma skin cancers [174]. The application of high-protection sunscreens to lip vermilion represents the third line of UV protection. A combination of a wide-brimmed hat and sunscreen is likely to be the optimal way for sun protection with minimal risk [173]. When the UV index is 3 or more, it is recommended that the blocker agent is applied every day on lip vermilion, ideally as a morning routine [172]. Despite it is advisable not to use tanning beds, if the individual decides to use them, it is logical to protect the lip with sunscreens, since it is an area in which aesthetic changes due to tanning that are not intended, thus damage should be avoided.

Sunscreens can be categorised broadly as *organic and inorganic*. In inorganic sunscreens, the active components are minerals, such as TiO2 and ZnO, and function by reflecting and scattering UVR. They tend to be opaque, and as a result, appear white on the lip. As sunscreens, this makes them cosmetically less acceptable [145, 165, 175]. Organic sunscreens reduce UV radiation by absorbing UV rays, and more than 60 kinds of organic sunscreens have been researched and developed internationally [145, 175]. A new category of sunscreens has emerged in recent years, plant-based sunscreens, whose main components are compounds with aromatic rings that show a broader absorption spectrum covering a wavelength range of 200–400 nm. Its main advantage seems to be less ecological damage in areas of high use, but its commercial development is still very scarce [176]. In any of the categories, the composition of lip balms can include organic or plant compounds that exhibit strong antioxidant properties.

It is advisable to use sunscreens specifically designed for use on the lip; as they contain a vehicle that makes it more resistant to fluids, they are usually more cosmetically acceptable, and have a more pleasant taste, characteristics that make it easier for the patient to use them. Because of the large variety of lip sunscreens available, it is recommended to try more than one brand to find the one they would be most likely to use consistently [145]. For patients with light phototypes, lip protectors with a sun protection factor (SPF) of at least 50 are recommended, with UVB and UVA filters, since both UVR can promote carcinogenesis and aging of the lip. In patients with darker phototypes, a lip protector with an SPF of 30 against UVB and UVA may be sufficient, but due to the lower protection of the lip compared to the skin, it would be advisable to use more than SPF 50 and should include a filter for visible light, to prevent dyschromia [18, 165]. Although there are tinted lip balms for cosmetic purposes, to our knowledge there are no lip balms specifically designed to filter visible light, so if such protection were necessary, products designed for the skin could be used, considering their disadvantages in duration and flavour. Using lip balms with a lower SPF than those mentioned would not make sense, since the aim is not usually to regulate lip tanning, but rather to obtain the greatest possible protection.

Sunscreens should be applied generously to all body surfaces, including the lips. However, they are often applied insufficiently, both in terms of quantity and frequency. Photoprotective lipsticks with high and ultrahigh SPF are recommended, especially for individuals at an increased risk of developing lip malignancies [145, 177, 178]. A significant percentage of commercially available lip sunscreens have lower UV absorption capacity than advertised and are notably photo unstable, degrading quickly [179]. This further emphasises the importance of using lip balm with the highest SPF available. In addition to providing immediate protection against ultraviolet radiation after application, it is advisable to wait 15–30 minutes if water resistance is necessary. Reapplication is recommended every 1–2 hours or whenever the likelihood of sunscreen being removed is high, such as after eating, swimming, licking the lips or exfoliation from sand [145, 165, 170, 174].

Adverse reactions to sunscreens are rare, but with increased sunscreen use, they are being reported more frequently, mainly in the skin. Most of these adverse effects do not occur when applying lip balms with sun protection. The almost exclusive effect on lips is reactions due to direct contact of its components with the lip surface. Contact dermatitis can occur with chemical sunscreens and is usually due to one of the preservatives or fragrances used in the formulation rather than the active ingredient. Allergic reactions to some UV filters are seen most often in patients taking medications that predispose them to photosensitivity or in individuals with photosensitivity disorders [145, 180]. Another risk of using lip sunscreen is that patients may spend more time in the sun because they feel protected, without reapplying it properly, and thus end up developing UVR-associated lesions [145].

Another adverse effect of organic sunscreens does not occur in humans but in the environment, where compounds such as octocrylene and octinoxate cause damage to aquatic ecosystems. These compounds are frequently used in lip balms, and it should be noted that despite the small amount used to protect the lip, this is added to the components of sunscreens for the skin [181, 182].

21.3.4 Oral or Systemic Photoprotection

Oral or systemic photoprotection refers to substances taken internally that offer protection against the effects of sunlight, including UVR [183]. UVR generates excessive free radical species, leading to oxidative stress, which is responsible for cellular and DNA damage [184]. Certain dietary compounds, such as carotenoids, flavonoids and non-flavonoid polyphenols, can inhibit the synthesis of inflammatory factors, thereby reducing free radical formation and preserving DNA integrity. These dietary compounds confer photoprotective effects by mitigating UV-induced inflammation, DNA damage and immunosuppression [175, 184]. Systemic photoprotective agents have multiple advantages: they are not affected by external factors such as water, sweat or rubbing; they distribute evenly; they act for an extended period; they protect the entire body surface and they are independent of cream properties and the amount applied. Current evidence indicates that systemic photoprotection should be used as an adjunctive measure rather than a replacement for topical photoprotection with skin sunscreens. However, evidence for the safety and efficacy of these supplements is limited [183]. Research into oral and systemic photoprotection is virtually non-existent regarding the prevention of UVR-induced lip diseases. However, it is reasonable to consider that if it has beneficial effects on the skin, it could also have beneficial effects on the vermilion of the lip.

21.3.5 Prevention of UVR Damage in Individuals or Risk Groups

Risk groups for UVR-induced injury can be categorised into those with high UVR exposure and those with high susceptibility to UVR damage. Among the former, it's easy to identify people who spend many hours outdoors due to work or recreational activities such as sports. Susceptible individuals include newborns, children, adolescents, the elderly, very fair-skinned people and those with genetic or autoimmune conditions like xeroderma pigmentosum, lupus erythematosus and vitiligo. In both instances, educating individuals and populations about UVR risks and protective measures is essential.

For susceptible individuals, the primary recommendation is to avoid UVR exposure by any means possible. In the event of exposure, it is advisable to maximise protection by wearing hats and using water-resistant lip balms with an SPF of 50 SPF or higher [18]. For those with high UVR exposure, it is essential to limit the number of hours of exposure, avoid being outside during midday hours, provide shade shelters and wear hats and lip balms with an SPF of 50 or higher [172], which should be reapplied more frequently than on the skin.

Those who work outdoors—such as farmers, fishermen, military personnel and bricklayers, among many other jobs—face elevated levels of UVR exposure, which often go unrecognised and are seldom discussed as a significant occupational hazard [185]. Although these measures can undoubtedly reduce solar UV exposure for workers using them, more than half of outdoor workers wear a hat or cap but rarely use lip balm. This is likely because such products are impractical, unsafe or uncomfortable or due to workplace culture [186, 187].

Among indoor workers exposed to UVR, those at the highest risk are arc welders and, to a lesser extent, employees who work with UVR-emitting lamps, such as those in tanning centres. These UVR sources affect the eyes directly, causing damage more rapidly than in outdoor workers, where UVR is often influenced by reflection. In these situations, prioritising eye safety is reasonable, but this can diminish the importance of protecting the skin and lips. Therefore, strict use of face masks with visors is recommended for these workers [17].

For those participating in outdoor sports, consideration must be given to athletes and their coaches. These sports include skiing, mountaineering, cycling, running, triathlon, kitesurfing, windsurfing, beach handball, beach volleyball and sailing. Despite the inherent risks, participants often fail to protect themselves adequately from the sun. The use of sunscreen is frequently undervalued, and reapplying sunscreen is notably rare [170]. Many athletes view a suntan as aesthetically desirable and socially acceptable. Group norms influence their compliance with sun protection, and they often remain unaware of the importance of using specific lip products [188].

Since LSCC and its precursor lesion, AC/AKL, are closely related to UVR, identifying individuals and risk groups is likely to be more specific. Skin cancer prevention campaigns are effective and cost-effective [189, 190], suggesting that LSCC prevention campaigns, especially targeting high-risk populations, could significantly impact the incidence and mortality from LSCC. However, while several studies analyse the association between sun exposure and UVR protection with lip diseases, no studies investigate the effect of prevention campaigns on the incidence and morbidity from AC/AKL and LSCC, or on mortality from LSCC. It is important to note that prevention campaigns specifically for LSCC are scarce, as these campaigns are generally included within those aimed at oral cancer in general.

21.3.6 UVR Control in the Prevention of AC/AKL Malignant Transformation

In studies of AC/AKL, 66–90% of patients reported never using sun protection, and among those who used lip balms, the application was infrequent [97, 191]. Individuals using any type of sun protection are less likely to have actinic cheilitis than those who do not use sun protection, and this effect is more pronounced in individuals with greater sun exposure [192]. In addition, patients who use lip balms have a lower risk of LSCC [193]. These data demonstrate the significant potential of UVR protection in preventing malignant transformation. Although the rate of malignant transformation of AC/AKL is still controversial, ranging from 3.07 to 16.9% [65, 72, 97], no studies are analysing the impact of UVR protection measures on the AC/AKL transformation rate.

References

1. Biernat K, Malinowski A, Gnat M, Biernat K, Malinowski A, Gnat M. The possibility of future biofuels production using waste carbon dioxide and solar energy. In: Biofuels – economy, environment and sustainability. IntechOpen; 2013. Available from: https://www.intechopen.com/chapters/42202. Accessed 5 Feb 2025.
2. Haigh PJ. Solar influences on climate. 2011.Available from: https://www.imperial.ac.uk/grantham/publications/briefing-papers/solar-influences-on-climate%2D%2D-grantham-briefing-paper-5.php. Accessed 5 Feb 2025.
3. Şen Z. Solar energy in progress and future research trends. Prog Energy Combust Sci. 2004;30:367–416. https://doi.org/10.1016/j.pecs.2004.02.004.
4. Stamnes K. Ultraviolet radiation. In: Holton JR, editor. Encyclopedia of atmospheric sciences. Oxford: Academic Press; 2003. p. 2467–73. Available from: https://www.sciencedirect.com/science/article/pii/B0122270908004449. Accessed 5 Feb 2025.
5. Corrêa M de P. Solar ultraviolet radiation: properties, characteristics and amounts observed in Brazil and South America. An Bras Dermatol. 2015;90:297–313. https://doi.org/10.1590/abd1806-4841.20154089.
6. Bais AF, Lucas RM, Bornman JF, Williamson CE, Sulzberger B, Austin AT, et al. Environmental effects of ozone depletion, UV radiation and interactions with climate change: UNEP Environmental Effects Assessment Panel, update 2017. Photochem Photobiol Sci. 2018;17:127–79. https://doi.org/10.1039/c7pp90043k.
7. Fioletov V, Kerr JB, Fergusson A. The UV index: definition, distribution and factors affecting it. Can J Public Health Rev Can Santé Publique. 2010;101:I5–9. https://doi.org/10.1007/BF03405303.
8. Lim HW, Cooper K. The health impact of solar radiation and prevention strategies. J Am Acad Dermatol. 1999;41:81–99. https://doi.org/10.1016/s0190-9622(99)70412-3.
9. Modenese A, Korpinen L, Gobba F. Solar radiation exposure and outdoor work: an underestimated occupational risk. Int J Environ Res Public Health. 2018;15:2063. https://doi.org/10.3390/ijerph15102063.
10. Bauer A, Diepgen TL, Schmitt J. Is occupational solar ultraviolet irradiation a relevant risk factor for basal cell carcinoma? A systematic review and meta-analysis of the epidemiological literature. Br J Dermatol. 2011;165:612–25. https://doi.org/10.1111/j.1365-2133.2011.10425.x.
11. Dessinioti C, Stratigos AJ. An epidemiological update on indoor tanning and the risk of skin cancers. Curr Oncol Tor Ont. 2022;29:8886–903. https://doi.org/10.3390/curroncol29110699.

12. Kimlin MG, Tenkate TD. Occupational exposure to ultraviolet radiation: the duality dilemma. Rev Environ Health. 2007;22:1–38. https://doi.org/10.1515/reveh.2007.22.1.1.
13. Mogensen M, Jemec GB. The potential carcinogenic risk of tanning beds: clinical guidelines and patient safety advice. Cancer Manag Res. 2010;2:277–82. https://doi.org/10.2147/CMR.S7403.
14. Zaffina S, Camisa V, Lembo M, Vinci MR, Tucci MG, Borra M, et al. Accidental exposure to UV radiation produced by germicidal lamp: case report and risk assessment. Photochem Photobiol. 2012;88:1001–4. https://doi.org/10.1111/j.1751-1097.2012.01151.x.
15. Heltoft KN, Slagor RM, Agner T, Bonde JP. Metal arc welding and the risk of skin cancer. Int Arch Occup Environ Health. 2017;90:873–81. https://doi.org/10.1007/s00420-017-1248-5.
16. Larese Filon F, Buric M, Fluehler C. UV exposure, preventive habits, risk perception, and occupation in NMSC patients: a case-control study in Trieste (NE Italy). Photodermatol Photoimmunol Photomed. 2019;35:24–30. https://doi.org/10.1111/phpp.12417.
17. International Commission on Non-Ionizing Radiation Protection (ICNIRP). ICNIRP statement–protection of workers against ultraviolet radiation. Health Phys. 2010;99:66–87. https://doi.org/10.1097/HP.0b013e3181d85908.
18. Passeron T, Lim HW, Goh CL, Kang HY, Ly F, Morita A, et al. Photoprotection according to skin phototype and dermatoses: practical recommendations from an expert panel. J Eur Acad Dermatol Venereol. 2021;35:1460–9. https://doi.org/10.1111/jdv.17242.
19. Shang J, Feng X, Chen Y, Gu Z, Liu Y. Human lip vermilion: physiology and age-related changes. J Cosmet Dermatol. 2024;23:2676–80. https://doi.org/10.1111/jocd.16317.
20. Fitzpatrick TB. The validity and practicality of sun-reactive skin types I through VI. Arch Dermatol. 1988;124:869–71. https://doi.org/10.1001/archderm.124.6.869.
21. Goon P, Banfield C, Bello O, Levell NJ. Skin cancers in skin types IV-VI: does the Fitzpatrick scale give a false sense of security? Skin Health Dis. 2021;1:e40. https://doi.org/10.1002/ski2.40.
22. Vachiramon V, McMichael AJ. Approaches to the evaluation of lip hyperpigmentation. Int J Dermatol. 2012;51:761–70. https://doi.org/10.1111/j.1365-4632.2011.05272.x.
23. Manimegalai S, Sundaram JM, Venkatachalam N. Age changes in human skin from 3 years to 75 years of age. Int J Anat Res. 2015;3:1578–84. https://doi.org/10.16965/ijar.2015.292.
24. Odorici G, Monfrecola G, Bettoli V. Tetracyclines and photosensitive skin reactions: a narrative review. Dermatol Ther. 2021;34:e14978. https://doi.org/10.1111/dth.14978.
25. Soler-Orenes JA, Rodríguez-Muñiz GM, Hernández-Gil J, Miranda MA, Andreu I, Lhiaubet-Vallet V. Photosensitizing properties of the topical retinoid drug Adapalene. Chem Res Toxicol. 2024;37:2013–21. https://doi.org/10.1021/acs.chemrestox.4c00384.
26. Alataş ÖD, Alataş ET. Isotretinoin-induced pruritic erythematous lesions and acute chest pain in a 15-year-old girl. Am J Emerg Med. 2020;38:1043.e1–3. https://doi.org/10.1021/acs.chemrestox.4c00384.
27. Zghal M, Fazaa B, Abdelhak S, Mokni M. Xeroderma pigmentosum. Ann Dermatol Venereol. 2018;145(11):706–22. https://doi.org/10.1016/j.annder.2018.09.004.
28. Kurz B, Klein B, Berneburg M, Meller S. Ultraviolet radiation in the pathogenesis of lupus erythematosus. Dermatol Heidelb Ger. 2024;75:528–38. https://doi.org/10.1007/s00105-024-05369-w.
29. Grigalavicius M, Juzeniene A, Baturaite Z, Dahlback A, Moan J. Biologically efficient solar radiation: vitamin D production and induction of cutaneous malignant melanoma. Dermatoendocrinol. 2013;5:150–8. https://doi.org/10.4161/derm.22941.
30. Knuschke P. Sun exposure and vitamin D. Curr Probl Dermatol. 2021;55:296–315. https://doi.org/10.1159/000517640.
31. Galima SV, Vogel SR, Kowalski AW. Seasonal affective disorder: common questions and answers. Am Fam Physician. 2020;102:668–72. https://www.aafp.org/pubs/afp/issues/2020/1201/p668.html
32. Gupta A, Sharma PK, Garg VK, Singh AK, Mondal SC. Role of serotonin in seasonal affective disorder. Eur Rev Med Pharmacol Sci. 2013;17:49–55. https://www.europeanreview.org/article/1251

33. Desotelle JA, Wilking MJ, Ahmad N. The circadian control of skin and cutaneous photodamage. Photochem Photobiol. 2012;88:1037–47. https://doi.org/10.1111/j.1751-1097.2012.01099.x.
34. Hart PH, Norval M, Byrne SN, Rhodes LE. Exposure to ultraviolet radiation in the modulation of human diseases. Annu Rev Pathol. 2019;14:55–81. https://doi.org/10.1146/annurev-pathmechdis-012418-012809.
35. Kudish AI, Evseev EG, Cohen G, Harari M. Ultraviolet measurements and Photoclimatotherapy for psoriasis at the Dead Sea: 25 years of experience. Int J Environ Res Public Health. 2022;19:12364. https://doi.org/10.3390/ijerph191912364.
36. Xerfan EMS, Facina AS, Tomimori J, Tufik S, Andersen ML. The influence of phototherapy on circadian melatonin and sleep regulation and potential benefits of these pathways in the management of vitiligo: a narrative review: vitiligo, phototherapy, sleep and melatonin. Arch Dermatol Res. 2024;316:632. https://doi.org/10.1007/s00403-024-03363-9.
37. Narayanan DL, Saladi RN, Fox JL. Ultraviolet radiation and skin cancer. Int J Dermatol. 2010;49:978–86. https://doi.org/10.1111/j.1365-4632.2010.04474.x.
38. Merin KA, Shaji M, Kameswaran R. A review on Sun exposure and skin diseases. Indian J Dermatol. 2022;67:625. https://doi.org/10.4103/ijd.ijd_1092_20.
39. Guan LL, Lim HW, Mohammad TF. Recognizing photoallergy, phototoxicity, and immune-mediated photodermatoses. J Allergy Clin Immunol. 2022;149:1206–9. https://doi.org/10.1016/j.jaci.2022.02.013.
40. Pai SB, Anchan VN. Phototoxicity and photoallergy—a brief review on pathogenesis, recent advances, and approach to a patient with photosensitivity. Indian J Skin Allergy. 2024;3:28–35. https://skinallergyjournal.com/view-pdf/?article=b1b70ebe56299518d6a945230f760617iBOb66VFdCg=
41. Zuba EB, Koronowska S, Osmola-Mańkowska A, Jenerowicz D. Drug-induced photosensitivity. Acta Dermatovenerol Croat. 2016;24:55–64. https://actadermatovenerologicacroatica.hr/acta-dermatovenerologica-croatica-vol-24-no-1-2016/
42. Nishisgori C. Current concept of photocarcinogenesis. Photochem Photobiol Sci. 2015;14:1713–21. https://doi.org/10.1039/c5pp00185d.
43. Kim I, He YY. Ultraviolet radiation-induced non-melanoma skin cancer: regulation of DNA damage repair and inflammation. Genes Dis. 2014;1:188–98. https://doi.org/10.1016/j.gendis.2014.08.005.
44. Dotto GP, Rustgi AK. Squamous cell cancers: a unified perspective on biology and genetics. Cancer Cell. 2016;29:622–37. https://doi.org/10.1016/j.ccell.2016.04.004.
45. Katiyar SK, Singh T, Prasad R, Sun Q, Vaid M. Epigenetic alterations in ultraviolet radiation-induced skin carcinogenesis: interaction of bioactive dietary components on epigenetic targets. Photochem Photobiol. 2012;88:1066–74. https://doi.org/10.1111/j.1751-1097.2011.01020.x.
46. Gallagher RP, Lee TK. Adverse effects of ultraviolet radiation: a brief review. Prog Biophys Mol Biol. 2006;92:119–31. https://doi.org/10.1016/j.pbiomolbio.2006.02.011.
47. IARC Working Group on the Evaluation of Carcinogenic Risks to Humans. Solar and ultraviolet radiation. Lyon (FR): International Agency for Research on Cancer; 1992. (Iarc Monographs on the Evaluation of Carcinogenic Risks to Humans, No. 55.) Available from: https://www.ncbi.nlm.nih.gov/books/NBK401588/
48. Salminen A, Kaarniranta K, Kauppinen A. Photoaging: UV radiation-induced inflammation and immunosuppression accelerate the aging process in the skin. Inflamm Res. 2022;71:817–31. https://doi.org/10.1007/s00011-022-01598-8.
49. Lan CCE. Effects and interactions of increased environmental temperature and UV radiation on photoageing and photocarcinogenesis of the skin. Exp Dermatol. 2019;28(Suppl 1):23–7. https://doi.org/10.1111/exd.13818.
50. Taylor SC, Alexis AF, Armstrong AW, Chiesa Fuxench ZC, Lim HW. Misconceptions of photoprotection in skin of color. J Am Acad Dermatol. 2022;86:S9–17. https://doi.org/10.1016/j.jaad.2021.12.020.

51. Bennett MF, Robinson MK, Baron ED, Cooper KD. Skin immune systems and inflammation: protector of the skin or promoter of aging? J Investig Dermatol Symp Proc. 2008;13:15–9. https://doi.org/10.1038/jidsymp.2008.3.
52. Gibbs NK, Norval M. Photoimmunosuppression: a brief overview. Photodermatol Photoimmunol Photomed. 2013;29:57–64. https://doi.org/10.1111/phpp.12021.
53. Narayanan D, Rogge M. Cheilitis: a diagnostic algorithm and review of underlying etiologies. Dermat Contact Atopic Occup Drug. 2024;35:431–42. https://doi.org/10.1089/derm.2023.0276.
54. Lugović-Mihić L, Špiljak B, Blagec T, Delaš Aždajić M, Franceschi N, Gašić A, et al. Factors participating in the occurrence of inflammation of the lips (Cheilitis) and perioral skin. Cosmetics. 2023;10(1):9. https://doi.org/10.3390/cosmetics1001000.
55. Lugović-Mihić L, Pilipović K, Crnarić I, Šitum M, Duvančić T. Differential diagnosis of Cheilitis – how to classify Cheilitis? Acta Clin Croat. 2018;57:342–51. https://doi.org/10.20471/acc.2018.57.02.16.
56. Due E, Wulf HC. Cheilitis – the only presentation of photosensitivity. J Eur Acad Dermatol Venereol JEADV. 2006;20:766–7. https://doi.org/10.1111/j.1468-3083.2006.01543.x.
57. Pereira ASTM, Xará J, Gonçalo M. Drug-induced photosensitivity. Port J Dermatol Venereol. 2022;80:104–17. https://www.scienceopen.com/document?vid=4dd28f3a-dfc6-4f96-8207-ca10be9b2abb
58. Navarro-Triviño FJ, Ruiz-Villaverde R. Photoallergic contact cheilitis from methylchloroisothiazolinone/methylisothiazolinone: where is the culprit product? Contact Derm. 2021;84:199–200. https://doi.org/10.1111/cod.13708.
59. Romita P, Barlusconi C, Mercurio CS, Hansel K, Stingeni L, Foti C. Photoallergic contact cheilitis from benzydamine hydrochloride contained in a mouthwash. Contact Derm. 2020;83:130–2. https://doi.org/10.1111/cod.13541.
60. Canelas MM, Cardoso JC, Gonçalo M, Figueiredo A. Photoallergic contact dermatitis from benzydamine presenting mainly as lip dermatitis. Contact Derm. 2010;63:85–8. https://doi.org/10.1111/j.1600-0536.2010.01707.x.
61. Freeman S, Stephens R. Cheilitis: analysis of 75 cases referred to a contact dermatitis clinic. Am J Contact Dermat. 1999;10:198–200. https://doi.org/10.1053/AJCD01000198.
62. Warnakulasuriya S. Clinical features and presentation of oral potentially malignant disorders. Oral Surg Oral Med Oral Pathol Oral Radiol. 2018;125:582–90. https://doi.org/10.1016/j.oooo.2018.03.011.
63. Seoane J, Warnakulasuriya S, Bagán JV, Aguirre-Urizar JM, López-Jornet P, Hernández-Vallejo G, et al. Assembling a consensus on actinic cheilitis: a Delphi study. J Oral Pathol Med. 2021;50:962–70. https://doi.org/10.1111/jop.13200.
64. Jadotte YT, Schwartz RA. Solar cheilosis: an ominous precursor: part I. Diagnostic insights. J Am Acad Dermatol. 2012;66:173–84. https://doi.org/10.1016/j.jaad.2011.09.040.
65. Markopoulos A, Albanidou-Farmaki E, Kayavis I. Actinic cheilitis: clinical and pathologic characteristics in 65 cases. Oral Dis. 2004;10:212–6. https://doi.org/10.1111/j.1601-0825.2004.01004.x.
66. Rodriguez-Archilla A, Irfan-Bhatti A. Risk factors for actinic cheilitis: a meta-analysis. J Dent Res Dent Clin Dent Prospects. 2021;15:285–9. https://doi.org/10.34172/joddd.2021.047.
67. Lopes-Cardoso C, Paes da Silva Ramos Fernandes LM, Ferreira-Rocha J, Teixeira-Soares C, Antônio-Barreto J, Humberto-Damante J. Xeroderma Pigmentosum – a case report with oral implications. J Clin Exp Dent. 2012;4:e248–51. https://doi.org/10.4317/jced.50727.
68. Wayli HA. Xeroderma pigmentosum and its dental implications. Eur J Dent. 2015;9:145–8. https://doi.org/10.4103/1305-7456.149664.
69. Schipani G, Del Duca E, Todaro G, Scali E, Dastoli S, Bennardo L, et al. Arsenic and chromium levels in hair correlate with actinic keratosis/non-melanoma skin cancer: results of an observational controlled study. Ital J Dermatol Venereol. 2021;156:703–8. https://doi.org/10.23736/S2784-8671.20.06600-6.

70. Rajiv SV, George M, Nandakumar G. Dermatological manifestations of arsenic exposure. J Skin Sex Transm Dis. 2023;5:14–21. https://jsstd.org/dermatological-manifestations-of-arsenic-exposure/
71. Mello FW, Miguel AFP, Dutra KL, Porporatti AL, Warnakulasuriya S, Guerra ENS, et al. Prevalence of oral potentially malignant disorders: a systematic review and meta-analysis. J Oral Pathol Med. 2018;47:633–40. https://doi.org/10.1111/jop.12726.
72. Dancyger A, Heard V, Huang B, Suley C, Tang D, Ariyawardana A. Malignant transformation of actinic cheilitis: a systematic review of observational studies. J Investig Clin Dent. 2018;9:e12343. https://doi.org/10.1111/jicd.12343.
73. Carneiro MC, Quenta-Huayhua MG, Peralta-Mamani M, Honório HM, Santos PS da S, Rubira-Bullen IRF, et al. Clinicopathological analysis of actinic Cheilitis: a systematic review with meta-analyses. Head Neck Pathol. 2023;17:708–21. https://doi.org/10.1007/s12105-023-01543-z.
74. Cavalcante ASR, Anbinder AL, Carvalho YR. Actinic Cheilitis: clinical and histological features. J Oral Maxillofac Surg. 2008;66:498–503. https://doi.org/10.1016/j.joms.2006.09.016.
75. de Oliveira Ribeiro A, da Silva LCF, Martins-Filho PRS. Prevalence of and risk factors for actinic cheilitis in Brazilian fishermen and women. Int J Dermatol. 2014;53:1370–6. https://doi.org/10.1111/ijd.12526.
76. Vasilovici A, Ungureanu L, Grigore L, Cojocaru E, Şenilă S. Actinic Cheilitis – from risk factors to therapy. Front Med. 2022;9:805425. https://doi.org/10.3389/fmed.2022.805425.
77. Villalba V, Valenzuela Y, Ramírez MC, Faúndez E. Lesiones pigmentadas de la mucosa oral. Rev Chilena Dermatol. 2011;27:203–11. https://www.sochiderm.org/web/revista/27_2/9.pdf
78. Santana T, Queiroz A, Gonçales LMC, Andrade NS, Trierveiler M. Focal melanocytic lesions of the oral mucosa: an epidemiological and morphological study. Oral Dis. 2023;29:2723–33. https://doi.org/10.1111/odi.14482.
79. Vieira RAMAR, Minicucci EM, Marques MEA, Marques SA. Actinic cheilitis and squamous cell carcinoma of the lip: clinical, histopathological and immunogenetic aspects. An Bras Dermatol. 2012;87:105–14. https://doi.org/10.1590/s0365-05962012000100013.
80. de Santana Sarmento DJ, da Costa Miguel MC, Queiroz LMG, Godoy GP, da Silveira EJD. Actinic cheilitis: clinicopathologic profile and association with degree of dysplasia. Int J Dermatol. 2014;53:466–72. https://doi.org/10.1111/ijd.12332.
81. Su ZZ, Tan YQ, Zhou G. Multiple noninvasive auxiliary tests-assisted photodynamic therapy in actinic cheilitis: a case report. Photodiagn Photodyn Ther. 2023;44:103832. https://doi.org/10.1016/j.pdpdt.2023.103832.
82. Zhang Y, Wu Y, Pan D, Zhang Z, Jiang L, Feng X, et al. Accuracy of narrow band imaging for detecting the malignant transformation of oral potentially malignant disorders: A systematic review and meta-analysis. Front Surg. 2023;9:1068256. https://doi.org/10.3389/fsurg.2022.1068256.
83. Walsh T, Macey R, Kerr AR, Lingen MW, Ogden GR, Warnakulasuriya S. Diagnostic tests for oral cancer and potentially malignant disorders in patients presenting with clinically evident lesions. Cochrane Database Syst Rev. 2021;7:CD010276. https://doi.org/10.1002/14651858.CD010276.pub3.
84. Mendonca P, Sunny SP, Mohan U, Birur NP, Suresh A, Kuriakose MA. Non-invasive imaging of oral potentially malignant and malignant lesions: a systematic review and meta-analysis. Oral Oncol. 2022;130:105877. https://doi.org/10.1016/j.oraloncology.2022.105877.
85. Grover C, Jakhar D. Hand-held dermatoscope or videodermatoscope: which one to buy? Indian J Dermatol Venereol Leprol. 2021;87:739–41. https://doi.org/10.25259/IJDVL_802_19.
86. Miranda AM, Ferrari T, Leite T, Domingos T, Cunha K, Dias E. Value of videoroscopy in the detection of alterations of actinic cheilitis and the selection of biopsy areas. Med Oral Patol Oral Cirugia Bucal. 2015;20:e292–7. https://doi.org/10.4317/medoral.20297.
87. Lallas A, Martínez G, Arceu M, Kyrgidis A, Liopyris K, Brancaccio G, et al. Clinical and dermatoscopic predictors of squamous cell carcinoma of the lips: a case-control, multicentric study. J Eur Acad Dermatol Venereol JEADV. 2022;36:222–7. https://doi.org/10.1111/jdv.17790.

88. Jha AK, Sławińska M, Vinay K, Akay BN, Kamińska-Winciorek G, Sobjanek M, et al. Dermoscopic features of actinic Cheilitis and other common inflammatory Cheilitis: a multicentric retrospective observational study by the International Dermoscopy Society. Dermatol Basel Switz. 2022;238:870–5. https://doi.org/10.1159/000522602.
89. Cosci A, Takahama A, Correr WR, Azevedo RS, Fontes KBF da C, Kurachi C. Automated algorithm for actinic cheilitis diagnosis by wide-field fluorescence imaging. J Med Imaging Bellingham Wash. 2016;3:044004. https://doi.org/10.1117/1.JMI.3.4.044004.
90. Takahama A Jr, Kurachi C, Cosci A, Pereira Faustino IS, Camisasca DR, da Costa Fontes KB, et al. Usefulness of tissue autofluorescence imaging in actinic cheilitis diagnosis. J Biomed Opt. 2013;18:76023. https://doi.org/10.1117/1.JBO.18.7.076023.
91. Lupu M, Caruntu A, Caruntu C, Boda D, Moraru L, Voiculescu V, et al. Non-invasive imaging of actinic cheilitis and squamous cell carcinoma of the lip. Mol Clin Oncol. 2018;8:640–6. https://doi.org/10.3892/mco.2018.1599.
92. Ulrich M, González S, Lange-Asschenfeldt B, Roewert-Huber J, Sterry W, Stockfleth E, et al. Non-invasive diagnosis and monitoring of actinic cheilitis with reflectance confocal microscopy. J Eur Acad Dermatol Venereol JEADV. 2011;25:276–84. https://doi.org/10.1111/j.1468-3083.2010.03777.x.
93. Zhang MY, Jiang WW. In vivo reflectance confocal microscopy diagnostic features of actinic cheilitis: a retrospective case series. J Eur Acad Dermatol Venereol JEADV. 2022;36:e545–8. https://doi.org/10.1111/jdv.18018.
94. Ferreira PS, Rocha L, Bezerra APC, Nico MMS, Lourenço SV. Reflectance confocal microscopy (RCM)-based criteria for progression of lower-lip squamous cell carcinoma: a prospective study. Oral Oncol. 2022;125:105674. https://doi.org/10.1016/j.oraloncology.2021.105674.
95. Menta Simonsen Nico M, Rivitti EA, Lourenço SV. Actinic cheilitis: histologic study of the entire vermilion and comparison with previous biopsy. J Cutan Pathol. 2007;34:309–14. https://doi.org/10.1111/j.1600-0560.2006.00606.x.
96. Santana T, Matuck B, Tenório JR, Braga MM. Can immunohistochemical biomarkers distinguish epithelial dysplasia degrees in actinic cheilitis? A systematic review and meta-analysis. Med Oral Patol Oral Cirugia Bucal. 2020;25:e106–16. https://doi.org/10.4317/medoral.23223.
97. Pierin EG, Sassi LM, Schussel JL. Malignant transformation of actinic Cheilitis: a decade-long retrospective study in southern Brazil. J Clin Exp Dent. 2024;16:e666–9. https://doi.org/10.4317/jced.61590.
98. Abreu MAMM de, Silva OMP da, Neto Pimentel DR, Hirata CHW, Weckx LLM, Alchorne MM de A, et al. Actinic cheilitis adjacent to squamous carcinoma of the lips as an indicator of prognosis. Braz J Otorhinolaryngol. 2006;72:767–71. https://doi.org/10.1016/s1808-8694(15)31043-0.
99. Câmara PR, Dutra SN, Takahama Júnior A, Fontes K, Azevedo RS. A comparative study using WHO and binary oral epithelial dysplasia grading systems in actinic cheilitis. Oral Dis. 2016;22:523–9. https://doi.org/10.1111/odi.12484.
100. de Castro Abrantes T, Fonsêca TC, Cabral MG, Agostini M, Benevenuto de Andrade BA, Romañach MJ, et al. Epithelial dysplasia in actinic Cheilitis: microscopic study of 70 cases from Brazil. Head Neck Pathol. 2021;15:566–71. https://doi.org/10.1007/s12105-020-01250-z.
101. Mello FW, Melo G, Modolo F, Rivero ERC. Actinic cheilitis and lip squamous cell carcinoma: literature review and new data from Brazil. J Clin Exp Dent. 2019;11:e62–9. https://doi.org/10.4317/jced.55133.
102. Lopes MLD de S, Silva Júnior FL da, Lima KC, Oliveira PT de, Silveira ÉJD da. Clinicopathological profile and management of 161 cases of actinic cheilitis. An Bras Dermatol. 2015;90:505–12. https://doi.org/10.1590/abd1806-4841.20153848.
103. Medeiros CK, Lopes ML, Silveira ÉJ, Lima KC, Oliveira PT. Actinic cheilitis: proposal of a clinical index. Med Oral Patol Oral Cirugia Bucal. 2022;27:e310–8. https://doi.org/10.4317/medoral.25243.

104. Garcia NG, González-Moles MA, Ruiz-Ávila I, Bravo M, Ramos-García P, Minicucci EM, et al. Asymmetrical proliferative pattern loss linked to cyclin D1 overexpression during malignant transformation of the lip epithelium. J Eur Acad Dermatol Venereol JEADV. 2016;30:1315–20. https://doi.org/10.1111/jdv.13671.
105. Salvadori G, Dos Santos JN, Martins MAT, Vasconcelos AC, Meurer L, Rados PV, et al. Ki-67, TGF-β1, and elastin content are significantly altered in lip carcinogenesis. Tumour Biol J Int Soc Oncodevelopmental Biol Med. 2014;35:7635–44. https://doi.org/10.1007/s13277-014-1989-7.
106. Xavier FCA, Takiya CM, Reis SRA, Ramalho LMP. p63 Immunoexpression in lip carcinogenesis. J Mol Histol. 2009;40:131–7. https://doi.org/10.1007/s10735-009-9223-4.
107. Varela-Centelles P, Gonzalez-Moles MÁ, Seoane-Romero J, Leira-Feijoo Y, Takkouche B, Seoane-Romero JM. Immunohistochemical analysis of epithelium adjacent to lip cancer: a meta-analysis. Oral Dis. 2022;28:57–65. https://doi.org/10.1111/odi.13643.
108. Peixoto da-Silva J, Lourenço S, Nico M, Silva FH, Martins MT, Costa-Neves A. Expression of laminin-5 and integrins in actinic cheilitis and superficially invasive squamous cell carcinomas of the lip. Pathol Res Pract. 2012;208:598–603. https://doi.org/10.1016/j.prp.2012.07.004.
109. Costa NL, Oton-Leite AF, Cheim-Júnior AP, Alencar R de CG, Bittar GOJ, Silva TA, et al. Density and migration of mast cells in lip squamous cell carcinoma and actinic cheilitis. Histol Histopathol 2009;24:457–65. https://doi.org/10.14670/HH-24.457.
110. Schussel JL, Pinto DDS, Martins MT. Altered β-catenin expression related to cancer progression on actinic cheilitis and squamous cell carcinoma of the lip. Ann Diagn Pathol. 2011;15:1–5. https://doi.org/10.1016/j.anndiagpath.2010.07.002.
111. Vageli D, Doukas PG, Zacharouli K, Kakanis V, Strataki M, Zioga A, et al. Laminin immunostaining in biopsies as a useful biomarker of early invasion in actinic Cheilitis and differential diagnosis between actinic Cheilitis and lip cancer: new insights. Head Neck Pathol. 2023;17:331–8. https://doi.org/10.1007/s12105-022-01504-y.
112. de Freitas M da CA, Ramalho LMP, Xavier FCA, Moreira ALG, Reis SRA. p53 and MDM2 protein expression in actinic cheilitis. J Appl Oral Sci Rev FOB. 2008;16:414–9. https://doi.org/10.1590/s1678-77572008000600011.
113. Malaspina TS de S, Gasparoto TH, Costa MRSN, de Melo EF, Ikoma MRV, Damante JH, et al. Enhanced programmed death 1 (PD-1) and PD-1 ligand (PD-L1) expression in patients with actinic cheilitis and oral squamous cell carcinoma. Cancer Immunol Immunother. 2011;60:965–74. https://doi.org/10.1007/s00262-011-1007-5.
114. Varela-Centelles P, Seoane-Romero J, García-Pola MJ, Leira-Feijoo Y, Seoane-Romero JM. Therapeutic approaches for actinic cheilitis: therapeutic efficacy and malignant transformation after treatment. Int J Oral Maxillofac Surg. 2020;49:1343–50. https://doi.org/10.1016/j.ijom.2020.02.014.
115. Bakirtzi K, Papadimitriou I, Andreadis D, Sotiriou E. Treatment options and post-treatment malignant transformation rate of actinic Cheilitis: a systematic review. Cancer. 2021;13:3354. https://doi.org/10.3390/cancers13133354.
116. Trager MH, Farmer K, Ulrich C, Basset-Seguin N, Herms F, Geskin LJ, et al. Actinic cheilitis: a systematic review of treatment options. J Eur Acad Dermatol Venereol JEADV. 2021;35:815–23. https://doi.org/10.1111/jdv.16995.
117. Satorres Nieto M, Gargallo Albiol J, Gay Escoda C. Surgical management of actinic cheilitis. Med Oral. 2001;6:205–17.
118. de Godoy Peres FF, Aigotti Haberbeck Brandão A, Rodarte Carvalho Y, Dória Filho U, Plapler H. A study of actinic cheilitis treatment by two low-morbidity CO2 laser vaporization one-pass protocols. Lasers Med Sci. 2009;24:375–85. https://doi.org/10.1007/s10103-008-0574-y.
119. Choi SH, Kim KH, Song KH. Efficacy of ablative fractional laser-assisted photodynamic therapy for the treatment of actinic cheilitis: 12-month follow-up results of a prospective, randomized, comparative trial. Br J Dermatol. 2015;173:184–91. https://doi.org/10.1111/bjd.13542.

120. Lai M, Pampena R, Cornacchia L, Pellacani G, Peris K, Longo C. Treatments of actinic cheilitis: a systematic review of the literature. J Am Acad Dermatol. 2020;83:876–87. https://doi.org/10.1016/j.jaad.2019.07.106.
121. Carvalho M de V, de Moraes SLD, Lemos CAA, Santiago Júnior JF, Vasconcelos BC do E, Pellizzer EP. Surgical versus non-surgical treatment of actinic cheilitis: a systematic review and meta-analysis. Oral Dis. 2019;25:972–81. https://doi.org/10.1111/odi.12916.
122. de Visscher JG, van der Waal I. Etiology of cancer of the lip. A review. Int J Oral Maxillofac Surg. 1998;27:199–203. https://doi.org/10.1016/s0901-5027(98)80010-6.
123. IARC Global cancer observatory. Lip, Oral Cavity. 2022. Available from https://gco.iarc.who.int/media/globocan/factsheets/cancers/1-lip-oral-cavity-fact-sheet.pdf. Accessed 5 Feb 2025.
124. Maruccia M, Onesti MG, Parisi P, Cigna E, Troccola A, Scuderi N. Lip cancer: a 10-year retrospective epidemiological study. Anticancer Res. 2012;32:1543–6. https://ar.iiarjournals.org/content/32/4/1543.long
125. Domínguez-Gordillo A, Esparza-Gómez G, García-Jiménez B, Cerero-Lapiedra R, Casado-Gómez I, Romero-Lastra P, et al. The pattern of lip cancer occurrence over the 1990-2011 period in public hospitals in Madrid, Spain. J Oral Pathol Med. 2016;45:202–10. https://doi.org/10.1111/jop.12340.
126. Salan AI, Camen A, Ciuca A, Patru A, Scrieciu M, Popescu SM, et al. Epidemiological aspects in lip tumors in Oltenia region of Romania during 2012–2016. Curr Health Sci J. 2018;44:39–47. https://doi.org/10.12865/CHSJ.44.01.07.
127. Tseng HW, Liou HH, Tsai KW, Ger LP, Shiue YL. Clinicopathological study of lip cancer: a retrospective hospital-based study in Taiwan. APMIS. 2017;125:1007–16. https://doi.org/10.1111/apm.12751.
128. Silva WR, Bortoli MM, Leite SR, Barros CC, Brito MD, Montenegro LT, et al. Squamous cell carcinoma and basal cell carcinoma of the lips: 25 years of experience in a northeast Brazilian population. Med Oral Patol Oral Cirugia Bucal. 2024;29:e476–82. https://doi.org/10.4317/medoral.26454.
129. Cabello BT, Sazo BN, Salgado FA, Martínez RB. Squamous cell carcinoma of the lip survival rate. Rev Med Chile. 2015;143:847–55. https://doi.org/10.4067/S0034-98872015000700004.
130. van Hof KS, Wakkee M, Sewnaik A, Herkendaal AF, Tans L, Mast H, et al. Long-term outcomes, quality of life, and costs of treatment modalities for T1-T2 lip carcinomas. Oral Dis. 2024;30:2063–74. https://doi.org/10.1111/odi.14723.
131. Silapunt S, Peterson SR, Goldberg LH, Friedman PM, Alam M. Basal cell carcinoma on the vermilion lip: a study of 18 cases. J Am Acad Dermatol. 2004;50:384–7. https://doi.org/10.1016/j.jaad.2003.08.027.
132. Miranda-Filho A, Bray F. Global patterns and trends in cancers of the lip, tongue and mouth. Oral Oncol de. 2020;102:104551. https://doi.org/10.1016/j.oraloncology.2019.104551.
133. Shield KD, Ferlay J, Jemal A, Sankaranarayanan R, Chaturvedi AK, Bray F, et al. The global incidence of lip, oral cavity, and pharyngeal cancers by subsite in 2012. CA Cancer J Clin. 2017;67:51–64. https://doi.org/10.3322/caac.21384.
134. Abreu L, Kruger E, Tennant M. Lip cancer in Western Australia, 1982–2006: a 25-year retrospective epidemiological study. Aust Dent J. 2009;54:130–5. https://doi.org/10.1111/j.1834-7819.2009.01105.x.
135. Bota JP, Lyons AB, Carroll BT. Squamous cell carcinoma of the lip-a review of squamous cell carcinogenesis of the mucosal and cutaneous junction. Dermatologic Surg. 2017;43:494–506. https://doi.org/10.1097/DSS.0000000000001020.
136. Perea-Milla López E, Miñarro-Del Moral RM, Martínez-García C, Zanetti R, Rosso S, Serrano S, et al. Lifestyles, environmental and phenotypic factors associated with lip cancer: a case-control study in southern Spain. Br J Cancer. 2003;88:1702–7. https://doi.org/10.1038/sj.bjc.6600975.
137. Makita E, Akasaka E, Sakuraba Y, Korekawa A, Aizu T, Kaneko T, et al. Squamous cell carcinoma on the lip arising from discoid lupus erythematosus: a case report and review of Japanese patients. Eur J Dermatol. 2016;26:395–6. https://doi.org/10.1684/ejd.2016.2780.

138. Borges JFP, Lanaro ND, Bernardo VG, Albano RM, Dias F, de Faria Pa.S, et al. Lower lip squamous cell carcinoma in patients with photosensitive disorders: analysis of cases treated at the Brazilian National Cancer Institute (INCA) from 1999 to 2012. Med Oral Patol Oral Cirugia Bucal. 2018(23):e7–12. https://doi.org/10.4317/medoral.21960.
139. Piemonte ED, Gilligan GM, Garola F, Lazos JP, Panico RL, Normando AGC, et al. Differences among oral carcinomas arising de novo from those associated with oral potentially malignant disorders: a systematic review and meta-analysis. Oral Surg Oral Med Oral Pathol Oral Radiol. 2024;137:613–31. https://doi.org/10.1016/j.oooo.2024.03.006.
140. Custódio M, Pelissari C, Santana T, Trierveiler M. Expression of cancer stem cell markers CD44, ALDH1 and p75NTR in actinic cheilitis and lip cancer. Eur Arch Otorrinolaringol. 2018;275:1877–83. https://doi.org/10.1007/s00405-018-5002-8.
141. Correa GTB, Bernardes VF, de Sousa SF, Diniz MG, Salles JMP, Souza RP, et al. Lip cancer and pre-cancerous lesions harbor TP53 mutations, exhibit allelic loss at 9p, 9q, and 17p, but no BRAFV600E mutations. Tumour Biol J Int Soc Oncodevelopmental Biol Med. 2015;36:9059–66. https://doi.org/10.1007/s13277-015-3659-9.
142. Ochsenius G, Ormeño A, Godoy L, Rojas R. A retrospective study of 232 cases of lip cancer and pre cancer in Chilean patients. Clinical-histological correlation. Rev Med Chil. 2003;131:60–6. https://doi.org/10.4067/S0034-98872003000100009.
143. Hasson O. Squamous cell carcinoma of the lower lip. J Oral Maxillofac Surg. 2008;66:1259–62. https://doi.org/10.1016/j.joms.2008.01.055.
144. Agostini T, Spinelli G, Arcuri F, Perello R. Metastatic squamous cell carcinoma of the lower lip: analysis of the 5-year survival rate. Arch Craniofacial Surg. 2017;18:105–11. https://doi.org/10.7181/acfs.2017.18.2.105.
145. Kaugars GE, Abbey LM, Page DG, Svirsky JA, Burns JC, Pillion T. Prevention and detection of lip cancer–the dentist's role. J Calif Dent Assoc. 1999;27:318–23. https://doi.org/10.1080/19424396.2016.12221124.
146. Anand N, Chaudhary N, Mittal MK, Prasad R. Comparison of the efficacy of clinical examination, ultrasound neck and computed tomography in detection and staging of cervical lymph node metastasis in head and neck cancers. Indian J Otolaryngol Head Neck Surg. 2007;59:19–23. https://doi.org/10.1007/s12070-007-0005-6.
147. Alsibani A, Alqahtani A, Almohammadi R, Islam T, Alessa M, Aldhahri SF, et al. Comparing the efficacy of CT, MRI, PET-CT, and US in the detection of cervical lymph node metastases in head and neck squamous cell carcinoma with clinically negative neck lymph node: a systematic review and meta-analysis. J Clin Med. 2024;13:7622. https://doi.org/10.3390/jcm13247622.
148. Onercl M, Yilmaz T, Gedikoğlu G. Tumor thickness as a predictor of cervical lymph node metastasis in squamous cell carcinoma of the lower lip. Otolaryngol–Head Neck Surg. 2000;122:139–42. https://doi.org/10.1016/S0194-5998(00)70162-8.
149. Betka J. Distant metastases from lip and oral cavity cancer. ORL J Oto-Rhino-Laryngol Its Relat Spec. 2001;63:217–21. https://doi.org/10.1159/000055744.
150. Holmkvist KA, Roenigk RK. Squamous cell carcinoma of the lip treated with Mohs micrographic surgery: outcome at 5 years. J Am Acad Dermatol. 1998;38:960–6. https://doi.org/10.1016/s0190-9622(98)70160-4.
151. Campbell JP. Surgical management of lip carcinoma. J Oral Maxillofac Surg. 1998;56:955–61. https://doi.org/10.1016/s0278-2391(98)90658-9.
152. Nadir U, Le K, Shi K, Srivastava D, Nijhawan RI. Outcomes of squamous cell carcinoma of the lip treated with Mohs micrographic surgery: a retrospective cohort study. Dermatologic Surg. 2023;49:1108–11. https://doi.org/10.1097/DSS.0000000000003992.
153. Pfister DG, Spencer S, Brizel DM, Burtness B, Busse PM, Caudell JJ, et al. Head and neck cancers, version 2.2014. Clinical practice guidelines in oncology. J Natl Compr Cancer Netw. 2014;12:1454–87. https://doi.org/10.6004/jnccn.2014.0142.
154. Thanh Pham T, Cross S, Gebski V, Veness MJ. Squamous cell carcinoma of the lip in Australian patients: definitive radiotherapy is an efficacious option to surgery in select patients. Dermatologic Surg. 2015;41:219–25. https://doi.org/10.1097/DSS.0000000000000240.

155. Shukla A, Loy K, Lu GN. Total lower lip reconstruction: a review of recent advances. Curr Opin Otolaryngol Head Neck Surg. 2023;31:441–51. https://doi.org/10.1097/MOO.0000000000000926.
156. Vanison C, Beckmann N, Smith A. Recent advances in lip reconstruction. Curr Opin Otolaryngol Head Neck Surg. 2019;27:219–26. https://doi.org/10.1097/MOO.0000000000000531.
157. Arnold M, Singh D, Laversanne M, Vignat J, Vaccarella S, Meheus F, et al. Global burden of cutaneous melanoma in 2020 and projections to 2040. JAMA Dermatol. 2022;158:495–503. https://doi.org/10.1001/jamadermatol.2022.0160.
158. Long GV, Swetter SM, Menzies AM, Gershenwald JE, Scolyer RA. Cutaneous melanoma. Lancet Lond Engl. 2023;402:485–502. https://doi.org/10.1016/S0140-6736(23)00821-8.
159. Caraban BM, Aschie M, Deacu M, Cozaru GC, Pundiche MB, Orasanu CI, et al. A narrative review of current knowledge on cutaneous melanoma. Clin Pract. 2024;14:214–41. https://doi.org/10.3390/clinpract14010018.
160. Jing G, Wu Y, Song H, Ren G, Wang R, Guo W. Primary malignant melanoma of the lip: a report of 48 cases. J Oral Maxillofac Surg. 2015;73:2232–40. https://doi.org/10.1016/j.joms.2015.05.021.
161. Raderman D, Rothem A, Giler S, Ben-Bassat M. Primary malignant melanoma of the vermilion of the lower lip. J Dermatol Surg Oncol. 1986;12:1106–10. https://doi.org/10.1111/j.1524-4725.1986.tb02090.x.
162. Betz SJ, Jelmini JJ, Kim RY. Early stage melanoma of the Vermillion with mucosal melanoma in situ: a clinical conundrum. Head Neck Pathol. 2023;17:815–20. https://doi.org/10.1007/s12105-023-01552-y.
163. Godoy GP, de Castro Gomes DQ, Pereira JV, de Queiroz Figueiredo RL, Nonaka CFW, da Costa Miguel MC. Desmoplastic melanoma of the lower lip: a case report. Oral Surg Oral Med Oral Pathol Oral Radiol Endod. 2009;108:e64–9. https://doi.org/10.1016/j.tripleo.2009.07.006.
164. Hui JI, Linden KG, Barr RJ. Desmoplastic malignant melanoma of the lip: a report of 6 cases and review of the literature. J Am Acad Dermatol. 2002;47:863–8. https://doi.org/10.1067/mjd.2002.124686.
165. Zhou C, Lee C, Salas J, Luke J. Guide to tinted sunscreens in skin of color. Int J Dermatol. 2024;63:272–6. https://doi.org/10.1111/ijd.16954.
166. Sexton FM, Maize JC. Melanotic macules and melanoacanthomas of the lip. A comparative study with census of the basal melanocyte population. Am J Dermatopathol. 1987;9:438–44. https://doi.org/10.1097/00000372-198710000-00012.
167. Kaugars GE, Heise AP, Riley WT, Abbey LM, Svirsky JA. Oral melanotic macules. A review of 353 cases. Oral Surg Oral Med Oral Pathol. 1993;76:59–61. https://doi.org/10.1016/0030-4220(93)90295-f.
168. Nagarajan A, Masthan MK, Sankar LS, Narayanasamy AB, Elumalai R. Oral manifestations of vitiligo. Indian J Dermatol. 2015;60:103. https://doi.org/10.4103/0019-5154.147844.
169. Asadi LK, Khalili A, Wang SQ. The sociological basis of the skin cancer epidemic. Int J Dermatol febrero de. 2023;62(2):169–76.
170. Kliniec K, Tota M, Zalesińska A, Łyko M, Jankowska-Konsur A. Skin cancer risk, sun-protection knowledge and behavior in athletes-a narrative review. Cancers. 2023;15:3281. https://doi.org/10.3390/cancers15133281.
171. Sharma K, Dixon KM, Münch G, Chang D, Zhou X. Ultraviolet and infrared radiation in Australia: assessing the benefits, risks, and optimal exposure guidelines. Front Public Health. 2024;12:1505904. https://doi.org/10.3389/fpubh.2024.1505904.
172. Garbe C, Forsea AM, Amaral T, Arenberger P, Autier P, Berwick M, et al. Skin cancers are the most frequent cancers in fair-skinned populations, but we can prevent them. Eur J Cancer Oxf Engl. 1990;2024(204):114074. https://doi.org/10.1016/j.ejca.2024.114074.
173. Lu JT, Ilyas E. An overview of ultraviolet-protective clothing. Cureus. 2022;14:e27333. https://doi.org/10.7759/cureus.27333.

174. Sander M, Sander M, Burbidge T, Beecker J. The efficacy and safety of sunscreen use for the prevention of skin cancer. CMAJ. 2020;192:E1802–8. https://doi.org/10.1503/cmaj.201085.
175. Tang X, Yang T, Yu D, Xiong H, Zhang S. Current insights and future perspectives of ultraviolet radiation (UV) exposure: friends and foes to the skin and beyond the skin. Environ Int. 2024;185:108535. https://doi.org/10.1016/j.envint.2024.108535.
176. Li L, Chong L, Huang T, Ma Y, Li Y, Ding H. Natural products and extracts from plants as natural UV filters for sunscreens: a review. Anim Models Exp Med. 2023;6:183–95. https://doi.org/10.1002/ame2.12295.
177. Maier H, Schauberger G, Brunnhofer K, Hönigsmann H. Assessment of thickness of photoprotective lipsticks and frequency of reapplication: results from a laboratory test and a field experiment. Br J Dermatol. 2003;148:763–9. https://doi.org/10.1046/j.1365-2133.2003.05032.x.
178. Young AR. The adverse consequences of not using sunscreens. Int J Cosmet Sci. 2023;45(Suppl 1):11–9. https://doi.org/10.1111/ics.12897.
179. Maier H, Schauberger G, Martincigh BS, Brunnhofer K, Hönigsmann H. Ultraviolet protective performance of photoprotective lipsticks: change of spectral transmittance because of ultraviolet exposure. Photodermatol Photoimmunol Photomed. 2005;21:84–92. https://doi.org/10.1111/j.1600-0781.2005.00143.x.
180. Pellacani G, Lim HW, Stockfleth E, Sibaud V, Brugués AO, Saint Aroman M. Photoprotection: current developments and controversies. J Eur Acad Dermatol Venereol JEADV. 2024;38(Suppl 5):12–20. https://doi.org/10.1111/jdv.19677.
181. Milutinov J, Pavlović N, Ćirin D, Atanacković Krstonošić M, Krstonošić V. The potential of natural compounds in UV protection products. Molecules (Basel, Switzerland). 2024;29:5409. https://doi.org/10.3390/molecules29225409.
182. Breakell T, Kowalski I, Foerster Y, Kramer R, Erdmann M, Berking C, et al. Ultraviolet filters: dissecting current facts and myths. J Clin Med. 2024;13:2986. https://doi.org/10.3390/jcm13102986.
183. Hartmann D, Valenzuela F. Sunproofing from within: a deep dive into oral photoprotection strategies in dermatology. Photodermatol Photoimmunol Photomed. 2024;40:e12985. https://doi.org/10.1111/phpp.12985.
184. Anbualakan K, Tajul Urus NQ, Makpol S, Jamil A, Mohd Ramli ES, Md Pauzi SH, et al. A scoping review on the effects of carotenoids and flavonoids on skin damage due to ultraviolet radiation. Nutrients. 2022;15:92. https://doi.org/10.3390/nu15010092.
185. Slavinsky V, Helmy J, Vroman J, Valdebran M. Solar ultraviolet radiation exposure in workers with outdoor occupations: a systematic review and call to action. Int J Dermatol. 2024;63:288–97. https://doi.org/10.1111/ijd.16877.
186. Cherrie JW, Cherrie MPC. Workplace exposure to UV radiation and strategies to minimize cancer risk. Br Med Bull. 2022;144:45–56. https://doi.org/10.1093/bmb/ldac019.
187. Lucena EE de S, Costa DCB, da Silveira ÉJD, Lima KC. Adoption of photoprotection measures on lip and perioral regions among beach workers in North Brazil. Int J Dermatol. 2014;53:e480–5. https://doi.org/10.1111/ijd.12218.
188. Morton SK, Harrison SL. Slip, slop, slap, slide, seek and sport: a systematic scoping review of Sun protection in sport in Australasia. Curr Oncol. 2022;30:401–15. https://doi.org/10.3390/curroncol30010033.
189. Brunssen A, Waldmann A, Eisemann N, Katalinic A. Impact of skin cancer screening and secondary prevention campaigns on skin cancer incidence and mortality: a systematic review. J Am Acad Dermatol. 2017;76:129–139.e10. https://doi.org/10.1016/j.jaad.2016.07.045.
190. Collins LG, Gage R, Sinclair C, Lindsay D. The cost-effectiveness of primary prevention interventions for skin cancer: an updated systematic review. Appl Health Econ Health Policy. 2024;22:685–700. https://doi.org/10.1007/s40258-024-00892-2.
191. Rodriguez-Blanco I, Florez Á, Paredes-Suárez C, et al. Use of lip photoprotection in patients suffering from actinic cheilitis. Eur J Dermatol. 2019;29:383–6. https://doi.org/10.1684/ejd.2019.3604.

192. Lucena IM de, Santos I da S, Daroit NB, Salgueiro AP, Cavagni J, Haas AN, et al. Sun protection as a protective factor for actinic cheilitis: cross-sectional population-based study. Oral Dis. 2022;28:1802–10. https://doi.org/10.1111/odi.13837.
193. Moon S, Sangha A, Ravichandran M, Samuela A, Tso S, Sharma D, Ariyawardana A. Use of lip protecting agents in the prevention of actinic Cheilitis, herpes Labialis and cancer of lip: a systematic review. Open Dent J. 2021:15. https://doi.org/10.2174/1874210602115010428.

22 Poor Oral Hygiene: A Risk Factor for Periodontal Disease

Jaya Seneviratne and John Rong Hao Tay

22.1 Introduction

Periodontal disease remains a pervasive challenge for oral healthcare providers. Its onset and progression are intricately linked to oral hygiene, a modifiable lifestyle factor that significantly impacts oral and overall health. Neglecting oral hygiene results in dental plaque accumulation, which initiates gingivitis within a few weeks. Gingivitis is reversible if addressed promptly [1], but if left unchecked, it may progress to periodontitis, culminating in tooth loss and elevating risks for systemic conditions such as diabetes and adverse pregnancy outcomes [2–4]. Both landmark studies and contemporary evidence consistently demonstrate that effective oral hygiene is fundamental in maintaining periodontal health, as it disrupts the microbial dysbiosis that leads to periodontal disease [1, 5, 6].

Understanding the interaction between oral hygiene, environmental risk factors and periodontal disease is essential for oral healthcare providers. Habits such as tobacco smoking significantly increase periodontal risk and can diminish the protective benefits of good oral hygiene [3, 7]. The European Federation of Periodontology (EFP) S3 clinical practice guidelines add clarity by offering a structured framework for preventive strategies [8]. This chapter explores why individuals fail to maintain consistent oral hygiene, examining lifestyle-related risk factors such as poor diet, tobacco smoking, alcohol abuse, obesity, lack of sleep, sedentary behaviour and areca nut chewing. It also addresses socioeconomic barriers such as poverty and lack of access to dental care, which exacerbate poor hygiene practices. Drawing on evidence-based strategies, we discuss how dentists, public health

J. Seneviratne (✉)
Periodontology, School of Dentistry, The University of Queensland, Brisbane, QLD, Australia
e-mail: jaya.seneviratne@uq.edu.au

J. R. H. Tay
National Dental Centre Singapore, Singapore, Singapore
e-mail: john.tay.r.h@singahealth.com

S. R. Prabhu et al. (eds.), *Lifestyle in Oral Health and Disease*,
https://doi.org/10.1007/978-3-032-05888-1_22

campaigns and the media can promote better oral hygiene to prevent periodontal disease.

22.2 Importance of Oral Hygiene and Current Standard Practices

Effective oral hygiene, primarily through twice-daily tooth brushing with fluoride toothpaste and interdental cleaning, can prevent plaque buildup and periodontal disease [9, 10]. However, compliance with these practices is often poor due to lifestyle factors and broader determinants such as socioeconomic status, education and cultural perceptions toward oral health. In a landmark study, Löe et al. (1965) demonstrated that suspending oral hygiene induces gingivitis within 10–15 days and that it is reversible when brushing is resumed, underscoring the critical role of consistent plaque control [1]. This seminal finding, corroborated by subsequent research [11–14], reinforces that plaque control is pivotal in preventing the progression of gingivitis. Despite this, many individuals neglect oral hygiene.

Dental plaque is a microbial biofilm, and poor oral hygiene can disrupt its balance, leading to dysbiosis, chronic inflammation, tissue destruction and, ultimately, tooth loss [15]. Self-performed oral hygiene, primarily through mechanical plaque disruption, remains the most reliable method for preventing and managing gingivitis [16]. Thorough plaque removal reduces its quantity and alters the composition of subgingival plaque [17].

Effective supragingival plaque control is fundamental in preventing and managing periodontal disease [18]. Longitudinal cohort studies demonstrate that maintaining high oral hygiene standards ensures periodontal tissue stability over decades [19]. Plaque control is essential at all levels of prevention. In primary prevention, it helps avert the onset of periodontal disease. In secondary prevention, it prevents its recurrence and halts the progression of gingivitis. In tertiary prevention, it prevents further tissue destruction in periodontitis. This is achieved by targeting the supragingival plaque, a dynamic microbial community whose bacterial composition shifts with disease, distinguishing healthy gingiva from gingivitis and advanced periodontitis.

Meticulous supragingival plaque also reduces and may prevent subgingival colonisation. Waerhaug (1981), in a 12-month split-mouth trial in monkeys, demonstrated that bass-method tooth brushing enabled bristles to penetrate approximately 0.9 mm subgingivally, effectively inhibiting plaque formation in inaccessible areas [20]. Furthermore, a single manual tooth brushing session achieves a weighted mean plaque reduction of 42%, with studies indicating a significant reduction in gingival inflammation [16]. Power toothbrushes have been shown to enhance plaque removal efficacy, achieving a 46% plaque reduction after a single use compared to 42% in manual brushing. When used consistently, they lead to plaque reductions of 11% after 1–3 months and 21% after more than 3 months, along with reductions in gingival inflammation of 6% and 11%, respectively [21].

The optimal toothbrushing frequency remains debated [18]. Lang et al. (1973) explored the minimum frequency required to prevent gingivitis, finding that dental students who meticulously removed plaque every 48 hours using toothbrushes, floss and toothpicks showed no clinical gingival inflammation over 6 weeks [22]. This suggests thoroughness and consistency outweigh frequency alone in plaque control efficacy. Brushing twice daily for 2 minutes with fluoride toothpaste, paired with interdental cleaning such as flossing, is endorsed by the American Dental Association and the World Health Organization (WHO) [23–25]. The use of fluoride-containing toothpaste increases fluoride levels in saliva, promoting tooth remineralisation and reducing the risk of caries. According to the EFP S3 clinical practice guidelines, professional mechanical plaque removal also targets subgingival plaque [8]. Chemical adjuncts such as chlorhexidine mouthwash enhance outcomes, reducing plaque by 33% and gingivitis by 26% when combined with toothbrushing, although long-term use risks staining of tooth surfaces [26].

Axelsson et al. (2004) conducted a 30-year study to monitor tooth loss, caries and periodontal attachment loss in adults who adhered to a well-managed plaque control programme [27]. The study highlighted the positive impact of preventive dental care in individuals who received regular professional support and were consistently encouraged to maintain high oral hygiene standards. Over three decades, tooth loss was minimal, ranging from 0.4 to 1.8 teeth lost depending on age group. Notably, most tooth loss was due to root fractures, with only 21 teeth lost due to progressive periodontitis or caries. In a separate study, daily mechanical plaque removal at 24-hour intervals was shown to effectively prevent the development of gingival inflammation over a 30-day period in individuals without a history of periodontitis [28]. Patient education enhances the effectiveness of mechanical plaque control. Jönsson et al. (2020) demonstrated that an individually tailored oral health educational programme was more effective in achieving proper long-term oral hygiene self-care behaviour and led to a greater reduction in gingival inflammation [29]. These findings reinforce mechanical plaque control as the gold standard for maintaining periodontal health.

22.3 Barriers to Consistent Oral Hygiene

Maintaining consistent oral hygiene is essential for preventing dental diseases such as caries and periodontitis. However, many intersecting barriers, including socioeconomic, behavioural, psychological and cultural factors, hinder the individual's ability to sustain effective oral hygiene routines.

(i) Socioeconomic Factors

Poverty, limited access to dental care and low health literacy are well-documented barriers to maintaining oral hygiene. Individuals from socioeconomically disadvantaged backgrounds often face financial constraints that lead them to prioritise essential needs like food, shelter and utilities over dental care or routine dental visits [30, 31]. Accessibility is also a concern in rural or underserved communities, where dental clinics may be scarce or too distant to reach without reliable transportation. Furthermore, low health literacy exacerbates these challenges; individuals may lack the knowledge or skills needed to understand oral health information or apply it to daily practice [32, 33]. For example, they may not recognise the early signs of periodontal disease or understand the importance of regular tooth brushing and interdental cleaning. Educational interventions targeting vulnerable populations have shown promise in improving both awareness and behaviour, but sustainable implementation remains a challenge [34, 35].

(ii) Behavioural and Psychological Factors

Beyond socioeconomic challenges, daily habits and mental health can significantly influence oral hygiene practices [36, 37]. Time constraints due to work or caregiving responsibilities may cause individuals to skip brushing or flossing, particularly at night when fatigue sets in. Oral hygiene is often not prioritised amid competing tasks, especially when it is not perceived as having immediate consequences [34]. Additionally, psychological conditions such as depression and anxiety are linked to poor self-care behaviours. Studies have shown that individuals experiencing these mental health issues often neglect personal hygiene routines, including oral hygiene, due to diminished motivation, energy and executive functioning [38, 39]. Addressing these barriers requires integrated approaches that consider mental health support alongside oral health promotion.

(iii) Cultural and Habitual Practices

Cultural norms and traditional practices also play a role in shaping oral hygiene behaviours. In certain regions, habits such as areca nut (betel quid) chewing are deeply ingrained and socially accepted, despite their known deleterious effects on oral health [40, 41]. This practice, common in South and Southeast Asia, not only contributes to tooth staining but also facilitates plaque retention and increases the risk for periodontal disease and oral cancer [42]. Furthermore, misconceptions about oral care such as the belief that vigorous brushing causes tooth abrasion or that tooth loss is a natural part of aging can deter individuals from engaging in preventive oral hygiene routines [43]. Tailored oral health education that respects cultural beliefs while addressing harmful practices is critical for fostering behaviour change.

Socioeconomic status, psychological well-being, behavioural priorities and cultural norms influence consistent oral hygiene. Addressing these barriers requires multifaceted, interdisciplinary strategies, including education, care access, mental health support and culturally sensitive public health messaging.

22.4 Local and Systemic Factors Are Influenced by Oral Health

Beyond its local effects of connective tissue destruction, poor oral hygiene-induced local inflammation can contribute to systemic health conditions [44, 45]. Interventional studies have demonstrated that non-surgical periodontal therapy enhances glycaemic control in diabetic patients, with reductions in haemoglobin A1c (HbA1c) levels ranging from 0.4% to 0.6% within 3 months, representing a clinically meaningful improvement [46, 47]. Moreover, periodontitis has been shown to be independently associated with cardiovascular diseases, chronic obstructive pulmonary disease, obstructive sleep apnoea and COVID-19 complications [48].

The oral-systemic link highlights the impact of periodontal disease on general health. Dysbiotic oral plaque and the resulting inflammation have been implicated in a range of conditions such as diabetes mellitus, rheumatoid arthritis, atherosclerosis, pancreatic cancer and adverse pregnancy outcomes [49]. In diabetes, some studies suggest that a dysbiotic subgingival microbiomes may aggravate hyperglycaemia, while poor glycaemic control worsens periodontitis. Bacterial genera commonly associated with both diabetes and periodontitis include *Fusobacterium, Parvimonas, Peptostreptococcus, Gemella, Streptococcus, Leptotrichia, Filifactor, Veillonella, Saccharibacteria (TM7)* and *Terrahemophilus* [50]. Another study identified *TM7, Aggregatibacter, Neisseria, Gemella, Eikenella, Selenomonas, Actinomyces, Capnocytophaga, Fusobacterium, Veillonella* and *Streptococcus* as the most prevalent genera in individuals with diabetes and periodontitis [51].

Patients with rheumatoid arthritis also exhibit distinct oral microbiomes, with deep pockets enriched in anaerobes such as Tannerella forsythia and shallow pockets harbouring facultative taxa. This suggests that bacterial genera commonly associated with both diabetes and periodontitis may exacerbate joint inflammation [52, 53]. Atherosclerosis has been linked to oral pathogens such as *Porphyromonas gingivalis* and *Actinobacillus actinomycetemcomitans* within atheromatous plaques, indicating a role in promoting systemic inflammation [54, 55]. In pregnancy, dynamic shifts in the oral microbiome may influence placental health and have been associated with an increased risk of preterm birth [56].

However, establishing causality in these associations remains challenging due to variability in study design, the presence of confounding factors and methodological inconsistencies [49]. Non-modifiable variables such as age, gender and ethnicity, along with modifiable factors such as smoking, diet and comorbidities, can skew microbiome signatures. In addition, inconsistencies in sample collection and sequencing biases further complicate findings. These limitations highlight the need for standardised protocols and comprehensive data collection to better elucidate the complex interplay between oral and systemic health.

22.5 An Update of Classification of Periodontal Disease and Risk Factors

It is important for healthcare providers to remain up to date with current professional standards to deliver tailored oral health programmes for their patients. In this section, we highlight the new classification of periodontitis and discuss how it can be effectively incorporated into clinical practice. The 2018 classification, jointly developed by the European Federation of Periodontology and American Academy of Periodontology (EFP/AAP), redefined periodontal diseases with clearer diagnostic distinctions [57]. It recognises gingivitis as a reversible inflammatory condition confined to the gingiva, primarily caused by plaque accumulation. With effective oral hygiene, gingivitis can be reversed within 2–3 weeks, especially when supported by patient education [58]. The classification further distinguishes plaque-induced from non-plaque-induced gingival diseases, with the former typically manageable through mechanical plaque control alone [59].

In contrast, periodontitis is defined as a chronic, irreversible inflammatory disease associated with a dysbiotic biofilm and characterised by progressive destruction of the periodontal ligament and alveolar bone [60]. The classification introduces a staging and grading system [15].

- Stages I–IV reflect the severity, complexity and extent of the disease based on clinical attachment loss, bone loss, tooth loss, periodontal probing depths, furcation involvement and functional impairment.
- Grades A–C reflect the rate of progression, anticipated treatment response and impact on systemic health, with modifications based on individual risk factors such as diabetes and smoking.

Among the modifiable risk factors, diabetes mellitus and smoking are the most consistently associated with poorer periodontal outcomes. Periodontitis is recognised as the sixth complication of diabetes [61, 62]. Periodontitis is more prevalent and severe in people with diabetes, with studies showing a two- to threefold increased risk compared to non-diabetics [16, 63]. The relationship is bidirectional—periodontal inflammation can worsen glycaemic control, while hyperglycaemia can impair immune response and healing of the periodontium [64]. Periodontal therapy has also been shown to improve metabolic outcomes, with reductions in HbA1c of approximately 0.4% within 3–4 months of treatment [65]. This improvement is clinically meaningful, comparable to adding a second-line pharmacological agent in diabetes management [66]. These findings support the inclusion of routine periodontal assessment and treatment as part of comprehensive diabetes care.

Numerous cross-sectional, longitudinal and intervention studies have demonstrated that smokers have a significantly higher risk of periodontitis, with odds ratios ranging from 2.0 to 7.0 compared to non-smokers [67–70]. For example, Bergström (1989) found a 2.5-fold increased risk in smokers in a 10-year follow-up study [67]. Bergström et al. (2000) showed that smokers exhibited greater periodontal bone loss and more diseased sites compared to non-smokers, whose periodontal health remained stable [68]. Encouragingly, smoking cessation has been shown to reduce the risk of periodontitis progression and improve treatment outcomes, with some studies reporting that former smokers exhibit periodontal stability comparable to never-smokers [71–73].

In summary, smoking and poor glycaemic control exacerbate periodontitis progression, but they are also modifiable. The 2018 EFP/AAP classification reflects this by embedding risk factor assessment into the grading system, encouraging tailored care. For instance, a Grade C diagnosis—indicating rapid progression due to heavy smoking or uncontrolled diabetes—requires more intensive interventions beyond routine oral hygiene. Recognising and managing these risk factors not only improve periodontal outcomes but also contribute to better systemic health.

22.6 Dysbiotic Plaque and Immune Dysregulation in Periodontitis

Having explained the lifestyle factors and clinical updates related to oral health and periodontitis, we will now focus on the pathophysiology of the disease. This will help readers understand the biological plausibility of periodontal disease and how they can modify lifestyle factors to improve oral health outcomes for their patients. Dental plaque is a structured microbial biofilm and the primary etiological factor in gingival inflammation and the development of periodontal disease [74, 75]. Within 2–4 days of undisturbed plaque accumulation, histological signs of inflammation begin to appear, including vasculitis beneath the junctional epithelium and infiltration of polymorphonuclear neutrophils. This is known as the initial lesion as described by Page and Schroeder (1976) [76]. If plaque persists, this progresses through the stages of gingivitis to an advanced lesion, ultimately resulting in periodontitis. This is characterised by connective tissue destruction and alveolar bone loss.

The development of gingival inflammation is closely tied to changes in the microbial composition of plaque as it matures. Dental plaque formation begins when a cleaned tooth surface interacts with saliva and gingival crevicular fluid, forming an acquired pellicle of salivary glycoproteins and bacterial fragments on hydroxyapatite. Gram-positive streptococci such as *Streptococcus oralis* and *S. mitis* colonise first as primary colonisers, followed by secondary colonisers like *Actinomyces* and *Fusobacterium*, which promote co-aggregation into characteristic 'corn-cob' and 'test-tube brush' structures [77]. If oral hygiene is neglected, tertiary pathogens such as *Porphyromonas gingivalis* emerge, shifting plaque towards dysbiosis and disease [78]. Current insights on dental plaque recognise that not all oral bacteria are pathogenic. For example, bacterial species like *Veillonella parvula* and *Actinomyces naeslundii* are considered beneficial or host-compatible, contributing to a stable and health-associated oral microbiome.

In health, supragingival plaque maintains a stable, homeostatic balance with the host, but accumulation can tip this balance into gingivitis, a confined lesion [79].

Progression to periodontitis reflects a dysregulated immune response driven by host, systemic and environmental factors, resulting in connective tissue loss, alveolar destruction and junctional epithelium migration. Lifestyle factors such as poor oral hygiene, a high-sugar diet and smoking exacerbate this dysbiotic shift, accelerating subgingival plaque growth. Hence, effective oral hygiene is essential to disrupt the maturation of dental plaque, thereby preventing periodontal disease [80]. Supragingival plaque, dominant in gingivitis, comprises overgrown commensals that trigger inflammation in susceptible individuals. The resulting host immune response can lead to collagen degradation, sulcular epithelial damage and bleeding on probing. Over time, this plaque extends subgingivally, creating an anaerobic niche in periodontal pockets that favours bacteria associated with disease [44]. Dysbiotic plaque releases outer membrane vesicles, such as lipopolysaccharide from Gram-negative bacteria, into the gingival sulcus, triggering inflammatory host responses. This microbial-host cross-talk shapes an inflammatory cascade and is often destructive when dysregulated.

In a landmark publication in 1998, Sigmund Socransky and coworkers described a study that analysed 13,321 subgingival plaque samples from 185 adult subjects using DNA-DNA hybridisation assays [81]. Principal components analysis and correspondence analysis were used to identify clusters of bacterial species. This led to the identification of five major microbial complexes, with the red and orange complexes showing the strongest associations with clinical signs of periodontal disease, such as pocket depth and bleeding on probing. This study has had a lasting impact on the field of periodontal microbiology over the past few decades. More recently, Hajishengallis (2011) identified *P. gingivalis* as a keystone pathogen, capable of dysregulating host immunity and amplifying periodontal inflammation despite its low abundance [82].

P. gingivalis is a Gram-negative, non-motile, asaccharolytic, obligately anaerobic rod that is strongly associated with periodontitis. Consequently, numerous studies have focused on elucidating its pathogenic traits. It produces various virulence factors, such as lipopolysaccharides and numerous proteolytic enzymes. Among the most notable is the 'trypsin-like' enzyme known as gingipains, which cleave polypeptides at the carboxyl side of arginine or lysine residues. These factors contribute to its capacity to evade host defences and disrupt immune homeostasis, reinforcing its role as a keystone pathogen in periodontitis [83].

An alternative theory emphasises the central role of inflammation in driving periodontal pathogenesis. This is reflected in the Inflammation-Mediated Polymicrobial-Emergence and Dysbiotic-Exacerbation (IMPEDE) model [84]. According to this model, gingivitis begins with an overgrowth of commensal plaque bacteria, which induces an inflammatory response. This inflammation, in turn, promotes increased microbial diversity and triggers a shift towards dysbiosis. The inflammation-driven exacerbation of dysbiosis ultimately contributes to the transition from gingivitis to periodontitis.

In the IMPEDE model, periodontitis develops when a dysbiotic subgingival microbiota becomes established, and the host immune response shifts from being protective to becoming destructive, resulting in significant tissue destruction and clinical attachment loss. At this stage, periodontal pathogens and their virulence factors induce chronic inflammation, which causes tissue damage and bone resorption. The host immune response is also dysregulated, leading to an imbalance between pro-inflammatory and anti-inflammatory cytokines, which further contributes to tissue destruction and dysbiosis. The periodontal pocket forms, creating a protected environment for the growth and survival of pathogenic bacteria, thus enhancing the perpetuation of the disease.

It has been demonstrated that periodontal tissue destruction originates from host immune dysregulation rather than direct bacterial action. Pro-inflammatory cytokines such as interleukin-1 (IL-1), interleukin-6 (IL-6), tumour necrosis factor-alpha (TNF-α) and prostaglandin E2 (PGE2) stimulate fibroblasts to produce matrix metalloproteinases (MMPs), which degrade extracellular matrix collagen. MMP activity, regulated by tissue inhibitors of metalloproteinases (TIMPs) and influenced by cytokines and bacterial lipopolysaccharide, drives connective tissue remodelling. Concurrently, bone resorption accelerates through osteoclast activation, upregulated by PGE2, IL-1 and receptor activator of nuclear factor kappa-B ligand (RANKL). Elevated levels of RANKL and reduced levels of osteoprotegerin (OPG) have been detected in the gingival crevicular fluid of periodontitis patients [85, 86].

Taken together, the current paradigm suggests that the inflammatory response and the oral microbiome exist in a bidirectional state of balance in health (homeostasis) and in a bidirectional state of imbalance in periodontitis [87]. Both dental plaque dysbiosis and a dysregulated host immune-inflammatory response are central to the pathogenesis of periodontitis. Inflammation not only responds to microbial shifts but can also drive changes in the microbiome and upregulate bacterial virulence. Actively controlling excessive inflammation may play a key role in managing both dysbiosis and periodontal disease.

22.7 Conclusion

In conclusion, oral hygiene serves as a cornerstone in mitigating both local and systemic consequences of poor oral health. By reversing gingivitis and preventing the progression of periodontitis, effective oral hygiene can reduce the impact of established risk factors such as smoking and diabetes mellitus, a relationship supported by both foundational and contemporary evidence. Healthcare providers have a critical responsibility to advocate for and promote these practices, ensuring the preservation of oral health and the enhancement of overall well-being.

References

1. Löe H, Theilade E, Jensen SB. Experimental gingivitis in man. J Periodontal Res. 1965;2(4):282–9.
2. Tonetti MS, Van Dyke TE, Working Group 1 of the Joint EFP/AAP Workshop. Periodontitis and atherosclerotic cardiovascular disease: consensus report of the Joint EFP/AAP Workshop

on Periodontitis and Systemic Diseases. J Periodontol. 2013;84(4 Suppl):S24–9. https://doi.org/10.1902/jop.2013.1340019.
3. Chapple IL, Genco R, Working Group 2 of Joint EFP/AAP Workshop. Diabetes and periodontal diseases: consensus report of the Joint EFP/AAP Workshop on Periodontitis and Systemic Diseases. J Clin Periodontol. 2013;40(Suppl 14):S106–12.
4. Ide M, Papapanou PN. Epidemiology of association between maternal periodontal disease and adverse pregnancy outcomes—systematic review. J Periodontol. 2013;84(4 Suppl):S181–94.
5. Lertpimonchai A, Rattanasiri S, Arj-Ong Vallibhakara S, Attia J, Thakkinstian A. The association between oral hygiene and periodontitis: a systematic review and meta-analysis. Int Dent J. 2017;67(6):332–43.
6. Lang NP, Bartold PM. Periodontal health. J Periodontol. 2018;89(Suppl 1):S9–S16.
7. Albandar JM. Global risk factors and risk indicators for periodontal diseases. Periodontology 2000. 2002;29:177–206.
8. Sanz M, Herrera D, Kebschull M, Chapple I, Jepsen S, Beglundh T, Sculean A, Tonetti MS, EFP Workshop Participants and Methodological Consultants. Treatment of stage I–III periodontitis-the EFP S3 level clinical practice guideline. J Clin Periodontol. 2020;47 Suppl 22(Suppl 22):4–60.
9. Needleman I, Suvan J, Moles DR, Pimlott J. A systematic review of professional mechanical plaque removal for prevention of periodontal diseases. J Clin Periodontol. 2005;32(Suppl 6):229–82.
10. Zimmermann H, Zimmermann N, Hagenfeld D, Veile A, Kim TS, Becher H. Is frequency of tooth brushing a risk factor for periodontitis? A systematic review and meta-analysis. Community Dent Oral Epidemiol. 2015;43(2):116–27.
11. Kinane DF, Zhang P, Benakanakere M, et al. Experimental gingivitis, bacteremia and systemic biomarkers: a randomized clinical trial. J Periodontal Res. 2015;50(6):864–9. https://doi.org/10.1111/jre.12280.
12. Aghazada R, Marini L, Zeza B, et al. Experimental gingivitis in patients with and without altered passive eruption. J Periodontol. 2020;91(7):938–46.
13. Trombelli L, Tatakis DN, Scapoli C, Bottega S, Orlandini E, Tosi M. Modulation of clinical expression of plaque-induced gingivitis. II. Identification of "high-responder" and "low-responder" subjects. J Clin Periodontol. 2004;31(4):239–52.
14. Trombelli L, Scapoli C, Orlandini E, Tosi M, Bottega S, Tatakis DN. Modulation of clinical expression of plaque-induced gingivitis. III. Response of "high responders" and "low responders" to therapy. J Clin Periodontol. 2004;31(4):253–9.
15. Tonetti MS, Greenwell H, Kornman KS. Staging and grading of periodontitis: framework and proposal of a new classification and case definition. J Periodontol. 2018;89(Suppl 1):S159–72.
16. Chapple IL, Van der Weijden F, Doerfer C, Herrera D, Shapira L, Polak D, Madianos P, Louropoulou A, Machtei E, Donos N, Greenwell H, Van Winkelhoff AJ, Eren Kuru B, Arweiler N, Teughels W, Aimetti M, Molina A, Montero E, Graziani F. Primary prevention of periodontitis: managing gingivitis. J Clin Periodontol. 2015;42(Suppl 16):S71–6.
17. Dahlén G, Lindhe J, Sato K, Hanamura H, Okamoto H. The effect of supragingival plaque control on the subgingival microbiota in subjects with periodontal disease. J Clin Periodontol. 1992;19(10):802–9.
18. van der Weijden F, Slot DE. Oral hygiene in the prevention of periodontal diseases: the evidence. Periodontology 2011. 2000;55(1):104–23.
19. van der Weijden GA, Hioe KP. A systematic review of the effectiveness of self-performed mechanical plaque removal in adults with gingivitis using a manual toothbrush. J Clin Periodontol. 2005;32(Suppl 6):214–28.
20. Waerhaug J. Effect of toothbrushing on subgingival plaque formation. J Periodontol. 1981;52(1):30–4.
21. Yaacob M, Worthington HV, Deacon SA, Deery C, Walmsley AD, Robinson PG, Glenny AM. Powered versus manual toothbrushing for oral health. Cochrane Database Syst Rev. 2014;(6):CD002281.

22. Lang NP, Cumming BR, Löe H. Toothbrushing frequency as it relates to plaque development and gingival health. J Periodontol. 1973;44(7):396–405. https://doi.org/10.1902/jop.1973.44.7.396.
23. Creeth JE, Gallagher A, Sowinski J, Bowman J, Barrett K, Lowe S, Patel K, Bosma ML. The effect of brushing time and dentifrice on dental plaque removal in vivo. J Dent Hyg. 2009;83(3):111–6.
24. Newby EE, Martinez-Mier EA, Zero DT, Kelly SA, Fleming N, North M, Bosma ML. A randomised clinical study to evaluate the effect of brushing duration on fluoride levels in dental biofilm fluid and saliva in children aged 4-5 years. Int Dent J. 2013;63 Suppl 2(Suppl 2):39–47.
25. Worthington HV, MacDonald L, Poklepovic Pericic T, Sambunjak D, Johnson TM, Imai P, Clarkson JE. Home use of interdental cleaning devices, in addition to toothbrushing, for preventing and controlling periodontal diseases and dental caries. Cochrane Database Syst Rev. 2019;4(4):CD012018.
26. Van Strydonck DA, Slot DE, Van der Velden U, Van der Weijden F. Effect of a chlorhexidine mouthrinse on plaque, gingival inflammation and staining in gingivitis patients: a systematic review. J Clin Periodontol. 2012;39(11):1042–55.
27. Axelsson P, Nyström B, Lindhe J. The long-term effect of a plaque control program on tooth mortality, caries and periodontal disease in adults. Results after 30 years of maintenance. J Clin Periodontol. 2004;31(9):749–57.
28. Pinto TM, de Freitas GC, Dutra DA, Kantorski KZ, Moreira CH. Frequency of mechanical removal of plaque as it relates to gingival inflammation: a randomized clinical trial. J Clin Periodontol. 2013;40(10):948–54.
29. Jönsson B, Ohrn K, Oscarson N, Lindberg P. The effectiveness of an individually tailored oral health educational programme on oral hygiene behaviour in patients with periodontal disease: a blinded randomized-controlled clinical trial (one-year follow-up). J Clin Periodontol. 2009;36(12):1025–34.
30. de Abreu MHNG, Cruz AJS, Borges-Oliveira AC, Martins RC, Mattos FF. Perspectives on social and environmental determinants of oral health. Int J Environ Res Public Health. 2021;18(24):13429.
31. Manski RJ, Moeller JF, Chen H. Dental care coverage and use: modeling limitations and opportunities. Am J Public Health. 2014;104(10):2002–9.
32. Baskaradoss JK. Relationship between oral health literacy and oral health status. BMC Oral Health. 2018;18:172.
33. Yu S, Huang S, Song S, et al. Impact of oral health literacy on oral health behaviors and outcomes among the older adults: a scoping review. BMC Geriatr. 2024;24:858.
34. Suvan JE, Sabalic M, Araújo MR, Ramseier CA. Behavioral strategies for periodontal health. Periodontology 2000. 2022;90(1):247–61.
35. Watt RG, Heilmann A, Listl S, Peres MA. London charter on oral health inequalities. J Dent Res. 2016;95(3):245–7.
36. Slack-Smith L, Hearn L, Scrine C, Durey A. Barriers and enablers for oral health care for people affected by mental health disorders. Aust Dent J. 2017;62(1):6–13.
37. Tiwari T, Kelly A, Randall CL, Tranby E, Franstve-Hawley J. Association between mental health and oral health status and care utilization. Front Oral Health. 2022;2:732882.
38. Kisely S, Quek LH, Pais J, Lalloo R, Johnson NW, Lawrence D. Advanced dental disease in people with severe mental illness: systematic review and meta-analysis. Br J Psychiatry. 2011;199(3):187–93.
39. Kisely S, Sawyer E, Siskind D, Lalloo R. The oral health of people with anxiety and depressive disorders – a systematic review and meta-analysis. J Affect Disord. 2016;200:119–32.
40. Hsiao C-N, Ko EC, Shieh T-Y, Chen H-S. Relationship between areca nut chewing and periodontal status of people in a typical aboriginal community in Southern Taiwan. J Dent Sci. 2015;10(3):300–8.
41. Warnakulasuriya S, Dietrich T, Bornstein MM, Casals Peidró E, Preshaw PM, Walter C, Wennström JL, Bergström J. Oral health risks of tobacco use and effects of cessation. Int Dent J. 2010;60(1):7–30.

42. Javed F, Warnakulasuriya S. Is there a relationship between periodontal disease and oral cancer? A systematic review of currently available evidence. Crit Rev Oncol Hematol. 2016;97:197–205.
43. Singh A, Gambhir RS, Singh S, Kapoor V, Singh J. Oral health: how much do you know? – a study on knowledge, attitude and practices of patients visiting a North Indian dental school. Eur J Dent. 2014;8(1):63–7.
44. Hajishengallis G. Periodontitis: from microbial immune subversion to systemic inflammation. Nat Rev Immunol. 2015;15(1):30–44.
45. Sanz M, Ceriello A, Buysschaert M, Chapple I, Demmer RT, Graziani F, Herrera D, Jepsen S, Lione L, Madianos P, Mathur M, Montanya E, Shapira L, Tonetti M, Vegh D. Scientific evidence on the links between periodontal diseases and diabetes: consensus report and guidelines of the joint workshop on periodontal diseases and diabetes by the International Diabetes Federation and the European Federation of Periodontology. J Clin Periodontol. 2018;45(2):138–49.
46. Chen YF, Zhan Q, Wu CZ, Yuan YH, Chen W, Yu FY, Li Y, Li LJ. Baseline HbA1c level influences the effect of periodontal therapy on glycemic control in people with type 2 diabetes and periodontitis: a systematic review on randomized controlled trails. Diabetes Ther. 2021;12(5):1249–78.
47. Umezaki Y, Yamashita A, Nishimura F, Naito T. The role of periodontal treatment on the reduction of hemoglobinA1c, comparing with existing medication therapy: a systematic review and meta-analysis. Front Clin Diabetes Healthc. 2025;6:1541145.
48. Herrera D, Sanz M, Shapira L, Brotons C, Chapple I, Frese T, Graziani F, Hobbs FDR, Huck O, Hummers E, Jepsen S, Kravtchenko O, Madianos P, Molina A, Ungan M, Vilaseca J, Windak A, Vinker S. Association between periodontal diseases and cardiovascular diseases, diabetes and respiratory diseases: consensus report of the Joint Workshop by the European Federation of Periodontology (EFP) and the European arm of the World Organization of Family Doctors (WONCA Europe). J Clin Periodontol. 2023;50(6):819–41.
49. Seneviratne CJ, Balan P, Suriyanarayanan T, Lakshmanan M, Lee DY, Rho M, Jakubovics N, Brandt B, Crielaard W, Zaura E. Oral microbiome-systemic link studies: perspectives on current limitations and future artificial intelligence-based approaches. Crit Rev Microbiol. 2020;46(3):288–99.
50. Ganesan SM, Joshi V, Fellows M, Dabdoub SM, Nagaraja HN, O'Donnell B, Deshpande NR, Kumar PS. A tale of two risks: smoking, diabetes and the subgingival microbiome. ISME J. 2017;11(9):2075–89.
51. Casarin RCV, Barbagallo A, Meulman T, Santos VR, Sallum EA, Nociti FH, Duarte PM, Casati MZ, Gonc¸alves RB. Subgingival biodiversity in subjects with uncontrolled type-2 diabetes and chronic periodontitis. J Periodontal Res. 2013;48(1):30–6.
52. Beyer K, Zaura E, Brandt BW, Buijs MJ, Brun JG, Crielaard W, Bolstad AI. Subgingival microbiome of rheumatoid arthritis patients in relation to their disease status and periodontal health. PLoS One. 2018;13(9):e0202278.
53. Eriksson K, Fei G, Lundmark A, Benchimol D, Lee L, Hu YOO, Kats A, Saevarsdottir S, Catrina AI, Klinge B, et al. Periodontal health and oral microbiota in patients with rheumatoid arthritis. J Clin Med. 2019;8(5):630.
54. Haraszthy VI, Zambon JJ, Trevisan M, Zeid M, Genco RJ. Identification of periodontal pathogens in atheromatous plaques. J Periodontol. 2000;71(10):1554–60.
55. Kozarov EV, Dorn BR, Shelburne CE, Dunn WA Jr, ProgulskeFox A. Human atherosclerotic plaque contains viable invasive Actinobacillus actinomycetemcomitans and Porphyromonas gingivalis. Arterioscler Thromb Vasc Biol. 2005;25(3):e17–8.
56. Offenbacher S, Lin D, Strauss R, McKaig R, Irving J, Barros SP, Moss K, Barrow DA, Hefti A, Beck JD. Effects of periodontal therapy during pregnancy on periodontal status, biologic parameters, and pregnancy outcomes: a pilot study. J Periodontol. 2006;77(12):2011–24.
57. Caton JG, Armitage G, Berglundh T, et al. A new classification scheme for periodontal and peri-implant diseases and conditions – introduction and key changes from the 1999 classification. J Clin Periodontol. 2018;45(Suppl 20):S1–8.

58. Salvi GE, Roccuzzo A, Imber JC, Stähli A, Klinge B, Lang NP. Clinical periodontal diagnosis. Periodontology 2000. 2023:1–19.
59. Chapple ILC, Mealey BL, Van Dyke TE, et al. Periodontal health and gingival diseases and conditions on an intact and a reduced periodontium: consensus report of Workgroup 1 of the 2017 World Workshop. J Periodontol. 2018;89(S1):S74–84.
60. Papapanou PN, Sanz M, Buduneli N, Dietrich T, Feres M, Fine DH, Flemmig TF, Garcia R, Giannobile WV, Graziani F, Greenwell H, Herrera D, Kao RT, Kebschull M, Kinane DF, Kirkwood KL, Kocher T, Kornman KS, Kumar PS, Loos BG, Machtei E, Meng H, Mombelli A, Needleman I, Offenbacher S, Seymour GJ, Teles R, Tonetti MS. Periodontitis: consensus report of workgroup 2 of the 2017 World Workshop on the Classification of Periodontal and Peri-Implant Diseases and Conditions. J Clin Periodontol. 2018;45(Suppl 20):S162–70.
61. Löe H. Periodontal disease. The sixth complication of diabetes mellitus. Diabetes Care. 1993;16(1):329–34.
62. Saini R, Saini S, Sugandha R. Periodontal disease: the sixth complication of diabetes. J Fam Community Med. 2011;18(1):31.
63. Casanova L, Hughes FJ, Preshaw PM. Diabetes and periodontal disease: a two-way relationship. Br Dent J. 2014;217(8):433–7.
64. Preshaw PM, Alba AL, Herrera D, Jepsen S, Konstantinidis A, Makrilakis K, Taylor R. Periodontitis and diabetes: a two-way relationship. Diabetologia. 2012;55(1):21–31.
65. Simpson TC, Clarkson JE, Worthington HV, MacDonald L, Weldon JC, Needleman I, Iheozor-Ejiofor Z, Wild SH, Qureshi A, Walker A, Patel VA, Boyers D, Twigg J. Treatment of periodontitis for glycaemic control in people with diabetes mellitus. Cochrane Database Syst Rev. 2022;4(4):CD004714.
66. Borgnakke WS, Ylostalo PV, Taylor GW, Genco RJ. Effect of periodontal disease on diabetes: systematic review of epidemiologic observational evidence. J Periodontol. 2013;84(4 Suppl):S135–52.
67. Bergström J. Cigarette smoking as risk factor in chronic periodontal disease. Community Dent Oral Epidemiol. 1989;17(5):245–7.
68. Kinane DF, Chestnutt IG. Smoking and periodontal disease. Crit Rev Oral Biol Med. 2000;11(3):356–65.
69. Kulkarni V, Uttamani JR, Bhatavadekar NB. Comparison of clinical periodontal status among habitual smokeless-tobacco users and cigarette smokers. Int Dent J. 2016;66(1):29–35. https://doi.org/10.1111/idj.12192.
70. Mullally BH. The influence of tobacco smoking on the onset of periodontitis in young persons. Tob Induc Dis. 2004;2(1):6.
71. Bergström J, Eliasson S, Dock J. A 10-year prospective study of tobacco smoking and periodontal health. J Periodontol. 2000;71(8):1338–47.
72. Alexandridi F, Tsantila S, Pepelassi E. Smoking cessation and response to periodontal treatment. Aust Dent J. 2018;63(2):140–9.
73. Leite FRM, Nascimento GG, Baake S, Pedersen LD, Scheutz F, López R. Impact of smoking cessation on periodontitis: a systematic review and meta-analysis of prospective longitudinal observational and interventional studies. Nicotine Tob Res. 2019;21(12):1600–8.
74. Darveau RP. Periodontitis: a polymicrobial disruption of host homeostasis. Nat Rev Microbiol. 2010;8(7):481–90.
75. Seneviratne CJ, Zhang CF, Samaranayake LP. Dental plaque biofilm in oral health and disease. Chin J Dent Res. 2011;14(2):87–94.
76. Page RC, Schroeder HE. Pathogenesis of inflammatory periodontal disease: a summary of current work. Lab Investig. 1976;34(3):235–49.
77. Kolenbrander PE, Palmer RJ Jr, Rickard AH, Jakubovics NS, Chalmers NI, Diaz PI. Bacterial interactions and successions during plaque development. Periodontology 2000. 2006;42:47–79.
78. Marsh PD, Devine DA. How is the development of dental biofilms influenced by the host? J Clin Periodontol. 2011;38(Suppl 11):28–35.
79. Lang NP, Schätzle MA, Löe H. Gingivitis as a risk factor in periodontal disease. J Clin Periodontol. 2009;36(Suppl 10):3–8.

80. Marsh PD, Zaura E. Dental biofilm: ecological interactions in health and disease. J Clin Periodontol. 2017;44(Suppl 18):S12–22.
81. Socransky SS, Haffajee AD, Cugini MA, Smith C, Kent RL Jr. Microbial complexes in subgingival plaque. J Clin Periodontol. 1998;25(2):134–44.
82. Hajishengallis G, Liang S, Payne MA, Hashim A, Jotwani R, Eskan MA, McIntosh ML, Alsam A, Kirkwood KL, Lambris JD, Darveau RP, Curtis MA. Low-abundance biofilm species orchestrates inflammatory periodontal disease through the commensal microbiota and complement. Cell Host Microbe. 2011;10(5):497–506.
83. Hajishengallis G, Darveau RP, Curtis MA. The keystone-pathogen hypothesis. Nat Rev Microbiol. 2012;10(10):717–25.
84. Van Dyke TE, Bartold PM, Reynolds EC. The nexus between periodontal inflammation and dysbiosis. Front Immunol. 2020;11:511.
85. Balli U, Aydogdu A, Dede FO, Turer CC, Guven B. Gingival crevicular fluid levels of sclerostin, osteoprotegerin, and receptor activator of nuclear factor-κB ligand in periodontitis. J Periodontol. 2015;86(12):1396–404.
86. Bostanci N, Ilgenli T, Emingil G, et al. Gingival crevicular fluid levels of RANKL and OPG in periodontal diseases: implications of their relative ratio. J Clin Periodontol. 2007;34(5):370–6.
87. Curtis MA, Diaz PI, Van Dyke TE. The role of the microbiota in periodontal disease. Periodontology 2020. 2000;83(1):14–25.

Polypharmacy and Its Impact on Oral Health

23

Sachin Kulkarni and Sue-Ching Yeoh

23.1 Introduction

23.1.1 Polypharmacy

The use of medicines is the most common healthcare intervention. Medicines are designed to benefit patients, which is why they are referred to as pharmacotherapeutics; however, they can also cause harm. Medication-related harm refers to any injury experienced by a patient due to failures in any of the various stages of the medication use process or because of adverse drug reactions (ADRs). Harm from medications and other therapeutic options accounts for approximately 50% of all avoidable harm in medical care [1]. Consequently, the World Health Organization (WHO) launched a Global Patient Safety Challenge: Medication Without Harm, to which several countries have responded since 2017 [2].

The prevalence of medication-related harm varies based on a country's income level gross national income (GNI), healthcare setting, stages of medication use, type of medicine, age group, frailty and polypharmacy. The highest rates were reported for individuals in geriatric care units, in low- to middle-income countries (LMIC), and for those with comorbidities, frailty and polypharmacy [2]. The rates were also stratified according to the stage of reporting medication-related harm across the five stages of medication use: ordering/prescribing, administering, dispensing, monitoring/reporting and transcribing/verifying, with errors at the ordering/prescribing stage attributed to the highest medication-related harm.

Polypharmacy is commonly defined as the routine, concurrent use of five or more medications. This includes over-the-counter (OTC) medications, prescriptions and/or traditional and complementary medicines [3]. It is particularly prevalent among older individuals, with an estimated 4 in 10 people aged 50 and older using

S. Kulkarni · S.-C. Yeoh (✉)
Dental School, Sydney University, Sydney, NSW, Australia
e-mail: sue-ching.yeoh@sydney.edu.au

S. R. Prabhu et al. (eds.), *Lifestyle in Oral Health and Disease*,
https://doi.org/10.1007/978-3-032-05888-1_23

five or more medications [1]. Rates of polypharmacy tend to be higher among those living in residential care, those with multiple prescribers, individuals with poor overall health and those with multi-morbidity, especially those with intellectual or developmental disabilities, neuropsychiatric conditions or hereditary disorders [4, 5]. Individuals with polypharmacy are at a higher risk of experiencing harm, adverse drug reactions or events (ADR or ADE) and hospitalisations, particularly among the elderly [6, 7]. Additionally, medication prescribing and monitoring errors tend to increase with polypharmacy. For instance, among those taking five to ten medications, errors were reported at 30%, rising to 47% for those taking 10 or more medications [8]. Furthermore, the high avoidable costs of polypharmacy on health systems worldwide are notable. For example, wasted medications cost the UK £200 million annually [5], while Australia incurs $1.4 billion in medication-related hospital admissions [1].

The 1984 'Nairobi Declaration' emphasised that prescribing medicines should be done for the right patient, with the appropriate drug, at the correct dose and at an affordable cost. Additionally, it has become imperative to shift the traditional medical research and practice model from a single-disease intervention to a multi-morbidity model of human health and interventions, including medicines. Therefore, polypharmacy may be deemed appropriate in cases where clinical indications, multi-morbidity, hypersensitivity and potential drug–drug and drug–disease interactions are considered. In vulnerable situations, adverse drug reactions (ADRs) and adverse drug events (ADEs) must be regarded, monitored and managed using a multidisciplinary approach. Vulnerable groups include older individuals (65 years or older) and those living in care arrangements, such as residential facilities [9–11].

23.1.2 Impact of Age on Prescribing

Although no universal numerical estimate exists, an increase in polypharmacy is anticipated due to the growth of older demographics worldwide (from 8% in 2010 to 16% in 2050) and the rising prevalence of multi-morbidity with age [12, 13]. In individuals aged 65 years and older, frailty—defined as reduced resilience to external stressors—can encompass five key 'geriatric giants': falls, immobility, delirium, incontinence and susceptibility to adverse drug reactions. The presence of frailty is associated with increased mortality, hospitalisation, institutionalisation and the risk of prescribing errors [5].

With age, several key changes occur in pharmacokinetic and pharmacodynamic properties. Absorption decreases due to a reduction in intestinal motility and blood flow. As total body water diminishes and body fat increases, the distribution of water-soluble and fat-soluble drugs is influenced. Enzymatic function, hepatic blood flow and renal function decline, altering metabolism and excretion. Additionally, pharmacodynamic effects become more pronounced. The management of polypharmacy and adherence also declines as the number of medications increases, particularly in individuals with cognitive impairment [14].

Table 23.1 APINCH classification of high-risk medicines [15]

A	Antimicrobials
P	Potassium and other electrolytes
I	Insulin
N	Narcotics (opioids) and other sedatives
C	Chemotherapeutic agents
H	Heparin and other anticoagulants

23.1.3 Polypharmacy with High-Risk Medications

Over the years, researchers from various countries have endeavoured to review medications linked to the most preventable medication-related harm. They discovered that approximately £100 million, 180,000 hospital bed days and 100,000 deaths were connected to these drugs in Australia, the United States and the United Kingdom [5]. While several tools are available to assess these medications, they are most commonly summarised by the mnemonic APINCH (Table 23.1). It is important to note that this is not an exhaustive list, as other antipsychotics and over-the-counter medicines also present risks.

23.2 Oral Health Impact of Polypharmacy

Several medications can potentially cause ADRs in the oral and maxillofacial region. These medications may induce various side effects in the oral cavity; for example, ACE inhibitors can trigger potentially life-threatening angioedema, manifesting as rapid swelling of the lips, tongue and pharynx. Other drugs, including chemotherapeutic agents, nicorandil and nonsteroidal anti-inflammatory drugs (NSAIDs), can cause painful oral ulcerations. Furthermore, certain medications like antimalarials, minocycline and amiodarone may lead to localised or diffuse pigmentation of the oral mucosa due to the deposition of melanin or drug metabolites. The associations of individual drug ADRs are summarised in Table 23.2.

It is understood that poor oral health status is associated with polypharmacy (odds ratio: 1.6–2.5); however, no clear evidence exists discussing the specific role of polypharmacy [16]. A literature search revealed several key associations.

23.2.1 Mouth Dryness

One of the primary oral health concerns associated with polypharmacy is dry mouth, which can lead to mucosal discomfort, a burning sensation and an increased risk of caries, sialadenitis, mucositis, ulceration, oral candidosis, dysgeusia, dysphagia and dysphonia [38, 39]. A dry mouth may indicate xerostomia (the subjective sensation of oral dryness) and salivary gland hypofunction (reduced salivary flow). An unstimulated salivary flow rate of <0.1 mL/min or a stimulated flow rate of <0.2 mL/min is considered abnormal [38]. It is important to note that the complex

Table 23.2 Drug-related adverse reactions manifesting in the oral cavity

Oral manifestation	Definition	Associated drug classes and incidence	Management
Drug-related movement disorder			
Orofacial dyskinesia	Repetitive, involuntary oral–facial movements such as lip-smacking, tongue protrusion and grimacing [17].	Antipsychotics, dopamine antagonists. Prevalence: 20% among chronic antipsychotic users [18].	Discontinue causative drug, introduce atypical antipsychotics and consider clonazepam or tetrabenazine [18].
Tardive dyskinesia	Late-onset involuntary movements of the face and tongue after prolonged exposure to dopamine-blocking agents [19].	First-generation antipsychotics (e.g. haloperidol), metoclopramide. Incidence: 15–20% with chronic use [20].	Use of vesicular monoamine transporter inhibitors (e.g. valbenazine), dose reduction and cessation of offending drugs [19].
Parkinsonism	Medication-induced parkinsonism involves tremors, rigidity and bradykinesia, often affecting oral function [21].	Antipsychotics, calcium channel blockers. Prevalence: 50% of drug-induced movement disorders [22].	Discontinuation or substitution of causative drugs, initiation of levodopa in severe cases and physiotherapy [21].
Neuropathic presentations			
Neurotoxicity	Toxic effects on the nervous system manifesting as pain, altered sensation or weakness [23].	Chemotherapy agents (e.g. cisplatin), immunosuppressants.	Dose adjustment of causative agents, symptomatic treatment (e.g. pain management) and vitamin supplementation [23].
Paraesthesia, hypoesthesia, anaesthesia	Abnormal, decreased or absent sensation in the oral cavity due to neurotoxic drugs [24].	Local anaesthetics, chemotherapy drugs. Incidence: chemotherapy-induced paraesthesia ~20% [25].	Symptom management with nerve desensitisation therapies, discontinuation of causative agents and vitamin B complex therapy [24].
Halitosis	Persistent, offensive breath odour caused by systemic or oral factors [26].	Antihypertensives, antihistamines and antidepressants. Incidence is anecdotal.	Treat underlying cause, improve oral hygiene, hydration and use antimicrobial rinses [26].
Drug-induced taste disorders (DITD)	Alterations in taste perception, including dysgeusia or ageusia, caused by medications [21].	ACE inhibitors, chemotherapeutics, metronidazole. Incidence: 5–10% for ACE inhibitors [27].	Discontinue or replace causative drugs, use zinc supplements and encourage saliva stimulation [21].

(continued)

Table 23.2 (continued)

Oral manifestation	Definition	Associated drug classes and incidence	Management
Hard tissue impact			
Tetracycline staining	Intrinsic tooth discoloration due to deposition of tetracycline antibiotics in developing teeth [28].	Tetracyclines. Incidence: up to 100% if taken during tooth development in children under 8 years old [29].	Prevention by avoiding tetracycline use in children under 8 years; cosmetic management with veneers or bleaching [28].
MRONJ	Medication-related osteonecrosis of the jaws involves bone necrosis following antiresorptive therapies [30].	Bisphosphonates, denosumab. Incidence: ~1–2% in high-risk groups [31].	Preventive dental assessments before therapy, conservative debridement and antimicrobial rinses [30].
Soft tissue impact			
Drug-induced gingival enlargement	Overgrowth of gingival tissues induced by specific drugs [32].	Calcium channel blockers (e.g. nifedipine), anticonvulsants (e.g. phenytoin), immunosuppressants (e.g. cyclosporine). Incidence: ~10–30%.	Improved oral hygiene, periodontal therapy, drug substitution and gingivectomy if severe [32].
Mucosal pigmentation	Drug-induced hyperpigmentation in the oral mucosa due to melanin deposition [21].	Antimalarials, minocycline and antipsychotics.	Discontinuation of causative drugs, cosmetic management if indicated [21].
Angioedema	Swelling of oral and facial tissues due to drug-induced hypersensitivity reactions [33].	ACE inhibitors, NSAIDs. Incidence: ~0.1–2% for ACE inhibitors [34].	Immediate drug cessation, antihistamines, corticosteroids and emergency airway management if needed [33].
Fixed drug eruption	Recurrent, localised lesions at the same site following drug exposure [21].	NSAIDs, antibiotics (e.g. sulfonamides).	Discontinuation of offending drugs, topical corticosteroids and antihistamines [21].
Drug-induced lupus erythematosus (DILE)	Autoimmune-like condition caused by prolonged drug use, manifesting as oral ulcers or lesions [35].	Hydralazine, procainamide, isoniazid. Incidence: ~5–20% depending on medication [36].	Discontinuation of offending drugs, NSAIDs and corticosteroids for symptom management [35].
Salivary gland hypofunction and xerostomia	Reduced salivary production leading to dry mouth [26].	Antidepressants, antihypertensives, antihistamines. Incidence: ~30–60% for tricyclic antidepressants [37].	Saliva substitutes, sugar-free chewing gum, good hydration and pilocarpine therapy for severe cases [26].

relationship between salivary flow rate and the subjective sensation of oral dryness is not fully understood; individuals with a 'normal' flow rate may still experience xerostomia, while those with a measurable reduction in flow may not [40].

Salivary glands consist of secretory end pieces made up of mucous and/or serous cells and a ductal system (excretory, intercalated and striated) that transports saliva to the oral cavity with specific modifications. The three major salivary glands—the parotid, submandibular and sublingual—are outside the oral cavity and release their secretions into the mouth through extensive duct systems. Additionally, numerous minor salivary glands are scattered throughout various areas of the oral cavity, including the labial, lingual, palatal, buccal, glossopalatine and retromolar regions, where they are typically situated within the submucosal layer. Saliva from each gland is a complex fluid that varies in its composition and volume [41].

The parotid glands produce a watery saliva rich in enzymes such as amylase, along with proteins like proline-rich proteins and glycoproteins. Submandibular saliva contains these components in addition to highly glycosylated substances known as mucins. The sublingual glands secrete a thicker, more viscous saliva that is also abundant in mucins. Oral fluid, often referred to as whole or mixed saliva, comprises secretions from the major and minor salivary glands, desquamated oral epithelial cells, microorganisms and their byproducts, food particles, serum components and inflammatory cells that enter through the gingival crevice. However, whole saliva is not merely a combination of these elements, as many proteins are removed when they adhere to tooth surfaces, oral mucosa, microorganisms or undergo degradation. Some salivary proteins form a thin layer known as the salivary pellicle on the teeth and oral mucosa. Certain proteins bind calcium, protecting the tooth surface, while others contain binding sites for oral bacteria, facilitating the initial attachment of organisms that contribute to plaque formation [41].

The parasympathetic nervous system promotes salivary secretion by activating muscarinic cholinergic receptors (M3 receptors) on the acinar cells of the salivary glands. This activation triggers an increase in intracellular calcium levels, which facilitates the release of water and electrolytes through aquaporins and ion channels. This results in the production of watery, enzyme-rich saliva, including amylase.

In contrast, sympathetic stimulation acts through adrenergic receptors, primarily β-adrenergic receptors. This results in the secretion of a smaller volume of saliva that is more viscous and richer in protein due to increased enzymatic output. Furthermore, sympathetic activation causes vasoconstriction, decreasing blood flow to the glands and limiting saliva production [42].

Polypharmacy often involves medications with anticholinergic, sympathomimetic or diuretic properties that disrupt the normal function of salivary glands.

23.3 Anticholinergic Medications

A range of commonly prescribed drugs, including tricyclic antidepressants (e.g. amitriptyline), antihistamines (e.g. diphenhydramine), antipsychotics (e.g. haloperidol) and specific antihypertensive agents, have anticholinergic effects. These medications inhibit parasympathetic activity by blocking M3 muscarinic receptors on salivary gland acinar cells, thereby reducing saliva production. Chronic use of anticholinergics has been linked to a reduction of up to 50% in salivary flow rates [37].

23.4 Sympathomimetic Medications

Drugs that stimulate the sympathetic nervous system, such as decongestants (e.g. pseudoephedrine) and beta-agonists, primarily affect the composition of saliva. While they do not entirely stop salivary flow, they produce a smaller volume of thicker, more protein-concentrated saliva. This change in quality contributes to the sensation of dry mouth and interferes with saliva's protective role in oral health.

23.5 Diuretics

Diuretics, such as furosemide, are frequently prescribed to manage hypertension and other cardiovascular conditions. By promoting fluid loss through increased urine output, diuretics cause systemic dehydration. This reduces blood volume and decreases perfusion to the salivary glands, ultimately leading to diminished saliva secretion [43].

23.6 The Combined Impact of Polypharmacy

The simultaneous use of multiple medications increases the risk of salivary dysfunction, particularly in older adults who are more likely to be on complex medication regimens. The incidence of salivary hypofunction rises sharply when individuals take more than four medications [43]. Specifically, overlapping anticholinergic effects from multiple drugs worsen salivary gland suppression, creating an additive or synergistic impact on oral dryness and its related complications [16]. Furthermore, the presence of oral dryness is strongly associated with dysphagia and impaired swallowing efficiency, which is, in turn, linked to malnutrition [44, 45]. A recent cross-sectional study in New Zealand found that the risk of salivary hypofunction is higher in individuals taking a combination of tricyclic antidepressants with anticholinergic drugs or steroids [43, 46].

23.6.1 Bleeding Risk

Secondary prevention of atherosclerotic coronary disease is usually managed with antiplatelet therapy, which reduces the risk of myocardial infarction, stroke or ischaemia by approximately 20% [47, 48]. Aspirin is often used with a P2Y12 receptor antagonist, such as clopidogrel, further decreasing risk with minimal increase in bleeding risk [48]. However, in patients with coronary artery disease, including those with prosthetic heart valves, atrial fibrillation and venous thromboembolism, secondary prevention of in-stent or other thrombosis requires polypharmacy that includes one or more antiplatelet and anticoagulant medications [49].

In patients treated with warfarin, as well as those receiving additional aspirin (antiplatelet) therapy, regardless of the International Normalised Ratio (INR), there is no reduction in cardiac events but an increased risk of major bleeding [50]. Thus, newer anticoagulants like rivaroxaban have been trialled, demonstrating a similar increase in the risk of major bleeding (intracranial haemorrhage) [51]. Although the bleeding risk is lower in patients treated with rivaroxaban compared to warfarin under the same dual antiplatelet therapy, it remains significant when triple therapy (44% compared to 19%) is utilised (an anticoagulant with two antiplatelet drugs) compared to dual therapy [52, 53].

Additionally, OTC products have been linked to an increased risk of bleeding. Common OTC products that can independently heighten the risk of bleeding include fish oil (more than 3 g daily) and high-dose vitamin E. Furthermore, polypharmacy involving anticoagulants and antiplatelet therapy with arnica, chondroitin, garlic and ginkgo has also been reported to enhance bleeding risk [54].

In 2016, the United States Food and Drug Administration (FDA) issued a statement based on a retrospective analysis of their database of adverse events related to bleeding incidents that resulted in hospitalisation and transfusion due to blood loss. This occurred between 1 day and 3 years with the use of concurrent OTC antacid products containing aspirin, along with factors such as alcohol abuse, a history of gastric ulcers, anticoagulants, steroids or NSAIDs [55].

In a 2018 systematic review and meta-analysis, direct oral anticoagulants were associated with an increased risk of postoperative bleeding in the oral cavity (odds ratio: 4.12) [56]. However, a 2009 systematic review and meta-analysis found that warfarin alone did not increase this risk [57]. When single, dual or triple anticoagulant and antiplatelet therapy were compared for intra-oral postoperative bleeding risk, a significant increase was noted. Triple therapy was linked to an odds ratio of 1.56 for major bleeding, compared to clopidogrel and one anticoagulant [58]. The risk of bleeding-related adverse effects increases with multimorbidity, such as advanced age, liver disease and renal failure [59].

23.6.2 Medication-Related Osteonecrosis of the Jaw (MRONJ)

Medication-related osteonecrosis of the jaw (MRONJ) is characterised by an area of exposed bone in the maxillofacial region persisting for over 8 weeks in a patient undergoing antiresorptive therapy, which includes bisphosphonates, denosumab or antiangiogenic therapy for cancer, and in whom there is no history of radiation therapy to the jaws or evident metastatic disease in this area.

While single treatment with antiresorptive therapy has been linked to MRONJ, evidence indicates a heightened risk associated with chemotherapeutic agents, immune modulators or antiangiogenic medications. This risk is further stratified by factors such as dental extractions, smoking, trauma, poor dental health and individuals who are immunocompromised or immunosuppressed. It is known that the risk increases in those with periodontal disease due to bacterial invasion and delayed healing, as well as indirectly through a greater likelihood of dental extractions.

It is important to note that beyond polypharmacy, the use of antiresorptive medication has been associated with an increased risk for those undergoing treatment for malignancy. According to the literature, the prevalence of MRONJ is higher (average <5%, range: 0–18%) in cancer patients taking Zoledronate, which is comparable to those exposed to denosumab and is 2–10 times greater compared to cancer patients treated with a placebo [60].

The reported prevalence of MRONJ in individuals receiving antiresorptive therapy for osteoporosis is significantly lower compared to those with malignancy, ranging from 0.02% to 0.05%, or 1–70 cases per 100,000 patient-years. Notably, IV treatment shows a slightly higher prevalence, between 0 and 90 cases per 100,000 patient-years. The duration of antiresorptive treatment (4+ years) appears to influence MRONJ prevalence, as does the route of administration (intravenous > oral). However, the risk can be greater in a shorter duration due to polypharmacy with antiangiogenic medications [61].

Although osteonecrosis is defined as avascular necrosis, MRONJ is characterised solely by necrotic bone. Antiresorptive therapies, such as zoledronic acid (a bisphosphonate), have been shown in vitro to affect the arterial area, venous area and overall vascularity of periodontal tissues during both early and late MRONJ development [62–68]. Therefore, there seems to be a justification for the increased reported risk associated with concurrent antiangiogenic medications and antiresorptive drugs. Although the precise risk of concurrent antiangiogenic therapy remains undetermined, several studies have attempted to estimate it at twofold to fivefold [69–73].

Secondly, polypharmacy involving chemotherapeutic agents, steroid therapy and disease-modifying antirheumatic drugs (DMARDs), when combined with antiangiogenic medications and an antiresorptive agent, has increased the severity and prevalence of MRONJ by fourfold to sixfold, attributed to a compromised immune response in the tooth extraction area [74–78]. This effect is further amplified in individuals receiving multiple chemotherapeutic agents, such as those undergoing treatment for multiple myeloma [77, 78].

23.7 Conclusion

Polypharmacy is an increasing problem associated with older age, leading to a higher risk of hospitalisation, preventable medication-related harms and prescribing errors. It significantly impacts oral health in several ways. Many commonly used drugs, such as antihypertensives, analgesics and antidepressants, can cause individual adverse drug reactions, including oral lichenoid reactions, fixed drug eruptions and movement disorders. Polypharmacy also contributes to salivary hypofunction and xerostomia, as well as an increased risk of bleeding and MRONJ.

References

1. Australian Commission on Safety and Quality in Health Care. Status report medication without harm – WHO global patient safety challenge. Australia's response. Sydney: ACSQHC; 2024.
2. World Health Organization. Global burden of preventable medication-related harm in health care: a systematic review. Geneva: WHO; 2023. Licence: CC BY-NC-SA 3.0 IGO.
3. World Health Organization. Medication safety in polypharmacy. Geneva: WHO; 2019. (WHO/UHC/SDS/2019.11). Licence: CC BY-NC-SA 3.0 IGO.
4. National Disability Insurance Scheme (NDIS) Quality and Safeguards Commission. Polypharmacy. Sydney: NDIS Commission; 2020.
5. All Wales Medicines Strategy Group. Polypharmacy in older people: a guide for healthcare professionals. Cardiff: AWMSG; 2023.
6. Maher RL, Hanlon JT, Hajjar ER. Clinical consequences of polypharmacy in elderly. Expert Opin Drug Saf. 2014;13(1):57–65. Available from: https://www.ncbi.nlm.nih.gov/pmc/articles/PMC3864987/.
7. Nwadiugwu MC. Frailty and the risk of polypharmacy in the older person: enabling and preventative approaches. J Aging Res. 2020. Available from: https://www.hindawi.com/journals/jar/2020/6759521/.
8. Avery A, Barber N, Ghaleb M, Franklin BD, Armstrong S, Crowe S, et al. Investigating the prevalence and causes of prescribing errors in general practice: the PRACtICe study. London: General Medical Council; 2012. Available from: https://www.gmc-uk.org.
9. Davies EA, O'Mahony MS. Adverse drug reactions in special populations—the elderly. Br J Clin Pharmacol. 2015;80(4):796–807. https://doi.org/10.1111/bcp.12596. Available from: https://www.ncbi.nlm.nih.gov/pubmed/25619317.
10. Hubbard RE, O'Mahony MS, Woodhouse KW. Medication prescribing in frail older people. Eur J Clin Pharmacol. 2013;69(3):319–26. https://doi.org/10.1007/s00228-012-1387-2. Available from: https://www.ncbi.nlm.nih.gov/pubmed/22965651.
11. Molokhia M, Majeed A. Current and future perspectives on the management of polypharmacy. BMC Fam Pract. 2017;18:70. https://doi.org/10.1186/s12875-017-0642-0. Available from: https://www.ncbi.nlm.nih.gov/pubmed/28587644.
12. Barnett K, Mercer SW, Norbury M, Watt G, Wyke S, Guthrie B. Epidemiology of multimorbidity and implications for healthcare, research, and medical education: a cross-sectional study. Lancet. 2012;380(9836):37–43.
13. Organisation for Economic Co-operation and Development. Health at a glance 2017: OECD indicators. Paris: OECD Publishing; 2017. Available from: https://www.oecd-ilibrary.org/social-issues-migration-health/health-at-a-glance-2017_health_glance-2017-en.
14. Chippa V, Roy K. Geriatric cognitive decline and polypharmacy. [Updated 2023 Apr 16]. In: StatPearls [Internet]. Treasure Island: StatPearls Publishing; 2025. Available from: https://www.ncbi.nlm.nih.gov/books/NBK574575/.
15. New South Wales Government Clinical Excellence Commission (CEC). A PINCH. 2020. Available from: https://www.cec.health.nsw.gov.au/keep-patients-safe/medication-safety/high-risk-medicines/A-PINCH.
16. Nakamura J, Kitagaki K, Ueda Y, Nishio E, Shibatsuji T, Uchihashi Y, Adachi R, Ono R. Impact of polypharmacy on oral health status in elderly patients admitted to the recovery and rehabilitation ward. Geriatr Gerontol Int. 2021;21(1):66–70. https://doi.org/10.1111/ggi.14104. PMID: 33280240.
17. Bhidayasiri R, Fahn S, Weiner WJ, Gronseth GS, Sullivan KL, Zesiewicz TA. Evidence-based guideline: treatment of tardive syndromes: report of the Guideline Development Subcommittee of the American Academy of Neurology. Neurology. 2013;81(5):463–9. https://doi.org/10.1111/pcn.13785.
18. Kobayashi RM. Orofacial dyskinesia: clinical features, mechanisms, and drug therapy. West J Med. 1976;125(4):277–88. PMID: 23611; PMCID: PMC1237309.

19. Loughlin AM, Lin N, Abler V, Carroll B. Tardive dyskinesia among patients using antipsychotic medications in customary clinical care in the United States. PLoS One. 2019;14(6):e0216044. https://doi.org/10.1371/journal.pone.0216044. PMID: 31163035; PMCID: PMC6548364.
20. World Health Organization (WHO). Guidelines for pharmacovigilance: ensuring the safe use of medicines. Geneva: WHO; 2015.
21. Bhidayasiri R, Fahn S, Weiner WJ, Gronseth GS, Sullivan KL, Zesiewicz TA. Evidence-based guideline: treatment of tardive syndromes: report of the guideline development Subcommittee of the American Academy of Neurology. Neurology. 2013;81:463–9.
22. Shrimanker I, Tadi P, Schoo C, et al. Parkinsonism. [Updated 2024 Mar 13]. In: StatPearls [Internet]. Treasure Island: StatPearls Publishing; 2025. Available from: https://www.ncbi.nlm.nih.gov/books/NBK542224/.
23. Stone JB, DeAngelis LM. Cancer-treatment-induced neurotoxicity—focus on newer treatments. Nat Rev Clin Oncol. 2016;13(2):92–105. https://doi.org/10.1038/nrclinonc.2015.152. PMID: 26391778; PMCID: PMC4979320.
24. Tan YZ, Shi RJ, Ke BW, Tang YL, Liang XH. Paresthesia in dentistry: the ignored neurotoxicity of local anesthetics. Heliyon. 2023;9(7):e18031. https://doi.org/10.1016/j.heliyon.2023.e18031. PMID: 37539316; PMCID: PMC10395355.
25. Wang AB, Housley SN, Flores AM, et al. A review of movement disorders in chemotherapy-induced neurotoxicity. J Neuroeng Rehabil. 2021;18:16. https://doi.org/10.1186/s12984-021-00818-2.
26. Torsten M, Gómez-Moreno G, Aguilar-Salvatierra A. Drug-related oral malodour (halitosis): a literature review. Eur Rev Med Pharmacol Sci. 2017;21(21):4930–4. PMID: 29164566.
27. American Academy of Family Physicians (AAFP). [Clinical article on aafp.org]. 2020. Available from: https://www.aafp.org/pubs/afp/issues/2020/1115/p613.html.
28. Sánchez AR, Rogers RS 3rd, Sheridan PJ. Tetracycline and other tetracycline-derivative staining of the teeth and oral cavity. Int J Dermatol. 2004;43(10):709–15. https://doi.org/10.1111/j.1365-4632.2004.02108.x. PMID: 15485524.
29. Ravindra D, Huang G, Hallett K, Burgner DP, Gwee A, Silva MJ. Antibiotic exposure and dental health: a systematic review. Pediatrics. 2023;152(1):e2023061350. https://doi.org/10.1542/peds.2023-061350.
30. American Academy of Periodontology (AAP). Gingival enlargement guidelines. 2014.
31. European Academy of Allergy and Clinical Immunology (EAACI). Guidelines for the management of angioedema. Allergy. 2017;72(1):171–84.
32. Gabb GM, Mangoni AA, Anderson CS, Cowley D, Dowden JS, Golledge J, et al. Guidelines for the diagnosis and management of hypertension in adults—2016. Med J Aust. 2016;205(2):85–9.
33. American College of Rheumatology (ACR). Guidelines for the management of systemic lupus erythematosus. Arthritis Care Res. 2020;72(6):807–18.
34. Howarth DA. ACE inhibitor angioedema: a very late presentation. Aust Fam Physician. 2013;42(12):860–2. Available from: https://www.racgp.org.au/afp/2013/december/ace-inhibitor-angioedema.
35. Solhjoo M, Goyal A, Chauhan K. Drug-induced lupus erythematosus. [Updated 2023 Apr 3]. In: StatPearls [Internet]. Treasure Island: StatPearls Publishing; 2025. Available from: https://www.ncbi.nlm.nih.gov/books/NBK441889/.
36. Benn AML, Thomson WM. Saliva: an overview. N Z Dent J. 2014;110(3):92–6.
37. Thomson WM. Dry mouth and older people. Aust Dent J. 2015;60(1 Suppl):54–63.
38. Cannon I, Robinson-Barella A, McLellan G, Ramsay SE. From drugs to dry mouth: a systematic review exploring oral and psychological health conditions associated with dry mouth in older adults with polypharmacy. Drugs Aging. 2023;40(4):307–16. https://doi.org/10.1007/s40266-023-01017-5. PMID: 36943673.
39. Ten Cate AR. Ten Cate's oral histology: development, structure, and function. 9th ed. St. Louis: Elsevier; 2018.
40. Proctor GB. The physiology of salivary secretion. Periodontol 2000. 2016;70(1):11–25. https://doi.org/10.1111/prd.12116. PMID: 26662479.

41. Humphrey SP, Williamson RT. A review of saliva: normal composition, flow, and function. J Prosthet Dent. 2001;85(2):162–9. https://doi.org/10.1067/mpr.2001.113778. Available from: https://www.sciencedirect.com/science/article/pii/S0022391301540329.
42. Tobin G. Salivary secretion control. In: Binder MD, Hirokawa N, Windhorst U, editors. Encyclopedia of neuroscience. Berlin, Heidelberg: Springer; 2009. https://doi.org/10.1007/978-3-540-29678-2_5202.
43. Fernandes MS, Castelo PM, Chaves GN, Fernandes JPS, Fonseca FLA, Zanato LE, Gavião MBD. Relationship between polypharmacy, xerostomia, gustatory sensitivity, and swallowing complaints in the elderly: a multidisciplinary approach. J Texture Stud. 2021;52(2):187–96. https://doi.org/10.1111/jtxs.12573. PMID: 33191538.
44. Fávaro-Moreira NC, Krausch-Hofmann S, Matthys C, Vereecken C, Vanhauwaert E, Declercq A, Bekkering GE, Duyck J. Risk factors for malnutrition in older adults: a systematic review of the literature based on longitudinal data. Adv Nutr. 2016;7(3):507–22. https://doi.org/10.3945/an.115.011254. PMID: 27184278; PMCID: PMC4863272.
45. Venkatasalu MR, Murang ZR, Ramasamy DTR, Dhaliwal JS. Oral health problems among palliative and terminally ill patients: an integrated systematic review. BMC Oral Health. 2020;20(1):79. https://doi.org/10.1186/s12903-020-01075-w.
46. Thomson WM, Ferguson CA, Janssens BE, Kerse NM, Ting GS, Smith MB. Xerostomia and polypharmacy among dependent older New Zealanders: a national survey. Age Ageing. 2021;50(1):248–51. https://doi.org/10.1093/ageing/afaa099. PMID: 32706865.
47. Antithrombotic Trialists' Collaboration. Collaborative meta-analysis of randomized trials of antiplatelet therapy for prevention of death, myocardial infarction, and stroke in high-risk patients. BMJ. 2002;324:71–86. https://doi.org/10.1136/bmj.324.7329.71.
48. Yusuf S, Zhao F, Mehta SR, Chrolavicius S, Tognoni G, Fox KK, et al. Clopidogrel in Unstable Angina to Prevent Recurrent Events Trial Investigators. Effects of clopidogrel in addition to aspirin in patients with acute coronary syndromes without ST-segment elevation. N Engl J Med. 2001;345:494–502. https://doi.org/10.1056/NEJMoa010746.
49. Bhatt DL, Hulot JS, Moliterno DJ, Harrington RA. Antiplatelet and anticoagulation therapy for acute coronary syndromes. Circ Res. 2014;114(12):1929–43. https://doi.org/10.1161/CIRCRESAHA.114.302737.
50. Andreotti F, Testa L, Biondi-Zoccai GL, Crea F. Aspirin plus warfarin compared to aspirin alone after acute coronary syndromes: an updated and comprehensive meta-analysis of 25,307 patients. Eur Heart J. 2006;27(5):519–26. https://doi.org/10.1093/eurheartj/ehi485.
51. Alexander JH, Lopes RD, James S, Kilaru R, He Y, Mohan P, et al. APPRAISE-2 Investigators. Apixaban with antiplatelet therapy after acute coronary syndrome. N Engl J Med. 2011;365:699–708. https://doi.org/10.1056/NEJMoa1105819.
52. Dewilde WJ, Oirbans T, Verheugt FW, Kelder JC, De Smet BJ, Herrman JP, et al. WOEST study investigators. Use of clopidogrel with or without aspirin in patients taking oral anticoagulant therapy and undergoing percutaneous coronary intervention: an open-label, randomized, controlled trial. Lancet. 2013;381:1107–15. https://doi.org/10.1016/S0140-6736(12)62177-1.
53. Chilbert MR, Reidy SE, Clark CM, Guszkowski M, Gargala E, Woodruff AE. Comparison of bleeding rates between oral anticoagulants in combination with dual antiplatelet therapy (triple therapy) in a real-world cohort. Hosp Pharm. 2022;57(2):253–9. https://doi.org/10.1177/00185787211024602. PMID: 35601720; PMCID: PMC9117778.
54. Hamrick JW, Nykamp D. Drug-induced bleeding. US Pharmacist. 2023. Available from: https://www.uspharmacist.com/article/druginduced-bleeding.
55. U.S. Food and Drug Administration (FDA). FDA drug safety communication: FDA warns about serious bleeding risk with over-the-counter antacid products. 2018. Available from: https://www.fda.gov/drugs/drug-safety-and-availability/fda-drug-safety-communication-fda-warns-about-serious-bleeding-risk-over-counter-antacid-products.
56. Bensi C, Scarpelli G, Pavone P, et al. Postoperative bleeding risk in patients undergoing dental surgery while on direct oral anticoagulants: a systematic review and meta-analysis. BMC Oral Health. 2018;18(1):101. https://doi.org/10.1186/s12903-024-04738-0.

57. Nematullah A, Alabousi A, Blanas N, Douketis JD, Sutherland SE. Dental surgery for patients on anticoagulant therapy with warfarin: a systematic review and meta-analysis. J Can Dent Assoc. 2009;75(1):41. PMID: 19239742.
58. Yu JJ, Zou C, Liu WY, Yang GP. Dual versus single antiplatelet therapy for patients with long-term oral anticoagulation undergoing coronary intervention: a systematic review and meta-analysis. J Geriatr Cardiol. 2017;14(12):725–36. https://doi.org/10.11909/j.issn.1671-5411.2017.12.002. PMID: 29581711; PMCID: PMC5863050.
59. Zazzara MB, Palmer K, Vetrano DL, Carfì A, Onder G. Adverse drug reactions in older adults: a narrative review of the literature. Eur Geriatr Med. 2021;12(3):463–73. https://doi.org/10.1007/s41999-021-00481-9. PMID: 33738772; PMCID: PMC8149349
60. Ruggiero SL, Dodson TB, Fantasia J, et al. American Association of Oral and Maxillofacial Surgeons position paper on medication-related osteonecrosis of the jaw—2014 update. J Oral Maxillofac Surg. 2014;72(10):1938–56.
61. Kim HY. Review and update of the risk factors and prevention of antiresorptive-related osteonecrosis of the jaw. Endocrinol Metab. 2021;36(5):917–27.
62. Hellstein JW, Adler RA, Edwards B, et al. Managing the care of patients receiving antiresorptive therapy for prevention and treatment of osteoporosis: executive summary of recommendations from the American Dental Association Council on Scientific Affairs. J Am Dent Assoc. 2011;142(11):1243–51.
63. Lee ES, Tsai MC, Lee JX, Wong C, Cheng YN, Liu AC, Liang YF, Fang CY, Wu CY, Lee IT. Bisphosphonates and their connection to dental procedures: exploring bisphosphonate-related osteonecrosis of the jaws. Cancers (Basel). 2023;15(22):5366. https://doi.org/10.3390/cancers15225366. PMID: 38001626; PMCID: PMC10670230.
64. Wood J, Bonjean K, Ruetz S, et al. Novel antiangiogenic effects of the bisphosphonate compound zoledronic acid. J Pharmacol Exp Ther. 2002;302:1055.
65. Santini D, Vincenzi B, Dicuonzo G, et al. Zoledronic acid induces significant and long-lasting modifications of circulating angiogenic factors in cancer patients. Clin Cancer Res. 2003;9:2893.
66. Ishtiaq S, Edwards S, Sankaralingam A, et al. The effect of nitrogen-containing bisphosphonates, zoledronate and alendronate, on the production of pro-angiogenic factors by osteoblastic cells. Cytokine. 2015;71:154.
67. Kun-Darbois JD, Libouban H, Mabilleau G, et al. Bone mineralization and vascularization in bisphosphonate-related osteonecrosis of the jaw: an experimental study in the rat. Clin Oral Investig. 2018;22:2997.
68. Gao SY, Lin RB, Huang SH, et al. PDGF-BB exhibited therapeutic effects on a rat model of bisphosphonate-related osteonecrosis of the jaw by enhancing angiogenesis and osteogenesis. Bone. 2021;144:115117.
69. Bi Y, Gao Y, Ehirchiou D, et al. Bisphosphonates cause osteonecrosis of the jaw-like disease in mice. Am J Pathol. 2010;177:280.
70. Gkouveris I, Hadaya D, Soundia A, et al. Vasculature submucosal changes at early stages of osteonecrosis of the jaw (ONJ). Bone. 2019;123:234.
71. Rugani P, Walter C, Kirnbauer B, et al. Prevalence of medication-related osteonecrosis of the jaw in patients with breast cancer, prostate cancer, and multiple myeloma. Dent J (Basel). 2016;4:32.
72. Dimopoulos MA, Kastritis E, Anagnostopoulos A, et al. Osteonecrosis of the jaw in patients with multiple myeloma treated with bisphosphonates: evidence of increased risk after treatment with zoledronic acid. Haematologica. 2006;91:968.
73. Badros A, Weikel D, Salama A, et al. Osteonecrosis of the jaw in multiple myeloma patients: clinical features and risk factors. J Clin Oncol. 2006;24:945.
74. Raje N, Terpos E, Willenbacher W, et al. Denosumab versus zoledronic acid in bone disease treatment of newly diagnosed multiple myeloma: an international, double-blind, double-dummy, randomised, controlled, phase 3 study. Lancet Oncol. 2018;19:370.
75. Filleul O, Crompot E, Saussez S. Bisphosphonate-induced osteonecrosis of the jaw: a review of 2,400 patient cases. J Cancer Res Clin Oncol. 2010;136:1117.

76. Hayano H, Kuroshima S, Sasaki M, et al. Distinct immunopathology in the early stages between different antiresorptives-related osteonecrosis of the jaw-like lesions in mice. Bone. 2020;135:115308.
77. Rao NJ, Yu RQ, Wang JY, et al. Effect of periapical diseases in development of MRONJ in immunocompromised mouse model. Biomed Res Int. 2019:1271492.
78. Aghaloo TL, Tetradis S. Osteonecrosis of the jaw in the absence of antiresorptive or antiangiogenic exposure: a series of 6 cases. J Oral Maxillofac Surg. 2017;75:129.

Lifestyle and Orofacial Pain

24

Supeetha Suntharamoorthy, Lasanthini Weerakkody,
and Ramesh Balasubramaniam

24.1 Introduction

Chronic pain is a complex condition characterised by persistent pain in one or more areas of the body, often accompanied by emotional distress. It disrupts activities of daily living, interferes with sleep and frequently leads to reliance on medications that provide only partial relief [1, 2]. Globally, chronic pain affects over 1.5 billion people and contributes significantly to the disease burden, with approximately 10% of individuals being newly diagnosed each year [2–4]. The prevalence of chronic pain increases with age, driven by age-related conditions, degenerative diseases and the cumulative effects of lifestyle and injury [3, 4]. The prevalence also varies across different regions and demographics, with estimates ranging between 10 and 50% (Fig. 24.1). This variation is influenced by factors such as social inequalities in gender and income, government policies, cultural differences and personal health experiences [4].

The 11th version of the International Classification of Diseases (ICD-11) defines chronic pain as pain that persists or recurs for longer than three months and classifies it across seven key categories [1, 5–7]. The classification further distinguishes chronic pain as either primary or secondary based on the source of pain, and recognises primary chronic pain as a distinct condition in its own right [1, 6]. The experience of chronic pain varies widely across the global population and is closely

S. Suntharamoorthy (✉) · L. Weerakkody
Discipline of Oral Medicine, UWA Dental School, The University of Western Australia, Nedlands, WA, Australia
e-mail: 10404458@student.uwa.edu.au; 23776076@student.uwa.edu.au

R. Balasubramaniam
Discipline of Oral Medicine, UWA Dental School, The University of Western Australia, Nedlands, WA, Australia
e-mail: ramesh.balasubramaniam@uwa.edu.au

Dental and Maxillofacial Surgery Department, Perth Children's Hospital, Nedlands, WA, Australia

S. R. Prabhu et al. (eds.), *Lifestyle in Oral Health and Disease*,
https://doi.org/10.1007/978-3-032-05888-1_24

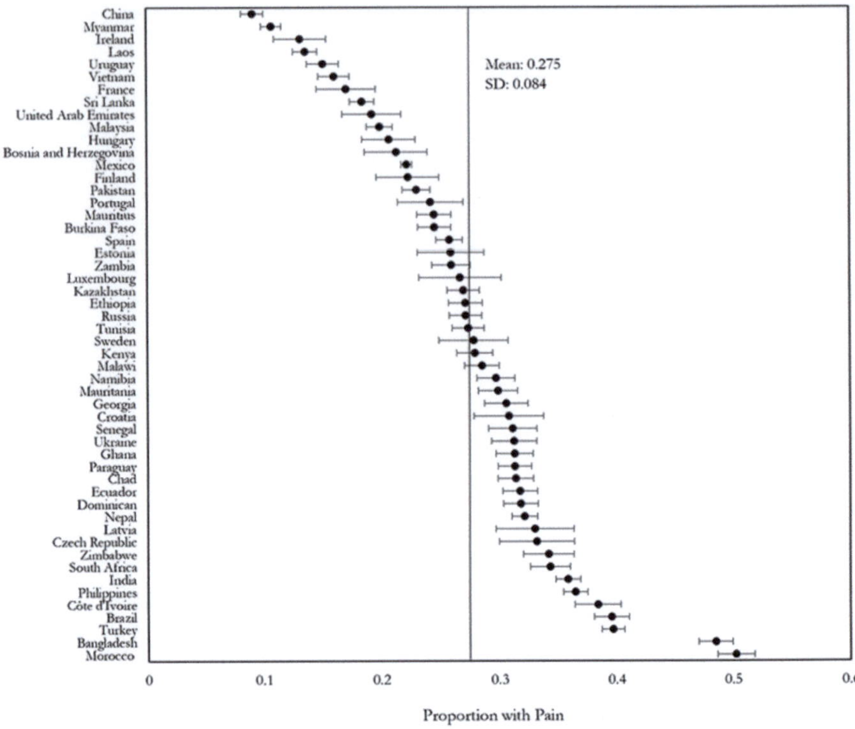

Fig. 24.1 Prevalence of pain in 52 countries standardised for age and gender (with 95% confidence interval). Based on the 2002–2004 World Health Survey. Vertical line represents the cross-country prevalence. (Reproduced with permission from Wolters Kluwer Health, Inc [4])

influenced by a range of biological, psychological and social factors collectively known as biopsychosocial factors. Environments in which a person is raised, resides, works, socialises and ages, along with their genetic susceptibility and mindset, play a considerable role in the onset and persistence of pain [8].

Chronic orofacial pain shares similar challenges with other chronic pain conditions, including emotional distress, impaired daily function and poor sleep quality, all of which can negatively affect psychosocial well-being and quality of life. Like other chronic pain conditions, it is driven by complex neurological processes and influenced by biopsychosocial factors. Chronic primary orofacial pain of non-odontogenic origin is defined by ICD-11 as pain in the face, jaw and oral cavity, occurring on at least 50% of days for a duration of at least three months and lasting at least two hours per day [7]. Headaches and temporomandibular disorders are among the most commonly reported chronic orofacial pain conditions and are often associated with pain in other areas of the body [9, 10]. It is estimated that chronic orofacial pain affects approximately 7–11% of the global adult population, with prevalence varying widely across different conditions, from 1% for burning mouth syndrome (BMS) to 81% for cancer therapy-related orofacial pain. Among children, the prevalence ranges from 0.2% for temporomandibular joint osteoarthrosis to 83% for headaches [10].

Managing chronic orofacial pain is both complex and challenging, and requires a personalised, multidimensional approach that addresses not only the physical aspects of pain but also the psychological and social factors that shape an individual's experience. Pharmacotherapy alone is inadequate to address these complexities, and a more holistic approach incorporating lifestyle and emotional well-being is essential for reprogramming the brain to manage pain, prevent its progression and improve outcomes and quality of life. Lifestyle factors, such as physical activity, nutrition, sleep patterns, stress levels, harmful substance use and social connection, can all influence pain, either exacerbating or alleviating it. This chapter will explore each lifestyle factor and provide guidance on how to assess patients and incorporate lifestyle strategies in pain management.

24.2 Nutrition

The role of nutrition in chronic pain is crucial, influencing processes such as inflammation, oxidative stress, glycolysis, lipolysis, the gut-brain axis, obesity and genetic and epigenetic mechanisms (Fig. 24.2) [11, 12]. In orofacial pain, similar biological processes are involved, and research suggests that an anti-inflammatory diet rich in key nutrients and antioxidants can improve pain management outcomes [13]. Foods rich in omega-3 fatty acids and antioxidants such as chicken bone broth [14], citrus fruits [15], grape seeds [16–18], purple corn [19], soy [20], unsweetened dark chocolate [21], red wine [22], legumes and nuts, as well as targeted nutraceuticals [23], can support brain health, reduce inflammation and provide pain relief in conditions like temporomandibular disorders and orofacial migraines [13, 24–26]. In the context of red wine, it is important to note that alcohol affects individuals differently, and excessive consumption can lead to adverse health outcomes, including increased inflammation. Thus, incorporating red wine into a pain management strategy should only be done under medical supervision and in moderation.

Despite this, individuals with chronic pain often adopt unhealthy dietary patterns characterised by the consumption of ultra-processed foods, caffeine, sugar and fats, while lacking nutrient-dense options like fruits and vegetables [27–32]. This imbalance can lead to nutrient deficiencies that impair the body's ability to regulate inflammation and oxidative stress, potentially worsening pain sensitivity [13]. Deficiencies in vitamins B12, C, D and E, as well as minerals like iron, magnesium, zinc, carotenoids and flavonoids, can disrupt nerve function and neurotransmitter regulation, exacerbating pain and conditions like BMS and neuropathic pain [12, 24]. In contrast, certain foods, such as fried and processed meats, dairy products, pickled food, caffeinated beverages, soft drinks, nuts, fava beans, citrus fruits, chocolate, canned foods, sauces, smoked fish and stored refrigerated food, can trigger migraines [31].

Dietary fats also play a key role in modulating pain perception. Omega-6 fatty acids promote inflammation, while omega-3 fatty acids help reduce it [24, 33–35].

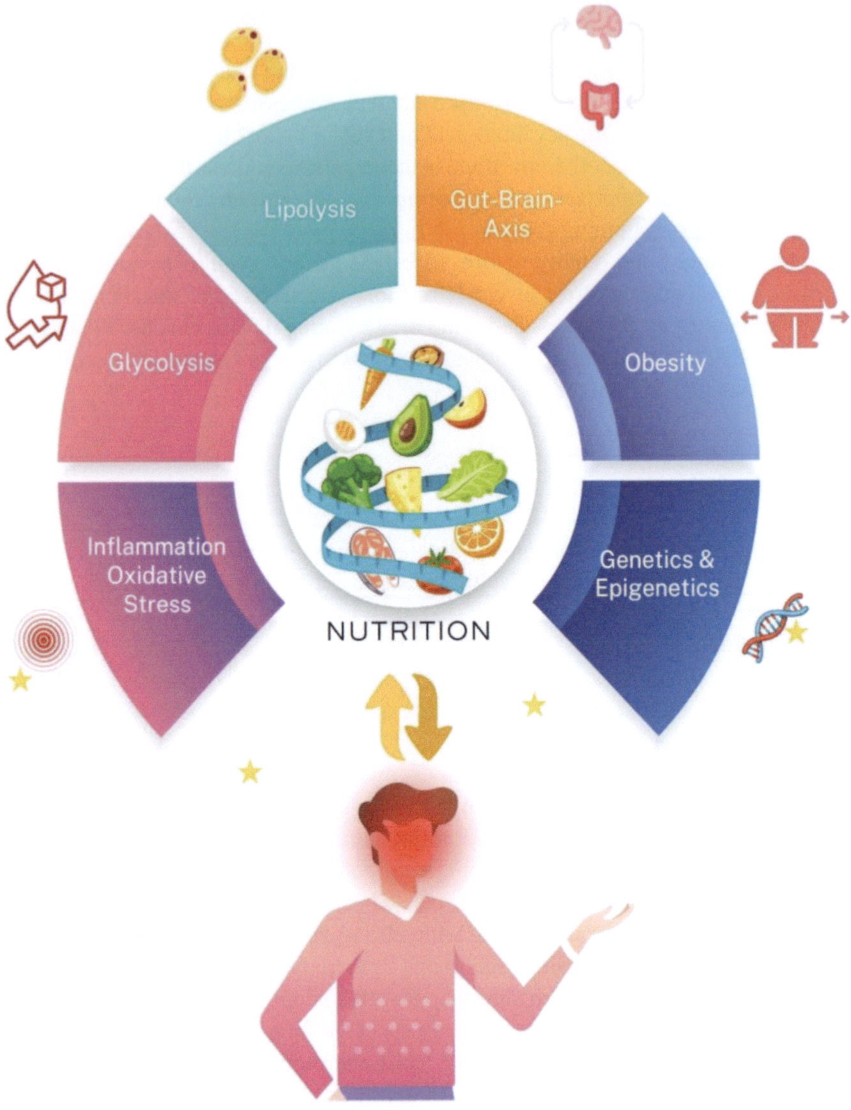

Fig. 24.2 The mechanisms and factors linking nutrition to chronic orofacial pain. Diet has a profound effect on inflammation, oxidative stress, glycolysis, lipolysis, gut–brain axis, obesity, genetic and epigenetic mechanisms, all of which play a significant role in the modulation of chronic orofacial pain, either exacerbating or alleviating its intensity. (Adapted under a CC BY 4.0 license from Elma et al. [11] Created using Canva)

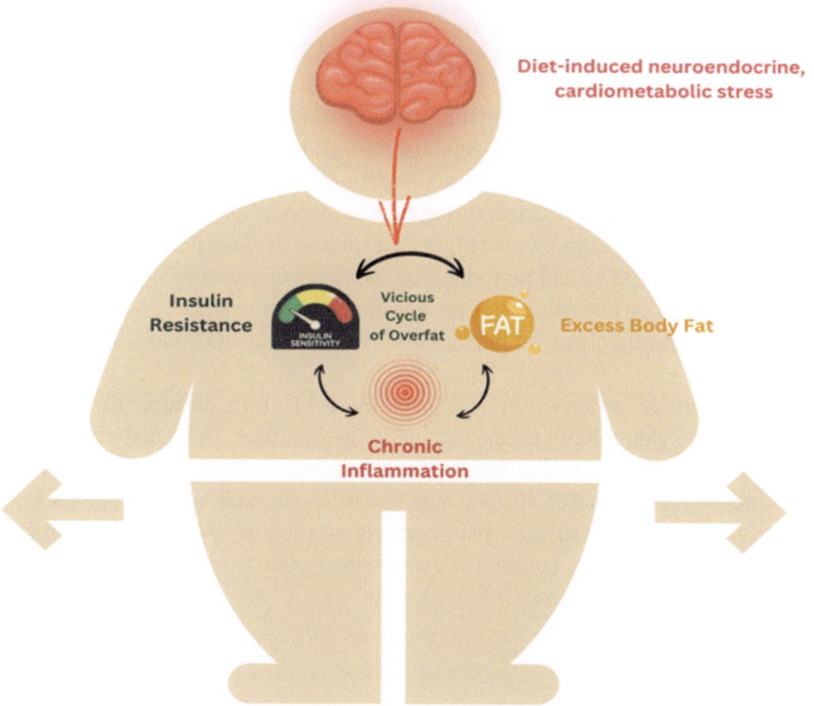

Fig. 24.3 The pro-inflammatory impact of obesity. Central nervous system dysregulation may begin as a vicious cycle where excess body fat promotes chronic inflammation and insulin resistance, which in turn exacerbates adiposity, creating a feedback loop that accelerates metabolic dysfunction, and neuroendocrine and cardiometabolic dysregulation. (Adapted under a CC BY 4.0 license from Maffetone et al. [38] Created using Canva)

A higher omega-6 to omega-3 ratio is linked to increased pain, particularly in temporomandibular disorders. Additionally, oleic acid in extra virgin olive oil has shown pain-relieving effects in trigeminal neuralgia [34, 36]. Gluten-free diets have also proven beneficial in managing chronic masticatory pain, positioning them as a valuable adjunct in comprehensive pain management [37].

Poor diet contributes to obesity, which impairs mobility, strength and central nervous system function, promoting pain sensitivity and central sensitisation [12]. Obesity also increases the risk of comorbidities such as type 2 diabetes mellitus, cardiovascular disease and non-alcoholic fatty liver disease, creating a feedback loop that exacerbates chronic pain and complicates its management (Fig. 24.3) [12, 38, 39].

Additionally, the gut microbiome significantly influences chronic pain, as diet-induced imbalances can cause dysbiosis, inflammation and altered pain signaling [40, 41]. A balanced diet supports gut health and can mitigate pain, emphasising the role of nutrition and lifestyle interventions in managing chronic pain [12].

24.3 Sleep

Chronic pain and sleep disturbances are closely linked, with each condition exacerbating the other. Between 67 and 88% of individuals with chronic pain report sleep issues, and at least 50% of those with insomnia experience chronic pain [42]. This bidirectional relationship is well-established—poor sleep contributes to the onset and intensification of chronic pain, while pain disrupts sleep [43–45]. Individuals with chronic pain often experience fragmented sleep, reduced sleep efficiency and less slow-wave sleep, along with a higher prevalence of sleep disorders like obstructive sleep apnoea (OSA) and periodic limb movements. Specific sleep disturbances, such as alpha-delta intrusions during non-rapid eye movement (non-REM) sleep phase, are commonly observed in conditions like fibromyalgia, worsening insomnia [43, 46, 47].

This reciprocal relationship is especially evident in chronic orofacial pain (Fig. 24.4). For example, in temporomandibular disorders, sleep disturbances often precede pain onset [48], and individuals with moderate-to-severe temporomandibular disorders report poorer sleep compared to those with mild or no pain [49]. Similarly, neuropathic orofacial pain conditions, such as trigeminal neuralgia and headaches, disrupt sleep, creating a cycle where pain worsens sleep quality, and poor sleep exacerbates pain [50, 51].

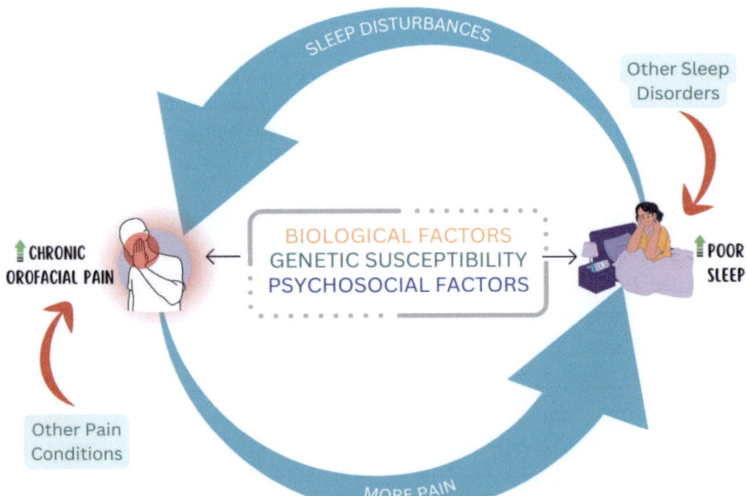

Fig. 24.4 The bi-directional relationship between sleep and chronic orofacial pain. Chronic orofacial pain can disrupt sleep quality and poor sleep, in turn, can exacerbate the pain, creating a harmful cycle. This cycle is often intensified by other pain conditions and sleep disorders. Moreover, biological, psychological and social factors can make individuals more susceptible to both chronic orofacial pain and poor sleep, further deepening the cycle and complicating treatment. (Created using Canva)

Beyond directly affecting pain, poor sleep can influence behaviours, contributing to unhealthy eating, inactivity and weakened mind–body connections [52]. Pain medications, such as opioids and benzodiazepines, can further disrupt sleep, complicating pain management [44, 53]. Individuals with chronic orofacial pain using a combination of opioids and benzodiazepines experienced more significant sleep disturbances than those using non-opioid medications (e.g. non-steroidal anti-inflammatories, analgesics, muscle relaxants, antidepressants, anticonvulsants and tricyclic antidepressants) or a combination of non-opioids, opioids and sleep medications [53]. Notably, individuals with chronic orofacial pain prescribed opioids experienced more significant sleep disturbances than those not using opioids [53].

Irregular sleep patterns, including sleeping less than six hours (short sleepers) or more than nine hours (long sleepers), are common in chronic pain sufferers [48]. Prolonged sleep, in particular, can trigger inflammation and metabolic imbalances, including insulin resistance, which may worsen or initiate chronic orofacial pain [54].

24.4 Physical Activity

A dose-dependent, inverse relationship exists between physical activity and chronic pain severity, meaning higher levels of physical activity generally correlate with reduced pain intensity (Fig. 24.5) [55]. However, factors such as discomfort, fatigue, perceived risks, personal beliefs, conflicting priorities, resource availability, co-existing health conditions and social support can influence one's willingness to engage in physical activity [56]. Individuals with chronic pain often adopt pain avoidance behaviours, leading to a sedentary lifestyle that increases the risk of obesity, musculoskeletal pain and worsened chronic pain symptoms [57].

Growing evidence supports the benefits of various physical activities such as general exercise, low-intensity exercises, strength training, aerobic exercises, aquatic exercises, Tai Chi, yoga and Pilates, in reducing pain severity. These activities activate endogenous analgesic pathways, modulate pain-related neurotransmitters, promote hypoalgesia, increase pain thresholds and reduce pain perception. They also improve physical function, reduce fatigue, enhance oxygen uptake and contribute to better mental health outcomes [28, 43, 44, 56, 58, 59].

For individuals with chronic orofacial pain, such as headaches and temporomandibular disorders, a combination of aerobic exercise, manual therapy and targeted jaw and neck exercises significantly improves pain intensity and quality of life [56–58, 60]. Yoga-based exercises are particularly effective for masticatory myofascial pain [61]. These findings underscore the importance of physical activity in managing chronic pain and alleviating orofacial symptoms.

While many studies highlight the positive effects of physical activity, fear of exacerbating symptoms (kinesophobia) can contribute to a more sedentary lifestyle [55]. In some cases, disrupted analgesic pathways may limit the benefits of exercise, potentially worsening pain, as seen in chronic masticatory myalgia, where exercise

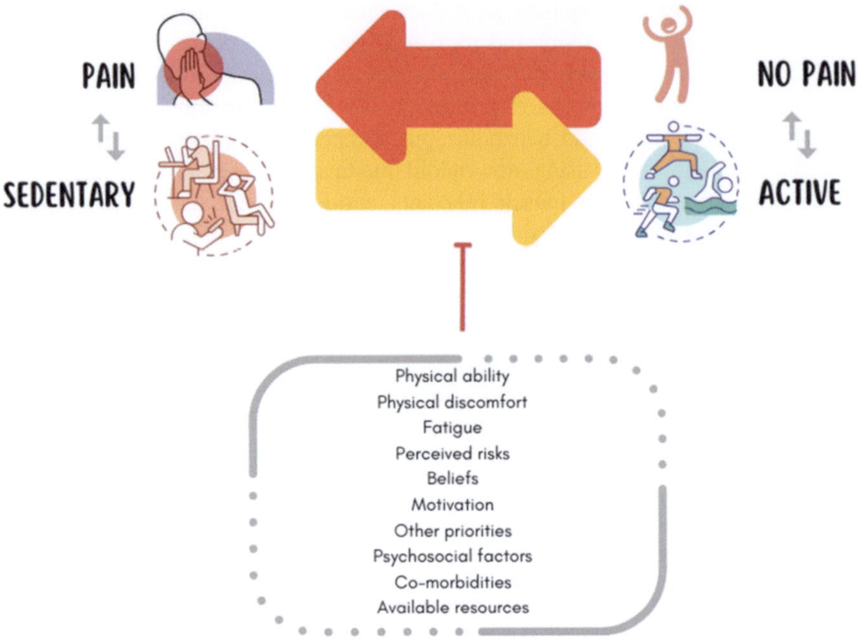

Fig. 24.5 The inverse relationship between chronic orofacial pain and the level of physical activity. As physical activity increases, the severity of chronic orofacial pain tends to decrease. However, individuals with chronic pain often engage in pain-avoidance behaviours and a sedentary lifestyle that can lead to worsening pain symptoms. (Created using Canva)

can increase rather than reduce pain [62]. Therefore, a tailored approach to physical activity is essential for effective pain management without exacerbating symptoms.

24.5 Stress

Chronic pain is strongly linked to mental health and social-learning experiences, particularly during childhood [63]. Psychological factors like unmanaged stress, anxiety and depression increase the sensitivity of the trigeminal system, intensifying pain [64, 65]. Individuals with chronic pain are two to three times more likely to experience these psychological conditions, which exacerbate pain behaviours and create a cycle of distress [43]. Traits like chronic stress, hypervigilance and catastrophising can further worsen orofacial pain [43, 66].

Early-life stress may lead to prolonged trigeminal sensitisation, potentially explaining the higher likelihood of developing migraines in adulthood [67]. Psychological distress, post-traumatic stress disorder (PTSD) and negative moods are strongly associated with temporomandibular disorders. Between 10% and 50% of individuals with chronic pain meet the Diagnostic and Statistical Manual of Mental Disorders (DSM-5) criteria for PTSD, with 15–23% of orofacial pain patients experiencing it. Trauma, including abuse and domestic violence, is also linked to treatment-resistant facial pain, poorer functional outcomes and reduced responses to medical treatments. The overlap of conditions like fibromyalgia, temporomandibular disorders and migraines supports the theory of central sensitivity syndrome, which connects heightened central nervous system sensitivity to chronic pain and psychiatric conditions like depression and anxiety [68, 69].

Mind–body practices, such as meditation, mindfulness, breathing exercises, yoga and Tai Chi, have shown promise in managing chronic pain and alleviating psychological stress. These practices reduce pain perception and stress by positively affecting neural activity, with long-term meditators showing a 40–50% reduction in brain activity related to pain [70]. Integrating movement, muscle coordination and controlled breathing through yoga and Tai Chi also help reduce stress and improve overall well-being [70]. These approaches offer effective strategies for managing both the psychological and physical aspects of chronic pain.

24.6 Harmful Substance Use

Unhealthy substance use, including tobacco, alcohol and recreational or illicit drugs, increases health risks and plays a significant role in the development of chronic pain [71]. Dysfunction in the brain's ventromedial prefrontal cortex, which regulates pain and stress, is influenced by substance use, potentially exacerbating and prolonging chronic pain [72]. Research shows high rates of substance use among individuals with chronic orofacial pain, with many using substances like tobacco, alcohol, cannabis, opioids and sedatives, often non-medically [72]. This underscores the complex relationship between substance use and chronic pain and highlights the need for comprehensive assessments and interventions for substance use in these individuals [73].

Tobacco smoking not only worsens chronic pain but also predisposes individuals to further substance use. Prolonged nicotine use enhances central sensitisation, a key factor in chronic pain [74]. Smokers with chronic pain experience greater pain and hypersensitivity, and smoking and alcohol use are strongly linked to temporomandibular disorder symptoms [75, 76]. Additionally, the combination of smoking and chronic pain increases the risk of opioid misuse, with non-medical opioid use being more common in individuals with chronic pain, especially those with chronic orofacial pain [77, 78].

Recreational and illicit drug use, such as methamphetamine and cocaine, can also contribute to orofacial pain. Methamphetamine use leads to temporomandibular joint pain and bruxism, while cocaine use alters dopaminergic neurotransmission [79]. As such, addressing substance use in orofacial pain management pain is essential for a comprehensive approach.

24.7 Social Connection

Chronic orofacial pain, such as trigeminal neuralgia, can significantly impact social interactions, leading to withdrawal, isolation and emotional distress, all of which reduce quality of life [80, 81]. Beyond physical discomfort, persistent pain often triggers chronic stress, depression, hypervigilance and catastrophising, which further complicate social dynamics and increase pain sensitivity [43, 66]. These emotional and social challenges intensify pain, leading to greater distress, disability and strained relationships [80, 81]. Individuals with musculoskeletal pain, in particular, are more vulnerable to feelings of loneliness and lack of support [82].

Barriers to effective self-management of chronic pain include insufficient social support, limited resources, time constraints, lack of personalised pain strategies and challenging interactions with healthcare providers [83, 84]. These obstacles often hinder treatment adherence and condition management.

To improve outcomes, interventions should focus on enhancing social connections and building resilience [85, 86]. Addressing social factors can improve well-being and potentially reduce the risk of chronic pain being passed down through generations. However, assessing social impacts is complex due to the subjective nature of pain, psychological factors and stigma, which can complicate both assessment and intervention development [81, 85].

24.8 Instruments Measuring Lifestyle

While there are no definitive gold standards for identifying all the lifestyle risk factors for chronic orofacial pain, using screening tools validated for chronic pain helps establish a baseline for recognising the most common risk factors. A selection of these validated assessment tools is listed below (Fig. 24.6).

24.8.1 Nutrition

Dietary risk factors for chronic orofacial pain can be identified through a food diary as well as the following validated screening tools:

1. *The Malnutrition Universal Screening Tool (MUST)*: The MUST is a widely used tool to identify individuals at risk of malnutrition or obesity. It evaluates body mass index (BMI), unintentional weight loss and the presence of acute disease. These factors are combined into a score to determine the level of nutritional risk [12, 87]. The tool is available online at: https://www.bapen.org.uk/pdfs/must/must_full.pdf.
2. *Malnutrition Screening Tool (MST)*: The MST is a simple, brief tool used to assess the risk of malnutrition based on factors such as weight loss, appetite changes and nutritional intake. It is quick to administer, making it suitable for routine clinical use. A higher score indicates a greater risk of malnutrition [12,

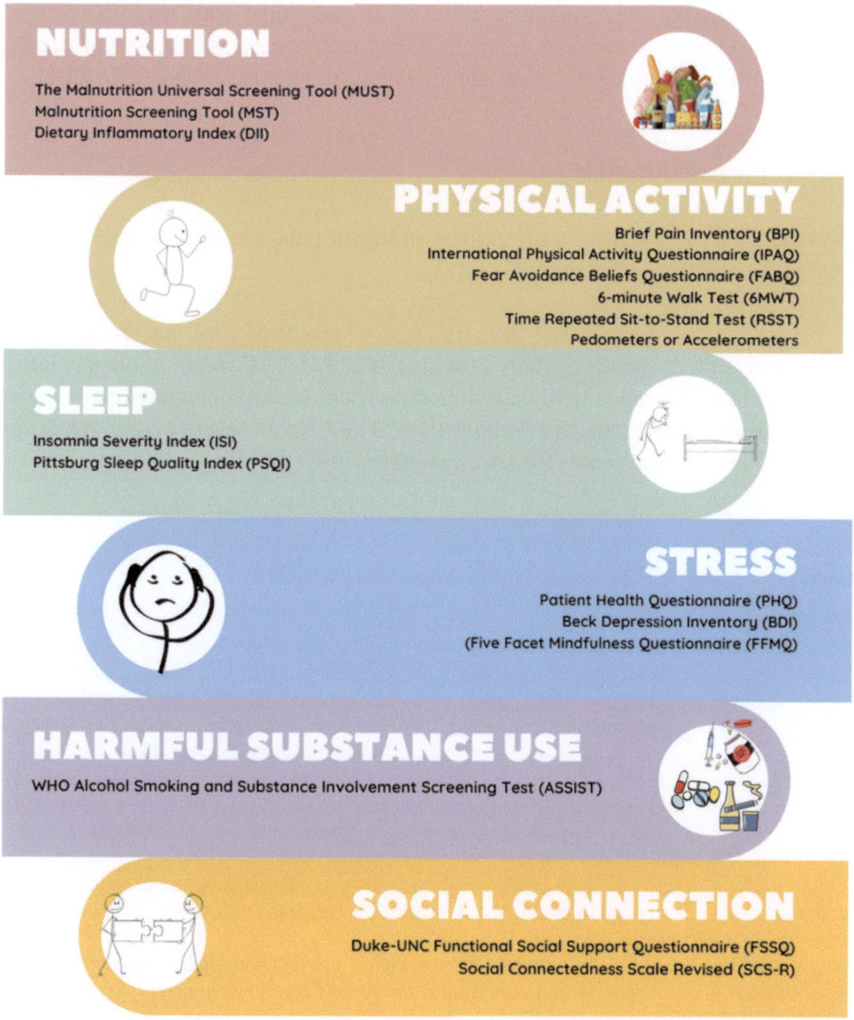

Fig. 24.6 Assessment tools for evaluating lifestyle factors in chronic pain that can be adapted for chronic orofacial pain. (Created using Canva)

87]. The tool is available online at: https://static.abbottnutrition.com/cms-prod/abbottnutrition-2016.com/img/Malnutrition%20Screening%20Tool_FINAL_tcm1226-57900.pdf

3. *Dietary Inflammatory Index (DII)*: The DII is a tool used to assess the inflammatory potential and dietary quality of an individual's diet, based on scientific evidence. A higher score indicates a more pro-inflammatory diet, while a lower score suggests an anti-inflammatory diet [88].

When assessing the nutritional status of an individual with chronic orofacial pain, it is important to consider their key dietary factors such as diet, weight change, comorbidities, functional disorders and biochemical abnormalities (Table 24.1).

24.8.2 Physical Activity

Physical activity risk factors for chronic orofacial pain can be assessed using the following validated screening tools:

1. *Brief Pain Inventory (BPI)*: The BPI is a widely used tool that assesses pain intensity and its impact on daily activities. It includes 11 questions on pain intensity, pain interference with daily functions, pain location and pain medications and pain relief over the past 24 hours. From this, a pain severity score (PSS) and a pain interference score (PIS) are calculated [89].

Table 24.1 Dietary factors associated with chronic orofacial pain

Dietary factor	Rationale
Current foods	Understanding an individual's regular diet helps identify foods that may exacerbate chronic pain or contribute to nutrient deficiencies.
Weight change	Tracking weight changes over time provides insights into potential undernutrition or overnutrition. Measures like the body mass index (BMI) and waist circumference can help identify these changes. However, BMI should be interpreted with caution, as it does not consider factors like muscle mass, bone density and fat distribution. A more approachable method may involve observing visible changes or asking about clothes fitting differently.
Presence of comorbid conditions	Metabolic disorders or comorbidities, such as diabetes mellitus or hypothyroidism, should be noted, as they can contribute to pain and affect nutritional status.
Appetite changes & inadequate dietary intake	Appetite changes, gastrointestinal issues and poor dietary intake can negatively impact nutritional health and contribute to chronic orofacial pain symptoms.
Functional gastrointestinal disorders (FGIDs)	Symptoms like abdominal pain, dysphagia, dyspepsia, diarrhoea, constipation and bloating may indicate underlying gastrointestinal issues that could be affecting nutritional absorption and contributing to pain.
Malnutrition	Malnutrition, especially in vulnerable populations like the elderly or those with chronic illness, can significantly worsen the experience of chronic orofacial pain and delay healing.
Abnormal biochemistry results	Abnormal biochemical markers, such as low levels of key vitamins, minerals or other nutrients, can indicate inadequate nutrition that may worsen chronic orofacial pain. Serum tests for *B-group vitamins, vitamin C, vitamin D, iron, zinc, lipids, glucose, insulin and thyroid function* can help identify deficiencies. Other tests like *serum albumin, C-reactive protein (CRP), complete blood count for total lymphocytes and haematocrit, electrolytes/urea/creatinine and liver function test* can provide additional insights [87].

Adapted under a CC BY 4.0 licence from Elma et al. [12] and Serón-Arbeloa et al. [87]

2. *International Physical Activity Questionnaire (IPAQ)*: The IPAQ is a tool that evaluates physical activity levels in adults and is available in a short-form version (7 questions) and a long-form version (27 questions). It assesses the frequency, duration and intensity of activities like walking and moderate-to-vigorous exercise over the past week, classifying individuals as having low, moderate or high physical activity levels [90, 91].
3. *Fear Avoidance Beliefs Questionnaire (FABQ)*: The FABQ is a tool to assess a person's fear-avoidance beliefs related to physical activity and work, particularly in association with musculoskeletal pain. It includes 16 questions in relation to physical activity and work [91, 92].
4. *6-minute walk test (6MWT)*: The 6MWT measures a person's endurance and functional capacity by having them walk as far as possible in 6 minutes. The test measures the distance covered and a low capacity evaluates the impact on conditions such as cardiovascular diseases and respiratory diseases [91, 93].
5. *Time repeated sit-to-stand test (RSST)*: The RSST measures a person's lower body strength and functional mobility by having them repeatedly stand up and sit down from a chair as quickly as possible for a set period. Variations in this test include the *Five Times Sit-to-Stand Test (5XSST)*, where individuals stand up and sit down five times as quickly as possible, and the *30-Second Sit-to-Stand Test*, which counts how many times a person can stand from a seated position in 30 seconds. A below average score indicates poorer functional mobility [91, 93].
6. *Pedometers or accelerometers*: While not a validated measure, pedometers or accelerometers are simple tools worn on an individual's body to capture the intensity of bodily movement [91].

24.8.3 Sleep

Sleep risk factors for chronic orofacial pain can be identified through assessments using the following validated screening tools:

1. *Insomnia Severity Index (ISI)*: The ISI is a simple and widely used tool to assess the severity of insomnia symptoms. It includes seven questions that evaluate the intensity of sleep difficulties including daytime impairment, over the past two weeks [94].
2. *Pittsburgh Sleep Quality Index (PSQI)*: The PSQI is a simple tool to assess the quality and patterns of sleep over the past month and helps identify sleep issues. It includes 19 questions across seven components: subjective sleep quality, sleep latency, sleep duration, habitual sleep efficiency, sleep disturbances, use of sleep medications and daytime dysfunction [95].

24.8.4 Stress

Psychological risk factors for chronic orofacial pain can be identified through assessments using the following validated screening tools:

1. *Patient Health Questionnaire (PHQ)*: The PHQ is a simple tool to assess mental health conditions such as depression, anxiety and somatic symptoms over the past two weeks. It is available in two short forms, PHQ-2 (2 questions), PHQ-4 (4 questions) and a long form, PHQ-9 (9 questions). The total score determines the severity of depression [96].
2. *Beck Depression Inventory (BDI)*: The BDI is a widely used tool to assess the severity of an individual's depression. It includes 21 questions on a specific symptom of depression such as mood, behaviour and physical symptoms [97].
3. *Five Facet Mindfulness Questionnaire (FFMQ)*: The FFMQ is a tool to assess an individual's overall mindfulness and how they engage with their thoughts, emotions and sensations across five key dimensions. It includes 39 questions, with each facet measuring different aspects of mindful awareness and behaviour [98].

24.8.5 Harmful Substance Use

To screen for risk factors related to harmful substance use in individuals with chronic orofacial pain, the validated *World Health Organization (WHO) Alcohol, Smoking, and Substance Involvement Screening Test (ASSIST)* can be used. This tool assesses the frequency, quantity and impact of substances such as alcohol, tobacco, cannabis, amphetamines and prescription medications like opioids, assigning a risk score to classify users as low, moderate or high risk for each substance [99, 100].

24.8.6 Social Connection

Social risk factors for chronic orofacial pain can be identified through assessments using the following validated screening tools:

1. *Duke-UNC Functional Social Support Questionnaire (FSSQ)*: The FSSQ is a widely used tool for assessing various aspects of social support and how supported a person feels in daily life. It comes in four versions: 5-item, 8-item, 11-item and the original 14-item version. The 11-item version effectively evaluates emotional, informational and practical support from family, friends and others in the community [101].
2. *Social Connectedness Scale Revised (SCS-R)*: The SCS-R is a widely used tool to assess a person's sense of social connectedness, social integration, quality of social relationships and belonging. It includes 20 questions that assess feelings of connection to others, community and society [102].

24.9 Managing Lifestyle Factors in Chronic Orofacial Pain

Barriers to effective chronic orofacial pain management include time constraints, lack of awareness of available resources, limited financial support, transportation issues, insufficient social support, ineffective pain management, depression, lack of personalised treatment plans, physical limitations, challenging patient-healthcare professional interactions and unrealistic patient expectations regarding treatments and recovery [83]. In contrast, facilitators that improve an individual's ability to manage their pain include encouragement from healthcare providers, effective depression treatment, a strong social support network and tailored self-management strategies [83].

To better manage chronic orofacial pain, individuals can make lifestyle changes with support from healthcare providers, services, family and friends. Healthcare professionals play a crucial role in ensuring a comprehensive approach to pain management, by integrating specialised care like dietitians, exercise physiologists and interdisciplinary pain management. Management plans should be reviewed regularly, with gradual changes and ongoing monitoring, recognising that retraining the brain and achieving pain relief take time [103, 104].

A tailored lifestyle management toolkit that includes assessment tools, management guidelines and progress tracking, can improve outcomes and treatment adherence. A progress diary can help patients and providers track improvements and adjust strategies as needed.

24.9.1 Education

Acknowledging the legitimacy of a patient's chronic orofacial pain, even without a clear cause, is crucial for effective management. Validating their experience fosters trust and encourages active participation in treatment and self-management. Educating patients about pain processing, neuroplasticity and influencing factors helps them understand that while chronic orofacial pain may not be completely curable, it can be effectively managed. A comprehensive approach, including pharmacotherapy, lifestyle changes, psychological support, physical therapy and self-management strategies, can reduce pain, improve function and enhance quality of life. Active engagement in daily pain management leads to the best outcomes [105–107]. Online resources, such as the video 'Tame the Beast', [106] can further support patient education.

24.9.2 Nutrition

Dietary modifications, guided by initial nutrition screening, are essential for managing chronic orofacial pain. Individuals on a pro-inflammatory diet should shift to an anti-inflammatory, minimally processed eating plan that is rich in fibre, low in sugar and glycaemic index and full of wholesome foods and nutraceuticals. The diet should be tailored to address specific pain triggers, such as avoiding fermented foods and dairy products for orofacial migraines and consuming softer foods for temporomandibular disorders [108]. Emphasising fruits, vegetables, wholegrains and healthy oils while reducing red meat can help reduce inflammation and alleviate pain [12, 27, 109]. Recommended foods and portion sizes are shown in Table 24.2 and Fig. 24.7.

24.9.3 Physical Activity

Physical activity and exercise interventions should be tailored to an individual's abilities, pain levels and participation barriers, guided by professionals such as physiotherapists, exercise physiologists or occupational therapists [56]. The goal

Table 24.2 Nutrition guidelines for the management of chronic orofacial pain. Glycaemic index (GI) is a ranking system for carbohydrate foods and is based on the speed of digestion and impact on the blood glucose levels over a period of time. Glucose has a GI of 100 and this is the reference used for other foods. Carbohydrates that break down quickly and cause a sharp increase in blood glucose levels are high GI foods. Conversely, carbohydrates that break down slowly and lead to a gradual and sustained increase of the blood glucose levels are low GI foods

Food group	Recommendation	Practical tips
Drinks	Drink 2–3 litres of water daily and limit caffeine intake	Carry a water bottle and set a daily drinking goal
Fruit and vegetables	Increase intake of a diverse selection fruits and vegetables with bright colours	Use frozen options to save time and reduce waste. Freezing helps preserve the nutrients Use pre-cut vegetables and canned goods for quick meals
Breads, cereals and grains	Choose wholegrain, fibre-rich, low glycaemic index (GI) options	Swap bread, pasta and rice for wholegrain alternatives
Meat and meat alternatives	Choose lean meats, oily fish, legumes, nuts and seeds	Replace processed meats with lean options or tinned fish/legumes
Dairy and alternatives	Choose high quality dairy foods	Opt for reduced fat or pre-sliced options, and individual tubs of natural or Greek yoghurt (without added sugar) for convenience
Healthy fats and oils	Focus on omega-3 and monounsaturated fats	Use olive or canola oil for cooking
Added sugar and ultra-processed food	Limit intake	Choose water over sugary drinks and minimally processed snacks like fruits, nuts, cheese or popcorn

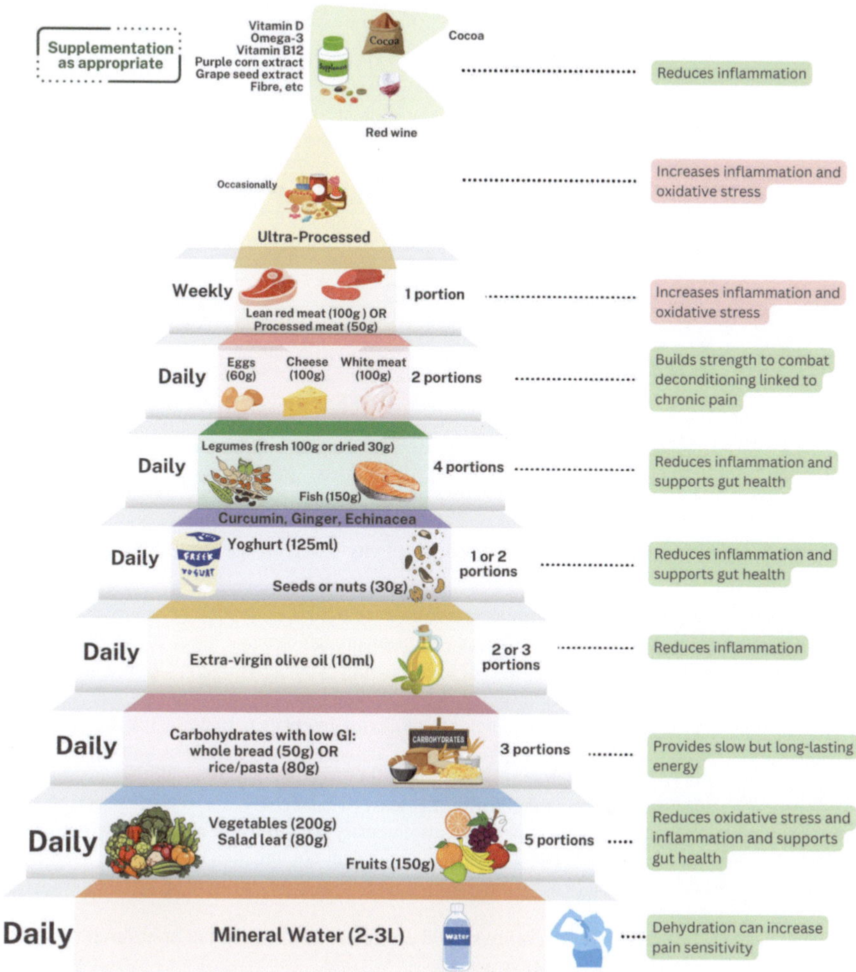

Fig. 24.7 Baseline food chart for the dietary management of chronic orofacial pain. (Adapted with permission from Cambridge University Press [32]. Created using Canva)

is to promote active self-management, improve daily activities and enhance overall well-being [104, 110]. The World Health Organization's guidelines on physical activity and sedentary behaviour for adults (Fig. 24.8, Table 24.3) emphasise that all physical activity is beneficial, sedentary time should be minimised and muscle-strengthening exercises are essential [112]. Even just 20 minutes of exercise, such as yoga, aerobic exercise or resistance training, can help manage chronic pain [113].

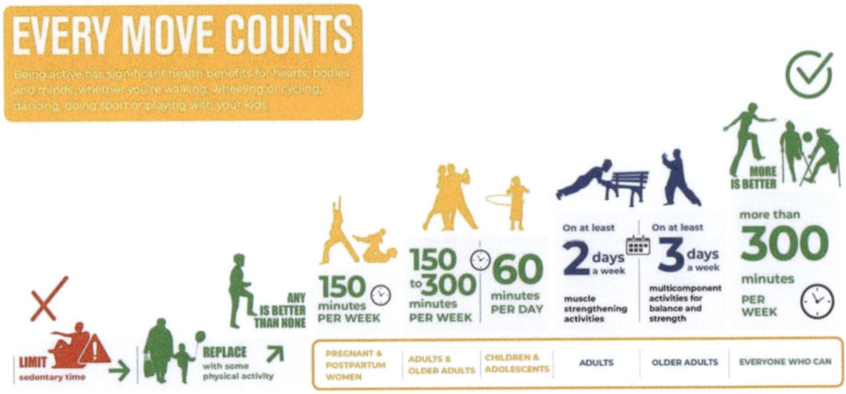
EVERY MOVE COUNTS
Being active has significant health benefits for hearts, bodies and minds, whether you're walking, wheeling or cycling, dancing, doing sport or playing with your kids
LIMIT
sedentary time
REPLACE
with some
physical activity
ANY
IS BETTER
THAN NONE
150 minutes PER WEEK
PREGNANT & POSTPARTUM WOMEN
150 to 300 minutes PER WEEK
ADULTS & OLDER ADULTS
60 minutes PER DAY
CHILDREN & ADOLESCENTS
On at least
2 days a week
muscle strengthening activities
ADULTS
On at least
3 days a week
multicomponent activities for balance and strength
OLDER ADULTS
MORE
IS BETTER
more than
300
minutes
PER
WEEK
EVERYONE WHO CAN

Fig. 24.8 WHO Guidelines on Physical Activity and Sedentary Behaviour. (Reproduced with permission from WHO [111])

Table 24.3 WHO recommendations for physical activity based on age group for chronic orofacial pain management

Age group	Physical activity recommendation
18–64 years	At least 150 minutes of moderate-intensity activity (e.g. brisk walking, golf, swimming) or 75 minutes of vigorous-intensity activity (e.g. jogging, aerobics, soccer) per week or an equivalent combination For additional benefits, increase moderate-intensity activity to 300 minutes weekly Perform muscle-strengthening activities targeting major muscle groups (e.g. push-ups, squats, weightlifting) at least twice weekly
65 years and above	At least 150 minutes of moderate-intensity activity or 75 minutes of vigorous-intensity activity per week, or an equivalent combination For additional benefits, increase moderate-intensity activity to 300 minutes weekly Those with poor mobility should engage in balance and fall prevention exercises at least 3 days a week Perform muscle-strengthening activities targeting major muscle groups at least twice weekly

Adapted under CC BY-NC-SA 3.0 IGO from WHO [3, 11, 112]

24.9.4 Sleep

To improve sleep, behavioural strategies such as sleep hygiene practices (Fig. 24.9) can be effective, particularly when poor sleep habits or insomnia are present [114]. If an underlying sleep disorder is suspected, referral to a sleep physician for comprehensive assessment is recommended.

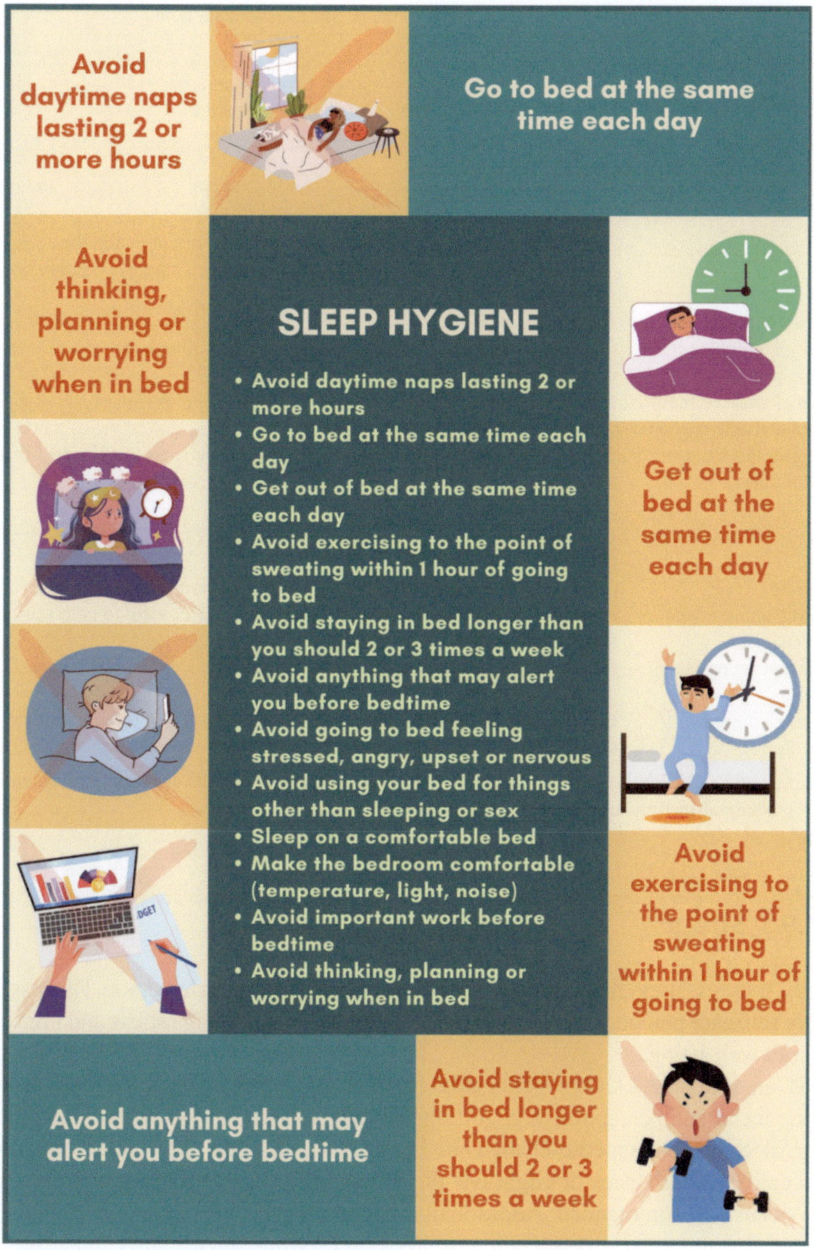

Fig. 24.9 Sleep hygiene strategies for the management of chronic orofacial pain. (Adapted under CC BY NC 4.0 from Gupta et al. [114] Created using Canva)

Table 24.4 Self-care practices for the management of chronic orofacial pain

Self-care practices	Recommendation
Stress reduction techniques	*Learn stress reduction techniques* to alleviate rapid breathing, muscle tension, nerve overstimulation and over-thinking: 1. *Breathing exercises*: Practice diaphragmatic and deep belly breathing [115] 2. *Movement therapies*: Engage in yoga [116], Tai Chi [117], Qi Gong and martial arts 3. *Mind–body therapies*: Practice mindfulness (e.g. using the headspace app or calm app), meditation [118], laughter therapy or imagery
Sleep hygiene	*Practice good sleep hygiene* for adequate rest
Social connection & support	*Connect with friends, family or support groups* to enhance emotional well-being and emotional resilience
Nutritional wellness	*Follow a balanced diet* to support overall health and stress management
Physical activity	*Movement and regular exercise* can reduce stress and improve mood
Pain desensitisation techniques	*Use desensitisation techniques* to not react negatively to pain, and help retrain the brain's response to pain, improving pain perception and intensity.
Distraction strategies	*Engage in enjoyable activities*, such as listening to music, to shift focus from pain
Pacing	*Balance periods of activity and rest* to reduce pain-related stress.
Limit social media and triggers	*Reduce exposure to social media and triggering content* to help lower stress and anxiety
Relaxation practices	*Engage in relaxing activities* such as, reading, listening to music or gardening to unwind
Complementary therapies	*Consider complementary approaches* such as, lavender aromatherapy to reduce pain perception and promote relaxation [119, 120]

Adapted under CC BY-NC-SA 3.0 IGO from WHO [121] and CC BY NC 4.0 from Pain Australia [104], National Institute of Mental Health (NIMH) [122]

24.9.5 Stress

Coping styles, stress response and symptoms vary from person to person. Discussing daily self-care practices (Table 24.4) can help individuals manage stress and improve overall well-being.

If an individual shows noticeable changes in appearance, behaviour, mood, thought content, perception or cognition, such as persistent stress-related symptoms (e.g. sleep issues, appetite changes or irritability), or signs like suicidal ideation, perceptual disturbances or cognitive alterations [123], a referral to a primary care physician is recommended. Additionally, patients facing mental health challenges can be directed to country-specific resources such as 988 Suicide and Crisis Lifeline (United States of America, USA) [124], Samaritans (United Kingdom, UK) [125] and Beyond Blue (Australia) [126] for further support.

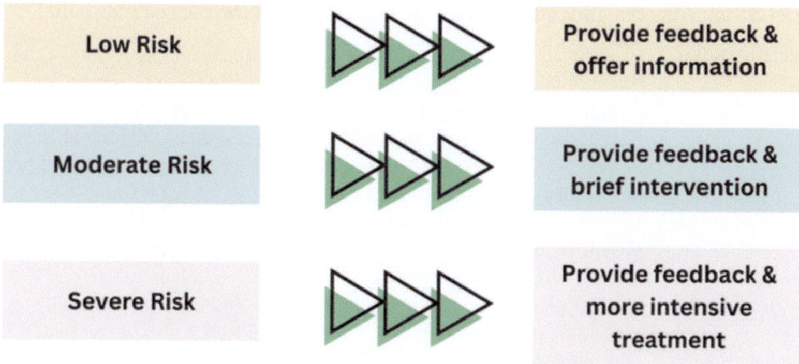

Fig. 24.10 Linking WHO ASSIST Score to appropriate intervention. (Adapted under CC BY-NC-SA 3.0 IGO from WHO [131]. Created using Canva)

24.9.6 Harmful Substance Use

Global guidelines for alcohol, smoking and substance use emphasise minimising risks, with the WHO stating no level of substance is safe and advising against initiation [127]. Alcohol consumption guidelines vary by country, shaped by cultural, health and policy differences [127]. For instance, the USA recommends up to 1 drink per day for women and 2 for men [128], the UK limits intake to 14 units per week with alcohol-free days [129] and Australia advises no more than 10 standard drinks per week, with a maximum of 4 drinks on any given occasion [130]. Across all these guidelines, there is a shared recommendation for pregnant and breastfeeding women to abstain from alcohol completely.

Primary care providers can support patients in managing substance use by following national guidelines, offering brief interventions based on the WHO ASSIST screening results, and encouraging healthier behaviours. Brief interventions, particularly when linked to screening outcomes, are effective for alcohol and tobacco use and increasingly applied to other substances. For low-risk individuals, providing feedback and support is recommended, while moderate-risk individuals should receive personalised guidance on reducing substance use (Fig. 24.10) [131].

Individuals with a history of substance use or dependence may need intensive treatment, starting with feedback and brief interventions (Fig. 24.10). High-risk patients, such as frequent injectors or multiple-substance users, require tailored care within the healthcare setting and should be referred for specialised services [131].

Smoking guidelines vary globally due to differences in public health priorities, cultural norms and economic factors. Nevertheless, there is a universal focus on reducing smoking rates and promoting cessation. The WHO advocates for a comprehensive approach to smoking cessation in both clinical and community settings. At a national level, individual governments offer a range of resources, such as counselling, treatment and support to aid cessation efforts. Key cessation strategies to use for individuals are summarised in Table 24.5.

Table 24.5 Smoking cessation strategies for the management of chronic orofacial pain

Smoking cessation strategy	Recommendation
Education	Explain smoking's impact on health and chronic orofacial pain. Emphasise that there is no evidence to suggest that switching to lower nicotine/tar cigarettes, filters or other forms of tobacco or e-cigarettes can help with quitting smoking.
Behavioural support	Encourage counselling, cognitive behavioural therapy (CBT), support groups (both in-person and online), quit-smoking apps and country-specific Quitlines and resources.
Pharmacotherapy	Discuss pharmacological options available through a primary care physician, including nicotine replacement therapy (NRT) like patches, gum, lozenges and inhalers, and prescription medication therapy options such as varenicline and bupropion.
Alternative therapies	Inform of alternative therapies such as hypnotherapy and acupuncture, although evidence supporting their effectiveness is limited.
Ongoing support	Offer continuous support through follow-up visits to motivate and guide patients throughout their quitting process, ensure long-term cessation and prevent relapse.

Adapted under CC BY-NC-SA 3.0 IGO from WHO [132] and Commonwealth of Australia [133]

24.9.7 Social Connection

Managing social connections is an essential aspect of chronic orofacial pain management, as strong social support can significantly reduce stress and enhance well-being. To address this, many countries have established professional bodies dedicated to supporting individuals with chronic pain. These organisations provide educational resources, online communities and access to local support groups, with the intention of reducing social isolation by connecting individuals with others facing similar challenges and fostering peer support. Notable examples of such organisations include Pain Connection (USA) [134], Pain Concern (UK) [135], Pain Australia (Australia) [136] and Pain BC (Canada) [137].

24.10 Conclusion

Lifestyle factors are an evolving and increasingly recognised aspect of chronic pain, including chronic orofacial pain, with much still to be explored and understood in the search for effective pain management. The complex relationship between nutrition, sleep, physical activity, stress, harmful substance use and social connection significantly influences the neurobiological mechanisms underlying pain perception and modulation. While lifestyle interventions offer promising benefits, their implementation can be challenging, particularly for individuals dealing with chronic stress and low motivation. A multidisciplinary approach that actively supports patients in adopting and maintaining lifestyle changes is essential, rather than placing the burden of self-management solely on the individual. As research in lifestyle medicine progresses, integrating evidence-based lifestyle modifications into a comprehensive pain management strategy will be key to improving long-term outcomes for those with chronic orofacial pain.

References

1. Treede RD, Rief W, Barke A, et al. Chronic pain as a symptom or a disease: the IASP classification of chronic pain for the international classification of diseases (ICD-11). Pain. 2019;160(1):19–27. https://doi.org/10.1097/j.pain.0000000000001384.
2. Cohen SP, Vase L, Hooten WM. Chronic pain: an update on burden, best practices, and new advances. Lancet. 2021;397(10289):2082–97. https://doi.org/10.1016/s0140-6736(21)00393-7.
3. Goldberg DS, McGee SJ. Pain as a global public health priority. BMC Public Health. 2011;11:770. https://doi.org/10.1186/1471-2458-11-770. Accepted manuscript. Published online 20111006
4. Zimmer Z, Fraser K, Grol-Prokopczyk H, Zajacova A. A global study of pain prevalence across 52 countries: examining the role of country-level contextual factors. Pain. 2022;163(9):1740–50. https://doi.org/10.1097/j.pain.0000000000002557. Accepted manuscript. Published online 20211215
5. Pain IAftSo. International classification of diseases, Eleventh Revision (ICD-11). 2021. https://icd.who.int/browse11
6. Korwisi B. Introduction to the ICD-11 chronic pain classification. 2023. https://www.who.int/news-room/events/detail/2023/06/14/default-calendar/who-webinar-on-unlocking-the-potential-of-icd-11-for-chronic-pain
7. Treede RD, Rief W, Barke A, et al. A classification of chronic pain for ICD-11. Pain. 2015;156(6):1003–7. https://doi.org/10.1097/j.pain.0000000000000160.
8. Bushnell MC, Case LK, Ceko M, et al. Effect of environment on the long-term consequences of chronic pain. Pain. 2015;156 Suppl 1(0 1):S42–s49. https://doi.org/10.1097/01.j.pain.0000460347.77341.bd.
9. Mills SEE, Nicolson KP, Smith BH. Chronic pain: a review of its epidemiology and associated factors in population-based studies. Br J Anaesth. 2019;123(2):e273–83. https://doi.org/10.1016/j.bja.2019.03.023. Accepted manuscript. Published online 20190510
10. Porporatti AL, Schroder ÂGD, Lebel A, et al. Prevalence of orofacial and head pain: an umbrella review of systematic reviews. J Oral Facial Pain Headache. 2024;38(3):1–14. https://doi.org/10.22514/jofph.2024.022.
11. Elma Ö, Brain K, Dong HJ. The importance of nutrition as a lifestyle factor in chronic pain management: a narrative review. J Clin Med. 2022;11(19) https://doi.org/10.3390/jcm11195950. Accepted manuscript. Published online 20221009
12. Elma Ö, Lebuf E, Marnef AQ, et al. Diet can exert both analgesic and pronociceptive effects in acute and chronic pain models: a systematic review of preclinical studies. Nutr Neurosci. 2022;25(10):2195–217. https://doi.org/10.1080/1028415x.2021.1934956. Accepted manuscript. Published online 20210607
13. Gianò M, Franco C, Castrezzati S, Rezzani R. Involvement of oxidative stress and nutrition in the anatomy of Orofacial Pain. Int J Mol Sci. 2023;24(17) Accepted manuscript. Published online 20230823. https://doi.org/10.3390/ijms241713128.
14. Hawkins JL, Durham PL. Enriched chicken bone broth as a dietary supplement reduces nociception and sensitization associated with prolonged jaw opening. J Oral Facial Pain Headache. 2018;32(2):208–15. https://doi.org/10.11607/ofph.1971. Accepted manuscript. Published online 20180306
15. Pereira EWM, Heimfarth L, Santos TK, et al. Limonene, a citrus monoterpene, non-complexed and complexed with hydroxypropyl-β-cyclodextrin attenuates acute and chronic orofacial nociception in rodents: evidence for involvement of the PKA and PKC pathway.

Phytomedicine. 2022;96:153893. https://doi.org/10.1016/j.phymed.2021.153893. Accepted manuscript. Published online 20211218
16. Antonopoulos SR, Garten DA, Durham PL. Dietary supplementation with grape seed extract from Vitus vinifera prevents suppression of GABAergic protein expression in female Sprague Dawley trigeminal ganglion in a model of chronic temporomandibular joint disorder. Arch Oral Biol. 2024;165:106014. https://doi.org/10.1016/j.archoralbio.2024.106014. Accepted manuscript. Published online 20240529
17. Cady RJ, Hirst JJ, Durham PL. Dietary grape seed polyphenols repress neuron and glia activation in trigeminal ganglion and trigeminal nucleus caudalis. Mol Pain. 2010;6:91. https://doi.org/10.1186/1744 8069 6 91. Accepted manuscript. Published online 20101210
18. Cornelison LE, Chelliboina N, Woodman SE, Durham PL. Dietary supplementation with grape seed extract prevents development of trigeminal sensitization and inhibits pain signaling in a preclinical chronic temporomandibular disorder model. J Oral Pathol Med. 2020;49(6):514–21. https://doi.org/10.1111/jop.13066. Accepted manuscript. Published online 20200625
19. Magni G, Marinelli A, Riccio D, et al. Purple corn extract as anti-allodynic treatment for trigeminal pain: role of microglia. Front Cell Neurosci. 2018;12:378. https://doi.org/10.3389/fncel.2018.00378. Accepted manuscript. Published online 20181105
20. Catunda IS, Vasconcelos BC, Andrade ES, Costa DF. Clinical effects of an avocado-soybean unsaponifiable extract on arthralgia and osteoarthritis of the temporomandibular joint: preliminary study. Int J Oral Maxillofac Surg. 2016;45(8):1015–22. https://doi.org/10.1016/j.ijom.2016.01.008. Accepted manuscript. Published online 20160326
21. Cady RJ, Denson JE, Durham PL. Inclusion of cocoa as a dietary supplement represses expression of inflammatory proteins in spinal trigeminal nucleus in response to chronic trigeminal nerve stimulation. Mol Nutr Food Res. 2013;57(6):996–1006. https://doi.org/10.1002/mnfr.201200630. Accepted manuscript. Published online 20130411
22. González-López-Arza MV, Triviño-Palomo JV, Montanero-Fernández J, et al. Benefits of the light consumption of red wine in pain, tender points, and anxiety in women with fibromyalgia: a pilot study. Nutrients. 2023;15(15) https://doi.org/10.3390/nu15153469. Accepted manuscript. Published online 20230805
23. Durham PL, Antonopoulos SR. Benefit of dietary supplementation of nutraceuticals as an integrative approach for management of migraine: evidence from preclinical and clinical studies. Curr Pain Headache Rep. 2024;28(5):373–81. https://doi.org/10.1007/s11916-024-01230-w. Accepted manuscript. Published online 20240302
24. Durham J, Touger-Decker R, Nixdorf DR, Rigassio-Radler D, Moynihan P. Oro-facial pain and nutrition: a forgotten relationship? J Oral Rehabil. 2015;42(1):75–80. https://doi.org/10.1111/joor.12226. Accepted manuscript. Published online 20140909
25. Kurowska A, Ziemichód W, Herbet M, Piątkowska-Chmiel I. The role of diet as a modulator of the inflammatory process in the neurological diseases. Nutrients. 2023;15(6) https://doi.org/10.3390/nu15061436. Accepted manuscript. Published online 20230316
26. Piriyaprasath K, Kakihara Y, Hasegawa M, et al. Nutritional strategies for chronic craniofacial pain and temporomandibular disorders: current clinical and preclinical insights. Nutrients. 2024;16(17) https://doi.org/10.3390/nu16172868. Accepted manuscript. Published online 20240827
27. Elma Ö, Yilmaz ST, Deliens T, et al. Chronic musculoskeletal pain and nutrition: where are we and where are we heading? PM R. 2020;12(12):1268–78. Accepted manuscript. Published online 20200320. https://doi.org/10.1002/pmrj.12346.
28. Dragan S, Şerban MC, Damian G, Buleu F, Valcovici M, Christodorescu R. Dietary patterns and interventions to alleviate chronic pain. Nutrients. 2020;12(9) https://doi.org/10.3390/nu12092510. Accepted manuscript. Published online 20200819
29. Tick H. Nutrition and pain. Phys Med Rehabil Clin N Am. 2015;26(2):309–20. https://doi.org/10.1016/j.pmr.2014.12.006.

30. Margină D, Ungurianu A, Purdel C, et al. Chronic inflammation in the context of everyday life: dietary changes as mitigating factors. Int J Environ Res Public Health. 2020;17(11):4135. https://doi.org/10.3390/ijerph17114135.
31. Meleger AL, Froude CK, Walker J 3rd. Nutrition and eating behavior in patients with chronic pain receiving long-term opioid therapy. PM R. 2014;6(1):7–12.e11. https://doi.org/10.1016/j.pmrj.2013.08.597. Accepted manuscript. Published online 20130822
32. Rondanelli M, Faliva MA, Miccono A, et al. Food pyramid for subjects with chronic pain: foods and dietary constituents as anti-inflammatory and antioxidant agents. Nutr Res Rev. 2018;31(1):131–51. https://doi.org/10.1017/s0954422417000270. Accepted manuscript. Published online 20180422
33. Calder PC. Omega-3 polyunsaturated fatty acids and inflammatory processes: nutrition or pharmacology? Br J Clin Pharmacol. 2013;75(3):645–62. https://doi.org/10.1111/j.1365-2125.2012.04374.x.
34. Sanders AE, Cai J, Daviglus ML, Garcia-Bedoya O, Slade GD. Long-chain PUFA and painful temporomandibular disorder in the Hispanic Community Health Study/Study of Latinos. Public Health Nutr. 2025;28(1):e41. https://doi.org/10.1017/S1368980025000102. Accepted manuscript. Published online 2025/02/03
35. Sanders AE, Weatherspoon ED, Ehrmann BM, et al. Circulating polyunsaturated fatty acids and Pain intensity in five chronic pain conditions. J Pain. 2023;24(3):478–89. https://doi.org/10.1016/j.jpain.2022.10.008. Accepted manuscript. Published online 20221020
36. Calder PC. Omega-3 fatty acids and inflammatory processes. Nutrients. 2010;2(3):355–74. https://doi.org/10.3390/nu2030355. Accepted manuscript. Published online 20100318
37. Araújo Oliveira Buosi J, Abreu Nogueira SM, Sousa MP, et al. Gluten-free diet reduces pain in women with myofascial Pain in masticatory muscles: a preliminary randomized controlled trial. J Oral Facial Pain Headache. 2021;35(3):199–207. https://doi.org/10.11607/ofph.2823.
38. Maffetone PB, Rivera-Dominguez I, Laursen PB. Overfat Adults and children in developed countries: the public Health importance of identifying excess body fat. Front Public Health. 2017:5. https://doi.org/10.3389/fpubh.2017.00190.
39. Brain K, Burrows TL, Rollo ME, et al. A systematic review and meta-analysis of nutrition interventions for chronic noncancer pain. J Hum Nutr Diet. 2019;32(2):198–225. https://doi.org/10.1111/jhn.12601.
40. Morreale C, Bresesti I, Bosi A, et al. Microbiota and pain: save your gut feeling. Cells. 2022;11(6):971. https://www.mdpi.com/2073-4409/11/6/971
41. Ceballos D, Hernández-Camba A, Ramos L. Diet and microbiome in the beginning of the sequence of gut inflammation. World J Clin Cases. 2021;9(36):11122–47. https://doi.org/10.12998/wjcc.v9.i36.11122.
42. Whale K, Gooberman-Hill R. The importance of sleep for people with chronic pain: current insights and evidence. JBMR Plus. 2022;6(7):e10658. https://doi.org/10.1002/jbm4.10658. Accepted manuscript. Published online 20220617.
43. Crandall JA. An introduction to orofacial pain. Dent Clin N Am. 2018;62(4):511–23. https://doi.org/10.1016/j.cden.2018.05.001. Accepted manuscript. Published online 20180727
44. Haack M, Simpson N, Sethna N, Kaur S, Mullington J. Sleep deficiency and chronic pain: potential underlying mechanisms and clinical implications. Neuropsychopharmacology. 2020;45(1):205–16. https://doi.org/10.1038/s41386-019-0439-z.
45. Herrero Babiloni A, De Koninck BP, Beetz G, De Beaumont L, Martel MO, Lavigne GJ. Sleep and pain: recent insights, mechanisms, and future directions in the investigation of this relationship. J Neural Transm. 2020;127(4):647–60. https://doi.org/10.1007/s00702-019-02067-z.
46. Dos Santos Bento AP, Filho NM, Ferreira AS, Cassetta AP, de Almeida RS. Sleep quality and polysomnographic changes in patients with chronic pain with and without central sensitization signs. Braz J Phys Ther. 2023;27(3):100504. https://doi.org/10.1016/j.bjpt.2023.100504. Accepted manuscript. Published online 20230426
47. Choiniere M, Racine M, Raymond-Shaw I. Epidemiology of pain and sleep disturbances and their reciprocal interrelationships. IASP Press; 2007. Sleep and pain

48. Edwards RR, Almeida DM, Klick B, Haythornthwaite JA, Smith MT. Duration of sleep contributes to next-day pain report in the general population. Pain. 2008;137(1):202–7. https://doi.org/10.1016/j.pain.2008.01.025. Accepted manuscript. Published online 20080422
49. Yap AU, Cao Y, Zhang MJ, Lei J, Fu KY. Temporomandibular disorder severity and diagnostic groups: their associations with sleep quality and impairments. Sleep Med. 2021;80:218–25. https://doi.org/10.1016/j.sleep.2021.01.063. Accepted manuscript. Published online 20210202
50. Lavigne GJ, Sessle BJ. The neurobiology of orofacial pain and sleep and their interactions. J Dent Res. 2016;95(10):1109–16. https://doi.org/10.1177/0022034516648264. Accepted manuscript. Published online 20160506
51. Orzeszek S, Martynowicz H, Smardz J, et al. Assessment of sleep quality in patients with orofacial pain and headache complaints: a polysomnographic study. Dent Med Probl. 2024;61(4):549–62. https://doi.org/10.17219/dmp/177008.
52. Husak AJ, Bair MJ. Chronic pain and sleep disturbances: a pragmatic review of their relationships, comorbidities, and treatments. Pain Med. 2020;21(6):1142–52. https://doi.org/10.1093/pm/pnz343.
53. Bavia PF, Khawaja S, Hernández-Nuño de la Rosa MF, Tseng LA, Keith DA. Association between pharmacotherapy and sleep quality in patients with chronic orofacial and chronic body pain: a cross-sectional study. J Pain Res. 2023;16:3433–40. https://doi.org/10.2147/jpr.S412459.
54. Jiang Y, Gong X, Yu M, Gao X. Relationships between orofacial pain and sleep: analysis of UK biobank and genome-wide association studies data. J Dent Sci. 2025;20(1):529–38. https://doi.org/10.1016/j.jds.2024.04.027. Accepted manuscript. Published online 20240506
55. Fjeld MK, Årnes AP, Engdahl B, et al. Consistent pattern between physical activity measures and chronic pain levels: the Tromsø study 2015 to 2016. Pain. 2023;164(4):838–47. https://doi.org/10.1097/j.pain.0000000000002773. Accepted manuscript. Published online 20220908
56. Vader K, Doulas T, Patel R, Miller J. Experiences, barriers, and facilitators to participating in physical activity and exercise in adults living with chronic pain: a qualitative study. Disabil Rehabil. 2021;43(13):1829–37. https://doi.org/10.1080/09638288.2019.1676834. Accepted manuscript. Published online 20191015
57. Mills EP, Keay KA, Henderson LA. Brainstem Pain-modulation circuitry and its plasticity in neuropathic Pain: insights from human Brain imaging investigations. Front Pain Res. 2021:2. https://doi.org/10.3389/fpain.2021.705345.
58. Daenen L, Varkey E, Kellmann M, Nijs J. Exercise, not to exercise, or how to exercise in patients with chronic pain? Applying science to practice. Clin J Pain. 2015;31(2):108–14. https://doi.org/10.1097/ajp.0000000000000099.
59. Shen J, Fox LE, Cheng J. Swim therapy reduces mechanical allodynia and thermal hyperalgesia induced by chronic constriction nerve injury in rats. Pain Med. 2013;14(4):516–25. https://doi.org/10.1111/pme.12057. Accepted manuscript. Published online 20130225
60. Geneen LJ, Moore RA, Clarke C, Martin D, Colvin LA, Smith BH. Physical activity and exercise for chronic pain in adults: an overview of Cochrane reviews. Cochrane Database Syst Rev. 2017;1(1):CD011279. https://doi.org/10.1002/14651858.CD011279.pub2. Accepted manuscript. Published online 20170114.
61. Atilgan E, Kurt H, Algun ZC. Effect of yoga-based exercise program in female patients with myofascial pain of temporomandibular disorders. Clin Oral Investig. 2024;28(12):642. https://doi.org/10.1007/s00784-024-06045-y. Accepted manuscript. Published online 20241116
62. Nasri-Heir C, Patil AG, Korczeniewska OA, et al. The effect of nonstrenuous aerobic exercise in patients with chronic masticatory myalgia. J Oral Facial Pain Headache. 2019;33(2):143–52. https://doi.org/10.11607/ofph.2342. Accepted manuscript. Published online 20190206
63. Karimi R, Mallah N, Scherer R, Rodríguez-Cano R, Takkouche B. Sleep quality as a mediator of the relation between depression and chronic pain: a systematic review and meta-analysis. Br J Anaesth. 2023; https://doi.org/10.1016/j.bja.2023.02.036. Accepted manuscript. Published online 20230412

64. Weerakkody L, Lau J, Vegunta K, Thomas D, Balasubramaniam R. Genetics, lifestyle and psychosocial considerations in orofacial pain. 2024:639–657. https://doi.org/10.1002/9781119989233.ch35.
65. Arnstein P. Chronic neuropathic pain: issues in patient education. Pain Manag Nurs. 2004;5:34–41. https://doi.org/10.1016/j.pmn.2004.10.003.
66. Adams LM, Turk DC. Psychosocial factors and central sensitivity syndromes. Curr Rheumatol Rev. 2015;11(2):96–108. https://doi.org/10.2174/1573397111666150619095330.
67. Hawkins JL, Moore NJ, Miley D, Durham PL. Secondary traumatic stress increases expression of proteins implicated in peripheral and central sensitization of trigeminal neurons. Brain Res. 2018;1687:162–72. https://doi.org/10.1016/j.brainres.2018.03.003. Accepted manuscript. Published online 20180306
68. Bavarian R, Schatman ME, Kulich RJ. Posttraumatic stress disorder and the role of psychosocial comorbidities in chronic orofacial pain. Dent Clin N Am. 2023;67(1):141–55. https://doi.org/10.1016/j.cden.2022.07.011. Accepted manuscript. Published online 20221027
69. Al-Abeedi F, Aldahish Y, Almotawa Z, Kujan O. The differential diagnosis of Desquamative gingivitis: review of the literature and clinical guide for dental undergraduates. J Int Oral Health. 2015;7(Suppl 1):88–92.
70. Chen L, Michalsen A. Management of chronic pain using complementary and integrative medicine. BMJ. 2017:357. https://doi.org/10.1136/bmj.j1284.
71. McNeely JHL, Whitley SD, et al. Substance use screening, risk assessment, and use disorder diagnosis in adults. Johns Hopkins University; 2024. https://www.ncbi.nlm.nih.gov/books/NBK565474/
72. Schaffer J, Fogelman N, Seo D, Sinha R. Chronic pain, chronic stress and substance use: overlapping mechanisms and implications. Front Pain Res (Lausanne). 2023;4:1145934. https://doi.org/10.3389/fpain.2023.1145934. Accepted manuscript. Published online 20230621
73. LaRowe LR, Bakhshaie J, Greenberg J. Substance use among adults with chronic orofacial pain. J Clin Psychol Med Settings. 2024. Accepted manuscript. Published online 20241225. https://doi.org/10.1007/s10880-024-10062-0.
74. Hawkins JL, Denson JE, Miley DR, Durham PL. Nicotine stimulates expression of proteins implicated in peripheral and central sensitization. Neuroscience. 2015;290:115–25. https://doi.org/10.1016/j.neuroscience.2015.01.034. Accepted manuscript. Published online 20150128
75. Ditre JW, Brandon TH, Zale EL, Meagher MM. Pain, nicotine, and smoking: research findings and mechanistic considerations. Psychol Bull. 2011;137(6):1065–93. https://doi.org/10.1037/a0025544.
76. Miettinen O, Anttonen V, Patinen P, Päkkilä J, Tjäderhane L, Sipilä K. Prevalence of temporomandibular disorder symptoms and their association with alcohol and smoking habits. J Oral Facial Pain Headache. 2017;31(31):30–6. https://doi.org/10.11607/ofph.1595.
77. Zvolensky MJ, Rogers AH, Garey L, Shepherd JM, Ditre JW. Opioid misuse among smokers with chronic pain: relations with substance use and mental health. Behav Med. 2021;47(4):335–43. https://doi.org/10.1080/08964289.2020.1742642. Accepted manuscript. Published online 20200617
78. Voon P, Karamouzian M, Kerr T. Chronic pain and opioid misuse: a review of reviews. Subst Abuse Treat Prev Policy. 2017;12(1):36. https://doi.org/10.1186/s13011-017-0120-7. Accepted manuscript. Published online 20170815
79. Teoh L, Moses G, McCullough MJ. A review and guide to drug-associated oral adverse effects-dental, salivary and neurosensory reactions. Part 1. J Oral Pathol Med. 2019;48(7):626–36. https://doi.org/10.1111/jop.12911. Accepted manuscript. Published online 20190628
80. Italia J. Living with chronic orofacial pain through a social relational lens: a qualitative phenomenological exploration. McGill University; 2017. Accessed 27/02/2025. https://escholarship.mcgill.ca/downloads/7p88ck07w.pdf
81. Ashton-James CE, Anderson SR, Mackey SC, Darnall BD. Beyond pain, distress, and disability: the importance of social outcomes in pain management research and practice. Pain. 2022;163(3):e426–31. https://doi.org/10.1097/j.pain.0000000000002404.

82. Nicolson PJA, Williamson E, Morris A, et al. Musculoskeletal pain and loneliness, social support and social engagement among older adults: analysis of the Oxford pain, activity and lifestyle cohort. Musculoskeletal Care. 2021;19(3):269–77. https://doi.org/10.1002/msc.1526. Accepted manuscript. Published online 20201117
83. Bair MJ, Matthias MS, Nyland KA, et al. Barriers and facilitators to chronic pain self-management: a qualitative study of primary care patients with comorbid musculoskeletal pain and depression. Pain Med. 2009;10(7):1280–90. https://doi.org/10.1111/j.1526-4637.2009.00707.x.
84. Penlington CO, Ohrbach R. Biopsychosocial assessment and management of persistent orofacial pain. Oral Surg. 2020;13:349–57. https://orofacialpain.org.uk/wp-content/uploads/2021/10/Link-6-Biopsychosocial-Mx-OFP.pdf
85. Yeung EW, Arewasikporn A, Zautra AJ. Resilience and chronic pain. J Soc Clin Psychol. 2012;31(6):593–617. https://doi.org/10.1521/jscp.2012.31.6.593.
86. Boggero IA, Rojas-Ramirez MV, de Leeuw R, Carlson CR. Satisfaction with life in Orofacial Pain disorders: associations and theoretical implications. J Oral Facial Pain Headache. 2016;30(2):99–106. https://doi.org/10.11607/ofph.1526.
87. Serón-Arbeloa C, Labarta-Monzón L, Puzo-Foncillas J, et al. Malnutrition screening and assessment. Nutrients. 2022;14(12) https://doi.org/10.3390/nu14122392. Accepted manuscript. Published online 20220609.
88. Shivappa N, Steck SE, Hurley TG, Hussey JR, Hébert JR. Designing and developing a literature-derived, population-based dietary inflammatory index. Public Health Nutr. 2014;17(8):1689–96. https://doi.org/10.1017/s1368980013002115. Accepted manuscript. Published online 20130814
89. Cleeland CS, Ryan KM. Pain assessment: global use of the brief Pain inventory. Ann Acad Med Singap. 1994;23(2):129–38.
90. Craig CL, Marshall AL, Sjöström M, et al. International physical activity questionnaire: 12-country reliability and validity. Med Sci Sports Exerc. 2003;35(8):1381–95. https://doi.org/10.1249/01.Mss.0000078924.61453.Fb.
91. Parker R, Bergman E, Mntambo A, Stubbs S, Wills M. Levels of physical activity in people with chronic pain. S Afr J Physiother. 2017;73(1):323. Accepted manuscript. Published online 20170331. https://doi.org/10.4102/sajp.v73i1.323.
92. Waddell G, Newton M, Henderson I, Somerville D, Main CJ. A fear-avoidance beliefs questionnaire (FABQ) and the role of fear-avoidance beliefs in chronic low back pain and disability. Pain. 1993;52(2):157–68. https://doi.org/10.1016/0304-3959(93)90127-b.
93. Du H, Newton PJ, Salamonson Y, Carrieri-Kohlman VL, Davidson PM. A review of the six-minute walk test: its implication as a self-administered assessment tool. Eur J Cardiovasc Nurs. 2009;8(1):2–8. https://doi.org/10.1016/j.ejcnurse.2008.07.001. Accepted manuscript. Published online 20080809
94. Morin CM, Belleville G, Bélanger L, Ivers H. The insomnia severity index: psychometric indicators to detect insomnia cases and evaluate treatment response. Sleep. 2011;34(5):601–8. https://doi.org/10.1093/sleep/34.5.601. Accepted manuscript. Published online 20110501
95. Buysse DJ, Reynolds CF, Monk TH, Berman SR, Kupfer DJ. The Pittsburgh Sleep Quality Index (PSQI): a new instrument for psychiatric research and practice. Psychiatry Res. 1989;28(2):193–213. https://www.sleep.pitt.edu/instruments/
96. Kroenke K, Spitzer RL, Williams JB. The PHQ-9: validity of a brief depression severity measure. J Gen Intern Med. 2001;16(9):606–13. https://doi.org/10.1046/j.1525-1497.2001.016009606.x.
97. Richter P, Werner J, Heerlein A, Kraus A, Sauer H. On the validity of the Beck depression inventory. A review. Psychopathology. 1998;31(3):160–8. https://doi.org/10.1159/000066239.
98. Bohlmeijer E, ten Klooster PM, Fledderus M, Veehof M, Baer R. Psychometric properties of the five facet mindfulness questionnaire in depressed adults and development of a short form. Assessment. 2011;18(3):308–20. https://doi.org/10.1177/1073191111408231. Accepted manuscript. Published online 20110517

99. Humeniuk REH-ES, Ali RL, Poznyak V, Monteiro M. The alcohol, smoking and substance involvement screening test (ASSIST). Manual for use in primary care 2010. Accessed 03/03/2025. https://iris.who.int/bitstream/handle/10665/44320/9789241599382_eng.pdf?sequence=1
100. Newcombe DA, Humeniuk RE, Ali R. Validation of the World Health Organization alcohol, smoking and substance involvement screening test (ASSIST): report of results from the Australian site. Drug Alcohol Rev. 2005;24(3):217–26. https://doi.org/10.1080/09595230500170266.
101. Lozano-Hernández CM, Cladellas YP, Gil Conesa M, Garin O, Forés MF, Del Cura-González I. Functional social support: a systematic review and standardized comparison of different versions of the DUFSS questionnaire using the EMPRO tool. PLoS One. 2023;18(9):e0291635. https://doi.org/10.1371/journal.pone.0291635. Accepted manuscript. Published online 20230915.
102. Watts R, Kettner H, Geerts D, et al. The Watts connectedness scale: a new scale for measuring a sense of connectedness to self, others, and world. Psychopharmacology. 2022;239(11):3461–83. https://doi.org/10.1007/s00213-022-06187-5.
103. IASP. Pain Management Center – Chapter 1. 2021. Accessed 03/03/2025. https://www.iasp-pain.org/resources/toolkits/pain-management-center/chapter1/
104. Self-managing chronic pain. 2016. Accessed 03/03/2025. http://painaustralia.staging3.webforcefive.com.au/static/uploads/files/painaust-factsheet10-final-wfecivdrvvtm.pdf.
105. Joypaul SKF, McMillan SS, King MA. Multi-disciplinary interventions for chronic pain involving education: a systematic review. PLoS One. 2019;14(10):e0223306. https://doi.org/10.1371/journal.pone.0223306.
106. Moseley LMD, Chisholm S. Tame the beast. Online 2024. Accessed 05/03/2025. https://www.tamethebeast.org
107. Kerns RD, Burgess DJ, Coleman BC, et al. Self-management of chronic pain: psychologically guided core competencies for providers. Pain Med. 2022;23(11):1815–9. https://doi.org/10.1093/pm/pnac083.
108. Trouvin AP, Attal N, Perrot S. Lifestyle and chronic pain: double jeopardy? Br J Anaesth. 2022;129(3):278–81. https://doi.org/10.1016/j.bja.2022.06.006. Accepted manuscript. Published online 20220706
109. Philpot U, Johnson MI. Diet therapy in the management of chronic pain: better diet less pain? Pain Manag. 2019;9(4):335–8. https://doi.org/10.2217/pmt-2019-0014. Accepted manuscript. Published online 20190619
110. Chronic Pain Management Strategies. 2023. Accessed 03/03/2025. https://aci.health.nsw.gov.au/__data/assets/pdf_file/0020/216308/Chronic_Pain_Management_Strategies.pdf
111. Organization WH. WHO guidelines on physical activity and sedentary behaviour. Geneva; 2025. Accessed 05/03/2025. https://www.who.int/multi-media/details/who-guidelines-on-physical-activity-and-sedentary-behaviour
112. Organization WH. Physical activity. Online 2025. Accessed 05/03/2025. https://www.who.int/initiatives/behealthy/physical-activity#:~:text=For%20additional%20health%20benefits%2C%20adults,or%20more%20days%20a%20week
113. IASP. Physical activity for pain prevention. Online 2025. Accessed 05/03/2025. https://www.iasp-pain.org/resources/fact-sheets/physical-activity-for-pain-prevention/
114. Gupta CC, Sprajcer M, Johnston-Devin C, Ferguson SA. Sleep hygiene strategies for individuals with chronic pain: a scoping review. BMJ Open. 2023;13(2):e060401. https://doi.org/10.1136/bmjopen-2021-060401. Accepted manuscript. Published online 20230202.
115. Hopper SI, Murray SL, Ferrara LR, Singleton JK. Effectiveness of diaphragmatic breathing for reducing physiological and psychological stress in adults: a quantitative systematic review. JBI Database System Rev Implement Rep. 2019;17(9):1855–76. https://doi.org/10.11124/jbisrir-2017-003848.
116. Büssing A, Ostermann T, Lüdtke R, Michalsen A. Effects of yoga interventions on pain and pain-associated disability: a meta-analysis. J Pain. 2012;13(1):1–9. https://doi.org/10.1016/j.jpain.2011.10.001. Accepted manuscript. Published online 20111216

117. Kong LJ, Lauche R, Klose P, et al. Tai Chi for chronic pain conditions: a systematic review and meta-analysis of randomized controlled trials. Sci Rep. 2016;6:25325. https://doi.org/10.1038/srep25325. Accepted manuscript. Published online 20160429
118. Jinich-Diamant A, Garland E, Baumgartner J, et al. Neurophysiological mechanisms supporting mindfulness meditation-based pain relief: an updated review. Curr Pain Headache Rep. 2020;24(10):56. Accepted manuscript. Published online 20200817. https://doi.org/10.1007/s11916-020-00890-8.
119. Koulivand PH, Khaleghi Ghadiri M, Gorji A. Lavender and the nervous system. Evid Based Complement Alternat Med. 2013;2013:681304. https://doi.org/10.1155/2013/681304. Accepted manuscript. Published online 20130314
120. Yoo O, Park SA. Anxiety-reducing effects of lavender essential oil inhalation: a systematic review. Healthcare (Basel). 2023;11(22) https://doi.org/10.3390/healthcare11222978. Accepted manuscript. Published online 20231117
121. Organization WH. Doing what matters in times of stress. Geneva; 2020. Accessed 10/03/2025. https://www.who.int/news-room/questions-and-answers/item/stress
122. Health NIoM. Caring for your mental Health. US 2025. Accessed 25/03/2025. https://www.nimh.nih.gov/health/topics/caring-for-your-mental-health
123. Organization WH. mhGAP Intervention Guide for mental, neurological and substance use disorders in non-specialized health settings. 2016. https://iris.who.int/bitstream/handle/10665/250239/9789241549790-eng.pdf?sequence=1
124. Lifeline. 988 Lifeline. Online 2025. Accessed 23/03/2025. https://988lifeline.org/
125. Samaritans. Samaritans. Online 2025. Accessed 23/03/2025. https://www.samaritans.org/
126. Blue B. Beyond Blue. Online 2024. Accessed 23/03/2025. https://www.beyondblue.org.au/
127. Organization WH. Global status report on alcohol and health and treatment of substance use disorders. 2024. https://iris.who.int/bitstream/handle/10665/377960/9789240096745-eng.pdf?sequence=1
128. Services USDoAaUSDoHaH. Dietary guidelines for Americans, 2020–2025. Services USDoAaUSDoHaH 2020. Accessed 25/03/2025. https://www.dietaryguidelines.gov/
129. Government UK. Chapter 12: Alcohol. United Kingdom. 2021. Accessed 25/03/2025. https://www.gov.uk/government/publications/delivering-better-oral-health-an-evidence-based-toolkit-for-prevention/chapter-12-alcohol#guidelines-on-alcohol
130. Australia Co. Australian alcohol guidelines revised. Online 2020. Accessed 05/03/2025. https://www.health.gov.au/news/australian-alcohol-guidelines-revised
131. Organization WH. Brief Intervention for Substance Use: A Manual For Use In Primary Care. 2005. Accessed 05/03/2025. https://swsphn.com.au/wp-content/uploads/2021/12/Draft_Brief_Intervention_for_Substance_Use.pdf
132. Organization WH. WHO clinical treatment guideline for tobacco cessation in adults. 2024. Accessed 24/03/2025. https://iris.who.int/bitstream/handle/10665/377825/9789240096431-eng.pdf?sequence=4
133. Australia Co. National Tobacco Strategy 2023–2030. 2023. Accessed 06/03/2025. https://www.health.gov.au/sites/default/files/2023-05/national-tobacco-strategy-2023-2030.pdf
134. Foundation USP. Pain Connection. Online 2022. Accessed 23/03/2025. https://painconnection.org/
135. Concern P. Pain Concern. Online 2025. Accessed 23/03/2025. https://painconcern.org.uk/
136. Australia P. Pain Australia. Online 2025. Accessed 23/03/2025. https://www.painaustralia.org.au/
137. Society PB. Pain BC. Online 2025. Accessed 23/03/2025. https://painbc.ca/

Future Opportunities: Telemedicine and Digital Technology for Lifestyle Shifts

25

Sanjana Bhardwaj and Sonali Kohli

25.1 Introduction

Lifestyle denotes the typical way of life of an individual, group, or culture. These patterns of living, encompassing choices in diet, physical activity, social interactions, and stress management, exert a significant influence on an individual's overall well-being, affecting their physical, mental, emotional, and spiritual health. Furthermore, it incorporates habits, which are regular activities and routines, and attitudes, reflecting beliefs and opinions, as well as preferences in areas such as food, music, art, and literature. Material possessions also serve as indicators of lifestyle choices, evident in the way individuals decorate their homes and the personal items they own.

The fundamental principles that guide an individual's behavior and the decisions they make daily are integral to their lifestyle. This is often reflected in regular engagement in physical exercise, adherence to a balanced diet, and the maintenance of consistent sleep patterns. Lifestyle shifts involve making sustained modifications to habits, routines, and overall ways of life with the primary goal of enhancing well-being. These changes typically focus on key areas such as dietary habits, sleep quality, exercise frequency, stress management techniques, and engagement in social activities.

The connection between oral health and lifestyle choices is undeniable. Dietary choices, particularly the consumption of sugary and acidic foods and beverages, along with habits such as alcohol consumption and smoking, are strongly associated with poor oral health and represent significant risk factors for the development of oral diseases [1]. The Global Burden of Disease 2021 report highlighted that untreated dental caries (tooth decay) in permanent teeth is the most prevalent health

S. Bhardwaj (✉)
Gates Foundation, Washington, USA

S. Kohli
Sir H N Reliance Foundation Hospital, Mumbai, India

S. R. Prabhu et al. (eds.), *Lifestyle in Oral Health and Disease*,
https://doi.org/10.1007/978-3-032-05888-1_25

condition worldwide. Oral diseases share a range of modifiable risk factors with many noncommunicable diseases (NCDs), including sugar intake, tobacco use, alcohol consumption, and inadequate oral hygiene practices, all of which are influenced by underlying social and commercial determinants [1].

The various facets of an individual's life are interwoven, and alterations in one area frequently trigger a sequence of effects in others. For instance, adopting a healthier diet not only benefits oral health by reducing sugar intake but can also lead to increased energy levels, which in turn may encourage more physical activity. This interconnectedness underscores the importance of considering lifestyle as a holistic entity when designing interventions for improving oral health.

25.2 The Current Landscape: Lifestyle Choices and Oral Health Outcomes

Current lifestyle trends are significantly impacting global oral health. The consumption of diets high in free sugars is a primary driver of dental caries, while tobacco use is a major cause of periodontal (gum) disease and a leading risk factor for oral cancer [2]. Alcohol consumption also contributes to poor oral health outcomes.

The WHO Global Oral Health Status Report (2022) estimated that approximately 3.5 billion people globally are affected by oral diseases, with a disproportionately high number residing in middle-income countries. Globally, an estimated 2 billion individuals suffer from caries in their permanent teeth, and 514 million children experience caries in their primary teeth.

As per the World Health Organization (WHO), the prevalence of oral diseases continues to rise globally, fueled by increasing urbanization and changes in living conditions. This rise is largely attributed to insufficient exposure to fluoride (in water supplies and oral hygiene products), the widespread availability and affordability of foods with high sugar content, and inadequate access to oral healthcare services within communities. The aggressive marketing of food and beverages high in sugar, as well as tobacco and alcohol products, has further exacerbated the problem by promoting increased consumption of these detrimental substances. Key oral health diseases resulting from these trends include dental caries (tooth decay), periodontal (gum) disease, edentulism (total tooth loss), oral cancer, and orodental trauma.

Research has demonstrated a clear link between oral health and overall wellbeing. A study involving a large group of patients attending general dental practices revealed that a decline in oral health often correlates with a decline in general health. This study also provided further evidence supporting the association between high-risk lifestyle factors such as smoking and heavy alcohol consumption and adverse oral health outcomes. Furthermore, another study indicated that providing health guidance on effective tooth brushing techniques, the importance of quitting smoking, and the management of obesity could be effective in preventing the development of periodontal disease in adults [3].

A global review of oral health highlighted that despite improvements in some countries, oral health problems persist, particularly among underprivileged groups in both developing and developed nations [4]. In developing countries, oral health services are often concentrated in urban centers, with limited emphasis on preventive or restorative dental care [5]. Many of these countries face a shortage of oral health professionals, and the capacity of their healthcare systems is largely limited to providing pain relief or emergency care. For instance, in Africa, the dentist-to-population ratio is approximately 1:150,000, compared to about 1:2000 in most industrialized countries [6].

The economic burden of oral diseases is substantial. Traditional treatment of these conditions is costly, ranking as the fourth most expensive disease to treat in most industrialized countries [5]. Numerous epidemiological surveys have highlighted the significant role of socio-behavioral and environmental factors in the development of oral diseases [4]. Modifiable risk factors such as high consumption of sugary foods, low fluoride exposure, and tobacco use are common to many chronic diseases, including cardiovascular diseases, cancer, diabetes, and oral diseases [5]. Tobacco use, for example, is estimated to cause over 90% of oral cavity cancers and is associated with worsened periodontal disease, poorer oral hygiene, and premature tooth loss [5]. The increasing prevalence of oral diseases and their detrimental impact on individuals and communities, causing pain, functional impairment, and reduced quality of life, is a significant concern. Given the high cost of treating oral diseases, a proactive approach focusing on preventing these conditions through lifestyle modifications could yield substantial economic benefits for both individuals and healthcare systems.

Over the decades, oral health providers have consistently offered preventative advice aimed at improving oral hygiene and addressing these risk factors. The common risk factor approach emphasizes addressing these shared risk factors within the broader socio-environmental context. Oral health is significantly influenced by diet, hygiene practices, smoking habits, alcohol consumption, stress levels, and trauma. Since these factors are also implicated in several other chronic diseases, a collaborative, integrated approach is more effective than addressing each disease in isolation. Considering the rising consumption of sugars and inadequate fluoride exposure, coupled with the increasing prevalence of chronic diseases like diabetes and cardiovascular illnesses associated with dietary habits, exercise patterns, and sleep routines, the incidence of dental caries is likely to increase. This challenge is compounded by the shortage of healthcare providers and the limitations of existing health systems in providing preventative care to populations.

25.3 Telemedicine and Digital Technology: A Transformative Force in Healthcare

Digital technology encompasses the use of electronic tools and systems for the creation, storage, processing, and communication of information. This includes a wide array of components such as software applications, hardware devices, Internet technologies, and various digital platforms. Telemedicine, or telehealth, represents the application of technology to deliver healthcare services remotely. This approach enables patients to connect with healthcare providers via video conferencing or telephone for consultations, diagnoses, and treatment plans, effectively bridging the geographical gap between the provider and the patient and addressing traditional barriers to accessing care.

Telemedicine offers several key advantages beyond mere accessibility. It often proves to be less expensive than traditional in-person visits, leading to increased cost-effectiveness and improved efficiency within the healthcare system. It provides the opportunity for real-time consultations via phone, including video interactions, allowing for immediate communication and assessment. Furthermore, telemedicine facilitates the secure transfer of photographs, reports, images, and other relevant data for review by specialists, enhancing diagnostic capabilities and collaborative care. Continuous remote monitoring of patients' health data, such as vital signs and medication adherence, is another significant benefit, enabling proactive management of chronic conditions and timely intervention when necessary.

The implementation of telemedicine significantly supports efforts to enhance the quality of healthcare by improving accessibility and efficiency. It reduces the need for patients to travel to healthcare facilities, provides crucial clinical support to remote areas, overcomes geographical limitations, offers various communication modalities, and ultimately contributes to improved patient outcomes [7]. Given the ongoing challenges related to health financing and competing priorities, and in the pursuit of greater equity in the quality and accessibility of healthcare for all segments of the population, telemedicine stands out as a vital tool [7].

There are four primary clinical applications of telemedicine: (1) real-time interactive mode, (2) store-and-forward mode, (3) remote monitoring, and (4) communication via telephone [8].

Real-time telemedicine enables patients and providers to connect and interact simultaneously, sharing data between locations. This might involve the use of specially equipped computers connected via telephone lines to facilitate live video and audio communication. The store-and-forward mode allows for the capture, storage, and electronic transmission of patient information to a specialist or provider at a different location for subsequent interpretation and feedback. This method is particularly useful for asynchronous consultations, such as dermatology or radiology reviews. Remote monitoring involves the use of devices that continuously record patient data in real-time and transmit this information to their healthcare providers. This can be invaluable for tracking conditions such as chest pain or shortness of breath in patients with cardiovascular illnesses. Finally, communication via telephone can be critical in emergency situations, allowing patients to immediately notify their physician and receive timely advice and treatment instructions. These diverse applications demonstrate the versatility of telemedicine in addressing a wide range of healthcare needs.

25.4 Future Opportunities: Leveraging Telemedicine and Digital Technology for Lifestyle Shifts in Oral Health

Telemedicine and digital technology present significant opportunities to revolutionize oral healthcare by fostering positive lifestyle shifts and improving oral health outcomes.

Virtual consultations with dental professionals and health coaches can offer tailored advice on essential oral hygiene techniques, such as proper tooth brushing and flossing [9]. Individuals can receive real-time feedback and demonstrations, ensuring they are employing effective methods to remove plaque and maintain healthy gums. Furthermore, personalized dietary recommendations specifically geared towards oral health can be delivered remotely. These recommendations can focus on strategies to reduce the intake of sugary and acidic foods and drinks [1], which are major contributors to dental caries. Telemedicine platforms can also be utilized to deliver support and resources for smoking cessation and alcohol reduction, addressing key lifestyle factors that negatively impact oral health.

The potential for remote monitoring and early intervention in oral healthcare is substantial. Wearable devices could be developed to track oral hygiene behaviors, such as the frequency and duration of tooth brushing, providing valuable data for both individuals and their dental professionals. Smartphone applications can be designed for self-assessment of oral health, allowing users to identify potential issues early on and prompting them with reminders for regular oral hygiene practices. Teledentistry platforms can facilitate the remote monitoring of high-risk patients, such as those with diabetes who are more susceptible to periodontal disease [10], or individuals undergoing orthodontic treatment, ensuring timely intervention and management. The integration of artificial intelligence (AI)-powered tools capable of analyzing images of the oral cavity, captured by smartphone cameras or other devices, holds promise for the early detection of potential oral health problems, enabling proactive care.

Digital platforms offer an engaging and accessible means of delivering educational content on oral health and its crucial link to lifestyle [11]. This can include informative videos, interactive modules, and personalized feedback mechanisms to enhance understanding and promote behavior change. Gamification and rewards systems integrated into oral health apps can serve as powerful motivators, encouraging users to adopt and maintain positive oral hygiene habits and track their progress. Virtual support groups and online communities can connect individuals facing similar challenges in adopting healthier oral health-related lifestyles, providing a platform for peer support, sharing experiences, and fostering a sense of accountability.

Integrating telemedicine-based oral health interventions with broader digital health initiatives targeting diet, exercise, sleep, and stress management can create synergistic benefits. Comprehensive digital platforms that offer a holistic approach to lifestyle modification, incorporating oral health components alongside other wellness features, can lead to more effective and sustainable behavior change. Furthermore, the opportunity for seamless collaboration between dental and medical professionals through shared digital platforms can facilitate a more comprehensive and integrated approach to patient care, recognizing the interconnectedness of oral and systemic health [12]. This shift towards a proactive, preventative model, empowered by personalized guidance, remote monitoring, and accessible education, has the potential to significantly improve long-term oral health outcomes and reduce overall healthcare costs. The integration of oral health into broader digital wellness programs can harness the combined effects of various lifestyle modifications, leading to more substantial improvements in both oral and overall health. For instance, dietary changes made for oral health benefits can also positively impact weight management and blood sugar control, while increased physical activity encouraged for overall well-being can also reduce stress levels, potentially mitigating habits like teeth grinding.

25.5 Research Evidence and Emerging Trends

The potential of telemedicine and digital technology to facilitate lifestyle shifts in oral health is supported by a growing body of research and emerging trends in healthcare. A systematic review by Ezeamii [13] highlighted the transformative role of telemedicine in chronic disease management, particularly in diabetes care. This finding has significant implications for managing oral health in individuals with diabetes, who are at a higher risk of developing periodontal disease and other oral health issues. The review by Jadhav and Choure [14] on remote healthcare using digital technology identified key emerging trends, including the integration of telemedicine with traditional healthcare through hybrid models, addressing global health disparities, prioritizing patient-centered care, and even environmental benefits. These trends are directly applicable to the future of oral healthcare delivery, suggesting the potential for reaching underserved populations and tailoring care to individual needs.

Research has also demonstrated the effectiveness of telemedicine in improving intervention programs focused on key lifestyle components such as eating habits, physical activity, and sleep [15, 16]. A study by Marquez (2022) investigated the impact of a telehealth-based educational intervention on the lifestyle, body mass index, and glucose concentration of university staff during the Coronavirus Disease-2019 (COVID-19) pandemic. The results indicated that such interventions can be effective in improving lifestyles and achieving adequate body mass index and glucose levels, suggesting its potential for promoting healthy oral health behaviors as well. Calcaterra (2021) explored the use of telehealth to support increased self-monitoring and behavioral change, providing opportunities for online nutritional support and exercise training programs to promote healthy lifestyles and reduce sedentary behaviors in children and adolescents. This approach can be particularly beneficial for individuals in rural areas with limited access to traditional lifestyle services targeting behavior change, including those related to oral health.

Table 25.1 summarizes key studies and their relevance to the integration of telemedicine and digital technology for lifestyle shifts in oral health.

Table 25.1 Key studies and their relevance to the integration of telemedicine and digital technology for lifestyle shifts in oral health

Study (Reference)	Focus	Key findings	Relevance to oral health and telemedicine
Ezeamii (2024) [13]	Telemedicine in chronic disease management (diabetes)	Improved patient outcomes, access to care, and role in evolving healthcare	Suggests potential for similar positive impacts on oral health management, especially for individuals with diabetes who are at higher risk of oral health issues
Jadhav and Choure (2024) [14]	Remote healthcare using digital technology	Integration with traditional healthcare, addressing health disparities, patient-centered care, and environmental benefits	Highlights the potential for hybrid models of oral healthcare delivery, reaching underserved populations with digital tools, and focusing on patient needs and convenience
Marquez (2022) [15]	Telehealth intervention for lifestyle improvement (university staff)	Effective in improving lifestyles, body mass index (BMI), and glucose levels; feasible and associated with positive outcomes in promoting healthy lifestyles	Demonstrates the potential of telehealth-based educational interventions for promoting healthy oral health behaviors and improving related health indicators in various populations
Calcaterra (2021) [16]	Telehealth for lifestyle interventions in children and adolescents	Supports self-monitoring, behavioral change, online nutritional support, and exercise training; improves access in rural areas	Shows promise for using telehealth to address challenges in providing oral health services, especially in promoting healthy habits and reaching individuals with limited access to traditional care
Kitigawa (2017) [3]	Health guidance for periodontal disease prevention	Guidance on tooth brushing, smoking cessation, and obesity control may be effective in preventing periodontal disease in adults	Suggests specific areas where telemedicine interventions can focus to prevent periodontal disease through remote education and support
Yu et al. (2024) [17]	Self-reported oral health and systemic comorbidities	Fair or poor self-rated oral health associated with increased risk of cardiovascular disease (CVD), diabetes, and osteoporosis, and increased all-cause mortality	Highlights the importance of monitoring self-reported oral health through digital tools and the potential for early identification of individuals at risk for systemic diseases
Li et al. (2022) [18]	Oral microbiota and cardiometabolic health	Periodontal disease significantly associated with CVD, with dysbiotic oral bacteria and systemic inflammatory responses as primary mechanisms	Emphasizes the systemic implications of poor oral health and the potential for telemedicine to facilitate early intervention and management of oral health to reduce cardiometabolic risk

(continued)

Table 25.1 (continued)

Study (Reference)	Focus	Key findings	Relevance to oral health and telemedicine
Xi et al. (2024) [19]	Periodontal bacteria influence systemic diseases via gut microbiota	Oral infections can occur in distant sites, including the gut, potentially contributing to inflammatory and cardiometabolic diseases	Further highlights the systemic impact of oral health and suggests that telemedicine interventions focusing on oral hygiene and lifestyle can have broader benefits for overall health by influencing the oral–gut axis
VanWormer et al. (2014) [20]	Oral hygiene and cardiometabolic risk reduction	Daily toothbrushing and interdental cleaning lowered the risk of developing type 2 diabetes or hypertension in adults	Reinforces the importance of promoting proper oral hygiene through telemedicine-based education and reminders as a strategy for reducing the risk of major chronic diseases

A significant emerging trend is the increasing recognition of the close and often bidirectional relationship between oral and systemic health. This understanding, coupled with the growing evidence supporting the effectiveness of telemedicine and digital interventions in managing chronic conditions and promoting healthy behaviors, creates a promising environment for innovation in oral healthcare delivery.

25.6 Addressing Risk Factors and Health Inequalities Through Digital Solutions

Telemedicine and digital tools offer unique capabilities to address the modifiable risk factors that contribute to poor oral health. Targeted digital interventions can be developed to support smoking cessation, utilizing apps that provide resources, track progress, and offer virtual counselling and remote monitoring. Personalized digital nutrition programs can focus on educating individuals about the impact of sugar on oral health and guide them in adopting a balanced diet that promotes oral well-being. Wearable activity trackers and exercise applications can encourage individuals to engage in regular physical activity which has indirect benefits for oral health by reducing inflammation and improving overall health. Furthermore, digital tools for stress management, such as mindfulness apps and platforms offering virtual therapy, can help individuals cope with stress, which can negatively impact oral health.

These technologies also hold immense potential for reaching underserved populations and thereby reducing health disparities in oral healthcare. Telemedicine can overcome geographical barriers, providing access to dental professionals and crucial health education for individuals residing in rural or remote areas where traditional dental services may be scarce [5]. Low-cost mobile health (mHealth) solutions, accessible via basic smartphones, can reach individuals with limited access to more sophisticated healthcare infrastructure. Multilingual digital resources can be developed to cater to the diverse linguistic needs of various populations, ensuring that information is accessible and understandable. Collaborations with community health workers and public health organizations can facilitate the dissemination of digital oral health information and help individuals in underserved communities access teledentistry services.

By providing personalized digital interventions that target modifiable risk factors, there is a significant opportunity to prevent the onset and progression of oral diseases. This proactive approach can ultimately reduce the burden on healthcare systems and lead to improved overall health and well-being for vulnerable populations [14].

25.7 The Oral–Systemic Health Connection: A Holistic Perspective

The relationship between oral health and overall systemic health is increasingly recognized as bidirectional and profoundly interconnected. Poor oral health has been shown to contribute to or worsen a range of systemic conditions, including diabetes, heart disease, stroke, respiratory illnesses, and even certain types of cancer. Conversely, systemic diseases can also manifest in the oral cavity, such as the development of oral lesions in individuals with HIV/AIDS or an increased susceptibility to gum disease in those with diabetes.

Positive lifestyle shifts in oral health, facilitated by telemedicine and digital technology, can have far-reaching benefits in the prevention and management of chronic diseases. Improving oral hygiene practices and reducing inflammation in the mouth through telemedicine-guided interventions may potentially lower the risk or improve the management of cardiovascular diseases and diabetes. Telemedicine can also play a crucial role in promoting smoking cessation and healthier dietary habits [1], which not only benefit oral health but also reduce the risk of multiple chronic diseases. Furthermore, telemedicine provides an effective platform for raising awareness among patients about the critical oral–systemic link, encouraging them to adopt healthier lifestyles for the sake of their overall well-being [21].

Recognizing and addressing the oral–systemic connection through telemedicine offers a more integrated and comprehensive approach to healthcare, moving beyond the traditional focus on treating isolated conditions. This holistic perspective acknowledges the intricate ways in which the body's systems interact and influence one another. By prioritizing lifestyle modifications for oral health through telemedicine, the potential exists to not only improve oral health outcomes but also prevent or mitigate the severity of a wide spectrum of chronic diseases, leading to significant advancements in public health and a reduction in the overall burden of disease.

25.8 Challenges, Ethical Considerations and the Future Roadmap

While the integration of telemedicine and digital technology into oral healthcare for lifestyle shifts presents numerous opportunities, several challenges and ethical considerations must be addressed to ensure widespread and effective adoption. One significant challenge is digital literacy, particularly among older adults and underserved populations who may lack the necessary skills or access to technology to fully utilize digital health tools. Data privacy and security are also paramount concerns, as the collection and transmission of personal health information require robust safeguards to protect patient confidentiality. The development of clear and comprehensive regulatory frameworks and guidelines for the delivery of teledentistry and digital oral health interventions is essential to ensure quality of care and patient safety. There is also a risk that the digital divide could exacerbate existing health inequalities if the implementation of these technologies does not prioritize accessibility and inclusivity for all. Finally, while telemedicine offers many benefits, it is important to acknowledge the limitations of remote examinations and to maintain a balanced approach that integrates virtual care with necessary in-person consultations and treatments.

Future research should focus on rigorously evaluating the long-term effectiveness and cost-effectiveness of telemedicine-based lifestyle interventions for oral health. Studies are needed to develop and validate AI-powered tools for accurate and reliable remote oral health assessment and monitoring. Understanding the experiences of both patients and providers with teledentistry and digital oral health platforms is crucial for optimizing their design and implementation. Research should also explore the seamless integration of oral health data with electronic health records to provide a more complete and holistic view of a patient's overall health status.

Successful implementation of telemedicine and digital technology in oral healthcare will require strategic investments in digital infrastructure and training programs to enhance digital literacy among both patients and healthcare providers. The development of user-friendly and accessible digital oral health tools that are intuitive and cater to diverse needs is essential. Establishing clear ethical guidelines and robust regulatory frameworks specifically for teledentistry will be critical for building trust and ensuring responsible use of these technologies. Collaborative efforts involving dental professionals, medical practitioners, technology developers, and policymakers are necessary to ensure the successful and sustainable integration of telemedicine and digital solutions into the broader healthcare system.

25.9 Conclusion

Telemedicine and digital technology hold immense transformative potential for fostering positive lifestyle shifts that can significantly improve oral health and overall well-being. This approach offers a unique and compelling vision for the future of healthcare, moving towards a model that is increasingly proactive, personalized, and accessible. By leveraging the power of digital tools, individuals can receive tailored guidance, engage in remote monitoring, access valuable educational resources, and connect with healthcare professionals from the convenience of their own homes. This shift towards digital innovation in oral healthcare promises to empower individuals to take greater control of their oral health, leading to healthier lifestyles and improved quality of life for all.

References

1. WHO Health Topics. Oral health – World Health Organization (WHO). 2024. https://www.who.int/health-topics/oral-health.
2. WHO Fact Sheet. Oral health – World Health Organization (WHO). https://www.who.int/news-room/fact-sheets/detail/oral-health.
3. Kitagawa M, et al. Relationship between general health, lifestyle, oral health and periodontal disease in adults: a large cross sectional study in Japan. Bull Tokyo Dent Coll. 2017;58:1–2.
4. Petersen PE. The World Oral Health Report 2003: continuous improvement of oral health in the 21st century – the approach of the WHO Global Oral Health Programme. Community Dent Oral Epidemiol. 2003;31(Suppl 1):3–24.
5. Petersen PE. Sociobehavioural risk factors in dental caries – an international perspective. Community Dent Oral Epidemiol. 2005;33:274–9.
6. Petersen PE, et al. The global burden of oral diseases and risks to oral health. Bull World Health Organ. 2005;83(9):661–9.
7. Maryam A. Telemedicine and its role in revolutionizing healthcare delivery. Popul Health Equity Outcomes. 2017;5(1):e1–5.
8. McGonigle D, Mastrian KG. Nursing informatics and the foundation of knowledge. 2nd ed. Burlington: Jones and Bartlett Learning; 2011.
9. Home Oral Care | American Dental Association. https://www.ada.org/resources/ada-library/oral-health-topics/home-care.
10. Healthy Mouth, Healthy Body | National Institute of Dental and Caraniofacial Research. https://www.nidcr.nih.gov/news-events/nidcr-news/2024/healthy-mouth-healthy-body.
11. Kumar BJ, et al. Influence of lifestyle on dental health behaviour. J Lifestyle Med. 2019;9(2):119–24. https://doi.org/10.15280/jlm.2019.9.2.119.
12. National Association of Chronic Disease Directors. The connection between poor oral health and chronic disease. https://nursing.nyu.edu/sites/default/files/inline-files/connection-poor-oral-health-chronic-disease.pdf.
13. Ezeamii VC, et al. Revolutionizing healthcare: how telemedicine is improving patient outcomes and expanding access to care. Cureus. 2024;16(7):e63881. PMCID: PMC11298029 PMID: 39099901.
14. Jadhav OP, Choure V. Telemedicine: transforming healthcare delivery in the digital age. Int J Acad Med Pharm. 2024;6(3):565–71.
15. Marquez Neidis M, et al. Telehealth based interventions on lifestyle, body mass index, and glucose concentration in university staff during the coronavirus disease 2019 pandemic: a pre experimental study. Digit Health. 2022;8:20552076221129719. https://doi.org/10.1177/20552076221129719. PMCID: PMC9537489 PMID: 36211802.
16. Calcaterra V, et al. Telehealth: a useful tool for the management of nutrition and exercise programs in pediatric obesity in the COVID 19 era. Nutrients. 2021;13(11):3689. https://doi.org/10.3390/nu13113689. PMCID: PMC8618189 PMID: 34835945.

17. Yu YH, et al. Self-reported oral health is associated with systemic health outcomes and all-cause mortality. J Am Dent Assoc. 2024;155(3):233–43.e8. https://doi.org/10.1016/j.adaj.2023.11.006. https://pmc.ncbi.nlm.nih.gov/articles/PMC10932849/.
18. Oral Microbiome and Cardiometabolic Conditions | The Institute for ... https://www.ifm.org/articles/oral-microbiome-and-cardiometabolic. Accessed on 18 Mar 2025.
19. Xi M, et al. Periodontal bacteria influence systemic diseases through the gut microbiota. Front Cell Infect Microbiol. 2024;14:1478362. https://doi.org/10.3389/fcimb.2024.1478362. eCollection 2024.
20. VanWormer JJ, et al. Oral hygiene and cardiometabolic disease risk in the survey of the health of Wisconsin. Community Dent Oral Epidemiol. 2012;41(4):374–84. https://doi.org/10.1111/cdoe.12015.
21. www.deltadental.com. https://www.deltadental.com/content/dam/ddpa/us/en/state-of-america%27s-oral-health-and-wellness-report/2024%20State%20of%20America%27s%20Oral%20Health%20and%20Wellness%20Report.pdf. Accessed on 18 Mar 2025.

The Role of Health Care Providers in Preventing Lifestyle Disorders

26

Sanjana Bhardwaj and Latasha Treger Slavin

26.1 Introduction

Lifestyle disorders are described as a set of chronic diseases caused by a variety of risk factors, including unhealthy behaviours. As highlighted by the United Nations chronicles, these diseases share risk factors such as long-term exposure to three modifiable lifestyle behaviours, namely, smoking, unhealthy diet and physical inactivity [1]. Other risk factors include excessive alcohol use, air pollution and stress.

Oral health is a key determinant of overall health and well-being. Poor and untreated oral health diseases have systemic lifestyle consequences and contribute to lifestyle diseases, including cardiovascular disease, diabetes and adverse pregnancy outcomes. In resource-constrained settings, lack of awareness of preventative care, exorbitant health care costs and limited access exacerbate the oral disease burden further. Individuals often seek treatment only when symptoms become severe. The bidirectional relationship between oral health and systemic conditions highlights the need to integrate oral health within the primary health care (PHC) system, which significantly prevents lifestyle disorders impacting oral health [2]. Integrating oral health with PHC and preventative lifestyle shifts can prioritise prevention, early detection and timely referrals, thereby preventing systemic lifestyle diseases.

This chapter highlights the critical linkages between lifestyle diseases and oral health and the role of health care workers (HCWs) in advancing oral health education and prevention through integration into PHC and task-sharing.

Health care workers (HCWs) (community health workers [CHWs], school health nurses, midwives and other frontline workers) are uniquely positioned to address

S. Bhardwaj (✉)
Gates Foundation, Washington, USA

L. T. Slavin
Global Health Visions, Gauteng, South Africa

S. R. Prabhu et al. (eds.), *Lifestyle in Oral Health and Disease*,
https://doi.org/10.1007/978-3-032-05888-1_26

lifestyle disorders and oral health. Task-sharing strategies, where non-dental health professionals provide basic oral health screenings and education, can expand access by combining oral health with education; water, sanitation and hygiene (WASH); and nutrition, which can address the root cause of lifestyle and oral diseases.

Aside from clinical management, behavioural factors—such as diet, alcohol and tobacco consumption and oral hygiene practices—are significant predictors of oral health outcomes. HCWs can change health behaviours through education and counselling. Using the Health Belief Model (HBM), this chapter explores how perceived risks, self-efficacy and enabling environments shape individual and community-level decisions about oral health. Integrating oral health into the broader health system and leveraging multisectoral collaboration will ensure that oral health is critical to overall health and well-being.

26.2 Theory of Change

The theory of change posits that integrating oral health into PHC will improve health outcomes and ensure equitable access to oral health care, task-sharing, multisectoral collaboration and behaviour change.

A multisectoral approach underpins an integrated approach to health and aligns oral health with other sectors (water, sanitation and hygiene [WASH], education and nutrition). Schools are an ideal setting for early intervention, where integrated school health programmes can promote oral hygiene practices, healthy eating and routine screenings. Collaboration with WASH ensures access to clean water, fluoride use and hygiene promotion become part of comprehensive health strategies.

A crucial element of the theory of change rests on the role that HCWs play in influencing behavioural change and lifestyle choices, such as diet, smoking, alcohol consumption and oral hygiene habits. Integrating two to three oral health screening questions into routine PHC visits can identify early risk factors and enable behaviour change.

Rooted in the Health Belief Model (HBM), an explanation of individual health decision-making suggests that individuals are more likely to change their behaviours when they understand the consequences and benefits of preventative activity [3]. The HBM hypothesises that people will adopt healthy behaviours when they:

- See themselves at risk
- Recognise consequences and severity
- Acknowledge the benefits of prevention
- Feel optimistic about their healthy decision-making capability
- Are prompted by HCWs (counselling, reminders, education)

The HBM places HCWs at the centre of behaviour change as 'agents of change', reinforcing oral health messages during routine care and guiding individuals towards healthier habits [4]. Through education, screening and community-based interventions, HCWs can tackle the social determinants of health and barriers.

Successful oral health PHC relies on policy adaptation, resource allocation, sustained cross-sector collaboration and HCWs as agents of behaviour change.

26.3 Health Care Workers as Agents of Change

HCWs influence behaviours through social influence, empowerment and ongoing interaction. In collaboration with educators, faith-based organisations and community leaders, health messages can be well conveyed, resulting in successful and sustained behaviour change [5].

26.4 Building Self-Efficacy and Empowering Communities

Behaviour change is most effective when individuals believe they can improve their health. HCWs reinforce this by providing actionable feedback, leveraging small victories and countering social barriers. For example, when promoting tobacco cessation, HCWs help in setting realistic and achievable goals, offer follow-up support and connect individuals to peer support networks [3]. This holds individuals responsible for their health and gives them the skills to act.

26.5 Sustained Engagement and Reinforcement

Ongoing support, follow-ups and reminders are critical for sustained behaviour change. Home visits, PHC consultations and mobile health interventions are avenues for ensuring sustained engagement [6].

26.6 Tailoring Health Messages to Local Contexts

Tailoring health messages to the local context, culture, society and economy is essential. Ensuring health education is practical and relatable improves the acceptance and adherence to preventive messages [7]. In resource-constrained settings, CHWs bridge gaps by directly bringing health education, preventive care and referrals to communities [8]. By providing culturally sensitive guidance on disease prevention, hygiene, nutrition and maternal care, HCWs influence long-term healthy behaviours and health-seeking decisions [3]. Their personalised, patient-centred approach [9] strengthens trust and allows individuals to adopt and sustain healthy behaviours [7]. HCWs play a role in bridging health systems and communities by establishing trust, facilitating behaviour change and improving access to stronger health services. Expanding HCWs' roles through training, task-sharing and multisectoral collaboration is at the core of alleviating the burden of oral diseases globally [10].

26.7 Integrating Oral Health into Primary Health Care: A Holistic Approach

By focusing on early detection, prevention and routine care, HCWs can reduce the oral health burden, lower treatment costs and improve overall health outcomes [11].

Routine health checkups, health education, screening and referrals enable HCWs to identify early tooth decay, gum disease and oral infections. Simple interventions such as fluoride application, provision of oral hygiene kits and community education on brushing are low-cost and can prevent advanced oral diseases.

In rural Kenya, community health initiatives are improving oral hygiene among children. For example, in a 2019 project in Mamba village, Kwale County, trained teachers, parents, health workers and village elders promoted daily tooth brushing among 1200 primary school students, emphasising supervised brushing to prevent cavities.

Integrating oral health into maternal and child health services guarantees pregnant women and young children receive health education, screening and preventive care. Studies have shown midwives can successfully incorporate oral health education into prenatal care to improve pregnant women's attitudes and oral health habits. Research indicates that pregnant women are receptive to oral health education from midwives, highlighting the potential for integrating oral health promotion into prenatal visits [12–14].

While prevention is ideal, access to timely curative services remains critical. Strengthening referral pathways ensures dental treatment, advanced procedures, or speciality care is received on time. Task-sharing strategies allow HCWs to initiate essential interventions, provide first-line treatment and refer patients when necessary. In Brazil, CHWs perform initial dental screenings, identify dental issues early and refer patients for further treatment, thus reducing the burden on specialised dental services and expanding access to essential dental services.

Building HCWs' capacity for early detection and oral health promotion can significantly improve community health. For example:

- *Basic Oral Screenings*: In Tanzania, CHWs conduct simple dental screenings during routine visits to identify cavities and gum disease early and refer for further treatment [15].
- *Community Education*: In Mexico, school health nurses educate students and parents on the impact of sugary snacks and the benefits of regular brushing and flossing.
- *Routine Checkups*: In Uganda, midwives include oral health questions in antenatal care checklists to identify pregnant women at risk of gum disease [16].
- *Referrals for Specialist Care*: In South Africa, CHWs refer patients with severe dental issues to district-level hospitals for treatment by specialists [17].
- *Visual oral examination* of adults by primary health care workers during home visits for the early detection of oral cancer and precancer in Sri Lanka [18].
- *Noma*: PHC in early detection of Noma in young children in Africa [19].

Task-sharing models like these can potentially increase access to oral care, reduce the burden on dental professionals and screen and refer individuals for oral health services and treatments they need.

26.8 Multisectoral Collaboration: Strengthening Oral Health Through Cross-Sector Partnerships

In addition to individual action, multisectoral collaboration between health, education, nutrition and WASH is essential to sustain oral health outcomes.

26.8.1 Oral Health and Education

Schools are ideal settings for early intervention of oral health. Integrating oral health into school programmes can:

- *Teach Correct Techniques*: In the Philippines, correct brushing and flossing are taught to children using participatory demonstration and singing [20].
- *Promote Healthy Diets*: In Japan, school programmes encourage children to eat fruits and vegetables over sugary snacks [21].
- *Conduct Screenings*: In Nigeria, mobile dental clinics visit schools to conduct checkups and screenings to identify oral health issues early and provide fluoride treatments and toothbrushes [22].
- Supervised tooth cleansing every second week in Danish school children in the school setting resulted in lower rates of dental caries.

26.9 Oral Health and WASH

Access to clean water and sanitation is essential for oral health and infection prevention. WASH, including the provision of fluoride, clean water and hygiene education, plays a role in improving oral health.

- *Fluoride in Water*: In the United States, fluoridation of water has significantly reduced dental caries in children [23].
- *Clean Water Access*: In rural areas of Ethiopia, WASH programmes provide clean water to improve oral hygiene [24].
- *Hygiene Education*: In Bangladesh, hand hygiene and oral hygiene are promoted through oral health campaigns [25].

26.10 Oral Health and Nutrition

Excessive sugar is one of the leading causes of dental caries. HCWs and nutritionists play a role in:

- *Educating Communities*: In Brazil, nutritionists and dental health professionals are working with families and communities through health education on food choices and oral health [26].

- *Promoting Nutritious Foods*: In Thailand, community health programmes encourage the consumption of calcium- and vitamin-enriched foods like dairy products and leafy greens for healthy gums and teeth [27].
- *Advocating and Promoting Healthy School Lunches and Meals*: In the UK, school meal programmes have been reshaped to reduce sugar intake and ensure that healthy options, such as fruits and vegetables, are included [28].

Linking oral health interventions with public health activities ensures that the causative determinants of poor oral health are addressed.

26.11 Strengthening Health System and Policy

Strong policy frameworks and investment in strengthening health systems are central to integrating oral health into PHC sustainably. Governments and stakeholders should prioritise the following:

- Equipping HCWs with skills to deliver oral health services
- Advocating for national health policies that include oral health as a core component of PHC
- Resource allocation that provides essential supplies (fluoride toothpaste, mouthwash and screening tools)
- Improving referral pathways to ensure timely treatment for specialised dental care

Global health organisations, like the World Health Organization (WHO), United Nations International Children's Emergency Fund (UNICEF) and the Draft Global Oral Health Action Partnership [29], have emphasised stronger oral health policies integrating oral care into existing health systems. Investing in prevention, workforce training and policy reform will ensure sustained improvements in oral health worldwide.

26.12 Conclusion

Despite its criticality to overall health and well-being, oral health is neglected in most PHC systems. Emphasising early detection, prevention and cross-sector collaboration will address this deficit. HCWs can expand access through task-sharing strategies, closing education gaps, promoting WASH and nutrition and empowering individuals and communities to adopt healthier behaviours. Strengthening policy support, training and multisectoral collaboration will ensure equitable access and reduce the global burden of oral diseases.

Integrating oral health into broader PHC services can create sustainable, patient-centred health systems that prioritise prevention, improve health equity and promote long-term health outcomes.

References

1. Al-Maskari F. Lifestyle diseases: an economic burden on the health services. UN Chronicle; 2010.
2. Gavaza P, Kim W, Rogers T, Fry-Bowers E, Mosavin R. Knowledge and opinions regarding the interface between oral and overall health among California physicians, dentists, pharmacists and advanced practice registered nurse practitioners. Calif J Health Promot. 2017. https://doi.org/10.32398/cjhp.v15i2.1900.
3. Rosenstock IM. The health belief model and preventive health behavior. Health Educ Monogr. 1974;2(4):354–86. https://doi.org/10.1177/109019817400200405.
4. Gibson C, Smith D, Morrison AK. Improving health literacy knowledge, behaviors, and confidence with interactive training. Health Lit Res Pract. 2022;6(2):e113–120. https://doi.org/10.3928/24748307-20220420-01. Epub 2022 May 6. PMID: 35522855; PMCID: PMC9126053.
5. Ndambo MK, Munyaneza F, Aron M, Makungwa H, Nhlema B, Connolly E. The role of community health workers in influencing social connectedness using the household model: a qualitative case study from Malawi. Glob Health Action. 2022;15(1):2090123. https://doi.org/10.1080/16549716.2022.2090123. PMID: 35960168; PMCID: PMC9377265.
6. Matthews JA, Matthews S, Faries MD, Wolever RQ. Supporting sustainable health behavior change: the whole is greater than the sum of its parts. Mayo Clin Proc Innov Qual Outcomes. 2024;8(3):263–75. https://doi.org/10.1016/j.mayocpiqo.2023.10.002. PMID: 38807973; PMCID: PMC11130595.
7. Coulter A, Oldham J. Person-centred care: what is it and how do we get there? Future Hosp J. 2016;3(2):114–6. https://doi.org/10.7861/futurehosp.3-2-114. PMID: 31098200; PMCID: PMC6465833.
8. What do we know about community health workers? A systemic review of existing reviews. Geneva: World Health Organization; 2020 (Human Resources for Health Observer Series No. 19). Licence CC BY-NC-SA 3.0 IGO. https://creativecommons.org/licenses/by-nc-sa/3.0/igo.
9. The Health Foundation Person-centered care made simple: what everyone should know about person-centered care. 2016. https://www.health.org.uk/sites/default/files/PersonCentredCareMadeSimple.pdf.
10. Kok G, Peters GY, Kessels LTE, Ten Hoor GA, Ruiter RAC. Ignoring theory and misinterpreting evidence: the false belief in fear appeals. Health Psychol Rev. 2018;12(2):111–25. https://doi.org/10.1080/17437199.2017.1415767. Epub 2017 Dec 28.
11. Love Kenya Foundation. Transforming oral health in Kenya's remote areas. Downloaded March 2025. https://www.lovekenyafoundation.org/oral-health-kenya.
12. Adeniyi A, Donnelly L, Janssen P, Jevitt C, Kardeh B, von Bergmann H, Brondani M. Pregnant women's perspectives on integrating preventive oral health in prenatal care. BMC Pregnancy Childbirth. 2021;21(1):271. https://doi.org/10.1186/s12884-021-03750-4. PMID: 33794806; PMCID: PMC8016156.
13. Vamos CA, Cayama MR, Mahony H, Griner SB, Quinonez RB, Boggess K, Beckstead J, Daley EM. Oral health during pregnancy: an analysis of interprofessional guideline awareness and practice behaviors among prenatal and oral health providers. BMC Pregnancy Childbirth. 2023;23(1):721. https://doi.org/10.1186/s12884-023-06032-3. PMID: 37821843; PMCID: PMC10566079.
14. Braimoh M, Ogunbodede E, Adeniyi A. Integration of oral health into primary health care system: views of primary health care workers in Lagos State, Nigeria. J Public Health Afr. 2014. https://doi.org/10.4081/jphia.2014.328.
15. Tanzania's community-based health program. Downloaded March 2025 https://chwcentral.org/tanzanias-community-based-health-program/.
16. Lulu PM, Nanyingi M. Factors influencing adoption of oral health promotion by antenatal care providers in Moyo district, North-Western Uganda. PLoS ONE. 2023;18(4):e0272238. https://doi.org/10.1371/journal.pone.0272238.

17. South African Department of Health. National oral health policy and strategy. 2024–2023. Downloaded March 2025. https://www.health.gov.za/wp-content/uploads/2025/03/National-Oral-Health-Policy-and-Strategy-2024-2034.pdf.
18. Warnakulasuriya KA, Ekanayake AN, Sivayoham S, Stjernswärd J, Pindborg JJ, Sobin LH, Perera KS. Utilization of primary health care workers for early detection of oral cancer and precancer cases in Sri Lanka. Bull World Health Organ. 1984;62(2):243–50. PMID: 6610492; PMCID: PMC2536304.
19. Ahlgren M, Funk T, Marimo C, Ndiaye C, Alfvén T. Management of noma: practice competence and knowledge among healthcare workers in a rural district of Zambia. Glob Health Action. 2017;10(1):1340253. https://doi.org/10.1080/16549716.2017.1340253. PMID: 28678680; PMCID: PMC5533138.
20. Philippine Information Agency. Gene Ace Sapit. Bye-bye tooth decay: Palawan schoolchildren join tooth brushing drill in dental health drive. 2024. Downloaded March 2024. https://pia.gov.ph/bye-bye-tooth-decay-palawan-schoolchildren-join-toothbrushing-drill-in-dental-health-drive/?utm_source=chatgpt.com.
21. Tanaka N, Miyoshi M. School-based "Shokuiku" program in Japan: application to nutrition education in Asian countries. Asia Pac J Clin Nutr. 2012;21(1):159–62.
22. Amedari M, Adedigba MA. Enhancing oral health care access for school children: a perspective. Niger Dent J. 2024;32:30–36.
23. Centers for Disease Control and Prevention. Community water fluoridation. 2022. https://www.cdc.gov/fluoridation/index.html.
24. UNICEF. WASH in Ethiopia. 2021. https://www.unicef.org/ethiopia/water-sanitation-and-hygiene.
25. World Health Organization. Promoting oral health in South-East Asia. 2020. https://www.who.int/bangladesh/news/detail/20-03-2020-promoting-oral-health-in-south-east-asia.
26. Pan American Health Organization. Brazil strengthens actions to promote oral health in primary care. 2021. https://www.paho.org/en/news/17-6-2021-brazil-strengthens-actions-promote-oral-health-primary-care.
27. World Health Organization. Oral health in Thailand: promoting nutrition and healthy behaviors. 2020. https://www.who.int/thailand.
28. Public Health England. Improving the nutritional quality of school meals. 2019. https://www.gov.uk/government/publications.
29. Draft Global Oral Health Action Plan (2023–2030). WHO. 2023. https://cdn.who.int/media/docs/default-source/ncds/mnd/oral-health/eb152-draft-global-oral-health-action-plan-2023-2030-en.pdf?sfvrsn=2f348123_19&download=true.

Index

S. R. Prabhu et al. (eds.), *Lifestyle in Oral Health and Disease*,
https://doi.org/10.1007/978-3-032-05888-1

B

C